Essentials of
Pharmacology for Dentistry

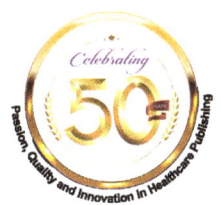

Essentials of *Pharmacology for Dentistry*

4th Edition

KD Tripathi MD
Ex-Director-Professor and Head of Pharmacology
Maulana Azad Medical College and associated
LN and GB Pant Hospitals
New Delhi, India

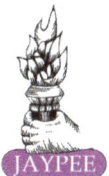

JAYPEE BROTHERS MEDICAL PUBLISHERS
The Health Sciences Publisher
New Delhi | London

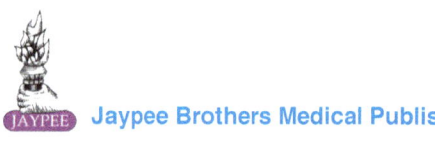 **Jaypee Brothers Medical Publishers (P) Ltd**

Headquarters
Jaypee Brothers Medical Publishers (P) Ltd
EMCA House
23/23-B, Ansari Road, Daryaganj
New Delhi - 110 002, India
Landline: +91-11-23272143, +91-11-23272703
+91-11-23282021, +91-11-23245672
Email: jaypee@jaypeebrothers.com

Corporate Office
Jaypee Brothers Medical Publishers (P) Ltd
4838/24, Ansari Road, Daryaganj
New Delhi 110 002, India
Phone: +91-11-43574357
Fax: +91-11-43574314
Email: jaypee@jaypeebrothers.com

Overseas Office
J.P. Medical Ltd
83 Victoria Street, London
SW1H 0HW (UK)
Phone: +44 20 3170 8910
Fax: +44 (0)20 3008 6180
Email: info@jpmedpub.com

Website: www.jaypeebrothers.com

Website: www.jaypeedigital.com

© 2021, KD Tripathi

Managing Editor: M Tripathi

The views and opinions expressed in this book are solely those of the original contributor(s)/author(s) and do not necessarily represent those of editor(s) of the book.

All rights reserved. No part of this publication may be reproduced, stored or transmitted in any form or by any means, electronic, mechanical, photocopying, recording or otherwise, without the prior permission in writing of the publishers.

All brand names and product names used in this book are trade names, service marks, trademarks or registered trademarks of their respective owners. The publisher is not associated with any product or vendor mentioned in this book.

Medical knowledge and practice change constantly. This book is designed to provide accurate, authoritative information about the subject matter in question. However, readers are advised to check the most current information available on procedures included and check information from the manufacturer of each product to be administered, to verify the recommended dose, formula, method and duration of administration, adverse effects and contraindications. It is the responsibility of the practitioner to take all appropriate safety precautions. Neither the publisher nor the author(s)/editor(s) assume any liability for any injury and/or damage to persons or property arising from or related to use of material in this book.

This book is sold on the understanding that the publisher is not engaged in providing professional medical services. If such advice or services are required, the services of a competent medical professional should be sought.

Every effort has been made where necessary to contact holders of copyright to obtain permission to reproduce copyright material. If any has been inadvertently overlooked, the publisher will be pleased to make the necessary arrangements at the first opportunity.

Inquiries for bulk sales may be solicited at: jaypee@jaypeebrothers.com

Essentials of Pharmacology for Dentistry

First Edition: 2005
Second Edition: 2011
Third Edition: 2016
Fourth Edition: **2021**

ISBN 978-93-5090-420-6

Preface to the Fourth Edition

Pharmacology, the science of drugs (medicines), is a highly dynamic discipline with concepts and priority drugs changing rapidly. Its relevance to all health professionals (including dentists) cannot be over emphasized. Practice of dentistry utilizes drugs both as primary treatment modality, as well as facilitator of/adjuvant to dental procedures. Dentists routinely prescribe analgesics and antibiotics, apply antiseptics and other locally acting drugs, and inject local anaesthetics. Further, many dental patients could be receiving other medication that may have orodental implications, or may interact with drugs prescribed by the dentist. Occasionally, dentists have to manage a medical emergency which may arise during a dental procedure or in their clinic. As such, a broad knowledge of pharmacology along with focus on particular aspects is needed by the dentist. This book has been produced to specifically meet the above outlined needs.

The book is divided into three sections. The first describes the general pharmacological principles with which all professionals involved in drug therapy must be conversant. The second on systemic pharmacology presents a brief account of drugs acting on various organ systems and used in the treatment of common disorders affecting these systems, but are generally not prescribed by dentists. Each chapter is organised systematically. The opening sentence defines the class of drugs, followed by their classification presented in hierarchical chart form for better pictorial impression and easy remembrance. The 'prototype' approach has been adopted by describing the representative drug of the class followed by few salient features of the others. Matters particularly relevant to dental therapeutics have been highlighted. Wherever applicable, the implications in dentistry are prominently elaborated, e.g. drugs and diseases affecting postextraction haemostasis, dental procedures in patients on corticosteroid therapy or in diabetics, orodental complications of cancer chemotherapy and chronic alcoholism, etc.

The third section covers antimicrobials and other drugs which the dentists usually prescribe or administer themselves. However, the allocation of topics in sections two and three does not indicate water-tight distinction, which is impossible, but has been done with a view to focus attention on drugs that have greater relevance in dentistry. To mention a few, the application of analgesics and NSAIDs in dental pain, local anaesthetics for dental anaesthesia, role of each class of antimicrobials in orodental infections, prophylaxis of postextraction wound infection and endocarditis in patients at special risk are emphasized. Since dentists are constantly exposed to the risk of accidental HIV infection by sharp injury while performing dental procedures, the latest NACO recommended guidelines for prophylaxis of HIV infection are provided. Drugs and aids having specific application in dental disorders and in dental care, e.g. drugs for dental plaque, caries tooth, dentine sensitivity alongwith aids like dentifrices, bleaching agents, disclosing agents, etc. are described in a separate chapter, pointing out their role in current practice. Management of medical emergencies like fainting, hypoglycaemia, allergic/anaphylactic reaction, angina pectoris or myocardial infarction, asthmatic attack or seizures that may occur in a dental office are outlined in another chapter, along with a list of medicines that should be kept in the emergency tray. The last chapter on drug interactions highlights those that may be encountered in dental practice. Care has been taken that the syllabus prescribed by the Dental Council of India is fully covered.

All chapters in the present edition have been thoroughly updated to include latest information and new drugs, while nonrelevant material has been deleted. Presentation and illustrations have been improved. Leading trade names and dosage forms of drugs generally prescribed by dentists are mentioned distinctively. Thus, the book is oriented to provide core and contemporary pharmacological knowledge which can be easily assimilated by dental students, as well as serve to help dental practitioners in treating orodental conditions.

I am thankful to readers of the earlier editions for their comments and suggestions which helped in preparing the present edition. The motivational influence of Shri J.P. Vij (Group Chairman), M/s Jaypee Brothers Medical Publishers, was crucial. The meticulous preparation of the manuscript by the staff of M/s Jaypee Brothers Medical Publishers is highly appreciated. The participation and cooperation of my wife is sincerely acknowledged.

Nov. 2020 **KD Tripathi**

Contents

Section I: General Pharmacological Principles

1. **Introduction, Routes of Drug Administration** 3
   Introduction 3
   Sources of Drugs 5
   Dosage forms of Drugs 7
   Routes of Drug Administration 10

2. **Pharmacokinetics** 15
   Transport of Drugs 16
   Absorption of Drugs 19
   Distribution of Drugs 22
   Biotransformation (Metabolism) of Drugs 26
   Excretion of Drugs 32
   Kinetics of Drug Elimination 35

3. **Pharmacodynamics** 40
   Principles of Drug Action 40
   Mechanism of Drug Action 40
   Drug Synergism and Antagonism 56
   Drug Dosage; Fixed Dose Drug Combinations (FDCs) 59
   Factors Modifying Drug Action 61

4. **Adverse Drug Effects** 68
   Side Effects, Toxic Effects and Poisoning 69
   Drug Allergy 70
   Drug Dependence and Addiction 73
   Teratogenicity 74

Section II: Systemic Pharmacology

5. **Drugs Acting on Autonomic Nervous System-1** 79
   (General Considerations, Cholinergic and Anticholinergic Drugs)
   General Considerations 79
   Cholinergic Drugs (Cholinomimetic, Parasympathomimetic) 85
   Anticholinesterases 86
   Anticholinergic Drugs (Parasympatholytic) 89

6. **Drugs Acting on Autonomic Nervous System-2** 94
   (Adrenergic and Antiadrenergic Drugs)
   Adrenergic Transmission 94
   Adrenergic Drugs (Sympathomimetics) 98
   α-Adrenergic Blocking Drugs 104
   β-Adrenergic Blocking Drugs 107

7. **Autacoids and Related Drugs** 112
   Histamine 112
   H_1 Antagonists (Conventional Antihistaminics) 115
   5-Hydroxytryptamine (5-HT, Serotonin) 119
   Prostaglandins and Leukotrienes (Eicosanoids) 120

8. **General Anaesthetics and Skeletal Muscle Relaxants** 128
   General Anaesthetics 128
   Skeletal Muscle Relaxants 137

9. **Drugs Acting on Central Nervous System-1** 144
   (Sedative-Hypnotics, Ethyl Alcohol, Antiepileptics and Antiparkinsonian Drugs)
   Sedative-hypnotics 144
   Ethyl Alcohol (Ethanol) 151
   Antiepileptic Drugs 154
   Antiparkinsonian Drugs 161

10. **Drugs Acting on Central Nervous System-2** 165
    (Psychopharmacological Agents)
    Antipsychotic Drugs (Neuroleptics) 166
    Drugs for Mania and Bipolar Disorder 171
    Antidepressant Drugs 174
    Antianxiety Drugs 181

11. **Cardiovascular Drugs-1** 183
    (Drugs Affecting Renin-Angiotensin System, Calcium Channel Blockers,
    Drugs for Hypertension, Angina Pectoris and Myocardial Infarction)
    Drugs Affecting Renin-Angiotensin System 183
    Angiotensin Converting Enzyme Inhibitors 185
    Angiotensin Receptor Blockers 187
    Calcium Channel Blockers 188
    Antihypertensive Drugs 191
    Antianginal Drugs 197
    Drug Therapy in Myocardial Infarction 203

12. **Cardiovascular Drugs-2** 205
    (Drugs for Heart Failure and Cardiac Arrhythmia)
    Cardiac Glycosides 205
    Treatment of Congestive Heart Failure 209
    Antiarrhythmic Drugs 211

Contents ix

13. **Diuretics** 217
    Relevant Physiology of Urine Formation 217
    Diuretics 219

14. **Hormones and Related Drugs-1** 228
    (Anterior Pituitary Hormones, Antidiabetic Drugs, Corticosteroids)
    Introduction 228
    Anterior Pituitary Hormones 229
    Antidiabetic Drugs (Insulin; Oral Antidiabetic Drugs) 233
    Corticosteroids 244

15. **Hormones and Related Drugs-2** 251
    (Androgens, Anabolic Steroids, Estrogens, Progestins and Contraceptives)
    Androgens 251
    Anabolic Steroids 252
    Estrogens 253
    Progestins 256
    Hormonal Contraceptives 258

16. **Hormones and Related Drugs-3** 262
    (Thyroid Hormone and Thyroid Inhibitors, Hormones Regulating Calcium Balance)
    Thyroid Hormone 262
    Thyroid Inhibitors (Antithyroid Drugs) 265
    Hormones Regulating Calcium (Calcium; Vitamin D; Parathormone; Calcitonin) 267
    Bisphosphonates 272

17. **Drugs Affecting Blood** 274
    Haematinics 274
    Coagulants 279
    Haemostasis in Dentistry 281
    Anticoagulants 283
    Fibrinolytic Drugs (Thrombolytics) 287
    Antifibrinolytic Drugs 288
    Antiplatelet Drugs (Antithrombotic Drugs) 288
    Hypolipidaemic Drugs 291

18. **Drugs for Gastrointestinal Disorders** 294
    Drugs for Peptic Ulcer and Reflux Disease 294
    Antiemetic Drugs 301
    Laxatives (Aperients, Purgatives, Cathartics) 305
    Treatment of Diarrhoeas 309

19. **Drugs for Respiratory Disorders** 314
    Drugs for Cough 314
    Drugs for Bronchial Asthma 316

20. **Vitamins** 322
    Fat-soluble Vitamins 322
    Water-soluble Vitamins 325

21. **Anticancer and Immunosuppressant Drugs** 329
   Anticancer Drugs 329
   Immunosuppressant Drugs 339

Section III: Antimicrobials and Drugs Important in Dental Therapeutics

22. **Nonsteroidal Anti-inflammatory Drugs and Antipyretic-Analgesics** 347
   NSAIDs and Prostaglandin Synthesis Inhibition 348
   Properties and Uses of NSAIDs/Analgesics 350
   Analgesics/NSAIDs in Dentistry 262

23. **Opioid Analgesics and Antagonists** 364
   Opioid Analgesics 364
   Opioid Receptors 371
   Complex Action Opioids 373
   Pure Opioid Antagonists 375

24. **Local Anaesthetics** 377
   Mechanism of Action and Properties of Local Anaesthetics 378
   Uses and Techniques of Local Anaesthesia 384
   Local Anaesthesia in Dentistry 386

25. **Antimicrobial Drugs: General Considerations** 388
   Classification of Antimicrobials 389
   Drug Resistance 391
   Superinfection 393
   Choice of an Antimicrobial Agent 394
   Combined use of Antimicrobials 398
   Prophylactic Use of Antimicrobials 400
   Prophylaxis of Dental Wound Infection 400

26. **Sulfonamides, Cotrimoxazole, Quinolones and Nitroimidazoles** 403
   Sulfonamides 403
   Cotrimoxazole 405
   Quinolones 406
   Nitroimidazoles 411

27. **Beta-Lactam Antibiotics** 414
   Penicillins 414
   Beta-lactamase Inhibitors 422
   Cephalosporins 423
   Monobactams 429
   Carbapenems 429

28. **Tetracyclines, Chloramphenicol and Aminoglycoside Antibiotics** 431
    Tetracyclines and Tigecycline 431
    Chloramphenicol 436
    Aminoglycoside Antibiotics 439

29. **Macrolide and Other Antibacterial Antibiotics** 445
    Macrolide Antibiotics 445
    Lincosamide Antibiotics 449
    Glycopeptide Antibiotics 449
    Oxazolidinone 451
    Miscellaneous Antibiotics: Quinupristin/Dalfopristin,
      Daptomycin, Polypeptide Antibiotics 451

30. **Antitubercular and Antileprotic Drugs** 453
    Antitubercular Drugs 453
    Treatment of Tuberculosis 458
    Antileprotic Drugs 460
    Treatment of Leprosy 462

31. **Antifungal Drugs** 464
    Polyene Antibiotics 465
    Griseofulvin 467
    Imidazole and Triazole Antifungals 467
    Terbinafine 470
    Topical Antifungals 471

32. **Antiviral Drugs (Non-retroviral)** 472
    Anti-herpes Virus Drugs 472
    Anti-influenza Virus Drugs 474
    Anti-hepatitis Virus Drugs 475

33. **Anti-retrovirus Drugs** 479
    Nucleoside Reverse Transcriptase Inhibitors (NRTIs) 480
    Nonnucleoside Reverse Transcriptase Inhibitors (NNRTIs) 481
    Retroviral Protease Inhibitors (PIs) 481
    Integrase Inhibitors 482
    Treatment of HIV Infection 483
    Post-exposure Prophylaxis (PEP) of HIV Infection 484

34. **Antiprotozoal Drugs** 486
    Antimalarial Drugs 486
    Antiamoebic Drugs 494

35. **Antiseptics, Disinfectants and Other Locally Acting Drugs** 497
    Antiseptics and Disinfectants 497
    Locally Acting Drugs 504

36. **Drugs and Aids with Specific Application in Dental Disorders** 506
    Antiplaque and Antigingivitis Agents 506
    Antibiotics in Periodontal Disease 508
    Anticaries Drugs 509
    Desensitizing Agents 512
    Obtundants 513
    Mummifying Agents 514
    Bleaching Agents 514
    Disclosing Agents 515
    Dentifrices 515

37. **Management of Medical Emergencies in Dental Office** 517
    Emergency Drug Tray/Kit 517
    Management of Syncope (Fainting) 519
    Management of Acute Allergic Reaction 519
    Management of Angina Pectoris/Myocardial Infarction 520
    Management of Cardiac Arrest/Ventricular Fibrillation 521
    Management of Asthmatic Attack/Bronchospasm 521
    Management of Hypoglycaemia 521
    Management of Seizures/Status Epilepticus 522

38. **Drug Interactions** 523
    Mechanisms of Drug Interactions 524
    Drug Interactions in Dentistry 525

Index 531

List of Abbreviations

Ang-I/II/III	Angiotensin I/II/III	BSA	Body surface area
AA	Amino acid	BuChE	Butyryl cholinesterase
AB	Antibody	BW	Body weight
abc	ATP binding cassettee (trasporter)	BZD	Benzodiazepine
AC	Adenylyl cyclase		
ACE	Angiotensin II converting enzyme	C-10	Decamethonium
ACh	Acetylcholine	CA	Catecholamine
AChE	Acetylcholinesterase	CaBP	Calcium binding protein
ACT	Artemisinin combination therapy	CAD	Coronary artery disease
ACTH	Adrenocorticotropic hormone	CAM	Calmodulin
AD	Alzheimer's disease	cAMP	3', 5' Cyclic adenosine monophosphate
ADP	Adenosine diphosphate	cap	Capsule
Adr	Adrenaline	CAse	Carbonic anhydrase
AF	Atrial fibrillation	CBS	Colloidal bismuth subcitrate
AFl	Atrial flutter	CCB	Calcium channel blocker
AG	Antigen	CD	Collecting duct
AIDS	Acquired immunodeficiency syndrome	cGMP	3', 5' Cyclic guanosine monophosphate
AIP	Aldosterone induced protein	CGRP	Calcitonin gene-related peptide
ALA	Alanine	CH	Cholesterol
AMA	Antimicrobial agent	ChE	Cholinesterase
AMB	Amphotericin B	CHE	Cholesterol ester
amp	Ampoule	CHF	Congestive heart failure
AMP	Adenosine monophosphate	CI	Cardiac index
ANC	Acid neutralizing capacity	CL	Clearance
ANS	Autonomic nervous system	CLcr	Creatinine clearance
ANUG	Acute necrotizing ulcerative gingivitis	Clo	Clofazimine
AP	Action potential	CMI	Cell-mediated immunity
APD	Action potential duration	CMV	Cytomegalovirus
APF	Acidulated phosphate fluoride	CNS	Central nervous system
aPTT	Activated partial thromboplastin time	c.o.	Cardiac output
ARB	Angiotensin receptor blocker	CoEn-A	Coenzyme-A
ARC	AIDS related complex	COMT	Catechol-O-methyl transferase
ART	Antiretroviral therapy	COX	Cyclooxygenase
ARV	Antiretrovirus	CPS	Complex partial seizures
5-ASA	5-Amino salicyclic acid	CPZ	Chlorpromazine
AT-III	Antithrombin III	CRF	Corticotropin releasing factor
ATP	Adenosine triphosphate	CSF	Cerebrospinal fluid
ATPase	Adenosine triphosphatase	CTZ	Chemoreceptor trigger zone
A-V	Atrioventricular	CVS	Cardiovascular system
AVP	Arginine vasopressin	CWD	Cell wall deficient
AZT	Zidovudine	CYP450	Cytochrome P450
B_{12}	Vitamin B_{12}	DA	Dopamine
BCRP	Breast cancer resistance protein	DA-B_{12}	Deoxyadenosyl cobalamin
BD	Twice daily	DAG	Diacyl glycerol
BHP	Benign hypertrophy of prostate	DAT	Dopamine transporter
BMD	Bone mineral density	DCI	Dichloroisoproterenol
BMR	Basal metabolic rate	DDS	Diamino diphenyl sulfone (Dapsone)
BP	Blood pressure	DHFA	Dihydro folic acid
BPN	Bisphosphonate	DHFRase	Dihydrofolate reductase

DHP	Dihydropyridine		H	Isoniazid (Isonicotinic acid hydrazide)
DIT	Diiodotyrosine		Hb	Haemoglobin
dl	Decilitre		HBV	Hepatitis B virus
DLE	Disseminated lupus erythematosus		HCG	Human chorionic gonadotropin
DMCM	Dimethoxyethyl-carbomethoxy-β-carboline		HCV	Hepatitis C virus
			HDL	High density lipoprotein
DMPA	Depot medroxyprogesterone acetate		5-HIAA	5-Hydroxyindole acetic acid
DMPP	Dimethyl phenyl piperazinium		HETE	Hydroxyeicosa tetraenoic acid
DNA	Deoxyribonucleic acid		HIV	Human immunodeficiency virus
DOCA	Desoxy corticosterone acetate		HMG-CoA	Hydroxymethyl glutaryl coenzyme A
dopa	Dihydroxyphenyl alanine		HPA axis	Hypothalamo-pituitary-adrenal axis
DOSS	Dioctyl sulfosuccinate		HPETE	Hydroperoxy eicosatetraenoic acid
DOTS	Directly observed treatment short course		hr	Hour
DPP-4	Dipeptidyl peptidase-4		HR	Heart rate
DRC	Dose-response curve		HRT	Hormone replacement therapy
DT	Distal tubule		HSV	Herpes simplex virus
d-TC	d-Tubocurarine		5-HT	5-Hydroxytryptamine
			5-HTP	5-Hydroxytryptophan
E	Ethambutol		HVA	Homovanillic acid
EACA	Epsilon amino caproic acid			
e.c.f.	Extracellular fluid			
ECG	Electrocardiogram		ICSH	Interstitial cell stimulating hormone
EDRF	Endothelium dependent relaxing factor		IDL	Intermediate density lipoprotein
EDTA	Ethylene diamine tetraacetic acid		IGF	Insulin-like growth factor
EEG	Electroencephalogram		IL	Interleukin
EFV	Efavirenz		ILEU	Isoleucine
β-END	β-Endorphin		i.m.	Intramuscular
EPEC	Enteropathogenic E. coli		INH	Isonicotinic acid hydrazide
ERP	Effective refractory period		INR	International normalized ratio
EPSP	Excitatory postsynaptic potential		i.o.t.	Intraocular tension
ER	Estrogen receptor		IP_3	Inositol trisphosphate
ES	Extrasystole		IPSP	Inhibitory postsynaptic potential
ESR	Erythrocyte sedimentation rate		IU	International unit
ETEC	Enterotoxigenic E. coli		i.v.	Intravenous
Etm	Ethionamide			
			JAK	Janus-kinase
FA	Folic acid			
FEV_1	Forced expiratory volume in 1 second		KTZ	Ketoconazole
FFA	Free fatty acid			
FQ	Fluoroquinolone		LA	Local anaesthetic
FSH	Follicle stimulating hormone		L-AMB	Liposomal amphotericin B
5-FU	5-Fluorouracil		LC-3-KAT	Long chain 3-ketoacyl-CoA thiolase
			LDL	Low density lipoprotein
GABA	Gamma amino butyric acid		LES	Lower esophageal sphincter
GC	Guanylyl cyclase		leu-ENK	Leucine enkephalin
GDP	Guanosine diphosphate		LH	Luteinizing hormone
GERD	Gastroesophageal reflux disease		liq	Liquid
g.f.r.	Glomerular filtration rate		LMW	Low molecular weight
GH	Growth hormone		LOX	Lipoxygenase
g.i.t.	Gastrointestinal tract		LT	Leukotriene
GITS	Gastrointestinal therapeutic system			
GLP-1	Glucagon-like peptide-1		MAC	Minimal alveolar concentration
GLUT	Glucose transporter		MAC	*Mycobacterium avium* complex
GnRH	Gonadotropin releasing hormone		MAO	Monoamine oxidase
G-6-PD	Glucose-6-phosphate dehydrogenase		MAPKinase	Mitogen activated protein kinase
GTCS	Generalised tonic-clonic seizures		max	Maximum
GTN	Glyceryl trinitrate		MBC	Minimum bactericidal concentration
GTP	Guanosine triphosphate			

MBL	Multibacillary leprosy	PABA	Paraamino benzoic acid
MDR	Multidrug resistant	PAE	Postantibiotic effect
MDT	Multidrug therapy (of leprosy)	2-PAM	Pralidoxime
met-ENK	Methionine enkephalin	PAS	Paraamino salicylic acid
mEq	milliequivalent	PBPs	Penicillin binding proteins
MFP	Monofluorophosphate (sodium)	PBL	Paucibacillary leprosy
MHC	Major histocompatibility complex	PD	Parkinson's disease
MI	Myocardial infarction	PDE	Phosphodiesterase
MIC	Minimal inhibitory concentration	PEP	Postexposure prophylaxis (of HIV)
min	Minimum	PF	Purkinje fibre
MIT	Monoiodo tyrosine	PFOR	Pyruvate: ferredoxin oxidoreductase
MLCK	Myosin light chain kinase	PG	Prostaglandin
6-MP	6-Mercaptopurine	PGI_2	Prostacyclin
MRP2	Multidrug resistance associated protein 2	P-gp	P-glycoprotein
		PI	Protease inhibitor
MRSA	Methicillin resistant *Staphylococcus aureus*	PIP_2	Phosphatidyl inositol-4, 5-bisphosphate
		PKA	Protein kinase: cAMP dependent
Mtx	Methotrexate	PKC	Protein kinase C
MW	Molecular weight	PL_A	Phospholipase A
		PL_C	Phospholipase C
NA	Noradrenaline	PnG	Penicillin G
NABQI	N-acetyl-p-benzoquinoneimine	POMC	Pro-opio melanocortin
NACO	National AIDS Control Organization	PP	Partial pressure
NADP	Nicotinamide adenine dinucleotide phosphate	PPARγ	Paroxysome proliferator-activated receptor γ
NADPH	Reduced nicotinamide adenine dinucleotide phosphate	PPH	Postpartum haemorrhage
		PPI	Proton pump inhibitor
NAG	N-acetyl glucosamine	ppm	Part per million
NAM	N-acetyl muramic acid	PPNG	Penicillinase producing *N. gonorrhoeae*
NANC	Nonadrenergic noncholinergic	PSVT	Paroxysmal supra-ventricular tachycardia
NaSSA	Noradrenergic and specific serotonergic antidepressant	PT	Proximal tubule
NAT	N-acetyl transferase	PTCA	Percutaneous transluminal coronary angioplasty
NEE	Norethindrone enanthate		
NET	Norepinephrine transporter	PTH	Parathyroid hormone
NFAT	Nuclear factor of activated T-cell	PTP	Post-tetanic potentiation
NIS	Na^+ iodide symporter	PTSD	Post-traumatic stress disorder
NLEP	National leprosy eradication programme	QID	Four times a day
NMDA	N-methyl-D-aspartate		
NNRTI	Nonnucleoside reverse transcriptase inhibitor	R	Rifampin (Rifampicin)
		RAS	Renin-angiotensin system
NPV	Nevirapine	RBP	Retinol binding protein
NPY	Neuropeptide-Y	REM	Rapid eye movement (sleep)
NR	Nicotinic receptor	RIMA	Reversible inhibitor of MAO-A
N-REM	Non-rapid eye movement (sleep)	rINN	Recommended international nonproprietary name
NRTI	Nucleoside reverse transcriptase inhibitor	RMP	Resting membrane potential
NSAID	Nonsteroidal antiinflammatory drug	RNA	Ribonucleic acid
NTS	Nucleus tractus solitarius	RNTCP	Revised National Tuberculosis Control Programme
OATP	Organic anion transporting polypeptide	RP	Refractory period
OC	Oral contraceptive	RTF	Resistance transfer factor
OCD	Obsessive-compulsive disorder		
OCT	Organic cation transporter	S	Streptomycin
OD	Once daily	SA	Sinoatrial (node)
ORS	Oral rehydration salt (solution)	SABE	Subacute bacterial endocarditis
ORT	Oral rehydration therapy	s.c.	Subcutaneous

SCh	Succinylcholine	THFA	Tetrahydro folic acid
SERM	Selective estrogen receptor modulator	THR	Threonine
SERT	Serotonin transporter	TIAs	Transient ischaemic attacks
SGA	Second generation antihistaminic	TNF-α	Tumour necrosis factor α
s.l.	Sublingual	t-PA	Tissue plasminogen activator
SLC	Solute carrier (transporter)	t.p.r.	Total peripheral resistance
SLE	Systemic lupus erythematosus	TR	Thyroid hormone receptor
SMON	Subacute myelo-optic neuropathy	TRH	Thyrotropin releasing hormone
SNRI	Serotonin and noradrenaline reuptake inhibitor	TSH	Thyroid stimulating hormone
		TTS	Transdermal therapeutic system
s.o.s.	as required	TX	Thromboxane
SPS	Simple partial seizures		
SR	Sustained release	U	Unit
SRS-A	Slow reacting substance of anaphylaxis	UDP	Uridine diphosphate
SSRIs	Selective serotonin reuptake inhibitors	UFH	Unfractionated heparin
STAT	Signal transducer and activator of transcription	UGT	UDP-glucuronosyl transferase
		UT	Urea transporter
susp	Suspension		
SWS	Slow wave sleep	V	Volume of distribution
syr	Syrup	VAL	Valine
		VF	Ventricular fibrillation
$t_{1/2}$	Half-life	Vit	Vitamin
T_3	Triiodothyronine	VLDL	Very low density lipoprotein
T_4	Thyroxine	VMA	Vanillyl mandelic acid
tab	Tablet	VRE	Vancomycin resistant enterococci
TAL	Thick ascending limb of loop of Henle	VRSA	Vancomycin resistant *Staphylococcus aureus*
TB	Tubercle bacilli		
3-TC	Lamivudine	VT	Ventricular tachycardia
TCAs	Tricyclic antidepressants		
TDF	Tenofovir disoproxil fumarate		
TDS	Three times a day	WPW	Wolff-Parkinson-White syndrome
TG	Triglyceride		
6-TG	6-Thioguanine	Z	Pyrazinamide
THC	Tetrahydrocannabinol	ZE syndrome	Zollinger-Ellison syndrome

Section 1

General Pharmacological Principles

Section Outline

1. Introduction, Routes of Drug Administration
2. Pharmacokinetics
3. Pharmacodynamics
4. Adverse Drug Effects

CHAPTER 1

Introduction, Routes of Drug Administration

INTRODUCTION

Pharmacology

Pharmacology is the science of drugs (Greek: Pharmacon—drug; logos—discourse in). In a broad sense, it deals with interaction of exogenously administered chemical molecules (drugs) with living systems, and any chemical substance which can produce a biological response is a 'drug.' Pharmacology encompasses all aspects of knowledge about drugs, but most importantly those that are relevant to effective and safe use of drugs for medicinal purposes.

In the context of dental practice, a broad understanding of pharmacology with emphasis on certain aspects is imperative because:
- Dentists have to prescribe/use drugs, albeit from a limited range, for the treatment of dental conditions.
- Many dental patients concurrently suffer from other medical conditions, e.g. diabetes, hypertension, arthritis, etc. for which they may be taking drugs that may have dental implications or may interact with drugs prescribed by the dentist.
- The dentist may have to deal with a medical emergency arising in the dental office during the course of a procedure.

For thousands of years most drugs were crude natural products of unknown composition and limited efficacy. Only the overt effects of these substances on the body were known, that too rather imprecisely; but how the same were produced was entirely unknown. Over the past 150 years or so, drugs have been purified, chemically characterized and a vast variety of highly potent and selective new drugs have been developed. The mechanism of action including molecular target of many drugs has been elucidated. This has been possible due to prolific growth of pharmacology which forms the backbone of rational therapeutics.

The two main divisions of pharmacology are *pharmacodynamics* and *pharmacokinetics*.

Pharmacodynamics (Greek: *dynamis*—power)—What the drug does to the body.

This includes physiological and biochemical effects of drugs and their mechanism of action at organ system/subcellular/macromolecular levels, e.g. adrenaline → interaction with adrenoceptors → G-protein mediated stimulation of cell membrane bound adenylyl cyclase → increased intracellular cyclic 3',5'AMP → cardiac stimulation, hepatic glycogenolysis and hyperglycaemia, etc.

Pharmacokinetics (Greek: *Kinesis*—movement)—What the body does to the drug.

This refers to movement of the drug in and alteration of the drug by the body; includes absorption, distribution, binding/localization/storage, biotransformation and excretion of the drug, e.g. paracetamol is rapidly and almost completely absorbed orally attaining peak blood levels at 30–60 min; 25% bound to plasma proteins, widely and almost uniformly distributed in the body (volume of distribution ~ 1 L/kg); extensively metabolized in the liver, primarily by glucuronide and sulfate conjugation into inactive metabolites which are excreted in urine; has a plasma half-life (t½) of 2–3 hours and a clearance value of 5 ml/kg/min.

Drug (French: *Drogue*—a dry herb) *It is the single active chemical entity present in a medicine that is used for diagnosis, prevention, treatment/cure of a disease.*

The WHO (1966) has given a more comprehensive definition—*"Drug is any substance or product that is used or is intended to be used to modify or explore physiological systems or pathological states for the benefit of the recipient."*

The term 'drugs' is being also used to mean addictive/abused substances. However, this restricted and derogatory sense usage is unfortunate degradation of a time honoured term, and 'drug' should refer to a substance that has some therapeutic/health promoting/diagnostic application.

Some other important aspects of pharmacology are:

Pharmacotherapeutics It is the application of pharmacological information together with knowledge of the disease for its prevention, mitigation or cure. Selection of the most appropriate drug, dosage and duration of treatment in accordance with the stage of disease and the specific features of a patient are a part of pharmacotherapeutics.

Clinical pharmacology It is the scientific study of drugs (both new and old) in man. It includes pharmacodynamic and pharmacokinetic investigation in healthy volunteers as well as in patients; evaluation of efficacy and safety of drugs and comparative trials with other forms of treatment; surveillance of patterns of drug use, adverse effects, etc.

The aim of clinical pharmacology is to generate data for optimum use of drugs and for practice of medicine to be 'evidence based'.

Chemotherapy It is the treatment of systemic infection/malignancy with specific drugs that have selective toxicity for the infecting organism/malignant cell with no/minimal effects on the host cells.

Drugs, in general, can thus be divided into:

Pharmacodynamic agents These are designed to have pharmacodynamic effects in the recipient.

Chemotherapeutic agents These are designed to inhibit/kill invading parasites/malignant cell, but have no/minimal pharmacodynamic effects in the recipient.

Pharmacy It is the art and science of compounding and dispensing drugs or preparing suitable dosage forms for administration of drugs to man or animals. It includes collection, identification, purification, isolation, synthesis, standardization and quality control of medicinal substances. The large scale manufacture of drugs is called *Pharmaceutics*, which is primarily a technological science.

Toxicology It is the study of poisonous effect of drugs and other chemicals (household, environmental pollutant, industrial, agricultural, homicidal) with emphasis on detection, prevention and treatment of poisonings. It also includes the study of adverse effects of drugs, since the same substance can be a drug or a poison, depending on the dose.

Sources of drugs

Drugs are obtained from a variety of sources:
1. *Plants* Many plants contain biologically active substances and are the oldest source of drugs. Chemically, the active ingredients of plants fall in several categories:
   a. *Alkaloids:* These are alkaline nitrogenous bases having potent activity, and are the most important category of vegetable origin drugs. Prominent examples are: morphine, atropine, ephedrine, nicotine, ergotamine, reserpine, quinine, vincristine, etc. They are mostly used as their water soluble hydrochloride/sulfate salts.
   b. *Glycosides:* These compounds consist of a heterocyclic nonsugar moiety (aglycone) linked to a sugar moiety through ether linkage. Cardiac glycosides (digoxin, ouabain) are the best known glycosidic drugs. The active principle of senna and similar plant purgatives are anthraquinone glycosides. Aminoglycosides (gentamicin, etc.) are antibiotics obtained from microorganisms, and have an aminosugar in place of a sugar moiety.
   c. *Oils:* These are viscous, inflammable liquids, insoluble in water. *Fixed* (nonvolatile) oils are calorie yielding triglycerides of higher fatty acids; mostly used for food and as emollients, e.g. groundnut oil, coconut oil, sesame oil, etc. Castor oil is a stimulant purgative. *Essential* (volatile) oils, mostly obtained from flowers or leaves are aromatic (fragrant) terpene hydrocarbons that have no food value. They are used as flavouring agents, carminatives, counterirritants and astringents; examples are eucalyptus oil, pepermint oil, nilgiri oil, etc. Clove oil is used to allay dental pain. Menthol, thymol, camphor are volatile oils that are solids at room temperature and are included in mouth washes, tooth pastes.
   Mineral oils are not plant products, but obtained from petroleum; liquid paraffin is a lubricant laxative, soft and hard paraffin are used as emollient and as ointment bases.

   Other plant products like tanins are astringent; gums are demulcents and act as suspending agents in liquid dosage forms. Glycerine is a viscous, sweet liquid used as vehicle for gum/throat paint. Resins and balsams are used as antiseptic and in cough mixtures. The antimalarial drug artemisinin is a sesquiterpene endoperoxide obtained from a Chinese plant.
2. *Animals* Though animal parts have been used as cures since early times, it was exploration of activity of organ extracts in the late 19th and early 20th century that led to introduction of animal products into medicine, e.g. adrenaline, thyroxine, insulin, liver extract (vit. B_{12}). Antisera and few vaccines are also produced from animals.
3. *Microbes* Most antibiotics are obtained from fungi, actinomycetes and bacteria, e.g. penicillin, gentamicin, tetracycline, erythromycin, polymyxin B, actinomycin D (anticancer). Some enzymes, e.g. diastase from a fungus and streptokinase from streptococci have a microbial source. Vaccines are produced by the use of microbes.
4. *Minerals* Few minerals, e.g. iron salts, calcium salts, lithium carbonate, magnesium/aluminium hydroxide, iodine are used as medicinal substances.
5. *Synthetic chemistry* Synthetic chemistry made its debut in the 19th century, and is now the largest source of medicines. Not only diverse congeners

of naturally obtained drugs (atropine substitutes, adrenergic β_2 agonists, synthetic glucocorticoids/progestins/cephalosporins, etc.) have been introduced to achieve greater selectivity of action or even novel type of activity, but many entirely synthetic families of drugs, e.g. benzodiazepines, thiazides, benzimidazoles, fluoroquinolones, etc. have been produced. Many drugs are being synthesized to target specific biomolecules, e.g. ACE inhibitors, glycoprotein IIb/IIIa receptor antagonists, HIV-reverse transcriptase inhibitors, etc. Synthetic drugs that are *chiral* can be produced as single active enantiomer products, which may be therapeutically superior.

6. *Biotechnology* Several drugs, especially peptides and proteins are now produced by recombinant DNA technology, e.g. human growth hormone, human insulin, altaplase, interferon, etc. Monoclonal antibodies, regulator peptides, erythropoietin and other growth factors are the newer drugs of biotechnological origin.

Drug nomenclature

A drug generally has three categories of names:

(a) Chemical name It describes the substance chemically, e.g. 1-(Isopropylamino)-3-(1-naphthyloxy) propan-2-o1 for propranolol. This is cumbersome and not suitable for use in prescribing. A code name, e.g. RO 15-1788 (later named flumazenil) may be assigned by the manufacturer for convenience and simplicity before an approved name is coined.

(b) Nonproprietary name It is the name accepted by a competent scientific body/authority, e.g. the United States Adopted Name (USAN) or the British Approved Name (BAN). The nonproprietary names of newer drugs are kept uniform by an agreement to use the 'recommended International Nonproprietary Name (rINN)' only. However, many older drugs have more than one nonproprietary names, e.g. meperidine (USA) and pethidine (UK, India) for the same drug. Until the drug is included in a pharmacopoeia, the nonproprietary name may also be called the approved name. After its appearance in the official publication, it becomes the *official name*.

In common parlance, the term generic name is used in place of nonproprietary name. Etymologically this is incorrect: 'generic' should be applied to the chemical or pharmacological group (or genus) of the compound, e.g. aminoglycoside antibiotics, tricyclic antidepressants, etc.; but has become synonymous with nonproprietary name. A legitimate *'generic medicine'* should be chemically, pharmacokinetically and therapeutically equivalent to the reference 'branded medicine'.

(c) Proprietary (Brand) name It is the name assigned by the manufacturer(s) and is his property or trade mark. One drug may have multiple proprietary names, e.g. NOVAMOX, AMOXYLIN, SYNAMOX, AMOXIL, MOX for amoxicillin from different manufacturers. Brand names are designed to be catchy, short, easy to remember and often suggestive, e.g. LOPRESOR suggesting drug for lowering blood pressure. Brand names generally differ in different countries, e.g. timolol maleate eyedrops are marketed as TIMOPTIC in the USA but as GLUCOMOL in India. Even the same manufacturer may market the same drug under different brand names in different countries. In addition, combined formulations have their own multiple brand names. This is responsible for much confusion in drug nomenclature.

There are many arguments for using the nonproprietary name in prescribing:

uniformity, convenience, economy and better comprehension (propranolol, sotalol, timolol, pindolol, metoprolol, acebutolol, atenolol are all β blockers, but their brand names have no such similarity). Drugs marketed under nonproprietary name (called 'generic' products) are much cheaper than their 'branded' counterparts. However, when it is important to ensure consistency of the product in terms of quality and bioavailability, etc. and especially when official control over quality of manufactured products is not rigorous, it is better to prescribe by the dependable brand name.

Dosage forms of drugs

Dosage form is a product suitable for administration of a drug to a patient. Every active ingredient (drug) has to be formulated by adding other substances (excipients, diluents, preservatives, vehicles, etc.) according to a specific recipe and packaged into a specific 'dosage form' such as tablet, elixir, ointment, injection vial, etc. which is then administered to the subject. The dosage form provides body to the drug, demarcates single doses, protects the active ingredient(s), and makes it suitable for administration in various ways. The important dosage forms are briefly described below.

Solid dosage forms

1. *Powders* The drug is in a dry and finely pulverised state. If the drug is for oral administration, each dose has to be wrapped separately or packed in sachets; therefore this dosage form is inconvenient and unpopular except when the quantity is several grams, e.g. oral rehydration salts. Powders for topical application (tooth powders, dusting powders) are supplied as *bulk powders* in plastic or metallic containers with holes for sprinkling. *Effervescent powders* contain granulated sod. bicarbonate and citric or tartaric acid. They react when dissolved in water to liberate CO_2 causing bubbling.

2. *Tablets* The drug is powdered or granulated, mixed with binding agents, and other excipients, and compressed/moulded into discoid, oblong or other shapes suitable for swallowing. The tablet may be plain or sugar coated/film coated/enteric coated, etc. *Sustained release tablets* contain drug particles which are coated to dissolve at different rates. In *controlled release tablets* a semipermeable membrane controls release of the drug. Other specialized *gastrointestinal therapeutic systems* have also been developed.

3. *Pills* These are archaic dosage forms in which the drug powder is mixed with honey/syrup to make a sticky mass. This is then rolled into spherical/oval bodies meant to be swallowed. The term is often loosely applied to tablets as well.

4. *Capsules* These are water soluble cylindrical containers made of gelatin which are filled with powdered or liquid medicament. The container dissolves on swallowing so that the drug is released in the stomach. *Enteric coated* capsules are designed to dissolve only on reaching the ileum. *Spansules* are extended release capsules which are packed with granules of the drug having different coatings to dissolve over a range of time periods.

5. *Lozenges* These are tablet-like bodies of various shapes containing the drug along with a suitable gum, sweetening and flavouring agents. They are to be retained in the mouth and allowed to dissolve slowly providing the drug for local action in the mouth and throat.

6. *Suppositories* These are conical bullet-shaped dosage forms for insertion into the anal canal, in which the drug is mixed with a mouldable firm base that melts

at body temperature and releases the contained drug. Oval or suitably shaped bodies for vaginal insertion are called *'pessaries'*, while elongated pencil-like cones meant for insertion into male or female urethra are called *bougies*.

Liquid dosage forms

1. *Aqueous solutions* They contain the drug dissolved in water, which may be meant for oral, topical or parenteral administration. Oral drug solutions often contain sweetening and flavouring agents. Preservatives have to be mostly added because shelf-life of watery solutions is short.
2. *Suspensions* are dispersion of insoluble drugs in water with the help of a suspending agent. *Emulsions* are uniform mixtures of two immiscible liquids (mostly oil and water) in which droplets of one (dispersed phase) are suspended in the other (continuous phase) with the help of an amphiphilic emulsifying agent. Milk is a naturally occurring emulsion. Both suspensions and emulsions tend to settle down on keeping; should be shaken thoroughly before use.
3. *Elixirs* are hydro-alcoholic solutions of drugs, usually sweetened with syrup and flavoured by fruit extracts. *Syrups* have higher concentration of sugar and are thicker in consistency. Drugs that deteriorate in aqueous medium are dispensed in bottles as *dry syrups* which are reconstituted by adding measured quantity of water and shaking. The reconstituted suspension must be used within a few days. *Linctus* is a viscous syrupy liquid meant to be licked slowly for soothing the throat. It generally has menthol to impart cooling sensation, and an antitussive.
4. *Drops* These are relatively more concentrated solutions of medicaments meant for oral ingestion or external application to eye, nose or ear canal. Oral drops are the preferred dosage form for infants and young children. Eye/nasal drops should be isotonic. Eye drops need sterilization. Drops are supplied in vials with a nozzle, or alongwith a dropper for accurate dosing.
5. *Lotions* These are solutions, suspensions or emulsions meant for external application to the skin without rubbing. They generally have soothing, cooling, protective or emollient property. *Liniments* are similar preparations which generally contain counterirritants, and are to be rubbed on the skin to relieve pain and cause rubefaction.
6. *Injections* These are sterile solutions or suspensions in aqueous or oily medium for subcutaneous or intramuscular administration. Only aqueous solutions (not suspensions) are suitable for intravenous (i.v.) injection, because particles in suspension and oils injected i.v. can cause embolism. Injections are supplied in sealed glass *ampoules* or air tight rubber capped *vials*. Ampoules are broken just before injection, and usually contain a single dose. Drug from the vial is sucked in a syringe by piercing the rubber cap. Vials may be single-dose or multi-dose. Drugs which are unstable in solution are supplied as dry powder vials. Sterile solvent is injected in the vial and the dissolved/suspended drug is then sucked out into the syringe just before administration. Large volume i.v. infusions are marketed in glass/polypropylene bottles.

Semisolid dosage forms

1. *Ointments* These are greasy semisolid preparations meant for external application to the skin, eye, nasal mucosa, ear or anal canal. The drug is

incorporated in an oily base, such as soft or hard paraffin, wool fat, bee's wax, etc. Ointments are not suitable for oozing surfaces, because they do not allow evaporation of water. *Creams* are similar to ointment but the base is a water in oil emulsion.

2. *Pastes* These are nongreasy preparations of thick consistency containing hydrophilic adhesive powders such as starch, prepared chalk, aluminium/magnesium hydroxide, zinc oxide, carboxy methylcellulose, etc. which swell by absorbing water. Pastes may contain viscous nonoily liquids like glycerol or propylene glycol. Pastes can be applied to inflamed or excoriated skin, oozing surfaces, teeth and mucous membranes. Toothpastes are items of personal hygiene, and medicated toothpastes are extensively used in dentistry.

3. *Gels* The medicament is incorporated in a viscous colloidal solution of gelatin or similar material and is usually dispensed in collapsible tubes. They are meant for external application to the skin or mucosa and provide longer duration contact, but are nongreasy and washable with water. Gels are commonly applied to oral ulcers because they are better retained than aqueous solutions. Many toothpastes are gels.

Inhalations

Drugs which are gases or volatile liquids can be administered by inhalation carried into air or oxygen with the help of a mouth piece, face mask, hood or endotracheal tube. Nonvolatile liquids and fine particle solids can be aerosolized using a metered dose inhaler, jet nebulizer, rotahaler or spinhaler for inhalation through the mouth. *Pressurized metered dose inhalers* (PMDIs) are hand-held devices which use a propellant, mostly hydrofluoroalkane (HFA), and deliver a specified dose of the drug in aerosol form per actuation. *Jet nebulizers* produce a mist of the drug solution generated by pressurized air or oxygen. *Rotahaler* is also a portable device in which a capsule (rotacap) containing very fine powder of the drug is punctured during actuation and the released particles are aerosolized by the inspiratory airflow of the patient. A propellant can also be used in some *spin halers*. Efficacy of the aerosolized drug depends on the particle size: 1–5 μm diameter particles deposit on the bronchioles and effectively deliver the drug. Larger particles settle on the oropharynx, while <1 μm particles do not settle anywhere and are exhaled out.

Prescription and non-prescription drugs

As per drug rules, majority of drugs including all antibiotics must be sold in retail only against a prescription issued to a patient by a registered medical practitioner. These are called 'prescription drugs'. In India such drugs have been placed in the *schedule H* of the Drugs and Cosmetic Rules (1945) as amended from time to time. However, few drugs like simple analgesics (paracetamol, aspirin), antacids, laxatives (senna, lactulose), vitamins, ferrous salts, etc. are considered relatively harmless, and can be procured without a prescription. These are 'non-prescription' or 'over-the-counter' (OTC) drugs; can be sold even by grocery stores.

ROUTES OF DRUG ADMINISTRATION

Most drugs can be administered by a variety of routes. The choice of appropriate route in a given situation depends both on drug as well as patient-related factors. Mostly common sense considerations, feasibility and convenience dictate the route to be used.

Factors governing choice of route
1. Physical and chemical properties of the drug (solid/liquid/gas; solubility, stability, pH, irritancy).
2. Site of desired action—localized and approachable or generalized and not approachable.
3. Rate and extent of absorption of the drug from different routes.
4. Effect of digestive juices and first pass metabolism on the drug.
5. Rapidity with which the response is desired (routine treatment or emergency).
6. Accuracy of dosage required (i.v. and inhalational can provide fine tuning).
7. Condition of the patient (unconscious, vomiting).

Routes can be broadly divided into those for (a) local action and (b) systemic action.

LOCAL ROUTES

These routes can only be used for localized lesions at accessible sites and for drugs whose systemic absorption from these sites is minimal, slow or absent. Thus, high concentrations are attained at the desired site without exposing the rest of the body. Systemic side effects or toxicity are consequently absent or minimal. For drugs (in suitable dosage forms) that are absorbed from these sites/routes, the same can serve as a systemic route of administration. The local routes are:

1. Topical This refers to external application of the drug to the surface for localized action. It is often more convenient and efficient mode of delivering the drug to skin, oropharyngeal/nasal mucosa, eyes, ear canal, anal canal, vagina, etc. Nonabsorbable drugs given orally for action on g.i. mucosa (sucralfate, neomycin), inhalation of drugs for action on bronchi (salbutamol, fluticasone propionate) and irrigating solutions/jellies (povidone iodine, lidocaine) applied to urethra are other forms of topical medication. In dental practice antiseptics, astringents, haemostatics are often applied as paints, toothpastes, mouthwashes, gargles or lozenges.

2. Deeper tissues Certain deep areas can be approached by using a syringe and needle, but the drug should be in such a form that systemic absorption is slow, e.g. infiltration around a nerve or intrathecal injection (lidocaine, amphotericin B), intra-articular injection (hydrocortisone acetate), retrobulbar injection (hydrocortisone acetate).

3. Arterial supply Close intra-arterial injection is used for contrast media in angiography; anticancer drugs can be infused in femoral or brachial artery to localize the effect for limb malignancies.

SYSTEMIC ROUTES

The drug administered through systemic routes is intended to be absorbed into bloodstream and distributed all over, including the site of action, through circulation (Fig. 1.1).

1. Oral

Oral ingestion is the oldest and commonest mode of drug administration. It is safer, more convenient, does not need assistance, noninvasive, often painless, the medicament need not be sterile and so is cheaper. Both solid dosage forms (powders, tablets, capsules, spansules, dragees, moulded tablets, gastrointestinal therapeutic systems—GITs) and liquid dosage forms (elixirs, syrups, emulsions, mixtures) can be given orally.

> **Limitations of oral route of administration**
> - Action is slower and thus not suitable for emergencies.
> - Unpalatable drugs (chloramphenicol) are difficult to administer; drug may be filled in capsules to circumvent this.
> - May cause nausea and vomiting.
> - Cannot be used for uncooperative/unconscious/vomiting patient.
> - Certain drugs (e.g. gentamicin) are not absorbed. Absorption of some drugs is variable and not dependable.
> - Some drugs are destroyed by digestive juices (penicillin G, insulin) or in liver (glyceryl trinitrate, testosterone, lidocaine) by high first pass metabolism.

2. Sublingual (s.l.) or buccal

The tablet or pellet containing the drug is placed under the tongue or crushed in the mouth and spread over the buccal mucosa. Only lipid-soluble and non-irritating drugs can be so administered. Absorption is relatively rapid—action can be produced in minutes. Though it is somewhat inconvenient, one can spit the remaining drug after the desired effect has been obtained. The chief advantage is that liver is bypassed and drugs with high first pass metabolism can be absorbed directly into systemic circulation. Drugs given sublingually are—glyceryl trinitrate, buprenorphine, desamino-oxytocin.

3. Rectal

Certain drugs put into rectum as suppositories or retention enema get absorbed and produce systemic effect. This route is particularly utilized for irritant or unpleasant drugs, as well as for a patient having recurrent vomiting. However, rectal route is rather inconvenient and embarrassing; absorption is slower, irregular and often unpredictable, though diazepam solution and paracetamol suppository are dependably absorbed from the rectum in children. Drug absorbed into external haemorrhoidal veins (about 50%) bypasses liver, but not that absorbed into internal haemorrhoidal veins. Rectal inflammation can result from irritant drugs. Indomethacin, diazepam, ergotamine and a few other drugs are sometimes given rectally.

4. Cutaneous

Highly lipid-soluble drugs can be applied over the skin for slow and prolonged absorption. The liver is also bypassed. The drug can be incorporated in an ointment and applied over specified area of skin.

Transdermal therapeutic systems (TTS) These are devices in the form of adhesive patches of various shapes and sizes (5–20 cm^2) which deliver the contained drug at a constant rate into the systemic circulation via the stratum corneum (Fig. 1.2). The drug (in solution or bound to a polymer) is held in a reservoir between an occlusive backing film and a rate controlling micropore membrane, the undersurface of which is smeared with an adhesive impregnated with priming dose of the drug that is protected by another film to be peeled off just before application. The drug is delivered at the skin surface by diffusion for percutaneous absorption into circulation. The micropore membrane is such that rate of drug delivery to the skin surface is less than the slowest rate of absorption from skin. This offsets any variation in the rate of absorption according to the properties of different sites. As such, drug is delivered at constant and predictable rate irrespective of site of application, which is usually chest, abdomen, upper arm, lower back, buttock or mastoid region.

Transdermal patches of glyceryl trinitrate, fentanyl, nicotine and estradiol are available in India, while those of isosorbide dinitrate, hyoscine, and clonidine are marketed elsewhere. For different drugs, transdermal patches have been designed to last 1–3 days. They are relatively more expensive than oral dosage forms, but first pass metabolism is avoided. Local irritation and erythema occurs in some, but is generally mild; can be minimized by changing the site of application each time by rotation. Discontinuation has been necessary in 2 to 7% cases.

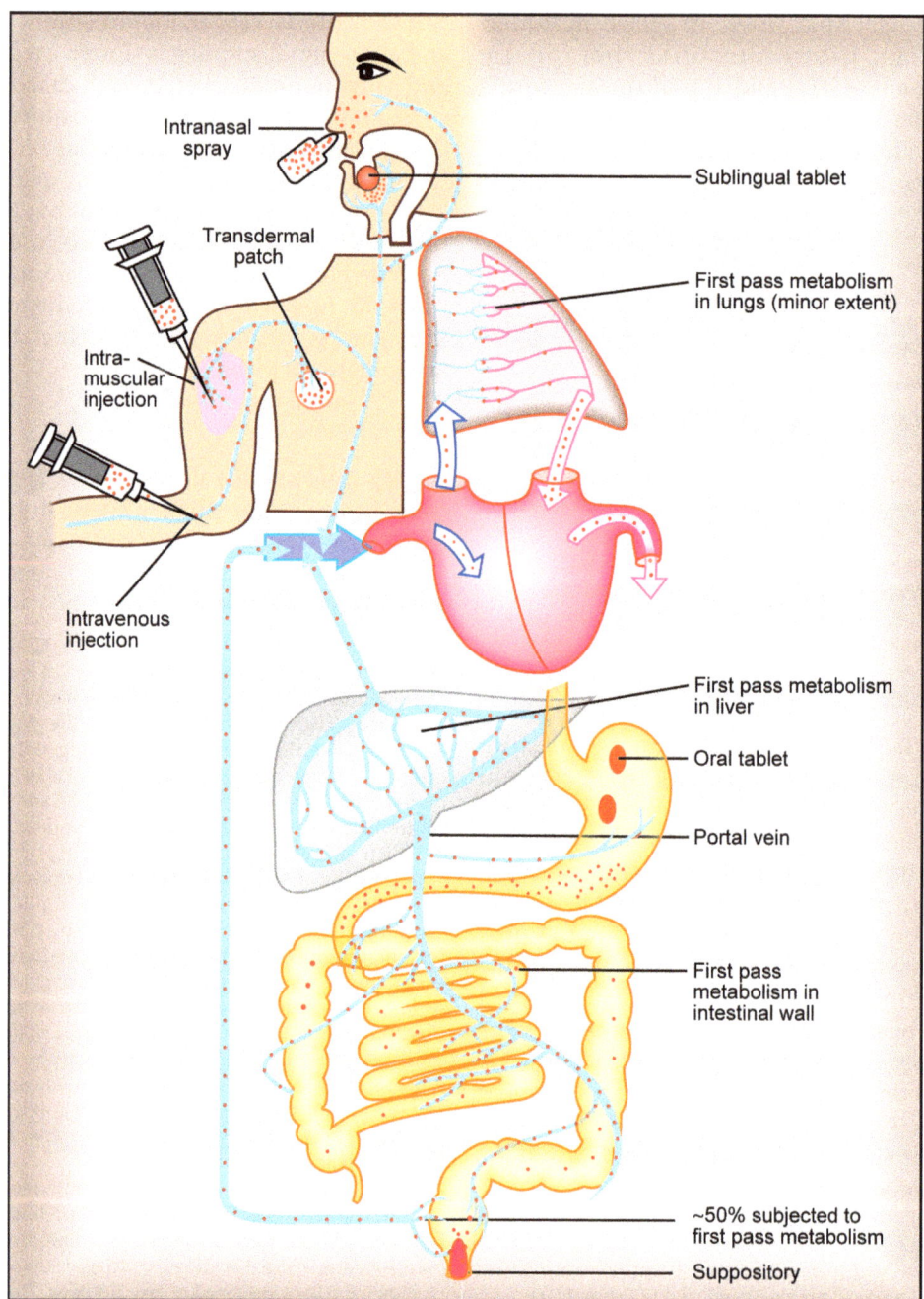

Fig. 1.1: Vascular pathway of drugs absorbed from various systemic routes of administration, and sites of first pass metabolism
Note: All the drug administered orally is subjected to first pass metabolism in intestinal wall and liver, while approximately half of that absorbed from rectum passes through liver. Drug entering from any systemic route is exposed to first pass metabolism in lungs, but its extent is minor for most drugs.

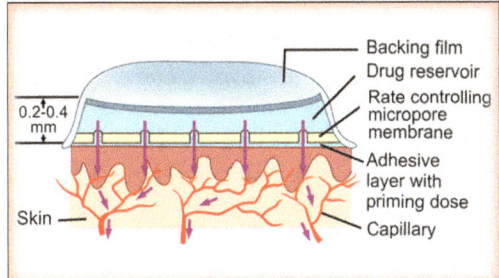

Fig. 1.2: Illustration of a transdermal drug delivery system

5. Inhalation

Volatile liquids and gases are given by inhalation for systemic action, e.g. general anaesthetics. Absorption takes place from the vast surface of alveoli—action is very rapid. When administration is discontinued, the drug diffuses back and is rapidly eliminated in expired air. Thus, controlled administration is possible with moment-to-moment adjustment. Irritant vapours (ether) cause inflammation of respiratory tract and increase secretion.

6. Nasal

The mucous membrane of the nose can readily absorb many drugs. Digestive juices and liver are bypassed. However, only certain drugs like GnRH agonists and desmopressin applied as a spray or nebulized solution have been used by this route.

7. Parenteral

(*Par*—beyond, enteral—intestinal) Conventionally, 'parenteral' refers to administration by injection which takes the drug directly into the tissue fluid or blood without having to cross the enteral mucosa. The limitations of oral administration are circumvented. Drug action is faster and surer (this is valuable in emergencies). Gastric irritation and vomiting are not provoked. Parenteral route can be employed even in unconscious, uncooperative or vomiting patient. There are no chances of interference by food or digestive juices. Liver is bypassed.

Disadvantages of parenteral routes are—the preparation has to be sterilized and is costlier, the technique is invasive and painful, assistance of another person is mostly needed (though self-injection is possible, e.g. insulin by diabetics), there are chances of local tissue injury, and in general it is more risky than oral. The important parenteral routes are:

(i) Subcutaneous (s.c.) The drug is deposited in the loose subcutaneous tissue which is richly supplied by nerves (irritant drugs cannot be injected) but is less vascular (absorption is slower). Self-injection is possible because deep penetration is not needed. This route should be avoided in shock patients who are vasoconstricted—absorption will be delayed. Repository (depot) preparations—oily solutions or aqueous suspensions can be injected for prolonged action.

Some special forms of this route are:

(a) *Dermojet* In this method needle is not used; a high velocity jet of drug solution is projected from a microfine orifice using a gun-like implement. The solution passes through the superficial layers and gets deposited in the subcutaneous tissue. It is essentially painless and suited for mass inoculations.

(b) *Pellet implantation* The drug as solid pellet is introduced with a trochar and cannula. This provides sustained release of the drug over weeks and months, e.g. DOCA, testosterone.

(c) *Sialistic (nonbiodegradable) and biodegradable implants* Crystalline drug is packed in tubes/capsules made of suitable materials and implanted under the skin. Slow and uniform leaching of the drug occurs over months providing constant blood levels. The nonbiodegradable implant has to be removed later on but not the biodegradable one. This has been tried for hormones and contraceptives (e.g. NORPLANT).

(ii) Intramuscular (i.m.) The drug is injected in one of the large skeletal muscles—deltoid, triceps, gluteus maximus, rectus femoris, etc. Muscle is less richly supplied with sensory nerves (mild irritants can be injected) and is more vascular (absorption is faster). It is less painful, but self-injection is often impracticable—deep penetration is needed. Depot preparations can be injected by this route. Intramuscular injection should be avoided in patients taking anticoagulant medication.

(iii) Intravenous (i.v.) The drug is injected as a bolus (Greek: bolos-lump) or infused slowly over hours in one of the superficial veins. The drug reaches directly into the bloodstream and effects are produced immediately. This is of great value in emergency. The intima of veins is insensitive and drug gets diluted with blood, therefore, even highly irritant drugs can be injected i.v., but the hazards of this route are—thrombophlebitis of the injected vein and necrosis of adjoining tissues if extravasation occurs. These complications can be minimized by diluting the drug or injecting it into a running i.v. line. Only aqueous solutions (not suspensions) can be injected i.v. and there are no depot preparations for this route. The dose of the drug required is smallest (bioavailability is 100%) and even large volumes can be infused. One big advantage with this route is—in case response is accurately measurable (e.g. BP) and the drug short acting (e.g. sodium nitroprusside), titration of the dose with the response is possible. However, this is the most risky route—vital organs like heart, brain, etc. get exposed to high concentrations of the drug. Possibility of causing air embolism is another risk.

(iv) Intradermal injection The drug is injected into the skin raising a bleb (e.g. BCG vaccine, sensitivity testing) or scarring/multiple puncture of the epidermis through a drop of the drug is done. This route is employed for specific purposes only.

Pharmacokinetics

Pharmacokinetics is the quantitative study of drug movement in, through and out of the body. The overall scheme of pharmacokinetic processes is depicted in Fig. 2.1. Intensity of response is related to concentration of the drug at the site of action, which in turn is dependent on its pharmacokinetic properties. Pharmacokinetic considerations, therefore, determine the route(s) of administration, dose, latency of onset, time of peak action, duration of action and thus frequency of administration of a drug.

All pharmacokinetic processes involve transport of the drug across biological membranes.

Biological membrane This is a bilayer (about 100 Å thick) of phospholipid and cholesterol molecules, the polar groups of these are oriented at the two surfaces and the nonpolar hydrocarbon chains are embedded in the matrix, along with adsorbed extrinsic and intrinsic protein molecules (Fig. 2.2). The proteins are able to freely float through the membrane: associate and organize or vice versa. Some of the intrinsic ones, which extend through the full thickness of the membrane, surround fine aqueous pores. Paracellular spaces or channels also exist between certain epithelial/endothelial cells. Other adsorbed proteins have enzymatic,

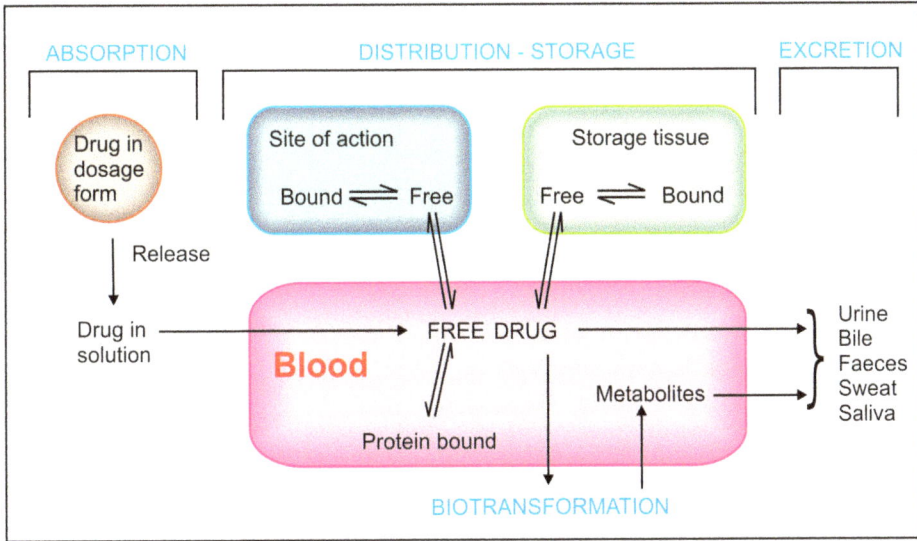

Fig. 2.1: Schematic depiction of pharmacokinetic processes

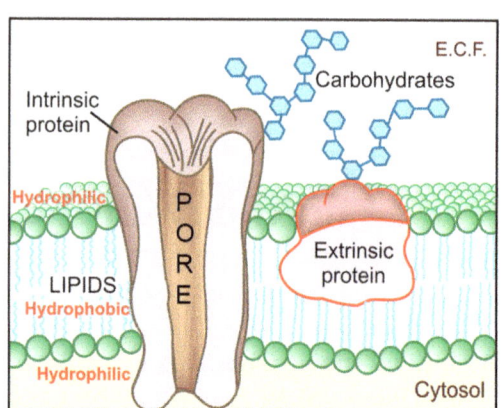

Fig. 2.2: Illustration of the organization of biological membrane

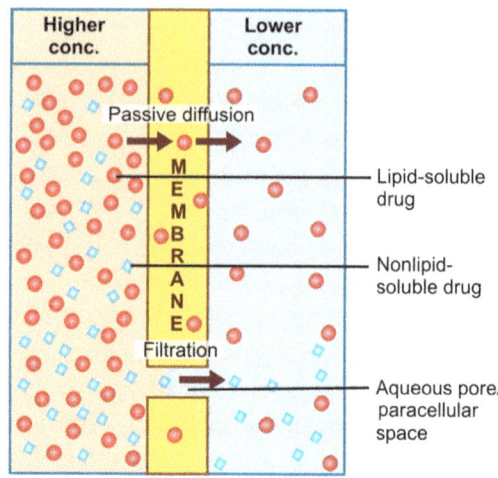

Fig. 2.3: Illustration of passive diffusion and filtration across the lipoidal biological membrane with aqueous pores

carrier, receptor or signal transduction properties. Lateral movement of lipid molecules also occurs. As such, biological membranes are highly dynamic structures. Drugs are transported across the membranes by:
(a) Passive diffusion and filtration.
(b) Specialized transport.

Passive diffusion

The drug diffuses across the membrane in the direction of its concentration gradient (high to low), the membrane playing no active role in the process. This is the most important mechanism for majority of drugs, because drugs are foreign substances and specialized mechanisms are developed by the body for normal metabolites only.

Lipid-soluble drugs diffuse by dissolving in the lipoidal matrix of the membrane (Fig. 2.3), the rate of transport being proportional to the lipid : water partition coefficient of the drug. A more lipid-soluble drug attains higher concentration in the membrane and diffuses quickly. Further, greater the difference in the concentration of the drug on two sides of the membrane, faster is its diffusion.

Influence of pH Most drugs are weak electrolytes, i.e. their ionization is pH dependent (contrast strong electrolytes which are nearly completely ionized at acidic as well as alkaline pH). The ionization of a weak acid HA is given by the equation:

$$pH = pKa + \log \frac{[A^-]}{[HA]} \quad \ldots(1)$$

pKa is the negative logarithm of acidic dissociation constant of the weak electrolyte. If the concentration of ionized drug $[A^-]$ is equal to the concentration of unionized drug $[HA]$, then—

$$\frac{[A^-]}{[HA]} = 1$$

since log 1 is 0, under this condition

$$pH = pKa \quad \ldots(2)$$

Thus, pKa is numerically equal to the pH at which the drug is 50% ionized.
If pH is increased by 1, then—
  $\log [A^-]/[HA] = 1$ or $[A^-]/[HA] = 10$
Similarly, if pH is reduced by 1, then—
  $[A^-]/[HA] = 1/10$

Thus, weakly acidic drugs, which form salts with cations, e.g. sod. phenobarbitone, sod. sulfadiazine, pot. penicillin-V, etc. ionize more at alkaline pH and 1 scale change in pH causes 10-fold change in ionization.

Weakly basic drugs, which form salts with anions, e.g. atropine sulfate, ephedrine HCl, chloroquine phosphate, etc. conversely ionize more at acidic pH. Ions being lipid insoluble, do not diffuse and a pH difference across a membrane can cause differential distribution of weakly acidic and weakly basic drugs on the two sides (Fig. 2.4).

Implications of this consideration are:
(a) Acidic drugs, e.g. aspirin (pKa 3.5) are largely unionized at acid gastric pH and are absorbed from the stomach, while bases, e.g. atropine (pKa 10) are largely ionized and are absorbed only when they reach the intestines.
(b) The unionized form of acidic drugs which crosses the surface membrane of gastric mucosal cell, reverts to the ionized form within the cell (where pH is 7.0) and then only slowly passes to the extracellular fluid. This is called ion trapping, i.e. a weak electrolyte crossing a membrane to encounter a pH from which it is not able to escape easily. This may contribute to gastric mucosal cell damage caused by aspirin.
(c) Basic drugs attain higher concentration intracellularly (pH 7.0 vs 7.4 of plasma).
(d) Acidic drugs are ionized more in alkaline urine—do not back diffuse in the kidney tubules and are excreted faster. Accordingly, basic drugs are excreted faster if urine is acidified.

Lipid-soluble nonelectrolytes (e.g. ethanol, diethyl-ether) readily cross biological membranes and their transport is pH independent.

Filtration

Filtration is passage of drugs through aqueous pores in the membrane or through paracellular spaces. This can be accelerated if hydrodynamic flow of the solvent is occurring under hydrostatic or osmotic pressure gradient, e.g. across most capillaries

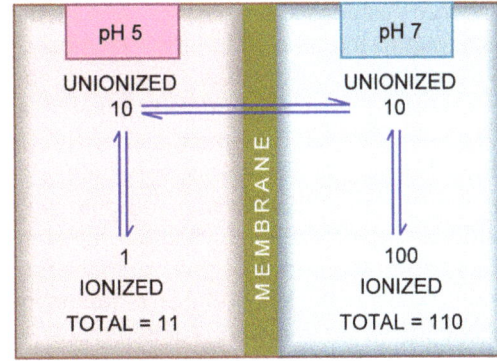

Fig. 2.4: Influence of pH difference on two sides of a biological membrane on the distribution of a weakly acidic drug with *pKa* = 6

including glomeruli. Lipid-insoluble drugs cross biological membranes by filtration if their molecular size is smaller than the diameter of the pores (Fig. 2.3). Majority of cells (intestinal mucosa, RBC, etc.) have very small pores (4 Å) and drugs with MW > 100 or 200 are not able to penetrate. However, capillaries (except those in brain) have large paracellular spaces (40 Å) and most drugs (even albumin) can filter through these (*see* Fig. 2.8A). As such, diffusion of drugs across capillaries is dependent on rate of blood flow through them rather than on lipid-solubility of the drug or pH of the medium.

Specialized transport

This can be carrier mediated or by vesicular transport (endocytosis and exocytosis).

Carrier transport

All cell membranes express a host of transmembrane proteins which serve as carriers or transporters for physiologically important ions, nutrients, metabolites, transmitters, etc. across the membrane. At some sites, certain transporters also translocate xenobiotics, including drugs and their metabolites. In contrast to channels, which open for a finite time and allow passage of specific ions, transporters combine transiently with their substrate (ion or organic compound)—

undergo a conformational change carrying the substrate to the other side of the membrane where the substrate dissociates and the transporter returns back to its original state (Fig. 2.5). Carrier transport is specific for the substrate (or the type of substrate, e.g. an organic anion), saturable, competitively inhibited by analogues which utilize the same transporter, and is much slower than the flux through channels. Depending on requirement of energy, carrier transport is of two types:

a. *Facilitated diffusion* The transporter, belonging to the super-family of solute carrier (SLC) transporters, operates passively without needing energy and translocates the substrate in the direction of its electrochemical gradient, i.e. from higher to lower concentration (Fig. 2.5A). It merely facilitates permeation of a poorly diffusible substrate, e.g. the entry of glucose into muscle and fat cells by the glucose transporter GLUT 4.

b. *Active transport* It requires energy, is inhibited by metabolic poisons, and transports the solute against its electrochemical gradient (low to high), resulting in selective accumulation of the substance on one side of the membrane. Drugs related to normal metabolites can utilize the transport processes meant for these, e.g. levodopa and methyl dopa are actively absorbed from the gut by the aromatic amino acid transporter. In addition, the body has developed some relatively nonselective transporters, like P-glycoprotein (P-gp), to deal with xenobiotics. Active transport can be primary or secondary depending on the source of the driving force.

i. *Primary active transport* Energy is obtained directly by the hydrolysis of ATP (Fig. 2.5B). The transporters belong to the superfamily of ATP binding cassette (ABC) transporters whose intracellular loops have ATPase activity.

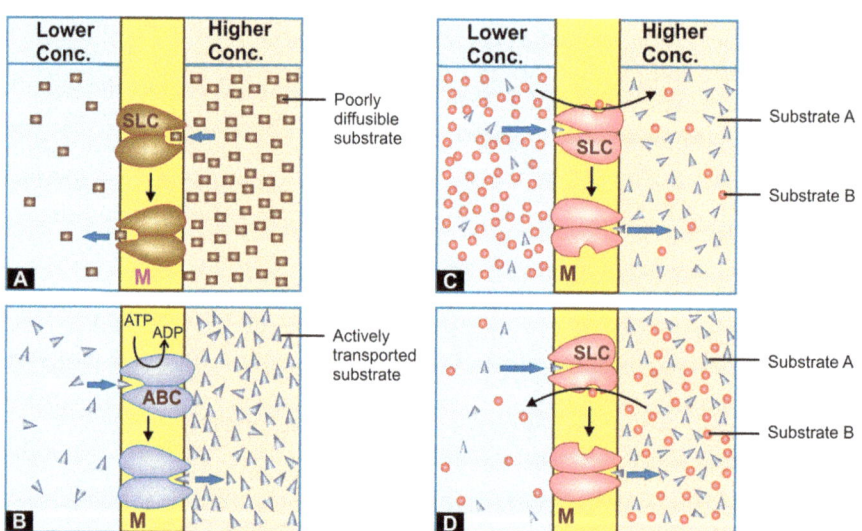

Fig. 2.5: Illustration of different types of carrier mediated transport across biological membrane
ABC—ATP-binding cassette transporter; SLC—Solute carrier transporter; M—Membrane
A. *Facilitated diffusion:* The carrier (SLC) binds and moves the poorly diffusible substrate along its concentration gradient (high to low) and does not require energy
B. *Primary active transport:* The carrier (ABC) derives energy directly by hydrolysing ATP and moves the substrate against its concentration gradient (low to high)
C. *Symport:* The carrier moves the substrate 'A' against its concentration gradient by utilizing energy from downhill movement of another substrate 'B' in the same direction
D. *Antiport:* The carrier moves the substrate 'A' against its concentration gradient and is energized by the downhill movement of another substrate 'B' in the opposite direction

P-glycoprotein is the most well-known primary active transporter. Others of pharmacological significance are multidrug resistance associated protein 2 (MRP 2) and breast cancer resistance protein (BCRP).

ii. **Secondary active transport** In this type of active transport effected by another set of SLC transporters, the energy to pump one solute is derived from the downhill movement of another solute (mostly Na⁺). When the concentration gradients are such that both the solutes move in the same direction (Fig. 2.5C), it is called *symport* or *cotransport*, but when they move in opposite directions (Fig. 2.5D), it is termed *antiport* or *exchange transport*. Metabolic energy (from hydrolysis of ATP) is spent in maintaining high transmembrane electrochemical gradient of the second solute.

The organic anion transporting polypeptide (OATP) and organic cation transporter (OCT), highly expressed in liver canaliculi and renal tubules, are secondary active transporters important in the metabolism and excretion of drugs and metabolites (especially glucuronides). The Na⁺,Cl⁻ dependent neurotransmitter transporters for norepinephrine, serotonin and dopamine (NET, SERT and DAT) are active SLC transporters that are targets for action of drugs like tricyclic antidepressants, selective serotonin reuptake inhibitors (SSRIs), cocaine, etc.

Vesicular transport (endocytosis, exocytosis)

Certain substances with very large or impermeable molecules are transported inside the cell (*endocytosis*) or extruded from it (*exocytosis*) by enclosing their particles into tiny vesicles. A binding protein located on the membrane complexes with the substance and initiates vesicle formation (Fig. 2.6). The vesicle then detaches from the membrane and may remain stored within the cell, or it may release the substance in the cytoplasm, or it may move to the opposite membrane, fuse with it to release the substance across the cell (exocytosis).

Vesicular transport is applicable to proteins and other big molecules, and contributes little to transport of most drugs, barring few like vit B₁₂ which is absorbed from the gut after binding to intrinsic factor (a protein). Most hormones (insulin, etc.) and neurotransmitters, like noradrenaline, are secreted/released from the cell/nerve ending by exocytosis.

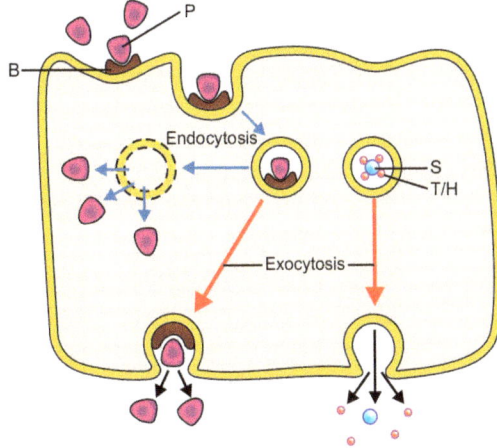

Fig. 2.6: Illustration of vesicular transport (endocytosis and exocytosis).
Endocytosis: The large molecular particle (P) binds to a binding protein (B) on the surface of the cell. The membrane invaginates to form a vesicle. The vesicle may remain stored within the cell, or it may disintegrate to release the substance in the cytoplasm, or be extruded across the cell by exocytosis.
Exocytosis: The particle or the transmitter/hormone (T/H) stored within intracellular vesicles, generally as a complex with a storage protein (S), is secreted by exocytosis.

ABSORPTION OF DRUGS

Absorption is the movement of drug from its site of administration into the circulation. Not only the fraction of the administered dose that gets absorbed, but also the rate of absorption is important. Except when given i.v., the drug has to cross biological membranes; absorption is governed by the above described principles. Other factors affecting absorption are:

Aqueous solubility Drugs given in solid form must dissolve in the aqueous biophase before they are absorbed. For poorly water-soluble drugs (aspirin, griseofulvin) rate of dissolution governs rate of absorption. Obviously, a drug given as watery solution is absorbed faster than when the same is given in solid form or as oily solution.

Concentration Passive transport depends on concentration gradient; drug given as concentrated solution is absorbed faster than from dilute solution.

Area of absorbing surface Larger it is, faster is the absorption.

Vascularity of the absorbing surface Blood circulation removes the drug from the site of absorption and maintains the concentration gradient across the absorbing surface. Increased blood flow hastens drug absorption just as wind hastens drying of clothes.

Route of administration This affects drug absorption, because each route has its own peculiarities.

Oral

The effective barrier to orally administered drugs is the epithelial lining of the gastrointestinal tract, which is lipoidal. Nonionized lipid-soluble drugs, e.g. ethanol are readily absorbed from stomach as well as intestine at rates proportional to their lipid : water partition coefficient. Acidic drugs, e.g. salicylates, barbiturates, etc. are predominantly unionized in the acid gastric juice and are absorbed from the stomach, while basic drugs, e.g. morphine, quinine, etc. are largely ionized and are absorbed only on reaching the duodenum. However, even for acidic drugs absorption from stomach is slower, because the mucosa is thick, covered with mucus and the surface area is small. Thus, faster gastric emptying accelerates drug absorption in general. Dissolution is a surface phenomenon, therefore, particle size of the drug in solid dosage form governs rate of dissolution and in turn rate of absorption.

Presence of food dilutes the drug and retards absorption. Moreover, certain drugs form poorly absorbed complexes with food constituents, e.g. tetracyclines with calcium present in milk. In addition, food delays gastric emptying. Thus, most drugs are absorbed better if taken in empty stomach. However, there are some exceptions, e.g. fatty food enhances absorption of lumefantrine. Highly ionized drugs, e.g. gentamicin, neostigmine, are practically not absorbed when given orally.

Certain drugs are degraded in the gastrointestinal tract, e.g. penicillin G by gastric acid, insulin by peptidases, and are ineffective orally. Enteric coated tablets (having acid resistant coating) and sustained release preparations (drug particles coated with slowly dissolving material) can be used to overcome acid lability, gastric irritancy and brief duration of action.

Oral absorption of certain drugs like digoxin, cyclosporine is limited, because a fraction of the absorbed drug is extruded back into the intestinal lumen by the efflux transporter P-gp located in the gut epithelium.

Absorption of a drug can be affected by other concurrently ingested drugs. This may be a *luminal effect*: formation of insoluble complexes, e.g. tetracyclines, iron preparations with calcium salts and antacids, or ciprofloxacin with sucralfate. This interaction can be minimized by administering the two drugs with a gap of 2–3 hours. Alteration of gut flora by antibiotics may disrupt the enterohepatic cycling of oral contraceptives and digoxin. Drugs can also alter absorption by *gut wall effects*: altering motility (anticholinergics, tricyclic antidepressants, opioids retard motility, while metoclopramide enhances it) or causing mucosal damage (neomycin, methotrexate, vinblastine).

Subcutaneous and intramuscular

By these routes the drug is deposited directly in the vicinity of the capillaries. Lipid-soluble drugs pass readily across the whole surface of the capillary endothelium. Capillaries being highly porous do not obstruct absorption of even large lipid-insoluble molecules or ions (*see* Fig. 2.9A). Very large molecules are absorbed through lymphatics. Thus, many drugs not absorbed orally are absorbed parenterally. Absorption from s.c. site is slower than that from i.m. site, but both are generally faster and more consistent/predictable than oral absorption. Application of heat and muscular exercise accelerate drug absorption by increasing blood flow, while vasoconstrictors, e.g. adrenaline injected with the drug (local anaesthetic) retard absorption. Many depot preparations, e.g. benzathine penicillin, depot progestins, etc. can be given by these routes.

Topical sites (skin, cornea, mucous membranes)

Systemic absorption after topical application depends primarily on lipid solubility of the drug. However, only few drugs significantly penetrate intact skin. Glyceryl trinitrate, fentanyl, nicotine, testosterone and estradiol (*see* p. 11) have been used in this manner. Absorption can be promoted by rubbing the drug incorporated in an olegenous base or by use of occlusive dressing which increases hydration of the skin. Organophosphate insecticides coming in contact with skin can produce systemic toxicity. Abraded surfaces readily absorb drugs.

Cornea is permeable to lipid soluble, unionized physostigmine but not to highly ionized neostigmine. Similarly, mucous membranes of mouth, rectum, vagina absorb lipophilic drugs.

Bioavailability

Bioavailability refers to the rate and extent of absorption of a drug from a dosage form administered by any route, as determined by its concentration-time curve in blood or by its excretion in urine (Fig. 2.7). It is a measure of the fraction (F) of administered dose of a drug that reaches the systemic circulation in the unchanged form. Bioavailability of drug injected i.v. is 100%, but is frequently lower after oral ingestion because—
(a) The drug may be incompletely absorbed.
(b) The absorbed drug may undergo first pass metabolism in intestinal wall/liver or be excreted in bile.
Incomplete bioavailability after s.c. or i.m. injection is less common, but may occur due to local binding of the drug.

Bioequivalence Oral formulation of a drug from different manufacturers or different batches from the same manufacturer may have the same amount of the drug

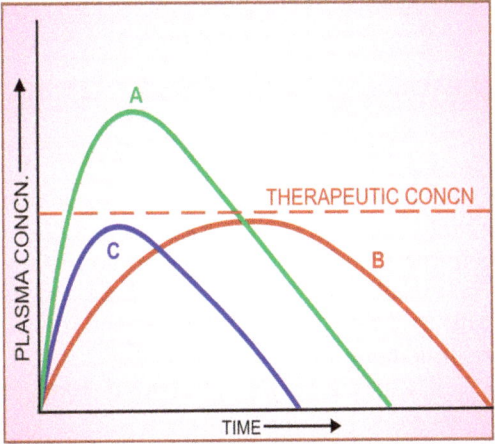

Fig. 2.7: Plasma concentration-time curves depicting bioavailability differences between three preparations of a drug containing the same amount
Note that formulation B is more slowly absorbed than A, and though ultimately both are absorbed to the same extent (area under the curve same), B may not produce therapeutic effect after a single dose. However, average blood levels may be similar with both A and B formulations when repeated doses are given. C is absorbed to a lesser extent—lower bioavailability.

(chemically equivalent) but may not yield the same blood levels—*biologically inequivalent*. Two preparations of a drug are considered bioequivalent when the rate and extent of bioavailability of the active drug from them is not significantly different under suitable test conditions.

Before a drug administered orally in solid dosage form can be absorbed, it must break into individual particles of the active drug (disintegration). Tablets and capsules contain a number of other materials—diluents, stabilizing agents, binders, lubricants, etc. The nature of these as well as details of the manufacture process, e.g. force used in compressing the tablet, may affect disintegration. The released drug must then dissolve in the aqueous gastrointestinal contents. The rate of dissolution is governed by the inherent solubility, particle size, crystal form and other physical properties of the drug. Differences in bioavailability may arise due to variations in disintegration and dissolution rates.

Differences in bioavailability are seen mostly with poorly soluble and slowly absorbed drugs. Reduction in particle size increases the rate of absorption of aspirin (microfine tablets). The amount of griseofulvin and spironolactone in the tablet can be reduced to half if the drug particle is microfined. There is no need to reduce the particle size of freely water-soluble drugs, e.g. paracetamol.

Bioavailability variation assumes practical significance for drugs with low safety margin (digoxin) or where dosage needs precise control (oral hypoglycaemics, oral anticoagulants). It may also be responsible for success or failure of an antimicrobial regimen.

However, in the case of a large number of drugs bioavailability differences are negligible and the risks of changing branded to generic product or to another brand of the same drug have often been exaggerated.

DISTRIBUTION OF DRUGS

Once a drug has gained access to the bloodstream, it diffuses to other tissues that initially had no drug, concentration gradient being in the direction of plasma to tissues. The extent of distribution of a drug and its pattern of tissue distribution depends on its:
- lipid solubility,
- ionization at physiological pH (dependent on pKa),
- extent of binding to plasma and tissue proteins and
- differences in regional blood flow.

Movement of drug from the vascular compartment proceeds until an equilibrium is established between unbound drug in the plasma and in the tissue fluids. Subsequently, there is a parallel decline in both due to elimination.

Apparent volume of distribution (V) Presuming that the body behaves as a single homogeneous compartment with volume V into which the drug gets immediately and uniformly distributed

$$V = \frac{\text{dose administered i.v.}}{\text{plasma concentration}} \quad \ldots(3)$$

Since in the example shown in Fig. 2.8 the drug does not actually distribute into 20 L of body water, with the exclusion of the rest of it, this is only an apparent volume of distribution which can be defined as "the volume that would accommodate all the drug in the body, if the concentration throughout was the same as in plasma." Thus, it describes the amount of drug present in the body as a multiple of that contained

Distribution of Drugs

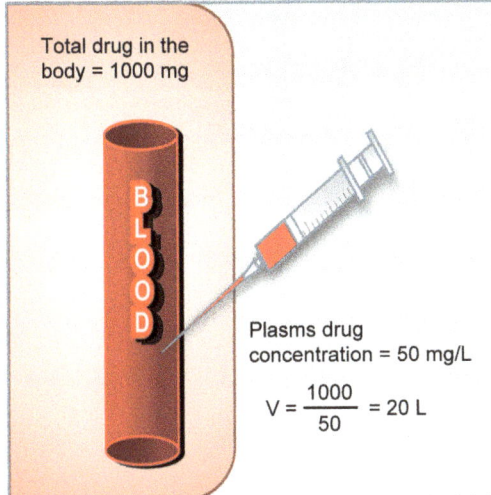

Fig. 2.8: Illustration of the concept of apparent volume of distribution (V)
In this example, 1000 mg of drug injected i.v. produces steady-state plasma concentration of 50 mg/L, apparent volume of distribution is 20 L.

Factors governing volume of drug distribution
- Lipid : water partition coefficient of the drug
- pKa value of the drug
- Degree of plasma protein binding
- Affinity for different tissues
- Fat : lean body mass ratio
- Diseases like CHF, uraemia, cirrhosis

in a unit volume of plasma. Considered together with drug clearance, this is a very useful pharmacokinetic concept.

Lipid-insoluble drugs do not enter cells—V approximates extracellular fluid volume, e.g. streptomycin, gentamicin 0.25 L/kg.

Distribution is not only a matter of dilution but also binding and sequestration. Drugs extensively bound to plasma proteins are largely restricted to the vascular compartment and have low values of V, e.g. diclofenac and warfarin (99% bound) V = 0.15 L/kg.

Drugs sequestrated in other tissues may have V much more than total body water or even body mass, e.g. digoxin 6 L/kg, chlorpromazine 25 L/kg, morphine 3.5 L/kg, because most of the drug is present in other tissues, and plasma concentration is low.

Pathological states, e.g. congestive heart failure, uraemia, cirrhosis of liver, etc. can alter the V of many drugs by altering distribution of body water, permeability of membranes, binding proteins or by accumulation of metabolites that displace the drug from binding sites.

Redistribution Highly lipid-soluble drugs get initially distributed to organs with high blood flow, i.e. brain, heart, kidney, etc. Later, less vascular but more bulky tissues (muscle, fat) take up the drug—plasma concentration falls and the drug is withdrawn from brain, etc. If the site of action of the drug was in one of the highly perfused organs, redistribution results in termination of drug action. Greater the lipid solubility of the drug, faster is its redistribution. Anaesthetic action of thiopentone injected i.v. is terminated in a few minutes due to redistribution. A relatively short (6-8 hr) hypnotic action due to redistribution is exerted by oral diazepam or nitrazepam despite their elimination half-life of > 30 hr. However, when the same drug is given repeatedly or by continuous i.v. infusion over long periods, the low perfusion high capacity sites get progressively filled up and the drug becomes longer acting.

Penetration into brain and CSF The capillary endothelial cells in brain have tight junctions and lack large paracellular spaces. Further, an investment of neural tissue (Fig. 2.9B) covers the capillaries. Together they constitute the so-called *blood-brain barrier* (BBB). A similar *blood-CSF barrier* is located in the choroid plexus where capillaries are lined by choroidal epithelium having tight junctions. Both these barriers are lipoidal, and limit the entry of nonlipid-soluble drugs, e.g. gentamicin, neostigmine, etc. Only lipid-soluble drugs, therefore, are able to penetrate and have action on the central nervous system. Efflux transporters like P-glycoprotein present in brain and choroidal vessels extrude many drugs that enter brain by other processes. Dopamine does not enter brain, but its

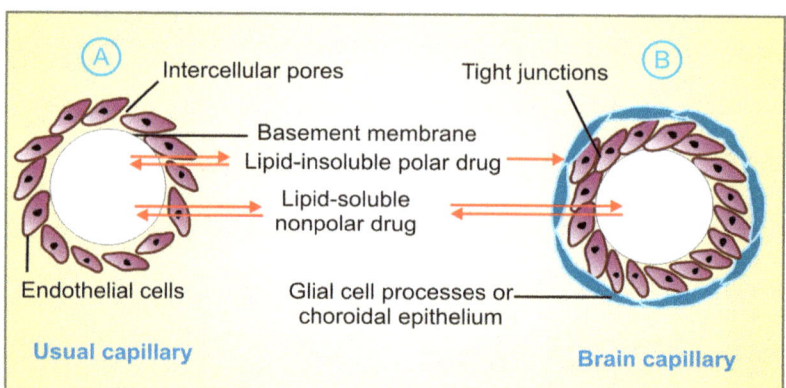

Fig. 2.9: Passage of drugs across capillaries
A. Usual capillary with large paracellular spaces through which even large lipid-insoluble molecules diffuse
B. Capillary constituting blood-brain or blood-CSF barrier. Tight junctions between capillary endothelial cells and investment of glial processes or choroidal epithelium do not allow passage of nonlipid-soluble molecules/ions

precursor levodopa does; as such, the latter is used in parkinsonism. Inflammation of meninges or brain increases permeability of these barriers.

There is also an enzymatic BBB: monoamine oxidase (MAO), cholinesterase and some other enzymes are present in the capillary walls or in the cells lining them. They do not allow catecholamines, 5-HT, acetylcholine, etc. to enter brain in the active form.

The BBB is deficient at the CTZ in the medulla oblongata (even lipid-insoluble drugs are emetic) and at certain periventricular sites—(anterior hypothalamus). Exit of drugs from the CSF and brain, however, is not dependent on lipid solubility and is rather unrestricted. This is due to bulk flow of CSF (along with the drug dissolved in it) back into the blood through the arachnoid villi. Further, nonspecific organic ion transport processes (similar to those in renal tubule) operate at the choroid plexus.

Passage across placenta Placental membranes are lipoidal and allow free passage of lipophilic drugs while restricting hydrophilic drugs. The placental efflux P-glycoprotein also serves to limit foetal exposure to maternally administered drugs. Placenta is a site for drug metabolism as well. However, restricted amounts of nonlipid-soluble drugs, when present in high concentration or for long periods in maternal circulation, gain access to the foetus. Thus, it is an incomplete barrier and almost any drug taken by the mother can affect the foetus or the new-born (drug taken just before delivery, e.g. morphine).

Plasma protein binding

Most drugs possess physicochemical affinity for plasma proteins. Acidic drugs generally bind to plasma albumin and basic drugs to α1 acid glycoprotein. Binding to albumin is quantitatively more important. Extent of binding depends on the individual compound; no generalization for a pharmacological or chemical class can be made (even small chemical change can markedly alter protein binding), for example:

Flurazepam 10%   Alprazolam 70%
Lorazepam 90%   Diazepam   99%

Increasing concentrations of the drug can progressively saturate the binding sites; fractional binding may be lower when large amounts of the drug are given. The generally expressed percentage binding refers to the

Drugs highly bound to plasma protein	
To Albumin	To α_1-acid glycoprotein
Barbiturates	β-blockers
Benzodiazepines	Bupivacaine
NSAIDs	Lidocaine
Valproic acid	Disopyramide
Phenytoin	Imipramine
Penicillins	Methadone
Sulfonamides	Prazosin
Tetracyclines	Quinidine
Warfarin	Verapamil

usual therapeutic plasma concentrations of a drug. The clinically significant implications of plasma protein binding are:

(i) Highly plasma protein bound drugs are largely restricted to the vascular compartment and tend to have lower volumes of distribution.

(ii) The bound fraction is not available for action. However, it is in equilibrium with the free drug in plasma and dissociates when the concentration of the latter is reduced due to elimination. Plasma protein binding thus tantamounts to temporary storage of the drug.

(iii) High degree of protein binding generally makes the drug long acting, because bound fraction is not available for metabolism or excretion, unless it is actively extracted by liver or kidney tubules. Glomerular filtration does not reduce the concentration of the free form in the efferent vessels because water is also filtered. Active tubular secretion, however, removes the drug without the attendant solvent → concentration of free drug falls → bound drug dissociates and is eliminated resulting in a higher renal clearance value of the drug than the total renal blood flow (See Fig. 2.12). The same is true of active transport of highly extracted drugs in the liver. Plasma protein binding in this situation acts as a carrier mechanism and hastens drug elimination, e.g. excretion of penicillin; metabolism of lidocaine. Highly protein bound drugs are not removed by haemodialysis and need special techniques for treatment of poisoning.

(iv) The generally expressed plasma concentrations of the drug refer to bound as well as free drug. Degree of protein binding should be taken into account while relating these to concentrations of the drug that are active in vitro, e.g. MIC of an antimicrobial.

(v) One drug can bind to many sites on the albumin molecule. Conversely, more than one drug can bind to the same site. This can give rise to displacement interactions among drugs bound to the same site(s); the drug bound with higher affinity will displace the one bound with lower affinity and tend to raise the concentration of its free form. This, however, is often transient because the displaced drug will diffuse into the tissues as well as get metabolized or excreted; the new steady-state free drug concentration is only marginally higher unless the displacement extends to tissue binding or there is concurrent inhibition of metabolism and/or excretion reducing drug clearance. The overall impact of many displacement interactions is minimal; except when the interaction is more complex. Moreover, two highly bound drugs do not necessarily displace each other—their binding sites may not overlap, e.g. probenecid and indomethacin are highly bound to albumin but do not displace each other. Similarly, acidic drugs do not generally displace basic drugs and vice versa.

(vi) In hypoalbuminaemia, binding may be reduced and high concentrations of free drug may be attained, e.g. phenytoin and furosemide. Other diseases may also alter drug binding, e.g. phenytoin and pethidine binding is reduced in uraemia; propranolol binding is increased in pregnant women and in patients with inflammatory disease (acute phase reactant α1 acid-glycoprotein increases).

Tissue storage Drugs may also accumulate in specific organs or get bound to specific tissue constituents (*see* box).

Drugs sequestrated in various tissues are distributed unequally, tend to have larger volume of distribution and longer duration of action. Some may exert local toxicity due to high concentration, e.g. tetracyclines on bone and teeth, chloroquine on retina, emetine on heart and skeletal muscle. Drugs may also selectively bind to specific intracellular organelle, e.g. tetracycline to mitochondria, chloroquine to nuclei.

Drugs concentrated in tissues	
Skeletal muscle, heart	— Digoxin, emetine (bound to muscle proteins)
Liver	— Chloroquine, tetracyclines, emetine, digoxin
Kidney	— Digoxin, chloroquine, emetine
Thyroid	— Iodine
Brain	— Chlorpromazine, acetazolamide, isoniazid
Retina	— Chloroquine (bound to nucleoproteins)
Iris	— Ephedrine, atropine (bound to melanin)
Bone and teeth	— Tetracyclines, heavy metals (bound to mucopolysaccharides of connective tissue), bisphosphonates (bound to hydroxyapatite)
Adipose tissue	— Thiopentone, ether, minocycline, DDT dissolve in neutral fat due to high lipid solubility; remain stored due to poor blood supply of fat

BIOTRANSFORMATION (Metabolism) OF DRUGS

Biotransformation means chemical alteration of the drug in the body. It is needed to render nonpolar (lipid soluble) compounds polar (lipid insoluble) so that they are not reabsorbed in the renal tubules and are excreted. Most hydrophilic drugs, e.g. gentamicin, neostigmine, etc. are not biotransformed and are excreted unchanged.

The primary site for drug metabolism is liver; others are—kidney, intestine, lungs and plasma. Biotransformation of drugs may lead to the following.

(i) Inactivation Most drugs and their active metabolites are rendered inactive or less active by metabolism, e.g. lidocaine, ibuprofen, paracetamol, chloramphenicol, propranolol and its active metabolite 4-hydroxypropranolol.

(ii) Active metabolite from an active drug Many drugs have been found to be partially converted to one or more active metabolite (*see* box); the effects observed are the sum total of that due to the parent drug and its active metabolite(s).

(iii) Activation of inactive drug Few drugs are inactive as such and need conversion in the body to one or more active metabolite(s).

Such a drug is called a *prodrug* (*see* box). The prodrug may offer advantages over the active form in being more stable, having better bioavailability or other desirable pharmacokinetic properties or less side effects and toxicity. Some prodrugs are activated selectively at the site of action.

Active drug	Active metabolite
Allopurinol	— Alloxanthine
Procainamide	— N-acetyl-procainamide
Primidone	— Phenobarbitone, phenylethylmalonamide
Cefotaxime	— Deacetyl cefotaxime
Diazepam	— Desmethyl-diazepam, oxazepam
Imipramine	— Desipramine
Amitriptyline	— Nortriptyline
Codeine	— Morphine
Morphine	— Morphine-6-glucuronide
Spironolactone	— Canrenone
Losartan	— E 3174

Biotransformation reactions can be classified into:

(a) Nonsynthetic/Phase I reactions: a functional group (–OH, –COOH, –CHO, –NH$_2$, –SH, etc.) may be generated/exposed. The metabolite may be active or inactive.

Prodrug	Active form
Levodopa	— Dopamine
Enalapril	— Enalaprilat
α-Methyldopa	— α-Methylnorepinephrine
Clopidogrel	— Thiol metabolite
Dipivefrine	— Epinephrine
Proguanil	— Cycloguanil
Sulfasalazine	— 5-Aminosalicylic acid
Acyclovir	— Acyclovir triphosphate
Cyclophos-phamide	— Aldophosphamide, phosphoramide mustard, acrolein
Mercaptopurine	— Methylmercaptopurine ribonucleotide

(b) Synthetic/Conjugation/Phase II reactions: an endogenous radical is conjugated to the drug. The metabolite is mostly inactive, except few drugs, e.g. morphine-6-glucuronide.

Nonsynthetic reactions

(i) Oxidation This reaction involves addition of oxygen/negatively charged radical or removal of hydrogen/positively charged radical. Oxidations are the most important drug metabolizing reactions. Various oxidation reactions are: hydroxylation; oxygenation at C, N or S atoms; N or O-dealkylation, oxidative deamination, etc.

In many cases, the initial insertion of oxygen atom into the drug molecule produces short lived highly reactive quinone/epoxide/superoxide intermediates which then convert to more stable compounds.

Oxidative reactions are mostly carried out by a group of monooxygenases in the liver, which in the final step involve a cytochrome P-450 haemoprotein, NADPH, cytochrome P-450 reductase and molecular O_2. More than 100 cytochrome P-450 (CYP-450) isoenzymes differing in their affinity for various substrates (drugs), have been identified. The CYP-450 isoenzymes important for drug metabolism in humans, along with their clinically relevant substrate drugs, inhibitors and inducers are listed in Table 2.1.

The relative amount of different cytochrome P-450s differs among species and among individuals of the same species. These differences largely account for the marked interspecies and interindividual differences in rate of metabolism of drugs.

(ii) Reduction This reaction is the converse of oxidation and involves cytochrome P-450 enzymes working in the opposite direction. Drugs primarily reduced are chloramphenicol, halothane and warfarin.

(iii) Hydrolysis This is cleavage of drug molecule by taking up a molecule of water.

$$Ester + H_2O \xrightarrow{esterase} Acid + Alcohol$$

Similarly, amides and polypeptides are hydrolyzed by amidases and peptidases. Hydrolysis occurs in liver, intestines, plasma and other tissues. Examples are choline esters, procaine, lidocaine, procainamide, indomethacin, pethidine, oxytocin.

Synthetic reactions

These reactions involve conjugation of the drug or its phase I metabolite with an endogenous substrate, usually derived from carbohydrate or amino acid, to form a polar highly ionized organic acid, which is easily excreted in urine or bile.

(i) Glucuronide conjugation This is the most important synthetic reaction carried out by a group of UDP-glucuronosyl transferases (UGTs). Compounds with a hydroxyl or carboxylic acid group are easily conjugated with glucuronic acid which is derived from glucose. Examples are chloramphenicol, aspirin, diazepam, morphine, metronidazole. Not only drugs but endogenous substrates like bilirubin, steroidal hormones and thyroxine utilize this pathway. Glucuronidation favours excretion of the drug in bile. Drug glucuronides excreted in bile can be hydrolyzed by bacteria in the gut—the liberated drug is

Table 2.1: Major drug metabolizing CYP450 isoenzymes in humans with their important substrate drugs, inhibitors and inducers

CYP-450 isoenzyme	Drugs metabolized	Inhibitors	Inducers
CYP3A4 CYP3A5	Losartan, Carbamazepine Hydrocortisone Paracetamol, Diazepam Buspirone, Mifepristone Ritonavir, Saquinavir Simvastatin, Quinidine Verapamil, Lidocaine Dapsone, Nevirapine	Erythromycin Clarithromycin Ketoconazole Itraconazole Verapamil Ritonavir Fluoxetine Grape fruit juice	Barbiturates Phenytoin Carbamazepine Rifampin Glucocorticoids Nevirapine
CYP2D6	Metoprolol, Debrisoquine Nebivolol, Amitryptyline Clomipramine, Fluoxetine Paroxetine, Venlafaxine Haloperidol, Clozapine Risperidone, Codeine Propafenone, Flecainide	Qunidine Fluoxetine Paroxetine	Phenobarbitone Rifampin
CYP2C8 CYP2C9	Phenytoin, Carbamazepine Warfarin, Tolbutamide Repaglinide, Pioglitazone Diclofenac, Ibuprofen Losartan	Fluvoxamine Fluconazole Gemfibrozil Trimethoprim	Phenobarbitone Carbamazepine Rifampin
CYP2C19	Omeprazole, Lansoprazole Amitriptyline, Citalopram Phenytoin, Diazepam Propranolol, Clopidogrel	Omeprazole Fluconazole	Carbamazepine Rifampin
CYP1A1 CYP1A2	Theophylline, Caffeine Paracetamol, Warfarin Carbamazepine	Fluvoxamine Fluoxetine	Polycyclic hydrocarbons Cigarette smoke Charbroiled meat Rifampin Carbamazepine
CYP2E1	Alcohol, Halothane Paracetamol*	Disulfiram Fomepizole	Chronic alcoholism Isoniazid
CYP2B6	Efavirenz, Nevirapine Cyclophosphamide, Methadone Sertraline, Clopidogrel	Paroxetine Sertraline Clopidogrel	Phenobarbitone Cyclophosphamide

* Generates toxic metabolite N-acetyl-p-benzoquinoneimine (NABQI)

reabsorbed and undergoes the same fate. This enterohepatic cycling of the drug prolongs its action, e.g., oral contraceptives.

(ii) *Acetylation* Compounds having amino or hydrazine residues are conjugated with the help of acetyl coenzyme-A, e.g. sulfonamides, isoniazid, PAS, dapsone, hydralazine. Multiple genes control the N-acetyl transferases (NATs) and rate of acetylation shows genetic polymorphism (slow and fast acetylators).

(iii) *Methylation* Amines and phenols can be methylated by methyl transferases; methionine and cysteine acting as methyl donors. Drugs methylated are adrenaline, histamine, nicotinic acid, methyldopa, etc.

(iv) *Sulfate conjugation* The phenolic compounds and steroids are sulfated by sulfotransferases (SULTs), e.g. chloramphenicol, adrenal steroids and sex steroids.

(v) *Glycine conjugation* Aspirin, nicotinic acid and other drugs having carboxylic acid group are conjugated with glycine, but this is not a major pathway of metabolism.

(vi) *Glutathione conjugation* Carried out by glutathione-S-transferase (GST) to form a mercapturate is normally a minor pathway. However, it serves to inactivate highly reactive quinone or epoxide intermediates formed during metabolism of certain drugs, e.g. paracetamol. When a large amount of such intermediates are formed (in poisoning or after enzyme induction), glutathione supply falls short—toxic adducts are formed with tissue constituents resulting in hepatic, renal and other tissue damage.

(vii) *Ribonucleoside/nucleotide synthesis* This reaction is important for the activation of many purine and pyrimidine antimetabolites used in cancer chemotherapy.

Most drugs are metabolized by multiple pathways, simultaneously or sequentially as illustrated in Fig. 2.10. As such, a variety of metabolities of a drug may be produced.

Only few drugs are metabolized by enzymes of intermediary metabolism, e.g. alcohol by dehydrogenase, allopurinol by xanthine oxidase, succinylcholine and procaine by plasma cholinesterase, adrenaline by monoamine oxidase. Majority of drugs are acted on by relatively nonspecific enzymes which are directed to types of molecules rather than to specific drugs. The same enzyme can metabolize many drugs. The drug metabolizing enzymes are divided into two types:

Microsomal enzymes These are located on smooth endoplasmic reticulum (a system of microtubules inside the cell), primarily in liver, also in kidney, intestinal mucosa and lungs. The monooxygenases, cytochrome P 450, UGTs, epoxide hydrolases are microsomal enzymes.

These enzymes catalyze most of the oxidations, reductions, hydrolysis and glucuronide conjugation. Microsomal enzymes are inducible by a number of drugs, certain dietary constituents and other agencies.

Nonmicrosomal enzymes These are present in the cytoplasm and mitochondria of hepatic cells as well as in other tissues including plasma. The esterases, amidases, some flavoprotein oxidases and most conjugases are nonmicrosomal. Reactions catalyzed are:

Some oxidations and reductions, many hydrolytic reactions and all conjugations except glucuronidation.

The nonmicrosomal enzymes are not inducible but many show genetic polymorphism (acetyl transferase, pseudocholinesterase).

Both microsomal and nonmicrosomal enzymes are deficient in the newborn, especially premature, making them more susceptible to many drugs, e.g. chloramphenicol, opioids. This deficit is made up in first few months, more quickly in case of oxidation and other phase I reactions than in case of glucuronide and other conjugations which take 3 or more months to reach adult levels.

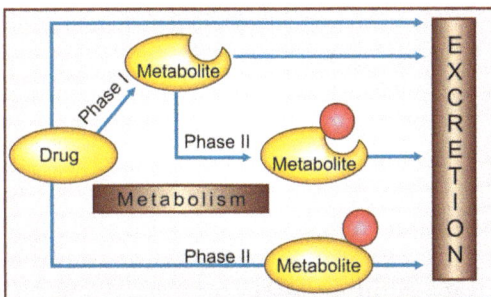

Fig. 2.10: Simultaneous and/or sequential metabolism of a drug by phase I and phase II reactions

The amount and kind of drug metabolizing enzymes is controlled genetically and is also altered by environmental factors. Thus, marked interspecies and interindividual differences are seen. Up to 6-fold difference in the rate of metabolism of a drug among normal human adults may be observed. This is one of the major causes of individual variation in drug response.

Hofmann elimination This refers to inactivation of the drug in the body fluids by spontaneous molecular rearrangement without the agency of any enzyme, e.g. atracurium.

INHIBITION OF DRUG METABOLISM

Few drugs, especially azole antifungals and macrolide antibiotics bind to the heme iron in CYP450 and inhibit the metabolism of several drugs. Moreover, one drug can competitively inhibit the metabolism of another if it utilizes the same enzyme or cofactors. However, such interactions are not as common as one would expect, because often different drugs are substrates for different CYP-450 isoenzymes. Moreover, a drug may inhibit one isoenzyme while being itself a substrate of another isoenzyme, e.g. quinidine is metabolized mainly by CYP3A4 but inhibits CYP2D6. Also most drugs, at therapeutic concentrations are metabolized by non-saturation kinetics, i.e. the enzyme is present in excess. Clinically significant inhibition of drug metabolism occurs in case of drugs having affinity for the same isoenzyme, especially if they are metabolized by saturation kinetics or if kinetics changes from first order to zero order over the therapeutic range (capacity limited metabolism). The 'boosted' HIV-protease inhibitor (PI) strategy utilizes the potent CYP3A4 inhibitory action of low-dose ritonavir to lower the dose of other PIs like atazanavir, lopinavir, etc. given concurrently. Inhibition of drug metabolism occurs in a dose-related manner and can precipitate toxicity of the object drug (whose metabolism has been inhibited).

Because enzyme inhibition occurs by direct effect on the enzyme, it has a fast time course (within hours) compared to enzyme induction (*see* below).

Metabolism of drugs with high hepatic extraction is dependent on liver blood flow, and is called blood flow limited metabolism. Propranolol reduces rate of lidocaine metabolism by decreasing hepatic blood flow.

Drugs that inhibit drug metabolizing enzymes	
Allopurinol	Amiodarone
Omeprazole	Propoxyphene
Erythromycin	Isoniazid
Clarithromycin	Cimetidine
Chloramphenicol	Quinidine
Ketoconazole	Metronidazole
Itraconazole	Disulfiram
Ciprofloxacin	Verapamil
Sulfonamides	Ritonavir
Fluoxetine	

MICROSOMAL ENZYME INDUCTION

Many drugs, insecticides and carcinogens interact with DNA and increase the synthesis of microsomal enzyme protein, especially cytochrome P-450 and glucuronyl transferase. As a result, the rate of metabolism of inducing drug itself and/or other coadministered drugs is increased.

Different inducers are relatively selective for certain CYP450 isoenzyme families, e.g.:
- Anticonvulsants (phenytoin, carbamazepine, phenobarbitone), rifampin, glucocorticoids induce CYP3A isoenzymes.
- Phenobarbitone and rifampin also induce CYP2B1, CYP2D6 and CYP2C8/9.
- Isoniazid and chronic alcohol consumption induce CYP2E1.
- Other important enzyme inducers are chronic alcoholism, nevirapine, griseofulvin, DDT.

Since different CYP isoenzymes are involved in the metabolism of different drugs, every inducer increases biotransformation of certain drugs but not that of others. However, phenobarbitone like inducers of CYP3A and CYP2D6 affect the metabolism of a large number of drugs, because these isoenzymes act on many drugs. On the other hand, induction by polycyclic hydrocarbons is limited to a few drugs (like theophylline, warfarin) because CYP1A isoenzyme metabolizes only few drugs.

Induction involves microsomal enzymes in liver as well as other organs and increases the rate of metabolism by 2–4-fold. Induction takes 4–14 days to reach its peak and is maintained till the inducing agent is being given. Thereafter, the enzymes return to their original value over 1 to 3 weeks.

Consequences of microsomal enzyme induction

1. Decreased intensity and/or duration of action of drugs that are inactivated by metabolism, e.g. failure of contraception with oral contraceptives and loss of anti-HIV action of nevirapine due to coadministration of rifampin.
2. Increased intensity of action of drugs that are activated by metabolism. Acute paracetamol toxicity is due to one of its metabolites—toxicity occurs at lower doses in patients receiving enzyme inducers.
3. Tolerance—if the drug induces its own metabolism (autoinduction), e.g. carbamazepine, rifampin. Nevirapine dose needs to be doubled after 2 weeks.
4. Some endogenous substrates (steroids, bilirubin) are also metabolized faster.
5. Precipitation of acute intermittent porphyria: enzyme induction increases porphyrin synthesis by derepressing d-aminolevulenic acid synthetase.
6. Intermittent use of an inducer may interfere with adjustment of dose of another drug prescribed on regular basis, e.g. oral anticoagulants, oral hypoglycaemics, antiepileptics, antihypertensives.

Drugs whose metabolism is significantly affected by enzyme induction are—phenytoin, warfarin, tolbutamide, oral contraceptives, chloramphenicol, doxycycline, theophylline, griseofulvin.

Possible uses of enzyme induction

1. Congenital nonhaemolytic jaundice: phenobarbitone causes rapid clearance of jaundice.
2. Cushing's syndrome: phenytoin may reduce the manifestations.
3. Chronic poisonings.
4. Liver disease.

FIRST PASS (PRESYSTEMIC) METABOLISM

This refers to metabolism of a drug during its passage from the site of absorption into the systemic circulation. All orally administered drugs are exposed to drug metabolizing enzymes in the intestinal wall and liver (where they first reach through the portal vein). This can be circumvented by administering the drug through sublingual, transdermal or parenteral routes. Presystemic metabolism of limited magnitude can also occur in the skin (transdermally administered drug) and in lungs (for drug reaching venous blood through any route). The extent of first pass metabolism differs for different drugs (Table 2.2) and is an important determinant of oral bioavailability.

Attributes of drugs with high first pass metabolism

(a) Oral dose is considerably higher than sublingual or parenteral dose.
(b) There is marked individual variation in the oral dose due to differences in the extent of first pass metabolism.
(c) Oral bioavailability is apparently increased in patients with severe liver disease.
(d) Oral bioavailability of a drug is increased if another drug competing with it in first pass metabolism is given concurrently, e.g. chlorpromazine and propranolol.

Table 2.2: Extent of hepatic first pass metabolism of some important drugs

Low	Intermediate	High	
		not given orally	high oral dose
Phenobarbitone	Aspirin	Isoprenaline	Propranolol
Tolbutamide	Quinidine	Lidocaine	Alprenolol
Theophylline	Desipramine	Hydrocortisone	Verapamil
Pindolol	Nortriptyline	Testosterone	Salbutamol
Isosorbide mononitrate	Chlorpromazine		Glyceryl trinitrate
	Pentazocine		Morphine
	Metoprolol		Pethidine

EXCRETION OF DRUGS

Excretion is the passage out of systemically absorbed drug. Drugs and their metabolites are excreted in:

1. Urine Through the kidney. It is the most important channel of excretion for majority of drugs (see below).

2. Faeces Apart from the unabsorbed fraction, most of the drug present in faeces is derived from bile. Organic acids (especially drug glucuronides), organic bases and steroids are actively transported into bile by liver through separate nonspecific active transporters (OATP, MRP2, OCT, P-gP, etc.). Relatively larger molecules (MW > 300) are preferentially eliminated in the bile. Most of the unconjugated drug present in the gut, including that released by deconjugation of glucuronides by gut bacteria is reabsorbed (enterohepatic cycling *see* Fig. 2.11) and ultimate excretion occurs in urine. Drugs that attain high concentrations in bile are erythromycin, ampicillin, rifampin, tetracycline, oral contraceptives.

Certain drugs are excreted directly in colon, e.g. anthracene purgatives, heavy metals.

3. Exhaled air Gases and volatile liquids (general anaesthetics, alcohol) are eliminated by lungs, irrespective of their lipid solubility. Alveolar transfer of the gas/vapour depends on its partial pressure in the blood. Lungs also serve to trap and extrude any particulate matter that enters circulation.

4. Saliva and sweat These are of minor importance for drug excretion. Lithium, pot. iodide, rifampin and heavy metals are present in these secretions. Most of the saliva along with the drug in it, is swallowed and meets the same fate as orally taken drug.

5. Milk The excretion of a drug in milk is not important for the mother, but the suckling infant inadvertently receives the drug. Most drugs enter breast milk by passive diffusion. As such, more lipid soluble and less protein bound drugs cross better. Milk has a lower pH (7.0) than plasma, basic drugs are somewhat more concentrated in it. However, the total amount of drug reaching the infant through breastfeeding is generally small. As such, majority of drugs can be given to lactating mothers without ill effects on the infant. Nevertheless, it is advisable to administer any drug to a lactating women only when essential.

RENAL EXCRETION

The kidney is responsible for excreting all water-soluble substances. The amount of unaltered drug or its metabolites ultimately present in urine is the sum total of glomerular filtration, tubular reabsorption and tubular secretion (Fig. 2.12).

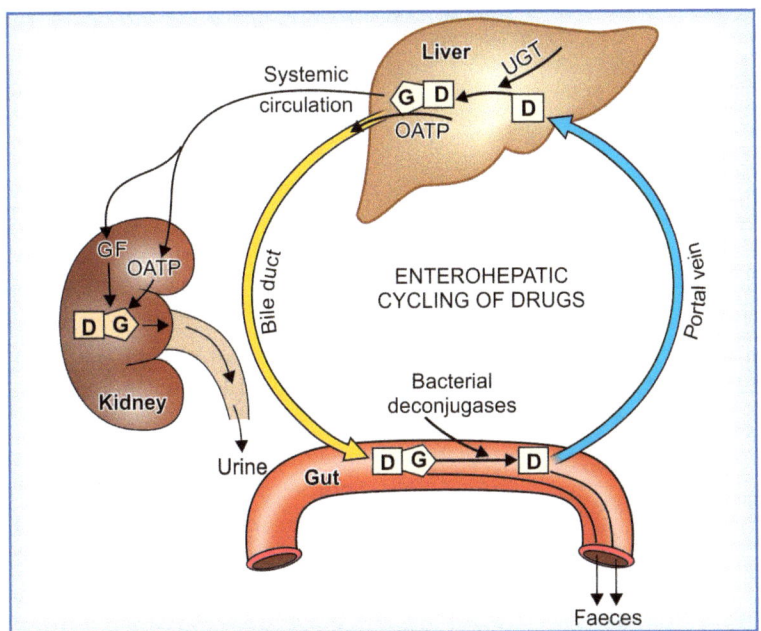

Fig. 2.11: Enterohepatic cycling of drugs
In the liver many drugs (D), including steroids, are conjugated by the enzyme UDP-glucuronosyl transferases (UGTs) to form drug-glucuronide (DG). Part of the DG enters systemic circulation and is excreted into urine by the kidney through both glomerular filtration (GF) as well as active tubular secretion involving renal organic-anion transporting peptide (OATP).
    Another part of DG is actively secreted into bile by the hepatic OATP. On reaching the gut lumen via bile, a major part of DG is deconjugated by bacterial hydrolytic enzymes (deconjugates) while the remaining is excreted into faeces. The released D is reabsorbed from the gut to again reach the liver through portal circulation and complete the enterohepatic cycle.

Net renal excretion = (glomerular filtration + tubular secretion) – tubular reabsorption

Glomerular filtration Glomerular capillaries have pores larger than usual; all nonprotein bound drug (whether-lipid soluble or insoluble) presented to the glomerulus is filtered. Thus, glomerular filtration of a drug depends on its plasma protein binding and renal blood flow. Glomerular filtration rate (g.f.r.), normally ~ 120 mL/min, declines progressively after the age of 50 and is low in renal failure.

Tubular reabsorption This depends on lipid solubility and ionization of the drug at the existing urinary pH. Lipid-soluble drugs filtered at the glomerulus back diffuse passively in the tubules because 99% of glomerular filtrate is reabsorbed, but nonlipid-soluble and highly ionized drugs are unable to do so. Thus, rate of excretion of such drugs, e.g. aminoglycoside antibiotics, quaternary ammonium compounds parallels g.f.r. (or creatinine clearance). Changes in urinary pH affect tubular reabsorption of drugs that are partially ionized—
- Weak bases ionize more and are less reabsorbed in acidic urine.
- Weak acids ionize more and are less reabsorbed in alkaline urine.

Tubular secretion Tubular secretion is the active transfer of organic acids and bases

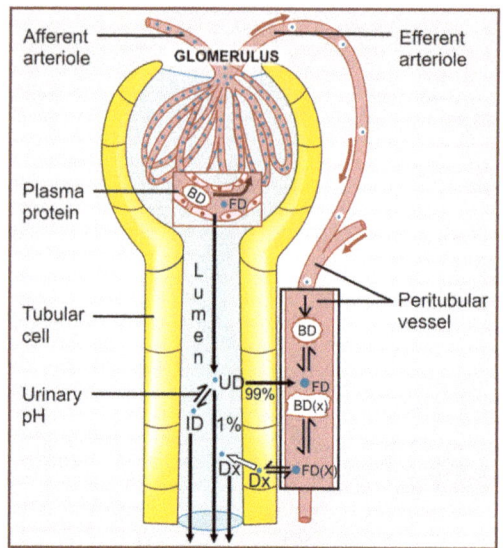

Fig. 2.12: Schematic depiction of glomerular filtration, tubular reabsorption and tubular secretion of drugs FD—free drug; BD—bound drug; UD—unionized drug; ID—ionized drug, Dx—highly secreted organic acid (or base) drug

by two separate classes of nonspecific transporters (OATP and OCT) which operate in the proximal tubules. In addition, efflux transporters P-gp and MRP2 are located in luminal membrane of proximal tubular cells. If renal clearance of a drug is greater than 120 mL/min or g.f.r., additional tubular secretion can be assumed to be occurring.

Active transport of the drug across the tubules reduces the concentration of its free form in the tubular vessels and promotes dissociation of protein bound drug, which again becomes available for secretion (Fig. 2.12). Thus, tubular secretion is very important for renal excretion of highly plasma protein bound drugs which are not removed by glomerular filtration.

(a) *Organic acid transport (by OATP)* It operates for penicillin, probenecid, uric acid, salicylates, sulfinpyrazone, nitrofurantoin, methotrexate, drug glucuronides, etc.

(b) *Organic base transport* (through OCT) This operates for thiazides, quinine, procainamide, choline, cimetidine, amiloride, etc.

Inherently both transport processes are bidirectional, i.e. they can transport their substrate from blood to tubular fluid and vice versa. However, for drugs and their metabolites (which are exogenous substances) secretion into the tubular lumen predominates, while an endogenous substrate like uric acid is predominantly reabsorbed.

Drugs utilizing the same active transport compete with each other. Probenecid is an organic acid which has high affinity for the tubular OATP. It blocks the active transport of both penicillin and uric acid, but whereas the net excretion of the former is decreased, that of the latter is increased. This is because penicillin is primarily secreted while uric acid is primarily reabsorbed. Many drug interactions occur due to competition for tubular secretion, e.g.

(i) Aspirin blocks uricosuric action of probenecid and sulfinpyrazone and decreases tubular secretion of methotrexate.

(ii) Probenecid decreases the concentration of nitrofurantoin in urine, increases the duration of action of penicillin/ampicillin and impairs secretion of methotrexate.

(iii) Quinidine decreases renal and biliary clearance of digoxin by inhibiting efflux carrier P-gp.

Tubular transport mechanisms are not well developed at birth. As a result, duration of action of many drugs, e.g. penicillin, cephalosporins, aspirin is longer in neonates. These systems mature during infancy. Renal function again progressively declines after the age of 50 years. The renal clearance of many drugs is substantially lower in the elderly above 75 years of age.

KINETICS OF DRUG ELIMINATION

The knowledge of kinetics of elimination of a drug provides the basis for, as well as serves to devise rational dosage regimens and to modify them according to individual needs. There are three fundamental pharmacokinetic parameters, viz. bioavailability (F), volume of distribution (V) and clearance (CL) which must be understood. The first two have already been considered.

Drug elimination is the sum total of metabolic inactivation and excretion. As depicted in Fig. 2.1, drug is eliminated only from the central compartment (blood) which is in equilibrium with peripheral compartments including the site of action. Depending upon the ability of the body to eliminate a drug, a certain fraction of the central compartment may be considered to be totally 'cleared' of that drug in a given period of time to account for elimination over that period.

Clearance (CL) The clearance of a drug is the theoretical volume of plasma from which the drug is completely removed in unit time (analogy creatinine clearance, Fig. 2.13). It can be calculated as

$$CL = \text{Rate of elimination}/C \quad \ldots(4)$$

where C is the plasma concentration.

For majority of drugs the processes involved in elimination are not saturated over the clinically obtained concentrations, they follow:

First order (exponential) kinetics The rate of elimination is directly proportional to drug concentration, CL remains constant; or a constant *fraction* of the drug present in the body is eliminated in unit time. This is the case with majority of drugs.

Few drugs, however, saturate eliminating mechanisms and are handled by—

Zero order (linear) kinetics The rate of elimination remains constant irrespective of drug concentration, CL decreases with increase in concentration; or a constant amount of the drug is eliminated in unit time, e.g. ethyl alcohol.

The elimination of some drugs approaches saturation over the therapeutic range, kinetics changes from first order to zero order at higher doses. As a result, plasma concentration increases disproportionately with increase in dose (*see* Fig. 2.15) as occurs in the case of phenytoin, tolbutamide, theophylline, warfarin.

Plasma half-life The plasma half-life (t½) of a drug is the time taken for its plasma concentration to be reduced to half of its original value.

Taking the simplest case of a drug which has rapid one compartment distribution, first order elimination, and is given i.v., a semilog plasma concentration-time plot as shown in Fig. 2.14 is obtained. The plot has two slopes:
(i) Initial rapidly declining (α) phase—due to distribution.
(ii) Later less declined (β) phase—due to elimination.
At least two half-lives (distribution t½ and elimination t½) can be calculated from the

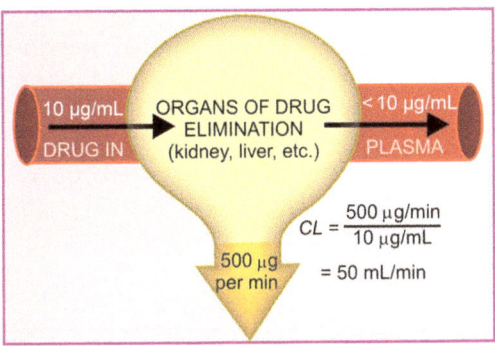

Fig. 2.13: Illustration of the concept of drug clearance. A fraction of the drug molecules present in plasma are removed on each passage through the organs of elimination. In the case shown, it requires 50 mL of plasma to account for the amount of drug being eliminated every minute: clearance is 50 mL/min

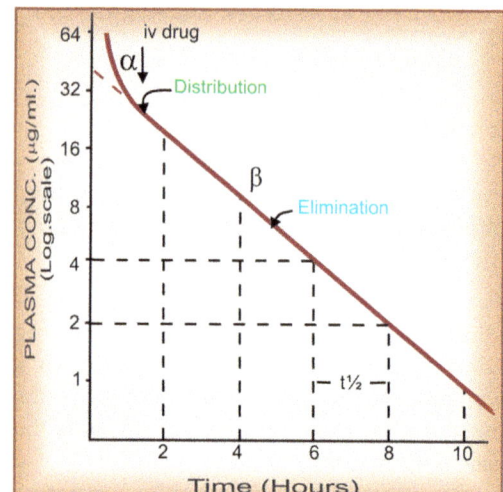

Fig. 2.14: Semilog plasma concentration-time plot of a drug eliminated by first order kinetics after intravenous injection

1 t½ – 50% drug is eliminated.
2 t½ – 75% (50 + 25) drug is eliminated.
3 t½ – 87.5% (50 + 25 + 12.5) drug is eliminated.
4 t½ – 93.75% (50 + 25 + 12.5 + 6.25) drug is eliminated.

Thus, nearly complete drug elimination occurs in 4–5 half-lives.
For drugs eliminated by—
First order kinetics—t½ remains constant because V and CL do not change with dose.
Zero order kinetics—t½ gets prolonged with increase in dose because CL progressively decreases as dose is increased.

Half-life of some representative drugs

Aspirin	4 hr	Digoxin	40 hr
Penicillin-G	30 min	Metronidazole	8 hr
Doxycycline	20 hr	Phenobarbitone	90 hr

two slopes. The elimination half-life derived from the β slope is simply called the 'half-life' of the drug. Since first order kinetics is an exponential process, the elimination t½ is

$$t_{1/2} = \frac{\ln 2}{k} \quad \ldots(5)$$

Where ln2 is the natural logarithm of 2 (or 0.693) and k is the *elimination rate constant* of the drug, i.e. the fraction of the total amount of drug in the body which is removed per unit time. For example, if 2 g of the drug is present in the body and 0.1 g is eliminated every hour, then $k = 0.1/2 = 0.05$. It is calculated as:

$$k = \frac{CL}{V} \quad \ldots(6)$$

therefore, $\quad t_{1/2} = 0.693 \times \dfrac{V}{CL} \quad \ldots(7)$

As such, half-life is a derived parameter from two variables V and CL, both of which may change independently. It, therefore, is not an exact index of drug elimination. Nevertheless, it is a simple and useful guide to the sojourn of the drug in the body, i.e. after

Repeated drug administration

When a drug is repeated at relatively short intervals, it accumulates in the body until elimination balances input and a steady-state plasma concentration (Cpss) is attained—

$$Cpss = \frac{\text{dose rate}}{CL} \quad \ldots(8)$$

From this equation it is implied that doubling the dose rate would double the average Cpss and so on. Further, if the therapeutic plasma concentration of the drug has been worked out and its CL is known, the dose rate needed to achieve the target Cpss can be determined—

$$\text{dose rate} = \text{target } Cpss \times CL \quad \ldots(9)$$

After oral administration, often only a fraction (F) of the dose reaches systemic circulation in the active form. In such a case—

$$\text{dose rate} = \frac{\text{target } Cpss \times CL}{F} \quad \ldots(10)$$

The dose rate-Cpss relationship is linear only in case of drugs eliminated by first order kinetics. For drugs (e.g. phenytoin) which follow Michaelis Menten kinetics, elimination changes from first order to zero order kinetics over the therapeutic range. Increase in their dose beyond saturation levels causes an increase in Cpss which is out of proportion to the change in dose rate (Fig. 2.15). In their case:

$$\text{Rate of drug elimination} = \frac{(V_{max})(C)}{K_m + C} \quad ...(11)$$

where C is the plasma concentration of the drug, Vmax is the maximum rate of drug elimination, and Km is the plasma concentration at which elimination rate is half maximal.

Plateau principle

When a constant dose of a drug is repeated before the expiry of 4 t½, it would achieve higher peak concentration, because some remnant of the previous dose will be present in the body. This continues with every dose until progressively increasing rate of elimination (which increases with increase in concentration) balances the amount administered over the dose interval. Subsequently, plasma concentration plateaus and fluctuates about an average steady-state level. This is known as the plateau principle of drug accumulation. Steady state is reached in 4–5 half-lives unless dose interval is very much longer than t½ (Fig. 2.16).

The amplitude of fluctuations in plasma concentration at steady state depends on the dose interval relative to t½, i.e. the difference between the maximum and minimum levels is less if smaller doses are repeated more frequently (dose rate remaining constant). Dosage intervals are generally a compromise between what amplitude of fluctuations is clinically acceptable (loss of efficacy at troughs and side effects at peaks) and what frequency of dosing is convenient. However, if the dose rate is changed, a new average Cpss is attained over the next 4–5 half-lives. When the drug is administered orally (absorption takes some time), average Cpss is approximately 1/3rd of the way between the minimal and maximal levels in a dose interval. Knowledge of half life of a drug in very helpful in devising its dosage regimen.

Target level strategy For drugs whose effects are not easily quantifiable and safety margin is not big, e.g. anticonvulsants, antidepressants, lithium, some antimicrobials, etc. or those given to prevent an event, it is best to aim at achieving a certain plasma concentration which has been defined to be in the therapeutic range;

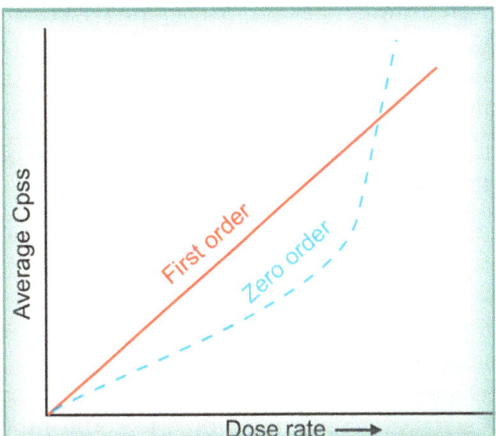

Fig. 2.15: Relationship between dose rate and average steady-state plasma concentration of drugs eliminated by first order and Michaelis Menten (zero order) kinetics

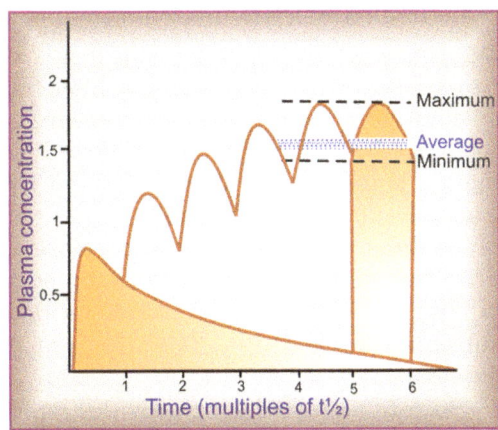

Fig. 2.16: Plateau principle of drug accumulation on repeated oral dosing
Note. The area of the two shaded portions is equal.

such data are now available for most drugs of this type.

Drugs with short t½ (up to 2–3 hr) administered at conventional intervals (6–12 hr) achieve the target levels only intermittently and fluctuations in plasma concentration are marked. In case of many drugs (penicillin, ampicillin, chloramphenicol, erythromycin, propranolol) this, however, is therapeutically acceptable.

For drugs with longer t½ a dose that is sufficient to attain the target concentration after a single administration, if repeated will accumulate according to plateau principle and produce toxicity later on. On the other hand, if the dosing is such as to attain target level at steady state, the therapeutic effect will be delayed by about 4 half-lives (this may be clinically unacceptable). Such drugs are often administered by initial loading and subsequent maintenance doses.

Loading dose This is a single or few quickly repeated doses given in the beginning to attain target concentration rapidly. It may be calculated as—

$$\text{Loading dose} = \frac{\text{target } Cp \times V}{F} \quad ...(12)$$

Thus, loading dose is governed only by V and not by CL or t½.

Maintenance dose This dose is one that is to be repeated at specified intervals after the attainment of target Cpss so as to maintain the same by balancing elimination. The maintenance dose rate is computed by equation (10) and is governed by CL (or t½) of the drug. If facilities for measurement of drug concentration are available, attainment of target level in a patient can be verified subsequently and dose rate adjusted if required.

Such two phase dosing provides rapid therapeutic effect with long-term safety. This is frequently applied to digoxin, chloroquine, doxycycline, etc. However, if there is no urgency, maintenance doses can be given from the beginning.

PROLONGATION OF DRUG ACTION

It is sometimes advantageous to modify a drug in such a way that it acts for a longer period. By doing so:
(i) Frequency of administration is reduced, which is more convenient.
(ii) Improved patient compliance—a single morning dose is less likely to be forgotten/omitted than a 6 or 8 hourly regimen.
(iii) Large fluctuations in plasma concentration are avoided—side effects related to high peak plasma level soon after a dose would be minimized (e.g. nifedipine); better round-the-clock control of blood sugar level, etc.
(iv) Drug effect could be maintained overnight without disturbing sleep, e.g. antiasthmatics, anticonvulsants, etc.

However, all drugs do not need to be made long acting, e.g. those used for brief therapeutic effect (sleep inducing hypnotic, headache remedy) or those with inherently long duration of action (digoxin, amlodipine, doxycycline, omeprazole). Drugs with t½ < 4 hr are suitable for controlled release formulations, while there is no need of such formulations for drugs with t½ >12 hr. Methods utilized for prolonging drug action are summarized below. Some of these have already been described.

1. By prolonging absorption from site of administration

(a) *Oral* Sustained release tablets, spansule capsules, etc.; drug particles are coated with resins, plastic materials or other substances which temporally disperse release of the active ingredient in the g.i.t. The controlled release tablet/capsule preparation utilizes a semipermeable membrane to control the release of drug from the dosage form. Such preparations prolong the action by 4 to 6 hours and no more because in that time drug particles reach the colon.

(b) *Parenteral* The s.c. and i.m. injection of drug in insoluble form (benzathine penicillin, lente insulin) or as oily solution (depot progestins); pellet implantation, sialistic and biodegradable implants can provide for its absorption over a couple of days to several months or even years. Inclusion of a vasoconstrictor with the drug also delays absorption (adrenaline with local anaesthetics).

(c) *Transdermal drug delivery systems* The drug impregnated in adhesive patches, strips or as ointment is applied on skin for prolonged absorption.

2. By increasing plasma protein binding

Drug congeners have been prepared which are highly bound to plasma protein and are slowly released in the free active form, e.g. sulfadoxine.

3. By retarding rate of metabolism Small chemical modification can markedly affect the rate of metabolism without affecting the biological action, e.g. addition of ethinyl group to estradiol makes it longer acting and suitable for use as oral contraceptive. Inhibition of specific enzyme by one drug can prolong the action of another drug, e.g. allopurinol inhibits degradation of 6-mercaptopurine; ritonavir boosts the action of atazanavir and lopinavir; cilastatin protects imipenem from degradation in kidney.

4. By retarding renal excretion The tubular secretion of drug being an active process, can be suppressed by a competing substance, e.g. probenecid prolongs duration of action of penicillin and ampicillin.

CHAPTER 3

Pharmacodynamics

Pharmacodynamics is the study of drug effects. It starts with describing what the drugs do, and goes on to explain how they do it. Thus, it attempts to elucidate the complete action-effect sequence and the dose-effect relationship. Modification of the effects of one drug by another drug and by other factors is also an aspect of pharmacodynamics.

PRINCIPLES OF DRUG ACTION

Drugs (except those gene based) do not impart new functions to any system, organ or cell; they only alter the pace of ongoing activity. The basic types of drug action can be broadly classed as:

1. Stimulation It refers to selective enhancement of the level of activity of specialized cells, e.g. adrenaline stimulates the heart, pilocarpine stimulates salivary glands.

2. Depression It means selective diminution of activity of specialized cells, e.g. barbiturates depress central nervous system (CNS), local anaesthetics depress nerve conduction.

Certain drugs stimulate one type of cells but depress the other, e.g. acetylcholine stimulates intestinal smooth muscle but depresses the SA node in heart.

3. Irritation This connotes a nonselective, often noxious effect, and is particularly applied to epithelium and connective tissue. Mild irritation may stimulate associated function, but strong irritation results in inflammation, corrosion, necrosis and morphological damage.

4. Replacement This refers to the use of natural metabolites, hormones or their congeners in deficiency states, e.g. levodopa in parkinsonism, insulin in diabetes mellitus, iron in anaemia.

5. Cytotoxic action Selective cytotoxic action for invading parasites or cancer cells, attenuating them without significantly affecting the host cells is utilized for cure/palliation of infections and neoplasms, e.g. penicillin, chloroquine, zidovudine, chlorhexidine, cyclophosphamide, etc.

MECHANISM OF DRUG ACTION

Only a handful of drugs act by virtue of their simple physical or chemical property; examples are:
- Bulk laxatives—physical mass
- Activated charcoal—adsorptive property
- Mannitol—osmotic activity
- ^{131}I and other radioisotopes—radioactivity
- Antacids—neutralization of gastric HCl

- Pot. permanganate—oxidizing property
- Dimercaprol—chelation of heavy metals.

Majority of drugs produce their effects by interacting with discrete target biomolecules, which usually are proteins. Such mechanism also confers selectivity of action to the drug. Functional proteins that are targets of drug action can be grouped into four basic categories, *viz.* enzymes, ion channels, transporters and receptors (Fig. 3.1). However, a few drugs do act on other proteins (e.g. colchicine, vinca alkaloids, taxanes bind to the structural protein tubulin) or on nucleic acids (alkylating agents).

I. ENZYMES

Almost all biological reactions are carried out under catalytic influence of enzymes; hence, enzymes are a very important target of drug action. Drugs can either increase or decrease the rate of enzymatically mediated reactions. However, in physiological systems enzyme activities are often optimally set. Thus, stimulation of enzymes by drugs, that are truly foreign substances, is unusual. Enzyme stimulation is relevant to some natural metabolites only, e.g. pyridoxine acts as a cofactor and increases decarboxylase activity. Several enzymes are stimulated through receptors and second messengers, e.g. adrenaline stimulates hepatic glycogen phosphorylase enzyme through β receptors and cyclic AMP (second messenger). Stimulation of an enzyme increases its affinity for the substrate so that rate constant (kM) of the reaction is lowered (Fig. 3.2).

Apparent increase in enzyme activity can also occur by enzyme induction, i.e. synthesis of more enzyme protein. This cannot be called stimulation because the kM does not change. Many drugs induce microsomal enzymes (*see* p. 30).

Inhibition of enzymes is a common mode of drug action.

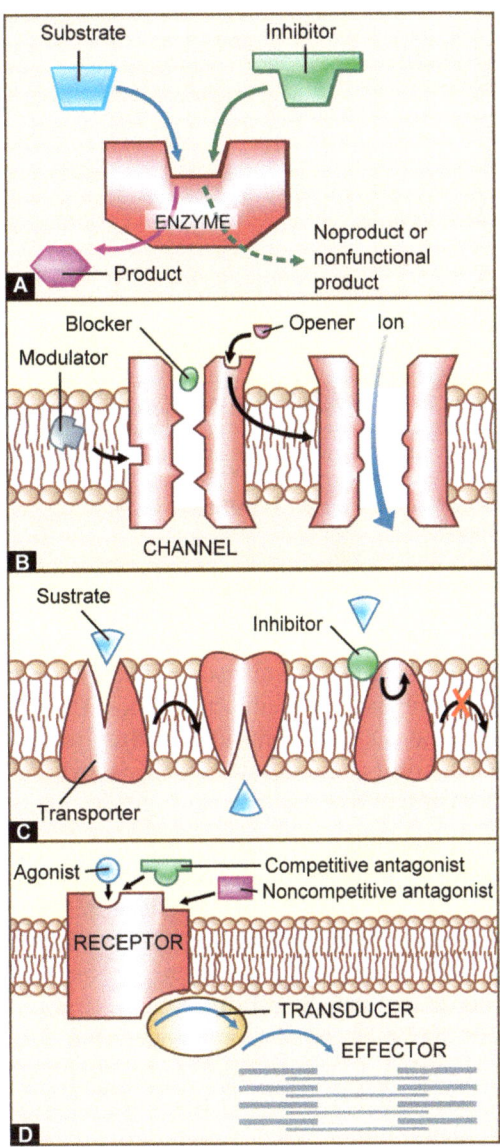

Fig. 3.1: Four major types of biomacromolecular targets of drug action
(A) Enzyme; (B) Transmembrane ion channel; (C) Membrane bound transporter; (D) Receptor (*see* text for description)

Enzyme inhibition

Some chemicals (heavy metal salts, strong acids and alkalies, formaldehyde, phenol, etc.) denature proteins and inhibit all enzymes nonselectively. They have limited medicinal

Chapter 3: Pharmacodynamics

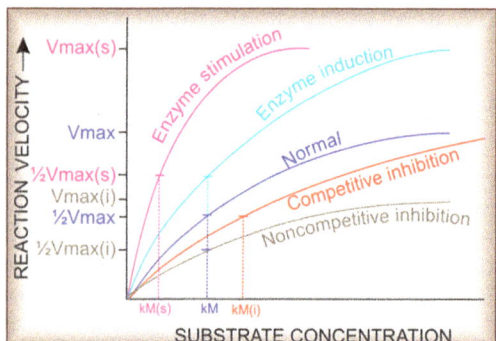

Fig. 3.2: Effect of enzyme induction, stimulation and inhibition on kinetics of the reaction
Vmax—Maximum velocity of reaction; *Vmax* (s) of stimulated enzyme; *Vmax* (i)—in presence of noncompetitive inhibitor; *k*M—rate constant of the reaction; *k*M (s)—of stimulated enzyme; *k*M (i)—in presence of competitive inhibitor
Note: Enzyme induction and noncompetitive inhibition do not change the affinity of the enzyme (*k*M is unaltered), whereas enzyme stimulation and competitive inhibition respectively decrease and increase the *k*M.

Enzyme	Endogenous substrate	Competitive inhibitor
Cholinesterase	Acetylcholine	Physostigmine, Neostigmine
Monoamine-oxidase A (MAO-A)	Catecholamines	Moclobemide
Dopa decarboxylase	Levodopa	Carbidopa, Benserazide
Xanthine oxidase	Hypoxanthine	Allopurinol
Angiotensin converting enzyme (ACE)	Angiotensin-1	Captopril
α-Reductase	Testosterone	Finasteride
Aromatase	Testosterone, Androstenedione	Letrozole, Anastrozole
Bacterial folate synthase	Para-amino benzoic acid (PABA)	Sulfadiazine

value restricted to external application only. However, selective inhibition of a particular enzyme is a common mode of drug action. Such inhibition is either competitive or noncompetitive.

(i) Competitive *(equilibrium type)* The drug being structurally similar competes with the normal substrate for the catalytic binding site of the enzyme (Fig. 3.1A), so that a new equilibrium is achieved in the presence of the drug. Such inhibitors increase the *k*M but the Vmax remains unchanged (Fig. 3.2), i.e. higher concentration of the substrate is required to achieve ½ maximal reaction velocity, but if substrate concentration is sufficiently increased, it can displace the drug and the same maximal reaction velocity can be attained. Examples are given in the box.
A *nonequilibrium type* of enzyme inhibition can also occur with drugs which react with the same catalytic site of the enzyme but either form strong covalent bonds or have such high affinity for the enzyme that the normal substrate is not able to displace the inhibitor, e.g.

- Organophosphates react covalently with the esteretic site of the enzyme cholinesterase.
- Methotrexate has 50,000 times higher affinity for dihydrofolate reductase than the normal substrate dihydrofolic acid.

In these situations, *k*M is increased and *Vmax* is reduced.

(ii) Noncompetitive The inhibitor reacts with an adjacent site and not with the catalytic site, but alters the enzyme in such a way that it loses its catalytic property. Thus, *k*M is unchanged but Vmax is reduced. Examples are given in the box:

Noncompetitive inhibitor	Enzyme
Acetazolamide	— Carbonic anhydrase
Aspirin, indomethacin	— Cyclooxygenase
Disulfiram	— Aldehyde dehydrogenase
Omeprazole	— $H^+ K^+$ ATPase
Digoxin	— $Na^+ K^+$ ATPase
Theophylline	— Phosphodiesterase
Propylthiouracil	— Peroxidase in thyroid
Lovastatin	— HMG-CoA reductase
Sildenafil	— Phosphodiesterase-5

II. ION CHANNELS

Proteins which act as ion selective channels participate in transmembrane signaling and regulate intracellular ionic composition. This makes them a common target of drug action (*see* Fig. 3.1B). Drugs can affect ion channels some of which actually are receptors, because they are operated by specific signal molecules, either directly (ligand gated channels, e.g. nicotinic receptor), or through G-proteins (G-protein regulated channels, e.g. β_1 adrenergic receptor activated cardiac calcium channel, *see* Table 3.1). Drugs can also act on voltage operated channels by binding directly to the channel and affecting ion movement through it, e.g. local anaesthetics which obstruct voltage sensitive Na^+ channels (*see* Ch. 24). In addition, certain drugs modulate the opening and closing of channels, e.g.:

- Nifedipine blocks L-type of voltage sensitive Ca^{2+} channel.
- Nicorandil opens ATP-sensitive K^+ channels.
- Sulfonylurea hypoglycaemics inhibit pancreatic ATP- sensitive K^+ channels (*see* Fig. 14.3).
- Amiloride inhibits renal epithelial Na^+ channels (*see* Fig. 13.5).

III. TRANSPORTERS

Several substrates are translocated across membranes by binding to specific transporters (carriers) which either facilitate diffusion in the direction of the concentration gradient or pump the metabolite/ion against the concentration gradient using metabolic energy (*see* Fig. 2.5). Many drugs produce their action by directly interacting with the carrier protein to inhibit the ongoing physiological transport of the metabolite/ion. Examples are:

- Cocaine and desipramine block neuronal reuptake of noradrenaline by inhibiting NET (*see* Fig. 6.4).
- Fluoxetine and other SSRIs selectively inhibits neuronal 5-HT transporter SERT.
- Reserpine blocks the vesicular reuptake of noradrenaline and 5-HT by vesicular monoamine transporter (VMAT-2) (*see* Fig. 6.4).
- Furosemide inhibits the Na^+-K^+-$2Cl^-$ cotransporter in the ascending limb of loop of Henle (*see* Fig. 13.3).
- Hydrochlorothiazide inhibits the Na^+-Cl^- symporter in the early distal tubule (*see* Fig. 13.4).
- Probenecid inhibits active transport of organic acids (uric acid, penicillin) in renal tubules by organic anion transporter (OAT).

IV. RECEPTORS

A large number of drugs do not bind directly to the effectors like enzymes, channels, transporters or structural proteins, etc. but act through specific regulatory macromolecules which control these effectors. These macromolecules or the sites on them which bind and interact with the drug are called 'receptors'.

Receptor It is defined as a macromolecule or binding site located on the surface or within the effector cell that serves to recognize the signal molecule/drug and initiate response to it, but itself has no other function. In this sense, effectors (enzymes, channels, transporters, etc.) which bind and interact directly with a drug are not referred to as receptors; e.g. xanthine oxidase is not called the receptor for allopurinol, or cholinesterase is not called the receptor for physostigmine.

The following terms are used in describing drug-receptor interaction.

Agonist An agent which activates a receptor to produce an effect similar to that of the physiological signal molecule.

Inverse agonist An agent which activates a receptor to produce an effect in the opposite direction to that of the agonist.

Antagonist An agent which prevents the action of an agonist on a receptor or the subsequent response but does not have any effect of its own.

Partial agonist An agent which activates a receptor to produce submaximal effect but antagonizes the action of a full agonist.

Ligand (Latin: *ligare*—to bind) Any molecule which attaches selectively to particular receptors or sites. The term only indicates affinity or ability to bind without regard to any functional change: agonists and competitive antagonists are both ligands of the same receptor.

Receptor occupation theory

After studying quantitative aspects of drug action, Clark (1937) propounded a theory of drug action based on occupation of receptors by specific drugs and that the pace of a cellular function can be altered by interaction of these receptors with drugs (small molecular ligands). He perceived the interaction between the two molecular species, viz. drug (D) and receptor (R) to be governed by the law of mass action, and the effect (E) to be a direct function of the drug-receptor complex (DR) formed:

$$D + R \underset{K_2}{\overset{K_1}{\rightleftharpoons}} DR \longrightarrow E \quad ...(1)$$

Subsequently, it has been realized that occupation of the receptor is essential but not itself sufficient to elicit a response; the agonist must also be able to activate (induce a conformational change in) the receptor. The ability to bind with the receptor designated as *affinity*, and the capacity to induce a functional change in the receptor designated as *intrinsic activity* (IA) or efficacy are independent properties. Competitive antagonists occupy the receptor but do not activate it. Moreover, certain drugs are partial agonists which occupy and submaximally activate the receptor. An all or none action is not a must at the receptor. A theoretical quantity(S) denoting strength of stimulus imparted to the cell was interposed in the Clark's equation:

$$D + R \underset{K_2}{\overset{K_1}{\rightleftharpoons}} DR \text{-\!\!\!\sim\!\!\!\sim\!\!\!\sim\!\!\!\sim\!\!\!\rightarrow} S \longrightarrow E \quad ...(2)$$

Depending on the agonist, DR could generate a stronger or weaker S, probably as a function of the conformational change brought about by the agonist in the receptor. Accordingly:

Agonists have both affinity and maximal intrinsic activity (IA = 1), e.g. adrenaline, histamine, morphine.

Competitive antagonists have affinity but no intrinsic activity (IA = 0), e.g. propranolol, atropine, chlorpheniramine, naloxone.

Partial agonists have affinity and submaximal intrinsic activity (IA between 0 and 1), e.g. dichloroisoproterenol on β adrenergic receptor and pentazocine on μ opioid receptor.

Inverse agonists have affinity but intrinsic activity with a minus sign (IA between 0 and –1).

Inverse agonism is manifest only in case of some receptors which manifest certain degree of *constitutive activation*, i.e. they are partially active even in the complete absence of any agonist (tonically active). Benzodiazepine receptor (*see* Fig. 9.2) is one such receptor, and DMCM is its inverse agonist.

Nature of receptors

Receptors are regulatory macromolecules, mostly proteins, though nucleic acids may also serve as receptors. Hundreds of receptor proteins have been isolated, purified, cloned and their primary amino acid (AA) sequence has been worked out. Molecular cloning has also helped in obtaining the receptor protein in larger quantity to study its structure and properties, and in subclassifying receptors. The surface receptors with their coupling and effector proteins are considered to be floating in a sea of membrane lipids; the folding, orientation and topography of the system being determined by interactions between the lipophilic and hydrophilic domains of the peptide chains with solvent molecules (water on one side and lipids on the other). Nonpolar portions of the AA chain tend to bury within the membrane, while polar groups tend to come out in the aqueous medium. In such a delicately balanced system, it is not difficult to visualize that a small molecular ligand binding to one site in the receptor molecule could be capable of tripping the balance (by altering distribution of charges, etc.) and bringing about conformational changes at distant sites. Majority of receptor molecules are made up of several non-identical subunits (heteropolymeric), and agonist binding has been shown to bring about changes in their quaternary structure or relative alignment of the subunits, e.g. on activation the subunits of nicotinic receptor move apart opening a centrally located cation channel (Fig. 3.3).

Many clinically useful drugs act upon *physiological receptors* which mediate responses to transmitters, hormones, autacoids and other endogenous signal molecules; examples are cholinergic, adrenergic, histaminergic, steroid, leukotriene and other receptors. In addition, now some truly *drug receptors* have been described for which there are no known physiological ligands, e.g. benzodiazepine receptor, sulfonylurea receptor.

Receptor subtypes

It has been found that most receptors exist in multiple types and subtypes, differing in their affinity for various agonists and antagonists, ligand binding, tissue distribution, transducer pathway used and molecular composition. Illustrative examples are muscarinic (M) and nicotinic (N) types of cholinergic receptors and their subtypes (M_1, M_2....M_5), α and β adrenergic receptors and their subtypes ($α_1$, $α_2$), ($β_1$, $β_2$, $β_3$). This receptor diversity has been exploited in producing more selective and more targeted newer drugs.

ACTION-EFFECT SEQUENCE

'Drug action' and 'drug effect' are often loosely used interchangeably, but are not synonymous.

Drug action It is the initial combination of the drug with its receptor resulting in a conformational change in the latter (in case of agonists), or prevention of conformational change through exclusion of the agonist (in case of antagonists).

Drug effect It is the ultimate change in biological function brought about as a consequence of drug action, through a series of intermediate steps (transducer).

Receptors subserve two essential functions, *viz, recognition* of the specific ligand molecule and *transduction* of the signal into a response. Accordingly, the receptor molecule has a *ligand binding domain* (spatially and energetically suitable for binding the specific ligand) and an *effector domain* (Fig. 3.3) which undergoes a functional conformational change. These domains have now actually been identified in some receptors. The perturbation in the receptor molecule is variously translated into the response. The sequential relationship between drug action, transducer and drug effect can be seen in Fig. 3.5.

TRANSDUCER MECHANISMS

Considerable progress has been made in the understanding of transducer mechanisms which, in most instances, have been found to be highly complex multistep processes that provide for amplification of the signal as well as integration of concurrently received

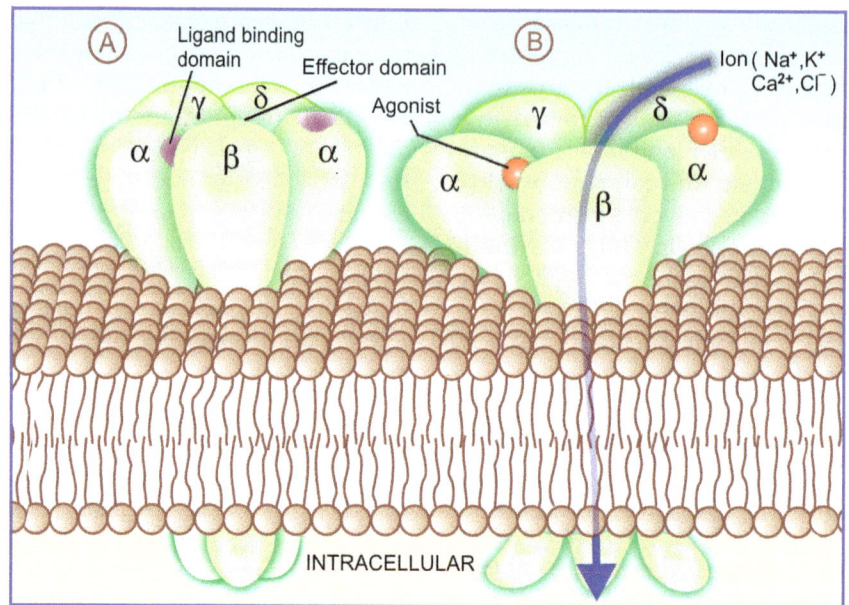

Fig. 3.3: Diagrammatic representation of direct receptor mediated operation of membrane ion channel
In case of nicotinic cholinergic receptor, the molecule (8 nm in diameter) is composed of 5 subunits ($2\alpha + \beta + \gamma + \delta$) enclosing a transmembrane ion channel within the α subunit. Normally the channel is closed (A). When two molecules of acetylcholine bind to the two α subunits (B), all subunits move apart opening the central pore to allow passage of partially hydrated Na^+ ions. Anions are blocked from passage through the channel by positive charges lining it.
In other cases, K^+, Ca^{2+} or Cl^- ions move through the channel depending on its ion selectivity.

extra- and intracellular signals at each step. These mechanisms of translation of receptor activation into functional response can be grouped into five major categories. Receptors falling in one category have also been found to possess considerable structural homology, and may be considered to belong to one super family of receptors.

1. G-protein coupled receptors These are a large family of cell membrane receptors which are linked to the effector (enzyme/channel/transporter protein) through one or more GTP-activated proteins (G-proteins) for response effectuation. All such receptors have a common pattern of structural organization (Fig. 3.4). The molecule has 7 α-helical membrane spanning hydrophobic amino acid (AA) segments which run into 3 extracellular and 3 intracellular loops. The agonist binding site is located

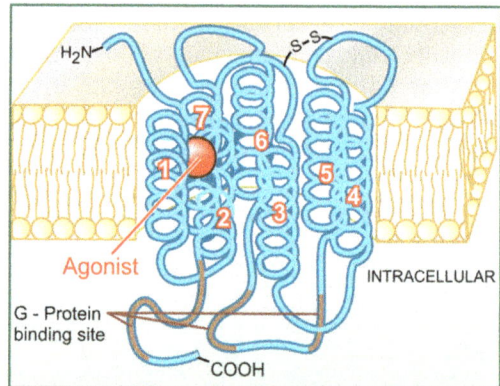

Fig. 3.4: Diagrammatic representation of G-protein coupled receptor molecule
The receptor consists of 7 membrane spanning helical segments of hydrophobic amino acids. The intervening segments connecting the helices form 3 loops on either side of the membrane. The amino terminus of the chain lies on the extracellular face, while the carboxy terminus is on the cytosolic side. The approximate location of the agonist and G-protein-binding sites is indicated.

somewhere between the helices on the extracellular face, while another recognition site formed by cytosolic segments binds the coupling G-protein. The G-proteins float in the membrane with their exposed domain lying in the cytosol, and are heterotrimeric in composition (α, β and γ subunits). In the inactive state GDP is bound to the exposed domain of the α subunit. Activation through the receptor leads to displacement of GDP by GTP. The activated α-subunit carrying GTP dissociates from the other two subunits and either activates or inhibits the effector. The βγ subunit diamer has also been shown to modulate certain effectors like receptor operated K⁺ channels, and to promote GPCR desensitization when overstimulated.

The α-subunit has GTPase activity: the bound GTP is slowly hydrolyzed to GDP: the α-subunit then dissociates from the effector to rejoin its other subunits, but not before the effector has been activated/inhibited for several seconds and the signal has been considerably amplified.

There are three major effector pathways (Table 3.1) through which G-protein coupled receptors function:

(a) *Adenylyl cyclase: cAMP pathway* Activation of AC results in intracellular accumulation of second messenger cAMP which functions mainly through cAMP-dependent protein kinase (PKA). The PKA phosphorylates and alters the function of many enzymes, ion channels, transporters and structural proteins to manifest as increased contractility/impulse generation (heart, Fig. 3.5), relaxation (smooth muscle), glycogenolysis, lipolysis, inhibition of secretion/mediator release, modulation of junctional transmission, hormone synthesis, etc. The reverse occurs when AC is inhibited through inhibitory Gi-protein.

(b) *Phospholipase C: IP_3-DAG pathway* Activation of phospholipase C (PLc) hydrolyzes the membrane phospholipid phosphatidyl inositol 4, 5-bisphosphate (PIP2) to generate the second messengers inositol 1,4,5-trisphosphate (IP_3) and diacylglycerol (DAG). While IP_3 mobilizes Ca^{2+} from endoplasmic reticular depots, DAG enhances protein kinase C (PKc) activation by Ca^{2+} (Fig. 3.6). The activated PKc phosphorylates many intracellular proteins and mediates various physiological responses. Triggered by IP_3, the released

Table 3.1: Major functional pathways of G-protein coupled receptor transduction

Adenylylcyclase: cAMP		Phospholipase IP_3-DAG	Channel regulation		
↑	↓		Ca^{2+} channel opening	Ca^{2+} channel closing	K^+ channel opening
Adrenergic-β	Adrenergic-$α_2$	Adrenergic-$α_1$	Adrenergic-$β_1$ (Heart, Sk. muscle)	Dopamine-D2	Adrenergic-$α_2$
Histamine-H_2	Muscarinic-M_2	Histamine-H_1		GABA-B	Muscarinic-M_2
Dopamine-D1	Dopamine-D2	Muscarinic-M_1, M_3		Opioid-κ	Dopamine-D2
Glucagon	$5-HT_1$	$5-HT_2$		Adenosine-A_1	$5-HT_{1A}$
FSH & LH	GABA-B	Vasopressin-Oxytocin		Somatostatin	GABA-B
ACTH	Opioid-μ, δ	Bradykinin-B_2			Opioid-μ, δ
TSH	Angiotensin	Angiotensin			Adenosine-A_1
Prostaglandin-EP_2	Prostaglandin-EP_3	Prostaglandin-FP, EP_1, EP_3			
Prostacyclin-IP	Somatostatin	Thromboxane-TP			
Adenosine-A_2	Adenosine-A_1	Leukotriene			
		Cholecystokinin-Gastrin			
		PAF			

↑ Activation; ↓ Inhibition

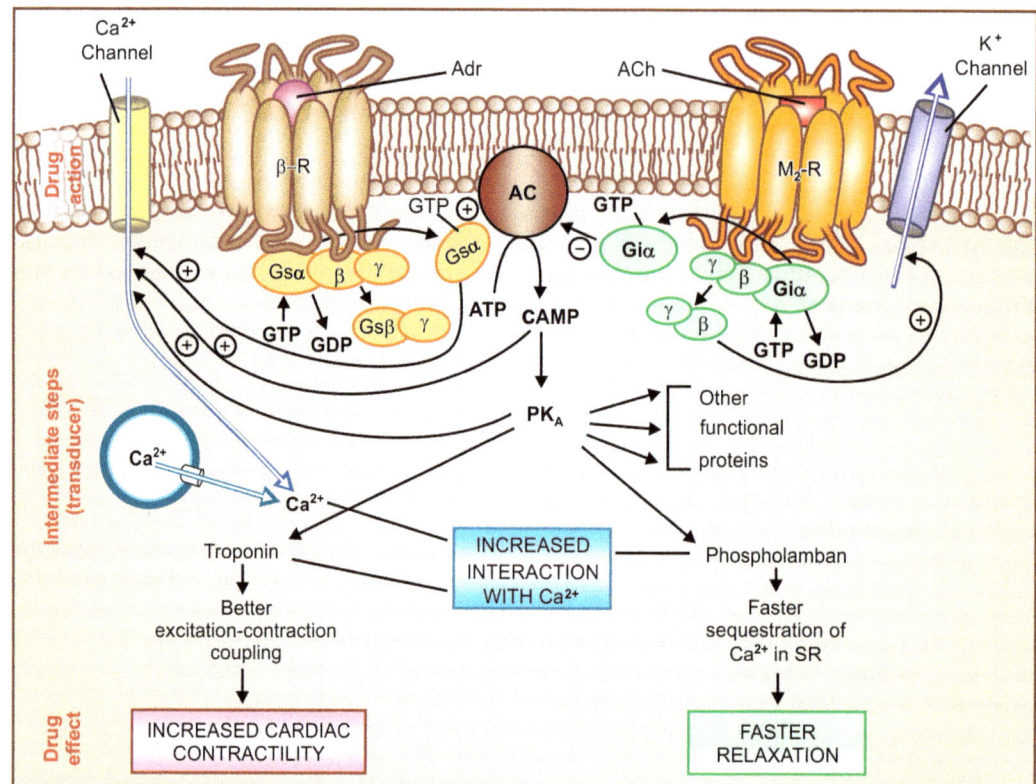

Fig. 3.5: The action-effect sequence of two G-protein coupled (β adrenergic and muscarinic M_2) receptor activation in myocardial cell

Adrenaline (Adr) binds to β-adrenergic receptor (β-R) on the cell surface inducing a conformational change which permits interaction of the G-protein binding site with the stimulatory G-protein (Gs). The activated α subunit of Gs now binds GTP (in place of GDP), and dissociates from the βγ diamer as well as the receptor. The Gsα carrying bound GTP associates with and activates the enzyme adenylyl cyclase (AC) located on the cytosolic side of the membrane: ATP is hydrolysed to cAMP which then phosphorylates and thus activates cAMP dependent protein kinase (PK_A). The PK_A in turn phosphorylates many functional proteins including troponin and phospholamban, so that they interact with Ca_{2+}, respectively resulting in increased force of contraction and faster relaxation. Calcium is made available by entry from outside (direct activation of myocardial membrane Ca^{2+} channels by Gsα and through their phosphorylation by PK_A) as well as from intracellular stores.

One of the other proteins phosphorylated by cAMP is phosphorylase kinase which then activates the enzyme phosphorylase resulting in breakdown of glycogen to be utilized as energy source for increased contractility.

Action of acetylcholine (ACh) on muscarinic M_2 receptor (M_2-R), also located in the myocardial membrane, similarly activates an inhibitory G-protein (Gi). The GTP carrying active Giα subunit inhibits AC, and opposes its activation by Gsα. The βγ diamer of Gi activates membrane K^+ channels causing hyperpolarization which depresses impulse generation.

cytosolic Ca^{2+} (third messenger in this setting) is a highly versatile regulator acting through calmodulin (CAM), PKc and other effectors; it mediates/modulates contraction, secretion/transmitter release, neuronal excitability, intracellular movements, membrane function, metabolism, cell proliferation, etc. Like AC, the PLc can also be inhibited through inhibitory G-protein resulting in directionally opposite responses.

(c) *Channel regulation* The activated G-proteins can also promote opening or closing of ionic channels specific for Ca^{2+}, or

Mechanism of Drug Action

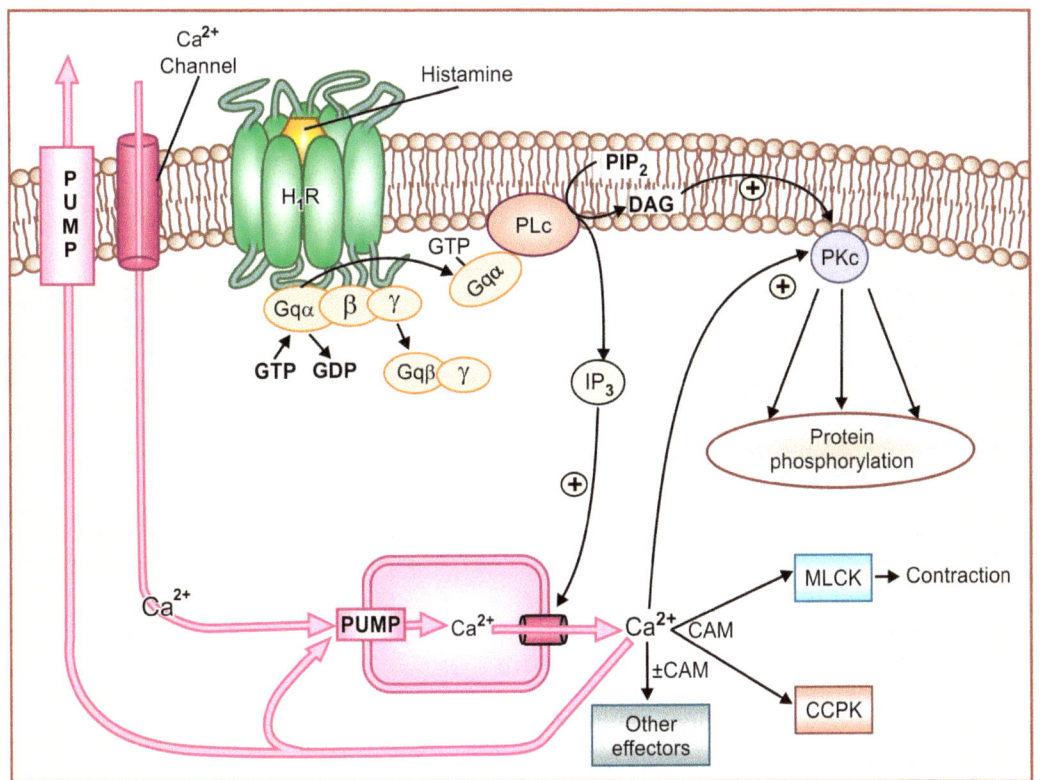

Fig. 3.6: The important steps of phospholipase cb (PLcβ) pathway of response effectuation (in smooth muscle) The agonist, e.g. histamine binds to its H_1 receptor (H_1 R) and activates the G-protein G_q. Its a subunit binds GTP in place of GDP, dissociates from the receptor as well as from βγ diamer to activate membrane bound PLcβ that hydrolyses phosphatidyl inositol 4, 5-bisphosphate (PIP_2), a membrane bound phospholipid. The products inositol 1, 4, 5-trisphosphate (IP_3) and diacylglycerol (DAG) act as second messengers. The primary action of IP_3 is facilitation of Ca^{2+} mobilization from intracellular organellar pools, while DAG in conjunction with Ca^{2+} activates protein kinase C (PKc) which phosphorylates and alters the activity of a number of functional and structural proteins. Cytosolic Ca^{2+} is a veritable messenger: combines with calmodulin (CAM) to activate myosin light chain kinase (MLCK) inducing contraction, and another important regulator calcium-calmodulin protein kinase (CCPK). Several other effectors are regulated by Ca^{2+} in a CAM dependent or independent manner. Cytosolic Ca^{2+} is recycled by uptake into the endoplasmic reticulum as well as effluxed by membrane Ca^{2+} pump.

K^+ without the intervention of any second messenger like cAMP or IP_3, and bring about hyperpolarization/depolarization/changes in intracellular Ca^{2+} levels. Physiological responses like changes in inotropy, chronotropy, transmitter release, neuronal activity and smooth muscle relaxation follow. Receptors found to regulate ionic channels through G-proteins are listed in Table 3.1.

2. Ion channel receptors These cell surface receptors enclose ion selective channels (for Na^+, K^+, Ca^{2+} or Cl^-) within their molecules. Agonist binding opens the channel (Fig. 3.3) and causes depolarization/ hyperpolarization/changes in cytosolic ionic composition, depending on the ion that flows through. The nicotinic cholinergic, GABA-A, glycine (inhibitory amino acid), excitatory amino acid (kainate, NMDA and AMPA) as well as $5-HT_3$ receptors fall in this category. A large number of clinically useful drugs act through this type of receptors.

The receptor is usually a pentameric protein; all subunits, in addition to large intra- and extracellular segments, generally have four membrane spanning helical domains. The subunits are mostly arranged round the channel like a rosette and the α subunits usually bear the agonist-binding sites.

Certain receptor operated ion channels also have secondary ligands which bind to an allosteric site and modulate the gating of the channel by the primary ligand, e.g. the benzodiazepine receptor modulates GABA-A gated Cl⁻channel.

Thus, in these receptors, agonists directly operate ion channels, without the intervention of any coupling protein or second messenger. The onset and offset of responses through this class of receptors is the fastest.

3. Transmembrane enzyme-linked receptors

This class of receptors are utilized primarily by peptide hormones, and are made up of a large extracellular ligand binding domain connected through a single transmembrane helical peptide chain to an intracellular subunit having enzymatic property. The enzyme at the cytosolic side is generally a protein kinase, but can also be guanylyl cyclase in few cases. The commonest protein kinases are the ones which phosphorylate tyrosine residues on the substrate proteins and are called 'receptor tyrosine kinases' (RTKs), (Fig. 3.7). Examples are—insulin, epidermal growth factor (EGF), and many other growth factor receptors.

In the unliganded monomeric state, the kinase remains inactive. Hormone binding induces dimerization of receptor molecules, brings about conformation changes which activate the kinase to autophosphorylate tyrosine residues on each other, increasing their affinity for binding substrate proteins which have SH_2 domains. These are then phosphorylated and released to carry forward the cascade of phosphorylations leading to the response. Receptor dimerization also promotes their internalization and degradation in lysosomes, leading to their down regulation, if activation is fast enough.

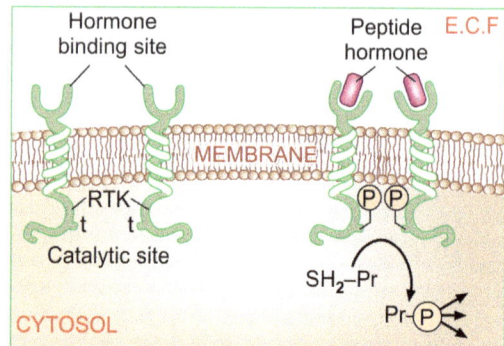

Fig. 3.7: Model of receptor tyrosine kinase, an enzyme-linked receptor:
On binding the peptide hormone to the extracellular domains, the monomeric receptors move laterally in the membrane and form diamers. Dimerization activates tyrosine-kinase (RTK) activity of the intracellular domains so that they phosphorylate tyrosine (t) residues on each other, as well as on several SH_2 domain substrate proteins (SH_2-Pr). The phosphorylated substrate proteins then perform downstream signaling function.

A large number of intracellular signaling proteins have SH_2 domains. Thus, the RTKs are able to regulate diverse cellular functions including metabolic reactions, cell growth and differentiation.

In place of protein kinase the enzyme can also be guanylyl cyclase (GC), as in the case of atrial natriuretic peptide (ANP). Agonist activation of the receptor generates cGMP in the cytosol as a second messenger, which in turn activates cGMP-dependent protein kinase (PK_G) and modulates cellular activity.

The transmembrane enzyme-linked receptors transduce responses in a matter of few minutes to few hours.

4. Transmembrane JAK-STAT binding receptors

These receptors differ from RTKs in not having any intrinsic catalytic domain (Fig. 3.8). Agonist induced dimerization alters the intracellular domain conformation to increase its affinity for a cytosolic tyrosine protein kinase JAK (Janus Kinase). On binding, JAK gets activated and phosphorylates tyrosine residues of the receptor, which now bind

Mechanism of Drug Action

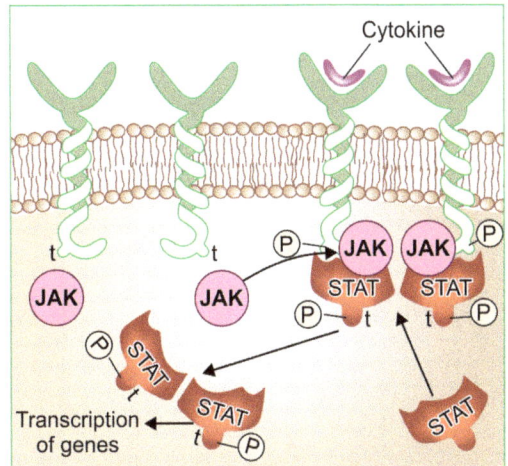

Fig. 3.8: Model of transmembrane JAK-STAT binding receptor.
The intracellular domain of these receptors lacks intrinsic protein kinase activity. Cytokines/hormones binding to the extracellular domain induce receptor dimerization which activates the intracellular domain to bind free moving JAK (Janus Kinase) molecules. The activated JAK phosphorylate tyrosine residues on the receptor which then binds another protein STAT (signal transducer and activator of transcription). Tyrosine residues of STAT also get phosphorylated by JAK. The phosphorylated STAT dimerize, dissociate from the receptor and move to the nucleus to regulate transcription of target genes.

another free moving protein STAT (signal transducer and activator of transcription). This is also phosphorylated by JAK. Pairs of phosphorylated STAT dimerize and translocate to the nucleus to regulate gene transcription resulting in a biological response. Growth hormone, prolactin, several cytokines and interferons act through this type of receptor.

5. Receptors regulating gene expression (Transcription factors, Nuclear receptors) In contrast to the above 4 classes of receptors, these are intracellular (cytoplasmic or nuclear) soluble proteins which respond to lipid soluble chemical messengers that penetrate the cell (Fig. 3.9). The receptor protein (specific for each hormone/regulator) is inherently capable of binding to specific genes, but its attached proteins HSP-90 and others prevent it from adopting the configuration needed for binding to DNA. When the hormone binds near the carboxy terminus of the receptor, the restricting proteins (HSP-90, etc.) are released, the receptor dimerizes and the DNA binding regulatory segment located in the middle of the molecule folds into the requisite configuration. The liganded receptor dimer moves to the nucleus and binds other co-activator/co-repressor proteins which have a modulatory influence on its capacity to alter gene function. The whole complex then attaches to specific DNA sequences (hormone response elements) of the target genes and facilitates or represses their expression so that specific mRNA is synthesized/repressed on the template of the gene. This mRNA moves to the ribosomes and directs synthesis of specific proteins which regulate activity of the target cells.

All steroidal hormones (glucocorticoids, mineralocorticoids, androgens, estrogens, progesterone), thyroxine, vit D and vit A function in this manner. This transduction mechanism is the slowest in its time course of action (takes hours).

Regulation of receptors

Receptors exist in a dynamic state; their density and efficacy to elicit the response is subject to regulation by the level of ongoing activity and other physiopathological influences. In tonically active systems, prolonged deprivation of the agonist (by denervation or continued use of an antagonist or a drug which reduces input) results in supersensitivity of the receptor as well as the effector system to the agonist. This has clinical relevance in clonidine/CNS depressant/opioid withdrawal syndromes, sudden discontinuation of propranolol in angina pectoris, etc. The mechanisms involved may be unmasking of receptors or their proliferation (*up regulation*) or accentuation of signal amplification by the transducer.

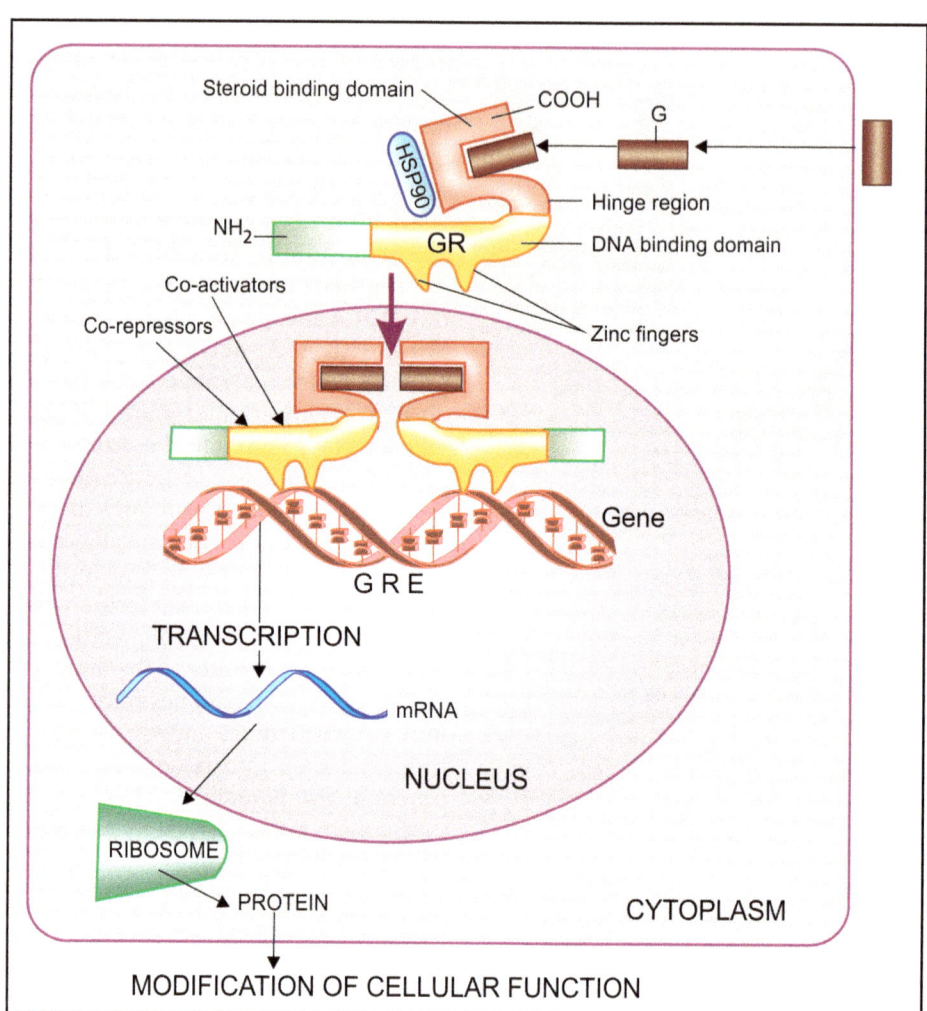

Fig. 3.9: Operational scheme of intracellular (glucocorticoid) receptor
The glucocorticoid (G) penetrates the cell membrane and binds to the glucocorticoid receptor (GR) protein that normally resides in the cytoplasm in association with heat shock protein 90 (HSP90) + other proteins. The GR has a steroid binding domain near the carboxy terminus and a mid-region DNA binding domain joined by a 'hinge region'. The DNA binding domain has two 'zinc fingers', each made up of a loop of amino acids with chelated zinc ion. Binding of the steroid to GR dissociates the complexed proteins (HSP90, etc) removing their inhibitory influence on it. A dimerization region that overlaps the steroid binding domain is exposed, promoting dimerization of the occupied receptor. The steroid bound receptor diamer translocates to the nucleus, binds coactivator/corepressor proteins and interacts with specific DNA sequences called 'glucocorticoid responsive elements' (GREs) within the regulatory region of appropriate genes. The expression of these genes is consequently altered resulting in promotion (or suppression) of their transcription. The specific mRNA thus produced is directed to the ribosome where the message is translated into a specific pattern of protein synthesis, which in turn modifies cell function.

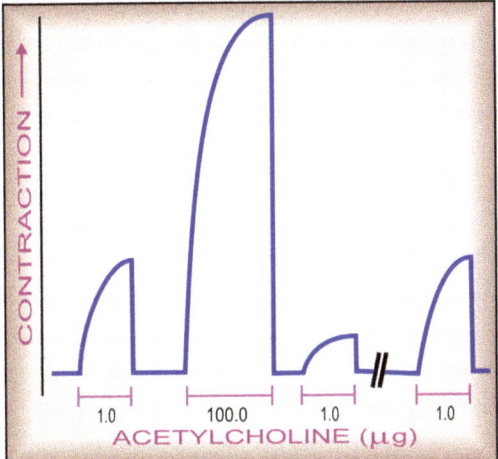

Fig. 3.10: Illustration of the phenomenon of desensitization Contractile responses of frog's rectus abdominis muscle to acetylcholine. Note that shortly after exposure to a high (100-fold) dose of the agonist, the response is markedly attenuated, but is regained if sufficient time is allowed to elapse.

Conversely, continued intense receptor stimulation causes desensitization or refractoriness: the receptor becomes less sensitive to the agonist. This can be easily demonstrated experimentally (Fig. 3.10); clinical examples are bronchial asthma patients treated continuously with β-adrenergic agonists and parkinsonian patients treated with high doses of levodopa. The changes may be brought about by:
(i) Masking or internalization of the receptor (the receptor becomes inaccessible to the agonist). In this case refractoriness develops as well as fades quickly.
(ii) Decreased synthesis/increased destruction of the receptor (down regulation): refractoriness develops over weeks or months and recedes slowly. Receptor down-regulation is particularly exhibited by the tyrosine protein kinase receptors.

Functions of receptors These can be summarized as:
(a) To propagate extracellular regulatory signals to inside the effector cell when the molecular species carrying the signal cannot itself penetrate the cell membrane.

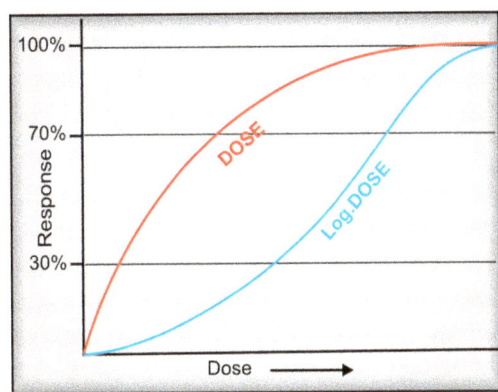

Fig. 3.11: Dose-response and log dose-response curves

(b) To amplify the signal.
(c) To integrate various extracellular and intracellular regulatory signals.
(d) To adapt to short-term and long-term changes in the regulatory melieu and maintain homeostasis.

DOSE-RESPONSE RELATIONSHIP

When a drug is administered systemically, the dose-response relationship has two components: *dose-plasma concentration* relationship and *plasma concentration-response* relationship. The former is determined by pharmacokinetic considerations and ordinarily, descriptions of dose-response relationship refer to the latter, which can be more easily studied *in vitro*.

Generally, the intensity of response increases with increase in dose (or more precisely concentration at the receptor) and the dose-response curve is a rectangular hyperbola (Fig. 3.11). This is because drug-receptor interaction obeys law of mass action, accordingly—

$$E = \frac{E max \times [D]}{K_D + [D]} \qquad ...(3)$$

where E is the observed effect at a dose [D] of the drug, *Emax* is the maximal response, K_D is the dissociation constant of the drug-receptor complex, which is equal to the dose of drug at which half maximal response is produced. If the dose is plotted on a logarithmic scale, the curve becomes sigmoid and a linear relationship between log of dose and the response is seen in the intermediate (30-70% response) zone, as can be predicted from equation (3). This is not peculiar to drugs. In fact, all stimuli are graded biologically by the fractional change in stimulus intensity, e.g. 1 kg and 2 kg weights held in two hands can be easily differentiated, but not 10 kg and 11 kg weights; though the absolute difference remains 1 kg, there is a 100% fractional change in the former case but only 10% change in the latter case. In other words, response is proportional to an exponential function (log) of the dose.

The log dose-response curve (DRC) can be characterized by its shape (slope and maxima) and position on the dose axis.

Drug potency and efficacy

The position of DRC on the dose axis is the index of *drug potency* which refers to the amount of drug needed to produce a certain response. A DRC positioned rightward indicates lower potency (Fig. 3.12). Relative potency is often more meaningful than absolute potency, e.g. if 10 mg of morphine = 100 mg of pethidine, morphine is 10 times more potent than pethidine. However, a higher potency, in itself, does not confer clinical superiority unless the potency for therapeutic effect is selectively increased over potency for adverse effect. Drug potency is clearly a factor in determining the dose of a drug.

The upper limit of DRC is the index of *drug efficacy* and refers to the maximal response that can be elicited by the drug, e.g. morphine produces a degree of analgesia not obtainable with any dose of aspirin—morphine is more efficacious than aspirin. Efficacy is a more decisive factor in the choice of a drug.

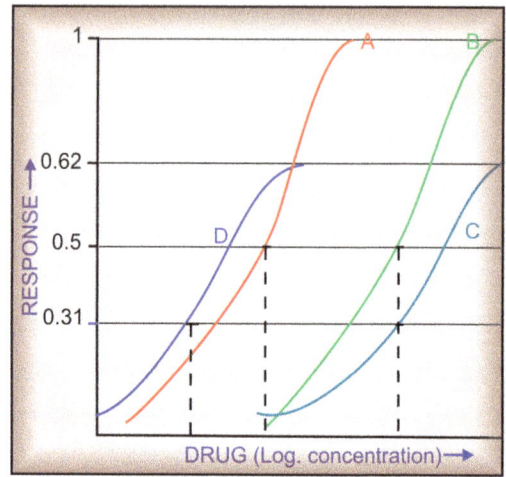

Fig. 3.12: Illustration of drug potency and drug efficacy. Dose-response curve of four drugs producing the same qualitative effect
Note: Drug B is less potent but equally efficacious as drug A.
Drug C is less potent and less efficacious than drug A, but equally potent and less efficacious than drug B.
Drug D is more potent than drugs A, B, & C, but less efficacious than drugs A & B, and equally efficacious as drug C.

Often, the terms 'drug potency' and 'drug efficacy' are used interchangeably, but these are not synonymous and refer to different characteristics of the drug. The two can vary independently:

(a) Aspirin is less potent as well as less efficacious analgesic than morphine.
(b) Pethidine is less potent but equally efficacious analgesic as morphine.
(c) Furosemide is less potent but more efficacious diuretic than metolazone.
(d) Diazepam is more potent but less efficacious CNS depressant than pentobarbitone.

Depending on the type of drug, both higher efficacy (as in the case of furosemide which acts even in renal failure), or lower efficacy (as in the case of diazepam: which is more safe in overdose) could be clinically advantageous.

The slope of the DRC is also important. A steep slope indicates that a moderate increase in dose will markedly increase the response (dose needs individualization), while a flat one implies that little increase in response will occur over a wide dose range (standard doses can be given to most patients). Hydralazine has a steep, while hydrochlorothiazide has a flat DRC of blood pressure lowering effect (Fig. 3.13).

Therapeutic efficacy

The 'therapeutic efficacy' or 'clinical effectiveness' is a composite attribute of a drug, different from the foregoing pharmacological description of 'potency' and 'efficacy'. It depends not only on the relative potency and efficacy of the drug, but also on many pharmacokinetic and pathophysiological variables. It is often expressed in terms of (a) degree of benefit/relief afforded by the drug (in the recommended dose range), i.e. *graded dose-response relationship*. For example, the degree of relief in postextraction pain and swelling afforded by diclofenac/etoricoxib is greater than that afforded by paracetamol: the former two have higher therapeutic efficacy than the latter.

The other method of expressing therapeutic efficacy is in terms of (b) success rate in achieving a defined therapeutic end point, i.e. *quantal dose-response relationship*, e.g. an antibiotic which cures 95% cases of periodontal abscess is a more efficacious drug than the one which cures only 75% patients.

Drug selectivity Drugs seldom produce just one action: the DRCs for different effects of a drug may be different. The extent of separation of DRCs of a drug for different effects is a measure of its selectivity, e.g. the DRCs for bronchodilatation and cardiac stimulation (Fig. 3.14) are quite similar in case of isoprenaline but far apart in case of salbutamol—the latter is a more selective bronchodilator drug.

The gap between the therapeutic effect DRC and the adverse effect DRC defines the *safety margin* or the *therapeutic index* of a drug. In experimental animals, therapeutic index is often calculated as:

$$\text{Therapeutic index} = \frac{\text{median lethal dose}}{\text{median effective dose}}$$

$$\text{or} \quad \frac{LD_{50}}{ED_{50}}$$

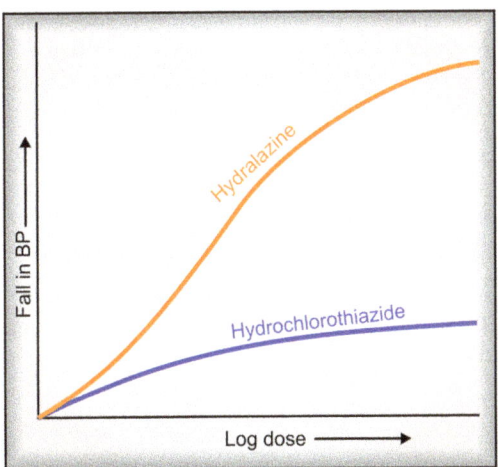

Fig. 3.13: Steep and flat dose-response curves, illustrated by blood pressure lowering effect of hydralazine and hydrochlorothiazide

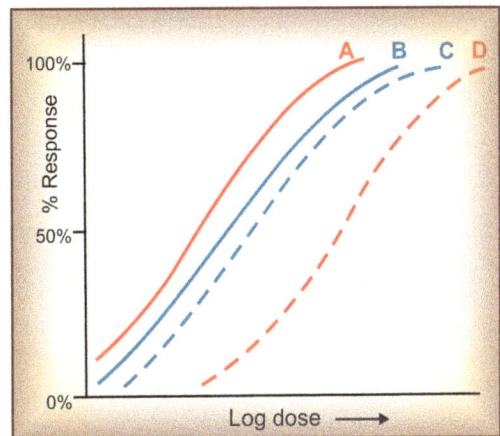

Fig. 3.14: Illustration of drug selectivity
Log dose-response curves of salbutamol for bronchodilatation (A) and cardiac stimulation (D)
Log dose-response curves of isoprenaline for bronchodilatation (B) and cardiac stimulation (C).

But this is irrelevant in the clinical set up where the *therapeutic range*, also called *therapeutic window* is bounded by the dose which produces minimal therapeutic effect and the dose which produces maximal acceptable adverse effect (Fig. 3.15). Because of inter-individual variability, the effective dose of a drug for one subject may be toxic for the other. A drug may be capable of inducing a higher therapeutic response (have higher efficacy), but development of intolerable adverse effects may preclude use of higher doses, e.g. prednisolone in bronchial asthma.

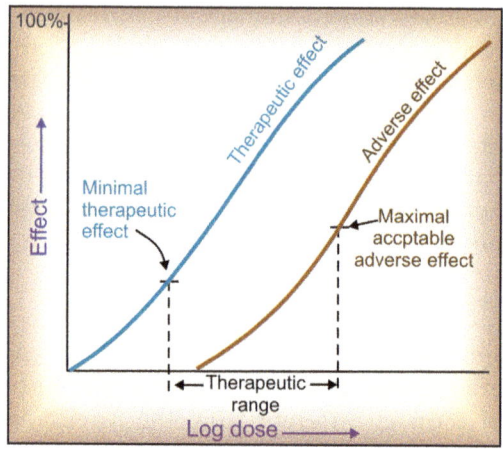

Fig. 3.15: Illustrative dose-response curves for therapeutic effect and adverse effect of the same drug

Risk-benefit ratio This term is very frequently used, and conveys a judgement on the estimated harm (adverse effects, inconvenience) vs expected advantages (relief of symptoms, cure, reduction of complications/mortality, improvement in quality of life). A drug should be prescribed only when the benefits outweigh the risks.

However, risk-benefit ratio can hardly ever be accurately measured for each instance of drug use. The physician has to rely on data from use of drugs in large populations (pharmacoepidemiology) and his own experience of the drug and the patient.

DRUG SYNERGISM AND ANTAGONISM

When two drugs are given simultaneously or in quick succession, they may be either indifferent to each other or exhibit *synergism* or *antagonism*. The interaction may take place at pharmacokinetic level (*see* Ch. 2) or at pharmacodynamic level.

SYNERGISM
(Greek: *Syn*—together; *ergon*—work)

When the action of one drug is facilitated or increased by the other, they are said to be synergistic. In a synergistic pair both the drugs can have action in the same direction or given alone one may be inactive but still enhance the action of the other when given together. Synergism can be:

(a) *Additive* The effect of the two drugs are in the same direction and simply add up:

effect of drugs A + B = effect of drug A + effect of drug B

Examples are given in the box:

Additive drug combinations	
Aspirin + paracetamol	as analgesic/antipyretic
Nitrous oxide + halothane	as general anaesthetic
Amlodipine + atenolol	as antihypertensive
Glibenclamide + metformin	as hypoglycaemic
Ephedrine + theophylline	as bronchodilator

Side effects of components of an additive pair may be different—do not add up. Thus, the combination is better tolerated than higher dose of one component.

(b) *Supra-additive (potentiation)* The effect of combination is greater than the individual effects of the components:

effect of drug A + B > effect of drug A + effect of drug B

This is always the case when one component given alone produces no effect, but enhances the effect of the other. Examples are given in the box.

Supraadditive drug combinations	
Drug pair	Basis of potentiation
Acetylcholine + physostigmine	Inhibition of break down of acetylcholine
Levodopa + carbidopa/ benserazide	Inhibition of peripheral metabolism of levodopa
Adrenaline + cocaine/ desipramine	Inhibition of neuronal uptake of adrenaline
Sulfamethoxazole + trimethoprim	Sequential blockade of folate metabolism
Antihypertensives (enalapril+ hydrochlorothiazide)	Tackling two contributory factors for rise in BP
Tyramine + MAO inhibitors	Increasing releaseable CA store

CA: catecholamine

ANTAGONISM

When one drug decreases or abolishes the action of another, they are said to be antagonistic:

effect of drugs A + B < effect of drug A + effect of drug B.

Usually, in an antagonistic pair one drug is inactive as such but decreases the response to the other. Depending on the mechanism involved, antagonism may be:

(a) Physical antagonism
Based on the physical property of the drugs, e.g. charcoal adsorbs alkaloids and can prevent their absorption—used in alkaloidal poisonings.

(b) Chemical antagonism
The two drugs react chemically and form an inactive product, e.g.
- $KMnO_4$ oxidizes alkaloids—used for gastric lavage in poisoning.
- Tannins + alkaloids—insoluble alkaloidal tannate is formed.
- Chelating agents (BAL, Cal. disod. edetate) complex metals (As, Pb).
- Nitrites form methaemoglobin which reacts with cyanide radical.

Drugs may react when mixed in the same syringe or infusion bottle:
- Thiopentone sod. + succinylcholine chloride
- Penicillin-G sod. + succinylcholine chloride
- Heparin + penicillin/tetracyclines/ streptomycin/hydrocortisone

(c) Physiological/functional Antagonism
The two drugs act on different receptors or by different mechanisms, but have opposite overt effects on the same physiological function, i.e. have pharmacological effects in opposite direction, e.g.
- Histamine and adrenaline on bronchial muscles and on BP.
- Hydrochlorothiazide and amiloride on urinary K^+ excretion.
- Glucagon and insulin on blood sugar level.

(d) Receptor antagonism
One drug (antagonist) blocks the receptor action of the other (agonist). This is a very important mechanism of drug action, because physiological signal molecules act through their receptors, blockade of which can produce specific and often profound pharmacological effects. Receptor antagonists are selective (though relatively), i.e. an anticholinergic will oppose contraction of intestinal smooth muscle induced by cholinergic agonists, but not that induced by histamine or 5-HT (they act through a different set of receptors). Receptor antagonism can be competitive or noncompetitive.

Competitive antagonism (equilibrium type)
The antagonist is chemically similar to the agonist, competes with it (Fig. 3.16A, D) and binds to the same site to the exclusion of the agonist molecules. Because the antagonist has affinity but no intrinsic activity, no response is produced. Since antagonist binding is reversible and depends on the relative concentration of the agonist and antagonist

Chapter 3: Pharmacodynamics

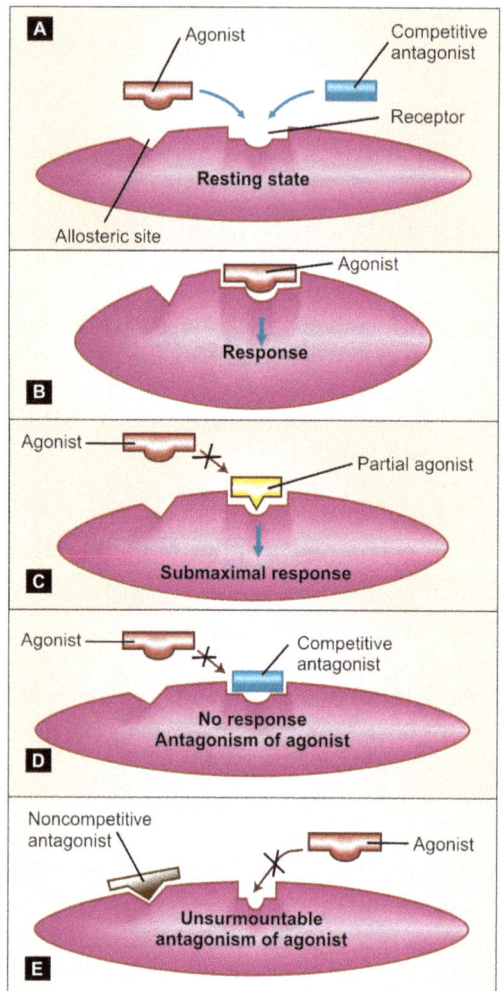

Fig. 3.16: Illustration of sites of action of agonists and antagonists (A), and the action of full agonist (B), partial agonist (C), competitive antagonist (D) and noncompetitive antagonist (E) on the receptor

molecules, higher concentration of the agonist progressively overcomes the block—a parallel shift to the right of the agonist DRC with no suppression of maximal response is obtained (Fig. 3.17a). The extent of shift is dependent on the affinity and concentration of the antagonist.

A partial agonist (Fig. 3.16C), having affinity for the same receptor, also competes with and antagonizes a full agonist, while producing a submaximal response of its own.

Noncompetitive antagonism The antagonist is chemically unrelated to the agonist, binds to a different *allosteric site* altering the receptor in such a way that it is either unable to combine with the agonist (Fig. 3.16E), or is unable to transduce the response, so that the downstream chain of events are uncoupled. Because the agonist and the antagonist are combining with different sites, there is no competition between them—even high agonist concentration is unable to reverse the block completely. Increasing concentrations of the antagonist progressively flatten the agonist DRC (Fig. 3.17b).

Nonequilibrium antagonism Certain antagonists bind to the receptor with strong (covalent) bonds or dissociate from it slowly (due to very high affinity) so that agonist molecules are unable to reduce receptor occupancy of the antagonist molecules—law

Competitive (equilibrium type)	Noncompetitive
1. Antagonist binds to the same receptor as the agonist	Binds to another site of receptor
2. Antagonist resembles chemically with the agonist	Does not resemble
3. Parallel rightward shift of agonist DRC	Flattening of agonist DRC
4. The same maximal response can be attained by increasing dose of agonist (surmountable antagonism)	Maximal response is suppressed (unsurmountable antagonism)
5. Intensity of response depends on the concentration of both agonist and antagonist	Maximal response depends only on the concentration of antagonist
6. Examples: ACh—Atropine Morphine—Naloxone	Diazepam—Bicuculline

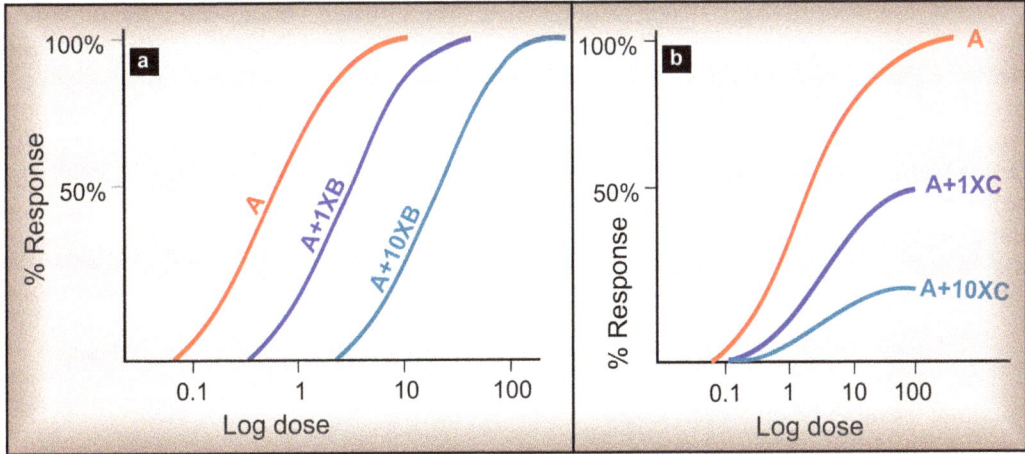

Fig. 3.17: Dose-response curves showing competitive (a) and noncompetitive (b) antagonism
A—agonist, B—competitive antagonist, C—noncompetitive antagonist

of mass action cannot apply—an irreversible or nonequilibrium antagonism is produced. The agonist DRC is shifted to the right and the maximal response is lowered (if spare receptors are few). Since in this situation agonist molecules are not able to compete with the antagonist molecules and flattening of agonist DRC is a feature of noncompetitive antagonism; the nonequilibrium antagonism has also been called 'a type of noncompetitive antagonism'. Phenoxybenzamine is a nonequilibrium antagonist of adrenaline at the α adrenergic receptors.

Features of competitive and noncompetitive antagonism are compared in the box on p. 58.

DRUG DOSAGE

'Dose' is the appropriate amount of a drug needed to produce a certain degree of response in a given subject.

Accordingly, dose of a drug has to be qualified in terms of the chosen response, e.g. the analgesic dose of aspirin for headache is 0.3–0.6 g, its antiplatelet dose is 75–150 mg/day, while its anti-inflammatory dose for rheumatoid arthritis is 3–5 g per day. Similarly, there could be *prophylactic dose*, a *therapeutic dose* or a *toxic dose* of the same drug.

The dose of a drug is governed by its inherent potency, i.e. the concentration at which it should be present at the target site, and its pharmacokinetic characteristics. In addition, it is modified by a number of factors (*see* later). The recommended doses are based on population data and cater to an 'average' patient. Therefore, different strategies are adopted for individualizing drug dosage.

1. *Standard dose* The same dose is appropriate for most patients—individual variations are minor or the drug has a wide safety margin so that enough can be given to cover them, e.g. oral contraceptives, penicillin, chloroquine, isoniazid, hydrochlorothiazide.

2. *Regulated dose* The drug modifies a finely regulated body function which can be easily measured. The dosage is accurately adjusted by repeated measurement of the affected physiological parameter, e.g. antihypertensives, hypoglycaemics, anticoagulants, diuretics, general anaesthetics.

3. *Target level dose* (see p. 37) The response is not easily measurable but has been demonstrated to be obtained at a certain range of drug concentration in plasma. An empirical dose aimed at attaining the target level is given in the beginning and adjustments are made later by measuring the plasma concentration or by observing the patient at relatively long intervals, e.g. antidepressants, antiepileptics, digoxin, lithium, theophylline.

4. *Titrated dose* The dose needed to produce maximal therapeutic effect cannot be given because of intolerable adverse effects. Optimal dose is arrived at by titrating it with an acceptable level of adverse effect. Low initial dose and upward titration (in most non-critical situations) or high initial dose and downward titration (in critical situations) can be practised. Often, a compromise between submaximal therapeutic effect but tolerable side effects can be struck, e.g. anticancer drugs, corticosteroids, levodopa.

Fixed dose combinations (FDCs) of drugs

A large number of pharmaceutical preparations (dosage forms) contain two or more drugs in a fixed dose ratio. *Advantages* offered by these are:

1. Convenience, better patient compliance and may be cost saving—when all the components present in the FDC are actually needed by the patient and their amounts are appropriate.
2. Certain drug combinations are synergistic, e.g. sulfamethoxazole + trimethoprim; levodopa + carbidopa/benserazide; combination oral contraceptives; isoniazid + rifampin.
3. The therapeutic effect of two components being same may add up while the side effects being different may not, e.g. amlodipine + atenolol as antihypertensive.
4. The side effect of one component may be counteracted by the other, e.g. a thiazide + a potassium sparing diuretic.
5. Combined formulation ensures that a single drug will not be taken. This is important in the treatment of tuberculosis, falciparum malaria and HIV-AIDS.

Before prescribing a combination, the physician must consider whether any of the ingredients is unnecessary; if it is, the combination should not be prescribed.

There are many inbuilt *disadvantages* of FDCs:

- The patient may not actually need all the drugs present in a combination. In that case, he is subjected to additional side effects and expense (often due to ignorance of the physician about the exact composition of the combined formulations).
- The dose of most drugs needs to be adjusted and individualized. When a combined formulation is used, this cannot be done without altering the dose of the other component(s).
- The time course of action of the components may be different.
- Altered renal or hepatic function of the patient may differently affect the pharmacokinetics of the components.
- Adverse effect, when it occurs, cannot be easily ascribed to the particular drug causing it.
- Contraindication to one component (allergy, other conditions) contraindicates the whole product.
- FDCs may create confusion of therapeutic aims. A false sense of superiority of two drugs over one is fostered, especially in case of antimicrobials when they are prescribed to cover up for diagnostic imprecision. Corticosteroids should never be combined with any other drug meant for internal use.

Thus, only a handful of FDCs are rational and justified, while far too many are produced and vigorously promoted by the pharmaceutical industry. In addition to the previously banned FDCs, 344 other irrational FDCs have been recently banned in India.

FACTORS MODIFYING DRUG ACTION

Variation in response to the same dose of a drug between different patients and even in the same patient on different occasions is a rule rather than exception. One or more of the following categories of differences among individuals are responsible for the variations in drug response:
(1) Individuals differ in pharmacokinetic handling of drugs; accordingly attain varying plasma/target site concentration of the drug. This is more marked for drugs disposed by metabolism (e.g. propranolol) than for drugs excreted unchanged (e.g. atenolol).
(2) Variations in number or state of receptors, coupling proteins or other components of response effectuation.
(3) Variations in neurogenic/hormonal tone or concentrations of specific constituents, e.g. atropine induced tachycardia depends on vagal tone, propranolol bradycardia depends on sympathetic tone, hypotension following captopril depends on body Na⁺ status.

A multitude of host and environmental factors influence drug response. Though individual variation cannot be totally accounted for by these factors, their understanding can guide choice of appropriate drug and dose for an individual patient. However, final adjustments have to be made by observing the response in a given patient on a given occasion.

These factors modify drug action either:
(a) *Quantitatively* The plasma concentration and/or the action of the drug is increased or decreased. Most of the factors introduce this type of change and can be dealt with by adjustment of drug dosage.

(b) *Qualitatively* The type of response is altered, e.g. drug allergy or idiosyncrasy. This is less common but often precludes further use of that drug in the affected patient.

The various factors are discussed below—

1. Body size It influences the concentration of the drug attained at the site of action. The average adult dose refers to individuals of medium built. For exceptionally obese or lean individuals and for children dose may be calculated on body weight (BW) basis:

$$\text{Individual dose} = \frac{\text{BW (kg)}}{70} \times \text{average adult dose}$$

In the case of few drugs, doses are calculated more appropriately on the basis of body surface area (BSA).

2. Age

Children The dose of a drug for children is often calculated from the adult dose using certain formulae. However, it is more accurate to calculate it on BW basis. For many drugs, manufacturers give dosage recommendations on mg/kg basis. Average figures for children are given in the box.

Age	Body weight (Kg)* Boys	Body weight (Kg)* Girls	% of Adult dose
Newborn	3.5	3.4	12.5
1 month	4.8	4.5	15
3 months	6.4	5.8	18
6 months	8.1	7.4	22
1 year	10.5	9.7	25
3 years	14.3	13.8	33
5 years	18.5	18.2	40
7 years	23.1	22.9	50
9 years	28.7	29.1	60
12 years	40.7	41.8	75

*50th percentile body weight of Indian boys and girls as per CDC 2000 guidelines.

It must be remembered that infants and children are not small adults. They have important physiological differences from adults. Children are growing and are susceptible to special adverse effects of drugs, e.g. suppression of growth can occur with corticosteroids; tetracyclines get deposited in growing teeth and discolour/deform them. Dystonic reactions to phenothiazines are more common in children.

Elderly In the elderly, renal function progressively declines (intact nephron loss) and drug doses have to be reduced, e.g. daily dose of streptomycin is 0.75 g after 50 years and 0.5 g after 70 years of age compared to 1 g for young adults. There is also a reduction in the hepatic microsomal drug metabolizing activity and liver blood flow: the oral bioavailability of drugs with high hepatic extraction is generally increased, but the overall effects on drug metabolism are not uniform. Other affected aspects of drug handling are:
- slower absorption due to reduced motility of and blood flow to intestines,
- lesser plasma protein binding due to lower plasma albumin,
- increased or decreased volume of distribution of lipophilic and hydrophilic drugs respectively.

The responsiveness of β adrenergic receptors to both agonists and antagonists is reduced in the elderly and sensitivity to other drugs also may be altered. Due to prostatism in elderly males, even mild anticholinergic activity of the drug can accentuate bladder voiding difficulty. Elderly are also likely to be on multiple drug therapy for hypertension, ischaemic heart disease, diabetes, arthritis, etc. which increases many fold the chances of drug interactions. They are more prone to develop postural instability (e.g. on standing up from dental chair) causing giddiness and fainting. In general, the incidence of adverse drug reactions is much higher in the elderly.

3. Sex Females have smaller body size and require doses that are on the lower side of the range. Subjective effects of drugs may differ in females because of their mental makeup. A number of antihypertensives (clonidine, methyldopa, β-blockers, diuretics) interfere with sexual function in males but not in females. Gynaecomastia is a side effect (of ketoconazole, metoclopramide, chlorpromazine, digitalis) that can occur only in men. Ketoconazole causes loss of libido in men but not in women. Obviously, androgens are unacceptable to women and estrogens to men. In women consideration must also be given to menstruation, pregnancy and lactation.

Drugs given during *pregnancy* can affect the foetus (*see* Ch. 4). There are marked physiological changes during pregnancy, especially in the third trimester, which can alter drug disposition.
- Gastrointestinal motility is reduced which may delay absorption of orally administered drugs.
- Plasma and extracellular fluid volume expands—volume of distribution of drugs may increase.
- While plasma albumin level falls, that of α_1 acid glycoprotein increases—the unbound fraction of acidic drugs increases but that of basic drugs decreases.
- Renal blood flow increases markedly—polar drugs are eliminated faster.
- Hepatic microsomal enzymes undergo induction—many drugs are metabolized faster.

Thus, the overall effect on drug disposition is complex and often difficult to predict.

4. Species and race There are many examples of differences in responsiveness to drugs among different species.

Among human beings some racial differences have been observed, e.g. blacks require higher and mongols require lower concentrations of atropine and ephedrine to dilate their pupil. β-blockers are less effective as antihypertensive in Afro-Caribbeans, and calcium channel blockers/diuretics are the first line antihypertensives in young blacks but not in young whites. Considering the widespread use of chloramphenicol in India and Hong Kong during 1950–1980 relatively few cases of aplastic anaemia have been reported compared to its incidence in the west. Similarly, quiniodochlor related cases of subacute myelooptic neuropathy (SMON) occurred in epidemic proportion in Japan, but there is no confirmed report of its occurrence in India despite extensive use.

5. Genetics The dose of a drug to produce the same effect may vary by 4 to 6-fold among different individuals. This is mainly because of differing rates of drug metabolism, because the amount and isoform pattern of drug metabolizing enzymes is genetically controlled. There are also differences in target organ sensitivity, transporters, ion channels, etc. The study of genetic basis for variability in drug response is called *Pharmacogenetics*

Pharmacogenomics It is the use of genetic information to guide the choice of drug and its dose on an individual basis.

It intends to identify individuals who are either more likely or less likely to respond to a drug and ultimately to provide 'personalized medicine'. A continuous variation with Gaussian frequency distribution is seen in the case of most drugs. However, there are some specific genetic defects which lead to discontinuous variation in drug responses, e.g.
1. Atypical pseudocholinesterase—prolonged succinylcholine apnoea.
2. G-6-PD deficiency—haemolysis with primaquine and other oxidizing drugs like sulfonamides, dapsone, quinine, nalidixic acid, nitrofurantoin and menadione, etc.
3. Acetylator polymorphism (fast and slow acetylators)—isoniazid neuropathy, procainamide and hydralazine induced lupus in slow acetylators.
4. CYP2D6 abnormality causes poor metoprolol/debrisoquin metabolizer status.
5. Precipitation of an attack of angle closure glaucoma by mydriatics in individuals with narrow iridocorneal angle.

6. Route of administration Route of administration governs the speed and intensity of drug response (*see* Ch. 1). Parenteral administration is often resorted to for more rapid, more pronounced and more predictable drug action.

7. Environmental factors and time of administration Several environmental factors affect drug responses. Exposure to insecticides, carcinogens, tobacco smoke and consumption of charcoal broiled meat are well known to induce drug metabolism. Type of diet and temporal relation between drug ingestion and meals can alter drug absorption, e.g. ampicillin absorption is reduced if taken after meals. Subjective effects of a drug may be markedly affected by the setup in which it is taken. It has been shown that corticosteroids taken as a single morning dose cause less pituitary-adrenal suppression. Statins cause greater suppression of cholesterol synthesis when taken in the evening. *Local anaesthetics have been found to produce more prolonged dental anaesthesia when injected in the afternoon than in the morning.*

8. Psychological factor Efficacy of a drug can be affected by the patient's beliefs, attitudes and expectations. This is particularly applicable to centrally acting drugs, e.g. a nervous and anxious patient requires more general anaesthetic; alcohol generally impairs performance, but if punishment (which induces anxiety) is introduced, it may actually improve performance by relieving anxiety.

Placebo This is an inert substance which is given in the garb of a medicine. It works by psychodynamic rather than pharmacodynamic means and often produces responses equivalent to the active drug. Some individuals are more suggestible and easily respond to a placebo: are called 'placebo reactors'. Placebos are used in two situations:
1. As a control device in clinical trial of drugs (dummy medication).
2. To treat a patient who, in the opinion of the physician, does not require an active drug.

Placebo is a Latin word meaning 'I shall please'. A patient responds to the whole therapeutic setting; placebo-effect largely depends on the physician-patient relationship.

Placebos do induce physiological responses, e.g. they can release endorphins in brain—causing analgesia. Naloxone, an opioid antagonist, blocks placebo analgesia. However, placebo effects are highly variable even in the same individual, e.g. a placebo may induce sleep on the first night but not subsequently. Thus, it has a very limited role in practical therapeutics. Substances commonly used as placebo are lactose tablets/capsules and distilled water injection.

9. Pathological states Not only drugs modify disease processes, several diseases can influence drug disposition and drug action:

Gastrointestinal (g.i.) diseases Certain g.i. diseases can alter absorption of orally administered drugs. The changes are complex and drug absorption may increase or decrease, e.g. in coeliac disease absorption of amoxicillin is decreased but that of cephalexin and cotrimoxazole is increased. Nonsteroidal antiinflammatory drugs (NSAIDS) can aggravate peptic ulcer disease.

Liver disease Liver disease (especially cirrhosis) can influence drug disposition in several ways:

(i) Bioavailability of drugs having high first pass metabolism (*see* Ch. 2) is increased due to loss of hepatocellular function and portocaval shunting.
(ii) Serum albumin is reduced—protein binding of acidic drugs (diclofenac, warfarin, etc.) is reduced and more drug is present in the free form.
(iii) Metabolism and elimination of some drugs (morphine, lidocaine, propranolol) is decreased: their dose should be reduced.
(iv) Prodrugs needing hepatic metabolism for activation, e.g. enalapril, prednisone are less effective and should be avoided.

The changes are complex and there is no simple test (like creatinine clearance for renal disease) to guide the extent of alteration in drug disposition; kinetics of different drugs is affected to different extents.

The action of certain drugs can also be altered in liver disease, e.g.
- The sensitivity of brain to depressant action of morphine and barbiturates is markedly increased in cirrhotics—normal doses can produce coma.
- Brisk diuresis can precipitate mental changes in patients with impending hepatic encephalopathy because diuretics cause hypokalemic alkalosis which favours conversion of NH_4^+ to NH_3. Ammonia enters brain easily causing mental derangement.
- Coumarin anticoagulants can markedly prolong prothrombin time because clotting factors are already low.

Hepatotoxic drugs should be avoided in liver disease.

Kidney disease It markedly affects pharmacokinetics of many drugs. Actions of certain drugs could also be altered.

Clearance of drugs that are primarily excreted unchanged (aminoglycoside antibiotics, digoxin, phenobarbitone) is reduced parallel to the decrease in creatinine clearance (CL_{cr}). Loading dose of such a drug is not altered (unless edema is present), but maintenance doses should be reduced or dose interval prolonged proportionately. A rough guideline is given in the box:

CL_{cr} (patient)	Dose rate to be reduced to
50–70 ml/min	70%
30–50 ml/min	50%
10–30 ml/min	30%
5–10 ml/min	20%

Dose rate of drugs only partly excreted unchanged in urine also needs reduction, but to lesser extents. If the t½ of the drug is prolonged, attainment of steady-state plasma concentration with maintenance doses is delayed proportionately.

Plasma proteins, especially albumin, are often low or altered in structure in patients with renal disease—binding of acidic drugs is reduced but that of basic drugs is not much affected.

The permeability of blood-brain barrier is increased in renal failure; opiates, barbiturates, phenothiazines, benzodiazepines, etc. produce more CNS depression. Pethidine should be avoided because its metabolite norpethidine can accumulate on repeated dosing and cause seizures. The target organ sensitivity may also be increased. Antihypertensive drugs produce greater postural hypotension in patients with renal insufficiency.

Certain drugs worsen the existing clinical condition in renal failure, e.g. tetracyclines have an antianabolic effect and accentuate uraemia; NSAIDs cause more fluid retention; potentially nephrotoxic drugs, e.g. aminoglycosides, tetracyclines (except doxycycline), sulfonamides (which cause crystalluria), vancomycin should be avoided.

Antimicrobials needing dose reduction in renal failure	
Even in mild failure	Only in severe failure
Aminoglycosides	Cotrimoxazole
Cephalexin	Carbenicillin
Ethambutol	Cefotaxime
Vancomycin	Norfloxacin
Amphotericin B	Ciprofloxacin
Acyclovir	Metronidazole

Thiazide diuretics tend to reduce g.f.r.; often fail to act in renal failure, and can worsen uraemia. Potassium-sparing diuretics are contraindicated; because they can cause hyperkalaemia → cardiac depression.

Congestive heart failure It can alter drug kinetics by—
- Decreasing drug absorption from g.i.t. due to mucosal edema and splanchnic vasoconstriction.
- Modifying volume of distribution which can increase for some drugs due to expansion of extracellular fluid volume or decrease for others as a result of reduced tissue perfusion.
- Retarding drug elimination as a result of decreased perfusion and congestion of liver, reduced glomerular filtration rate and increased tubular reabsorption; dosing rate of drugs may need reduction.
- The decompensated heart is more sensitive to digitalis action.

Thyroid disease The hypothyroid patients are more sensitive to digoxin, morphine and other CNS depressants. Hyperthyroid patients are relatively resistant to inotropic action of digoxin, but more prone to its arrhythmogenic action. The clearance of digoxin is roughly proportional to the thyroid function, but this only partially accounts for the observed changes in sensitivity.

Other examples of modification of drug response by pathological states are:
- Antipyretics lower body temperature only when it is raised (fever).
- Thiazides induce more marked diuresis in edematous patients.
- Myocardial infarction patients are more prone to adrenaline and digitalis induced cardiac arrhythmias.
- Myasthenics patients are very sensitive to curare.
- Schizophrenics tolerate large doses of phenothiazines.

- Head injury patients are prone to go into respiratory failure with normal doses of morphine.
- Atropine, imipramine, furosemide can cause urinary retention in individuals with prostatic hypertrophy.
- Hypnotics given to a patient in severe pain may cause mental confusion and delirium.
- Cotrimoxazole produces a much higher incidence of adverse reactions in AIDS patients.

10. Other drugs Drugs can modify the response to each other by pharmacokinetic or pharmacodynamic interaction between them. The number of reported interactions is already too large to remember. However, knowledge of drugs and patients at particular risk of being involved in drug interactions, and the mechanism underlying the interaction can avoid most iatrogenic disasters. Drug interactions are particularly likely to occur in elderly patients who often receive multiple drugs for several comorbidities like hypertension, diabetes, arthritis, ischaemic heart disease, etc. That two drugs interact does not necessarily mean that their concurrent use is contraindicated: many can be used together with dose adjustments or some other measures. Many drug interactions have already been considered (see pharmacokinetics and combined effect of drugs). Drug interactions relevant to dental practice are described in Ch. 38.

11. Cumulation Any drug will cumulate in the body if rate of intake is more than rate of elimination. However, slowly eliminated drugs are particularly liable to cause cumulative toxicity, e.g. prolonged use of chloroquine causes retinal damage.

Full loading dose of digoxin should not be given if patient has received it within the past week.

12. Tolerance It refers to the requirement of higher dose of a drug to produce a given response. Tolerance is a widely occurring adaptive biological phenomenon. Loss of therapeutic efficacy after prolonged/intensive use of a drug, e.g. of sulfonylureas in type 2 diabetes or of β_2 agonists in bronchial asthma, is generally called *refractoriness,* and is a form of tolerance. Drug tolerance may be:

Natural tolerance The species/individual is inherently less sensitive to the drug, e.g. rabbits are tolerant to atropine, black races are tolerant to mydriatics. Certain individuals in any population are hyporesponders to particular drugs, e.g. some subjects can consume large quantity of alcohol without getting inebriated.

Acquired tolerance This occurs by repeated use of a drug in an individual who was initially responsive. Body is capable of developing tolerance to most drugs, but the phenomenon is very easily recognized in the case of CNS depressants. An uninterrupted presence of the drug in the body favours development of tolerance. However, significant tolerance does not develop to atropine, digoxin, cocaine, sodium nitroprusside, etc. Tolerance need not develop equally to all actions of a drug; consequently, therapeutic index of a drug may increase or decrease with prolonged use, e.g.:
- Tolerance develops to sedative action of chlorpromazine but not to its antipsychotic action.
- Tolerance occurs to the sedative action of phenobarbitone but not to its antiepileptic action.
- Tolerance occurs to analgesic and euphoric action of morphine but not to its constipating and miotic actions.

Cross tolerance It is the development of tolerance to pharmacologically related drugs, e.g. alcoholics are relatively tolerant to barbiturates and general anaesthetics. Closer the two drugs are, more complete is the cross tolerance between them, e.g. there is partial cross tolerance between morphine and barbiturates but complete cross tolerance between morphine and pethidine.

Mechanism of tolerance The mechanisms responsible for development of tolerance are incompletely understood. However, tolerance may be:
  (i) Pharmacokinetic/drug disposition tolerance—the effective concentration of the drug at the site of action is decreased, mostly due to enhancement of drug elimination on chronic use, e.g. barbiturates, carbamazepine cause autoinduction of metabolism.
 (ii) Pharmacodynamic/cellular tolerance— drug action is lessened; cells of the target organ become less responsive, e.g. morphine, barbiturates, nitrates. This may be due to downregulation of receptors (*see* p. 53), weakening of response effectuation or other compensatory homeostatic mechanisms (e.g. antihypertensives).

Tachyphylaxis (*Tachy*—fast, *phylaxis*-protection) is rapid development of tolerance when doses of a drug are repeated in quick succession, and result in marked attenuation of response. This is usually seen with indirectly acting drugs, e.g. ephedrine, tyramine, nicotine. These drugs act by releasing catecholamines in the body, synthesis of which is unable to match the rate of release: stores get depleted. Other mechanisms like slow dissociation of the drug from its receptor, internalization of receptor, homeostatic adaptation, etc. may also be involved.

Drug resistance It refers to tolerance of microorganisms to inhibitory action of antimicrobials, e.g. *Staphylococci* to penicillin (*see* Ch. 25).

CHAPTER 4

Adverse Drug Effects

Adverse effect is 'any undesirable or unintended consequence of drug administration'. It is a broad term, includes all kinds of noxious effect—trivial, serious or even fatal.

All drugs are capable of producing adverse effects, and whenever a drug is given a risk is taken. The magnitude of risk has to be considered along with the magnitude of expected therapeutic benefit in deciding whether to use or not to use a particular drug in a given patient, e.g. even risk of bone marrow depression may be justified in treating cancer while mild drowsiness caused by an antihistaminic in treating common cold may be unacceptable.

Adverse effects may develop promptly or only after prolonged medication or even after stoppage of the drug. Adverse effects are not rare; an incidence of 10–25% has been documented in different clinical settings. They are more common with multiple drug therapy and in the elderly. Adverse effects have been classified in many ways. One may divide them into:

Predictable (Type A or augmented) reactions (mechanism based adverse reactions) These reactions are based on pharmacological properties of the drug, i.e. they are augmented but qualitatively normal response to the drug. This type of adverse effects include side effects, toxic effects and consequences of drug withdrawal. They are more common, dose related and are mostly preventable and reversible.

Unpredictable (Type B or Bizarre) reactions These reactions are based on peculiarities of the patient and not on the drug's known actions. Such reactions include allergy and idiosyncrasy. They are less common, often non-dose related, generally more serious and require withdrawal of the drug. Some of these reactions can be predicted and prevented if their genetic basis is known and suitable tests to characterize the individual's phenotype is performed.

Severity of adverse drug reactions has been graded as:

Minor: No therapy, antidote or prolongation of hospitalization is required.

Moderate: Requires change in drug therapy or specific treatment or prolongs hospital stay by at least one day.

Severe: Potentially life threatening, causes permanent damage or requires intensive medical treatment.

Lethal: Directly or indirectly contributes to death of the patient.

Prevention of adverse effects to drugs Adverse drug effects can be minimized but not altogether eliminated by observing the following practices:
1. Avoid all inappropriate use of drugs in the context of patient's clinical condition.
2. Use appropriate dose, route and frequency of drug administration based on patient's specific variables.

3. Elicit and take into consideration previous history of drug reactions.
4. Elicit history of allergic diseases and exercise caution (drug allergy is more common in patients with allergic diseases).
5. Rule out possibility of drug interactions when more than one drug is prescribed.
6. Adopt correct drug administration technique (e.g. NSAIDs not to be given on empty stomach).
7. Carry out appropriate laboratory monitoring (e.g. prothrombin time with warfarin, serum drug levels with lithium).

The adverse drug effects may be categorized into:

1. Side effects

These are unwanted but often unavoidable pharmacodynamic effects that occur at therapeutic doses. Generally, side effects are not serious, but may occasionally be hazardous, e.g. postural hypotension caused by prazosin as a side effect, may result in fall and fracture neck femur in the elderly patient. These effects can be predicted from the pharmacological profile of a drug and are known to occur in a given percentage of drug recipients. Reduction in dose usually ameliorates the symptoms.

A side effect may be based on the same action as the therapeutic effect, e.g. atropine is used in preanaesthetic medication for its antisecretory action, and the same produces dryness of mouth as a side effect; anti-inflammatory as well as gastric mucosal damaging effects of NSAIDs are due to inhibition of prostaglandin synthesis.

Side effect may also be based on a different facet of action, e.g. promethazine produces sedation which is unrelated to its antiallergic action. An effect may be therapeutic in one context but side effect in another context, e.g. codeine used for cough produces constipation as a side effect, but the latter is its therapeutic effect in traveller's diarrhoea.

2. Secondary effects

These are indirect consequences of a primary action of the drug, e.g. suppression of bacterial flora by tetracyclines paves the way for superinfections; corticosteroids weaken host defence mechanisms so that latent tuberculosis gets activated.

3. Toxic effects

These are the result of excessive pharmacological action of the drug due to overdosage or prolonged use. Overdosage may be absolute (accidental, homicidal, suicidal) or relative (i.e. usual dose of gentamicin in presence of renal failure). The manifestations are predictable and dose related. They result from functional alteration (high dose of atropine causing delirium) or drug induced tissue damage (hepatic necrosis from paracetamol overdosage). The CNS, CVS, kidney, liver, lung, skin and blood forming organs are most commonly involved in drug toxicity.

Toxicity may result from extension of the therapeutic effect itself, e.g. hypoglycaemia due to insulin, bleeding due to heparin.

Another action of the drug may be responsible for the toxicity, e.g.
- Morphine (analgesic) causes respiratory failure in overdosage.
- Gentamicin (antibacterial) in high dose causes vestibular damage.

Poisoning Poisoning may result from large doses of drugs because 'it is the dose which distinguishes a drug from a poison'. *Poison* is a 'substance which endangers life by severely affecting one or more vital functions'. Poisons derived from biologic sources are also called *'toxins'*. Not only drugs but other household and industrial chemicals, insecticides, etc. are frequently involved in poisonings. Specific antidotes, such as receptor antagonists, chelating agents (for heavy metal poisoning) or specific antibodies are available only for a few poisons. General supportive and symptomatic treatment is all that can be done for others, and this is also important for poisons which have a selective antagonist.

The general detoxification and supportive measures are:

1. *Resuscitation and maintenance of vital functions*
   a. Ensure patent airway, adequate ventilation, give artificial respiration/100% oxygen inhalation as needed.
   b. Maintain blood pressure and heart beat by fluid and crystalloid infusion, pressor agents, cardiac stimulants, external cardiac massage or cardiac pacing, etc, as needed.
   c. Maintain body temperature.
   d. Maintain blood sugar level by dextrose infusion, especially in patients with altered sensorium.
   e. Prevent and treat seizures by i.v. lorazepam injection.

2. *Termination of exposure (decontamination)* by removing the patient to fresh air (for inhaled poisons), washing the skin and eyes (for poisons entering from the surface), induction of emesis with syrup ipecac or gastric lavage (for ingested poisons). Emesis should not be attempted in comatose or haemodynamically unstable patient. Emesis/gastric lavage is not recommended if the patient presents > 2 hours after ingesting the poison, or if the patient has vomited after consuming the poison.

3. *Prevention of absorption of ingested poisons* A suspension of 20–40 g (1 g/kg) of activated charcoal, which has large surface area and can adsorb many chemicals, should be administered in 200 ml of water. However, strong acids and alkalies, metallic salts, iodine, cyanide, caustics, alcohol, hydrocarbons and other organic solvents are not adsorbed by charcoal.

4. *Hastening elimination* of the poison by inducing diuresis (furosemide, mannitol) or altering urinary pH (alkalinization for acidic drugs, e.g. barbiturates). However, excretion of many poisons is not enhanced by forced diuresis and this procedure is generally not employed now. Haemodialysis is more efficacious.

4. Intolerance

It is the appearance of characteristic toxic effects of a drug in an individual at therapeutic doses. Intolerance is the converse of tolerance, and indicates a low threshold of the individual to the action of a drug. These are individuals who fall on the extreme left side of the Gaussian frequency distribution curve for sensitivity to the drug. Examples are:
- A single dose of triflupromazine induces muscular dystonias in some individuals, especially children.
- Only few doses of carbamazepine may cause ataxia in some people.
- One tablet of aspirin may cause gastric bleeding.

5. Idiosyncrasy

Idiosyncrasy refers to genetically determined abnormal reactivity to a chemical producing an uncharacteristic reaction. Certain adverse effects of some drugs are largely restricted to individuals with a particular genotype (*see* p. 63). In addition, certain bizarre drug effects due to peculiarities of an individual (for which no definite genotype has been described) are included among idiosyncratic reactions, e.g.:
- Barbiturates cause excitement and mental confusion in some individuals.
- Chloramphenicol produces non-dose-related serious aplastic anaemia in rare individuals.

6. Drug allergy (hypersensitivity)

It is an immunologically mediated reaction producing stereotype symptoms which are unrelated to the pharmacodynamic profile of the drug. The symptoms may appear even with much smaller doses. This is also called *drug hypersensitivity*; but does not refer to increased response which is called supersensitivity.

Allergic reactions occur only in a small proportion of the population exposed to the drug and cannot be produced in other individuals at any dose. Prior sensitization is needed and a latent period of at least 1–2 weeks is required after the first exposure. The drug or its metabolite acts as antigen (AG) or more commonly hapten (incomplete antigen: drugs have small molecules which become antigenic only after binding with an endogenous protein) and induce production of antibody (AB) or sensitized lymphocytes. Presence of AB to a drug is not necessarily followed by allergy to it. Chemically related drugs often show cross sensitivity. One drug can produce different types of allergic reactions in different individuals, while widely different drugs can produce the same reaction. The course of drug allergy is variable; an individual previously sensitive to a drug may subsequently tolerate it without a reaction and *vice versa*.

Cardinal features of drug allergy

- Manifestations are unrelated to the pharmacodynamic actions of the drug.
- Manifestations are similar to food/protein allergy, allergic diseases.
- Severity of reaction is poorly correlated with dose of the drug; even small dose may trigger severe reaction.
- Occur only in few recipients, cannot be produced in other individuals.
- Prior sensitization (known/unknown) is needed.
- Positive dechallenge (on withdrawal of drug) and rechallenge (even with small dose).

Mechanism and Types of Allergic Reactions

A. Humoral

Type-I (anaphylactic) reactions Reaginic antibodies (IgE) are produced which get fixed to the mast cells and basophils. On exposure to the drug, AG: AB reaction takes place on the mast cell surface (*see* Fig. 7.2) releasing mediators like histamine, 5-HT, leukotrienes (especially LT-C4 and D4), prostaglandins, PAF, etc. resulting in urticaria, itching, angioedema, bronchospasm, rhinitis or anaphylactic shock. Anaphylaxis is usually heralded by flushing, paresthesia, generalized itching, swelling of lips, wheezing, palpitation followed by syncope. The manifestations occur quickly (within minutes to few hours) after challenge and are called *immediate hypersensitivity*. This is the only type of allergic drug reaction that the dentist may have to treat himself.

Type-II (cytolytic) reactions Drug + component of a specific tissue cell act as AG. The resulting antibodies (IgG, IgM) bind to the target cells; on reexposure AG: AB reaction takes place on the surface of these cells, complement is activated and cytolysis occurs, resulting in one or more of thrombocytopenia, agranulocytosis, aplastic anaemia, haemolysis, organ damage (liver, kidney, muscle), systemic lupus erythematosus.

Type-III (retarded, Arthus) reactions These are mediated by circulating antibodies (predominantly IgG, mopping AB). AG: AB complexes bind complement and precipitate on vascular endothelium and basement membrane in tissues, release chemotactic mediators and lytic enzymes giving rise to a destructive inflammatory response. Manifestations are rashes, serum sickness (fever, arthralgia, lymphadenopathy), polyarteritis nodosa, Stevens-Johnson syndrome (erythema multiforme, arthritis, nephritis, myocarditis, mental symptoms). The reaction usually develops in 3-4 days and subsides in 1–2 weeks.

B. Cell mediated

Type-IV (delayed hypersensitivity) reactions These are mediated through production of sensitized T-lymphocytes carrying receptors for the AG. On contact with AG, these T cells produce lymphokines which attract granulocytes and generate an inflammatory response, producing contact dermatitis, some types of rashes, fever, photosensitization. The reaction generally takes > 12 hours to develop. *Dentists may develop contact dermatitis by repeated handling of local anaesthetics*; though this is now rare due to replacement of procaine by lidocaine and use of surgical gloves.

Treatment of Drug Allergy

The offending drug must be immediately stopped. Most mild reactions (like skin rashes) subside by themselves and do not require specific treatment. Antihistamines (H_1) are beneficial in some type I reactions (urticaria, rhinitis, swelling of lips, etc.) and some skin rashes.

In case of *anaphylactic shock* or angioedema of larynx, the resuscitation council of UK has recommended the following measures:
- Put the patient in reclining position, administer oxygen at high flow rate and perform cardiopulmonary resuscitation if required.
- Inject adrenaline 0.5 mg (0.5 ml of 1 in 1000 solution) i.m.; repeat every 5–10 min in case the patient does not improve or improvement is transient. This is the only life-saving measure. Adrenaline should not be injected i.v. (can itself be fatal) unless shock is immediately life threatening. If adrenaline is to be injected i.v., it should be diluted to 1:10,000 or 1:100,000 and infused slowly with constant monitoring.
- Administer a H_1 antihistaminic (chlorpheniramine 10–20 mg) i.m./slow i.v. It may have adjuvant value.
- Intravenous glucocorticoid (hydrocortisone sod. succinate 200 mg) should be added in severe/recurrent cases. It acts slowly, but is especially valuable for prolonged reactions and in asthmatics.

Adrenaline followed by a short course of glucocorticoids is indicated for bronchospasm attending drug hypersensitivity. Glucocorticoids are the only drugs effective in type II, type III and type IV reactions.

Drugs frequently causing allergic reactions	
Penicillins	Local anaesthetics
Cephalosporins	Aspirin
Sulfonamides	Indomethacin
Tetracyclines	Carbamazepine
Quinolones	Allopurinol
Antitubercular drugs	ACE inhibitors
Phenothiazines	Methyldopa

Skin tests (intradermal injection, patch application) or intranasal tests may forewarn in case of Type I hypersensitivity but not in case of other types. However, these tests are not entirely reliable—false positive and false negative results are not rare.

7. Photosensitivity

It is a cutaneous reaction resulting from drug induced sensitization of the skin to UV radiation. The reactions are of two types:

(a) Phototoxic Drug or its metabolite accumulates in the skin, absorbs light and undergoes a photochemical reaction followed by a photobiological reaction resulting in local tissue damage (sunburn like), i.e. erythema, edema, blistering followed by hyperpigmentation and desquamation. The shorter wavelengths (290–320 nm, UV-B) are responsible. Drugs involved in acute phototoxic reactions are tetracyclines (especially demeclocycline) and tar products. Drugs causing chronic and low-grade sensitization are nalidixic acid, fluoroquinolones, dapsone, sulfonamides, phenothiazines, thiazides, amiodarone. This type of reaction is more common than photoallergic reaction.

(b) Photoallergic Drug or its metabolite induces a cell-mediated immune response which on exposure to light of longer

wavelengths (320–400 nm, UV-A) produces a papular or eczematous contact dermatitis like picture. Occasionally, antibodies may also mediate photoallergy, and the reaction takes the form of immediate flare and wheal on exposure to sun. Drugs involved are sulfonamides, sulfonylureas, griseofulvin, chloroquine, chlorpromazine.

8. Drug dependence and drug addiction

Drugs capable of altering mood and feelings (mind altering effects) are liable to repetitive use to derive euphoria, recreation, withdrawal from reality, social adjustment, etc. Some subjects who take the drug repeatedly for personal gratification, progress in indulgence with the drug and start according higher priority to taking the drug than to other basic needs, often in the face of known risks to health. They are said to be suffering from *'substance use disorder'*. Many of these drugs also induce adaptive physiological changes which result in escalation of the dose needed to produce the same effect. Thus *'tolerance'* develops and physiological equilibrium is disturbed when the drug is not present. Confusing terminology, *viz* 'dependence', physical dependence', 'psychological dependence', 'addiction', 'habituation', 'drug abuse' has been used over the past to describe the above phenomena. The terms as understood and applied currently are briefly explained below.

Drug dependence It is an altered physiological state produced by repeated administration of a drug which necessitates the continued presence of the drug to maintain physiological equilibrium. Discontinuation of the drug results in a characteristic *withdrawal (abstinence) syndrome*. This has been earlier termed *'physical dependence'*, but is now simply called 'dependence'. Since the essence of the process is adaptation of the nervous system to function normally in the presence of the drug, it has been also called *'neuroadaptation'*.

Drugs producing dependence are—opioids, barbiturates and other depressants including alcohol and benzodiazepines. Stimulant drugs, e.g. amphetamines, cocaine produce minimal or no dependence.

Drug addiction A person is said to have developed 'drug addiction' when he/she believes that optimal state of well being is achieved only through the actions of the drug. The subject feels emotionally distressed if the drug is not taken. It often starts as liking for the drug effects and progresses to compulsive drug use in some individuals who lose control and cannot stop taking the drug, even if they know it to be harmful. This was earlier termed *'psychological dependence'*. However, to avoid confusion, the widely understood term *'drug addiction'* is used now.

Drug addiction is a pattern of compulsive drug use characterized by overwhelming involvement with the use of a drug. Procuring the drug and using it takes precedence over other activities. Even after withdrawal, most addicts tend to relapse. Dependence, though a strong impetus for continued drug use, is not an essential feature of addiction. Amphetamines, cocaine, cannabis, LSD are drugs which produce addiction but little/no dependence. Moreover, drugs like nalorphine produce dependence without imparting addiction in the sense that there is little drug seeking behaviour.

Reinforcement It is the ability of the drug to produce effects that the user enjoys and which make him/her wish to take it again, or to induce *drug seeking behaviour*. Certain drugs (opioids, cocaine) are strong reinforcers, while others (benzodiazepines) are weak reinforcers. Faster the drug acts, more reinforcing it is. Thus, inhaled drugs and those injected i.v. are highly reinforcing—produce an intense 'high' in dependent individuals.

Drug habituation This term has been used to denote less intensive involvement with the drug, so that its withdrawal produces only mild discomfort. Dependence is absent. Consumption of tea, coffee, tobacco, social drinking are regarded habituating but not addicting. Thus, the difference between addiction and habituation is only quantitative. It is difficult to delineate when 'desire' turns into 'craving'. As such, it is better to avoid using the term 'habituation' as a distinct phenomenon.

Drug abuse This is another frequently used term which refers to use of a drug by self medication in a manner and amount that deviates from the approved medical and social patterns in a given culture at a given time. The term conveys social disapproval of the manner and purpose of drug use.

For regulatory agencies, *drug abuse* refers to any use of an ilicit drug.

The two major patterns of drug abuse are:
a. *Continuous use*: The drug is taken regularly, the subject wishes to continuously remain under the influence of the drug, e.g. opioids, alcohol, sedatives.
b. *Occasional use*: The drug is taken off-and-on to obtain pleasure or high, recreation (as in rave parties) or enhancement of sexual experience, e.g. cocaine, amphetamines, psychedelics, binge drinking (a pattern of excessive alcohol drinking), cannabis, solvents (inhalation), etc.

9. Drug withdrawal reactions

Apart from drugs that are usually recognised as producing dependence, sudden interruption of therapy with certain other drugs also results in adverse consequences, mostly in the form of worsening of the clinical condition for which the drug was being used, e.g.:

- Acute adrenal insufficiency may be precipitated by abrupt cessation of corticosteroid therapy.
- Severe hypertension, restlessness and sympathetic overactivity may occur shortly after discontinuing clonidine.
- Worsening of angina pectoris, precipitation of myocardial infarction may result from stoppage of β blockers.
- Frequency of seizures may increase on sudden withdrawal of an antiepileptic.

These manifestations are also due to adaptive changes, and can be minimized by gradual withdrawal.

10. Teratogenicity

It refers to the capacity of a drug to cause foetal abnormalities when administered to the pregnant mother. The placenta does not constitute a strict barrier, and any drug can cross it to a greater or lesser extent. The embryo is one of the most dynamic biological systems and in contrast to adults, drug effects are often irreversible. The thalidomide disaster (1958-61) resulting in thousands of babies born with *phocomelia* (seal like limbs) and other defects focused attention onto this type of adverse effect.

Drugs can affect the foetus at three stages–
(i) *Fertilization and implantation*—conception to 17 days. This generally results in failure of pregnancy which goes unnoticed.
(ii) *Organogenesis*—18 to 55 days of gestation. This is the most vulnerable period, deformities are produced.
(iii) *Growth and development*—56 days onwards. Effect at this stage produces developmental and functional abnormalities, e.g. ACE inhibitors can cause hypoplasia of organs, especially of lungs and kidneys; NSAIDs may induce premature closure of ductus arteriosus; antithyroid drugs and lithium cause foetal goiter.

Human teratogenic drugs

Drug	Abnormality
Thalidomide	Phocomelia, multiple defects of internal organs
Anticancer drugs (methotrexate)	Cleft palate, hydrocephalus, multiple defects, foetal death
Androgens	Virilization; limb, oesophageal, cardiac defects
Progestins	Virilization of female foetus
Stilboestrol	Vaginal carcinoma in teenage female offspring
Tetracyclines	Discoloured and deformed teeth, retarded bone growth
Warfarin	Depressed nose; eye and hand defects, growth retardation
Phenytoin	Hypoplastic phalanges, cleft lip/palate, microcephaly
Phenobarbitone	Various malformations
Carbamazepine	Neural tube defects, assorted abnormalities
Valproate sod.	Spina bifida and other neural tube defects, heart and limb abnormalities
Alcohol	Low IQ baby, growth retardation, foetal alcohol syndrome
ACE inhibitors	Hypoplasia of organs, growth retardation, foetal loss
Lithium	Foetal goiter, cardiac and other abnormalities
Antithyroid drugs	Foetal goiter and hypothyroidism
Indomethacin/aspirin	Premature closure of ductus arteriosus
Isotretinoin	Craniofacial, heart and CNS defects, hydrocephalus

The type of malformation depends on the drug as well as the stage at which exposure to the teratogen occurred.

The proven human teratogens are listed in the box above. However, only few mothers out of all those who receive these drugs during the vulnerable period will get a deformed baby, but the exact risk posed by a drug is difficult to estimate.

The US-FDA has graded the documentation of risk for causing birth defects into five categories *viz.* A, B, C, D and X indicating a range from A (safe) to X (contraindicated). Because evidence on teratogenic potential of drugs keeps accumulating, the FDA grading has become out-dated in many cases, and its utility is being questioned.

It is, therefore, wise to avoid all drugs during pregnancy, unless compelling reasons exist for their use, regardless of the assigned pregnancy category, or presumed safety. Only emergency dental treatment should be undertaken during the most vulnerable period of organogenesis.

11. Carcinogenicity and mutagenicity

It refers to capacity of a drug to cause cancer and genetic defects respectively. Usually, oxidation of the drug results in the production of reactive intermediates which affect genes and may cause structural changes in the chromosomes. Chemical carcinogenesis is a well-recognized phenomenon but generally takes several (10–40) years to develop. Drugs implicated in these adverse effects are—anticancer drugs, radioisotopes, estrogens, tobacco.

12. Drug-induced diseases

These are also called *iatrogenic* (physician-induced) diseases, and are functional disturbances (disease) caused by drugs which persist even after the offending drug has been withdrawn and largely eliminated, e.g.:

Peptic ulcer by NSAIDs and corticosteroids.
Parkinsonism by phenothiazines and other antipsychotics.
Hepatitis by isoniazid.
DLE by hydralazine.

Section 2

Systemic Pharmacology

Section Outline

5. Drugs Acting on Autonomic Nervous System (General Considerations, Cholinergic and Anticholinergic Drugs)
6. Drugs Acting on Autonomic Nervous System (Adrenergic and Antiadrenergic Drugs)
7. Autacoids and Related Drugs
8. General Anaesthetics and Skeletal Muscle Relaxants
9. Drugs Acting on Central Nervous System (Sedative-Hypnotics, Ethyl Alcohol, Antiepileptics and Antiparkinsonian Drugs)
10. Drugs Acting on Central Nervous System (Psychopharmacological Agents)
11. Cardiovascular Drugs (Drugs Affecting Renin-Angiotensin System, Calcium Channel Blockers, Drugs for Hypertension, Angina Pectoris and Myocardial Infarction
12. Cardiovascular Drugs (Drugs for Heart Failure and Cardiac Arrhythmia)
13. Diuretics
14. Hormones and Related Drugs (Anterior Pituitary Hormones, Antidiabetic Drugs, Corticosteroids)
15. Hormones and Related Drugs (Androgens, Anabolic Steroids, Estrogens, Progestins and Contraceptives)
16. Hormones and Related Drugs (Thyroid Hormone and Thyroid Inhibitors, Hormones Regulating Calcium Balance)
17. Drugs Affecting Blood
18. Drugs for Gastrointestinal Disorders
19. Drugs for Respiratory Disorders
20. Vitamins
21. Anticancer and Immunosuppressant Drugs

Drugs Acting on Autonomic Nervous System-1
General Considerations, Cholinergic and Anticholinergic Drugs

ORGANIZATION OF AUTONOMIC NERVOUS SYSTEM

The autonomic nervous system (ANS) functions largely below the level of consciousness and controls visceral functions. Like the somatic nervous system, the ANS consists of afferents, centre and efferents.

Autonomic afferents are carried in the visceral nerves, most of which are mixed nerves. They mediate visceral pain and visceral reflexes (cardiovascular, respiratory, vasomotor and other reflexes).

The highest seat regulating autonomic functions is in hypothalamus—posterior and lateral nuclei are primarily sympathetic while anterior and medial nuclei are primarily parasympathetic. Many autonomic centres (pupillary, vagal, respiratory, etc.) are located in the mid-brain and the medulla in relation to the cranial nerves. The lateral column in the thoracic spinal cord contains cells which give rise to the sympathetic outflow.

The motor limb of the ANS is anatomically divided into sympathetic and parasympathetic. In general, these subdivisions are functionally antagonistic and most organs receive both sympathetic and parasympathetic innervation. The level of activity of the innervated organ at a given moment is the algebraic sum of sympathetic and parasympathetic tone. However, most blood vessels, spleen, sweat glands and hair follicles receive only sympathetic, while ciliary muscle, bronchial smooth muscle, gastric and pancreatic glands receive only parasympathetic innervation. Thus, the two divisions of the ANS are not merely check-and-balance physiological antagonists of each other. The general layout of ANS is depicted in Fig. 5.1 and the important differences between its two subdivisions are given in Table 5.1.

Enteric nervous system The enteric nervous system (ENS) located in the gut wall consists of a submucosal and a myenteric plexus along with their afferent and efferent neurones. Their fibres travel anterograde, retrograde as well as in a circular manner. It receives inputs from both sympathetic and parasympathetic divisions of the ANS, but in addition functions independently to integrate bowel movements as well as regulate secretion and absorption. As such, it is now considered to be a distinct *'enteric nervous system'*, and not just a part of ANS.

NEUROHUMORAL TRANSMISSION

Neurohumoral transmission implies that nerves transmit their message across synapses and neuroeffector junctions by the release of humoral (chemical) messengers.

Steps in neurohumoral transmission

1. *Impulse conduction* The resting transmembrane potential (70 mV negative inside) is established by high K^+ permeability of axonal membrane and high axoplasmic concentration of this ion coupled with low

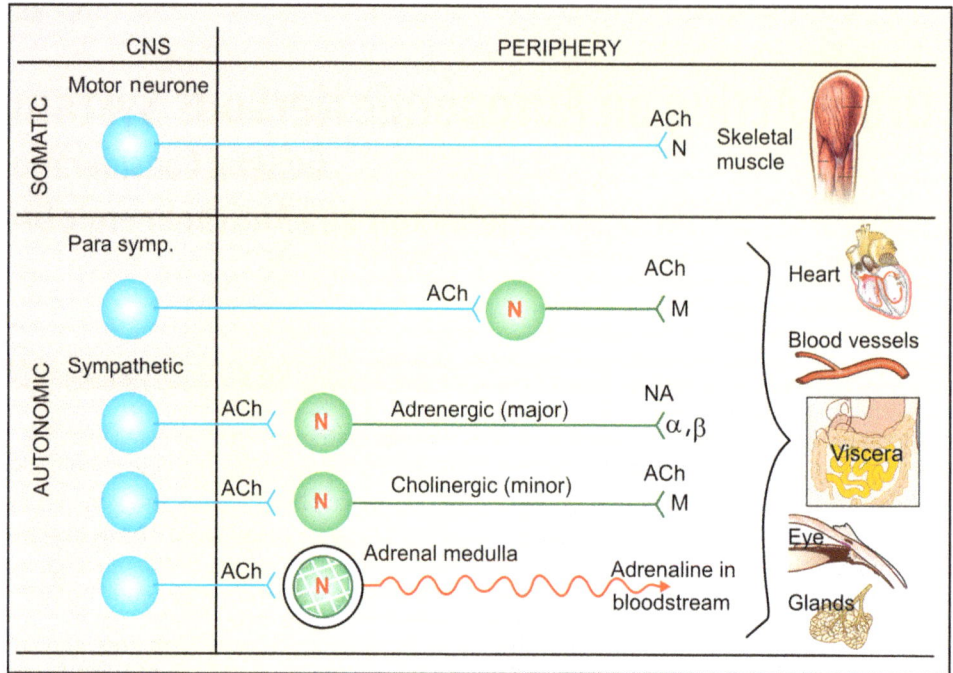

Fig. 5.1: The general outlay of efferent autonomic nervous system. The transmitter released and the primary postjunctional receptor subtype is shown at each synapse/neuroeffector junction
ACh—Acetylcholine; NA—Noradrenaline; N—Nicotinic; M—Muscarinic; α—α adrenergic; β—β adrenergic

Table 5.1: Differences between sympathetic and parasympathetic divisions of the autonomic nervous system

	Sympathetic	*Parasympathetic*
1. Origin	Dorso-lumbar (T1 to L2 or L3)	Cranio-sacral (III, VII, IX, X; S2–S4)
2. Distribution	Wide	Limited to head, neck and trunk
3. Ganglia	Away from the organs supplied	On or close to the organ supplied
4. Postganglionic fibre	Long	Short
5. Pre : post ganglionic fibre ratio	1: 20 to 1: 100	1: 1 to 1: 2 (except in enteric plexuses)
6. Neuroeffector transmitter	Major: NA Minor: ACh, ATP, NPY, DA	Major: ACh Minor: VIP, NO
7. Stability of major transmitter	NA stable, diffuses for wider actions	ACh—rapidly destroyed locally
8. Important function	Tackling stress and emergency	Assimilation of food, conservation of energy

NA—Noradrenaline; ACh—Acetylcholine; ATP—Adenosine triphosphate; NPY—Neuropeptide Y; DA—Dopamine; VIP—Vasoactive intestinal peptide; NO—Nitric oxide

Na^+ permeability and its active extrusion from the neurone. Stimulation or arrival of an electrical impulse causes a sudden increase in Na^+ conductance → depolarization and overshoot (reverse polarization: inside becoming 20 mV positive) occurs; K^+ ions then move out in the direction of their concentration gradient and repolarization is achieved. Ionic distribution is normalized during the refractory period by the activation of $Na^+ K^+$ pump. The action potential (AP) thus generated sets up local circuit currents which activate ionic channels at the next excitable part of the membrane (next node of Ranvier in myelinated fibre) and the AP is propagated without decrement.

II. *Transmitter release* The transmitter (excitatory or inhibitory) is stored in prejunctional nerve endings within 'synaptic vesicles' (Fig. 5.2). Nerve impulse promotes fusion of vesicular and axonal membranes, through Ca^{2+} entry which fluidizes membranes. All contents of the vesicle (transmitter, enzymes and other proteins) are extruded (*exocytosis*) in the junctional cleft.

The release process can be modulated by the transmitter itself and by other agents through activation of specific receptors located on the prejunctional membrane, e.g. noradrenaline (NA) release is inhibited by NA (through α_2 receptors), dopamine, adenosine, prostaglandins and enkephalins while isoprenaline (acting on β_2 receptors) and angiotensin (AT1 receptor) increase NA release. Similarly, α_2 and muscarinic agonists inhibit acetylcholine (ACh) release at autonomic neuroeffector sites (but not in ganglia and skeletal muscles).

III. *Transmitter action on postjunctional membrane* The released transmitter combines with specific receptors on the postjunctional membrane and depending on its nature induces an excitatory postsynaptic potential (EPSP) or an inhibitory postsynaptic potential (IPSP).

EPSP The excitatory transmitter selectively increases permeability to cations causing Na^+ or Ca^{2+} influx (through fast or slow channels). This results in *depolarization* followed by K^+ efflux. These ionic movements are passive as the flow is down their concentration gradients.

IPSP The inhibitory transmitter induced increase in permeability to anions, causes influx of Cl^- ions, because axonal Cl^- concentration is lower than its extracellular concentration. This tends to hyperpolarize the membrane → an IPSP is generated. Hyperpolarization can also result from selective increase in K^+ permeability, which move out carrying +ive charges.

In addition, a trophic influence on junctional morphology and functional status is exerted by the background basal release of the transmitter.

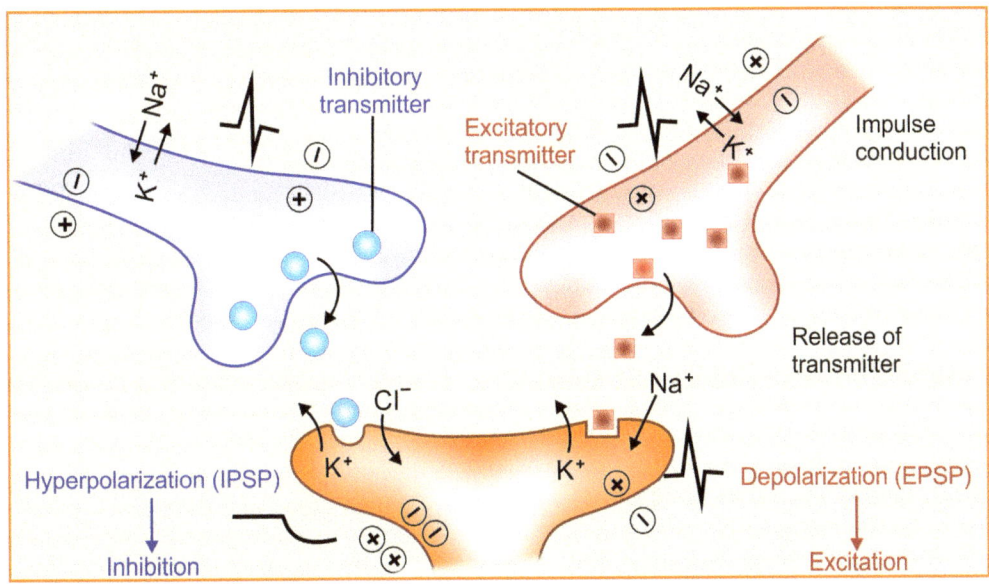

Fig. 5.2: Diagrammatic representation of steps in excitatory and inhibitory neurohumoral transmission
EPSP—Excitatory postsynaptic potential; IPSP—Inhibitory postsynaptic potential

IV. *Postjunctional activity* A suprathreshold EPSP generates a propagated postjunctional AP which results in nerve impulse (in neurone), contraction (in muscle) or secretion (in gland). An IPSP stabilizes the postjunctional membrane and resists depolarizing stimuli.

V. *Termination of transmitter action* Following its combination with the receptor, the transmitter is either locally degraded (e.g. ACh) or is taken back into the prejunctional neurone by active reuptake or diffuses away (e.g. NA). Peptide transmitters (VIP, NPY, enkephalins, etc.) only diffuse away and are not reuptaken, while amino acid transmitters (GABA, glutamate) are partly taken up into the neighbouring glial cells and partly diffuse away. Rate of termination of transmitter action governs the rate at which responses can be transmitted across a junction (1 to 1000/sec).

Cotransmission

It has become apparent that the classical 'one neurone—one transmitter' model is an over simplification. Most peripheral and central neurones on stimulation release more than one active substance. In the ANS, besides the primary transmitters ACh and NA, neurones have been found to elaborate purines (ATP, adenosine), peptides (vasoactive intestinal peptide or VIP, neuropeptide-Y or NPY, substance P, enkephalins, somatostatin, etc.), nitric oxide and prostaglandins as cotransmitters. The cotransmitter is stored in the same neurone but in distinct synaptic vesicles or locations (Fig. 5.3). However, ATP is stored along with NA in the same vesicle.

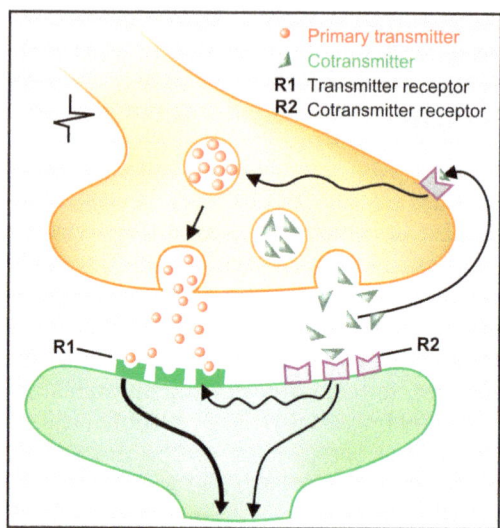

Fig. 5.3: Cotransmission
The cotransmitter is stored in the prejunctional nerve terminal along with the primary transmitter, but in separate vesicles (in some cases in the same vesicle itself). Nerve impulse releases both the transmitters concurrently. Acting on its own receptors, the cotransmitter modifies responsiveness of the effector to the primary transmitter or substitutes for it. Cotransmitter may also act on prejunctional receptors and modulate release of the transmitters

On being released by the nerve impulse, the cotransmitter may serve to regulate the presynaptic release of the primary transmitter and/or postsynaptic sensitivity to it (neuromodulator role). The cotransmitter may also serve as an alternative transmitter in its own right and/or exert a trophic influence on the synaptic structures. Nonadrenergic-noncholinergic (NANC) transmission has been shown in the innervation of the gut, urinary tract, vas deferens, salivary glands and in certain blood vessels.

CHOLINERGIC TRANSMISSION

Acetylcholine (ACh) is a major neurohumoral transmitter at autonomic, somatic as well as central sites as detailed in Table 5.2.

Synthesis, storage and destruction of ACh

The cholinergic neuronal mechanisms are summarized in Fig. 5.4.

Cholinergic Transmission

Table 5.2: Sites of cholinergic transmission and type of receptor involved

Site	Type of receptor	Selective agonist	Selective antagonist
1. a. All postganglionic parasymp. b. Few postganglionic symp (sweat glands, some blood vessels)	Muscarinic	Muscarine	Atropine
2. a. Ganglia (both symp. and parasymp). b. Adrenal medulla	Nicotinic (N_N)	DMPP*	Hexamethonium
3. Skeletal muscles	Nicotinic (N_M)	PTMA**	d-tubocurarine
4. CNS (cortex, basal ganglia, spinal cord and other sites)	Muscarinic Nicotinic	Muscarine/ Oxotremorine Carbachol	Atropine d-tubocurarine

*DMPP—Dimethyl phenyl piperazinium
**PTMA—Phenyl trimethyl ammonium

ATP + Acetate + CoEn-A
↓ Acetate activating reaction
Acetyl CoEn-A

CHOLINE ↘ ↓
    Choline acetyl transferase
ACETYLCHOLINE + CoEn-A

$$CH_3-\underset{\underset{CH_3}{|}}{\overset{\overset{CH_3}{|}}{N^+}}-CH_2-CH_2-O-\overset{\overset{O}{\|}}{C}-CH_3 \quad Cl^-$$

ACETYLCHOLINE CHLORIDE

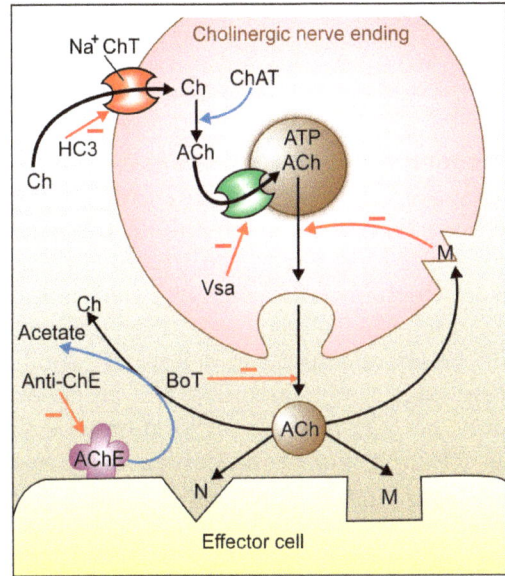

Fig. 5.4: Cholinergic neuronal mechanisms
Minus sign indicates inhibition while bold arrow indicates active transport
Ch—Choline; ACh—Acetylcholine; ChAT—Choline acetyl transferase; AChE—Acetylcholinesterase; Anti-ChE—Anticholinesterase; M—Muscarinic receptor; N—Nicotinic receptor; HC3—Hemicholinium; BoT—Botulinum toxin; Vsa—Vesamicol; Na+ChT—Na+–Choline Cotransporter.

Acetylcholine is synthesized locally in the cholinergic nerve endings by the following pathway—

Choline is actively taken up by the axonal membrane and acetylated with the help of ATP and coenzyme-A by the enzyme *choline acetyl transferase* (ChAT) present in the axoplasm. Hemicholinium (HC3) blocks choline uptake and depletes ACh. Most of the ACh is stored in ionic solution form within small synaptic vesicles with the help of a vesicle associated transporter (VAT) that is blocked by vesamicol.

Release of ACh from nerve terminals occurs in small quanta. The amount contained in few vesicles is extruded in pulses by exocytosis. In response to a nerve AP synchronous release of multiple quanta triggers postjunctional events. Botulinum toxin inhibits ACh release causing long-lasting loss of cholinergic transmission at the injection site and paralysis of the supplied muscle.

Cholinesterase Immediately after release, ACh is hydrolyzed by the enzyme cholinesterase and choline is recycled. A specific (*Acetylcholinesterase*—AChE or true cholinesterase) and a nonspecific (*Butyrylcholinesterase*—BuChE or pseudocholinesterase) type of enzyme occurs in the body.

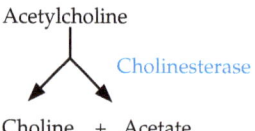

The true cholinesterase or acetylcholinesterase is strategically located at all cholinergic sites and serves to hydrolyze ACh instantaneously (in μS). The pseudocholinesterase is a relatively nonspecific esterase present in plasma, liver and some other tissues; hydrolyzes ACh slowly and probably serves to metabolize ingested esters.

Cholinoceptors

Two classes of receptors for ACh are recognized—muscarinic and nicotinic; the former is a G protein coupled receptor, while the latter is a ligand gated cation channel.

Muscarinic These receptors are selectively stimulated by muscarine and selectively blocked by atropine. They are located primarily on autonomic effector cells in heart, blood vessels, eye, smooth muscles and glands of gastrointestinal, respiratory and urinary tracts, sweat glands, etc. and in the CNS. Subsidiary muscarinic receptors are also present in autonomic ganglia (in addition to primary nicotinic N_N receptors) where they appear to play a modulatory role by inducing a long-lasting late EPSP.

Subtypes of muscarinic receptor The muscarinic receptors have been divided into 5 subtypes M_1, M_2, M_3, M_4 and M_5. Out of these, the major first 3 have been functionally characterized.

M_1: The M_1 is primarily a neuronal receptor located on ganglion cells and central neurones: especially in cortex, hippocampus and corpus striatum. It plays a major role in mediating gastric secretion and relaxation of lower esophageal sphincter (LES) caused by vagal stimulation.

M_2: Cardiac muscarinic receptors are predominantly M_2 and mediate vagal bradycardia. Autoreceptors on cholinergic nerve endings are also of M_2 subtype.

M_3: Visceral smooth muscle contraction and glandular secretions are elicited through M_3 receptors, which also mediate vasodilatation through EDRF release. Together the M_2 and M_3 receptors mediate most of the well-recognized muscarinic actions including contraction of LES.

Nicotinic These receptors are selectively activated by nicotine and blocked by tubocurarine or hexamethonium. These are rosette-like pentameric structures (*see* Fig. 3.3) which enclose a ligand gated cation channel. Their activation causes opening of the channel and rapid flow of cations resulting in depolarization and an action potential. On the basis of location as well as selective agonists and antagonists, two subtypes N_M and N_N are recognized.

N_M: These are present at skeletal muscle endplate. They are selectively stimulated by phenyl trimethyl ammonium (PTMA), blocked by tubocurarine, and mediate skeletal muscle contraction.

N_N: These are present on ganglionic cells (sympathetic as well as parasympathetic), adrenal medullary cells, in spinal cord and certain areas of brain. They are selectively stimulated by dimethyl phenyl piperazinium (DMPP), blocked by hexamethonium, and constitute the primary pathway of transmission in ganglia.

CHOLINERGIC DRUGS
(Cholinomimetic, Parasympathomimetic)

These are drugs which produce actions similar to that of ACh, either by directly interacting with cholinergic receptors (*cholinergic agonists*) or by increasing availability of ACh at these sites (*anticholinesterases*).

CHOLINERGIC AGONISTS

Choline esters	*Alkaloids*
Acetylcholine	Muscarine
Methacholine	Pilocarpine
Carbachol	Arecoline
Bethanechol	

Actions (of ACh as prototype)
Depending on the type of receptor through which it is mediated the peripheral actions of ACh may be classified as muscarinic or nicotinic. The central actions are not so classifiable and are described separately.

A. Muscarinic actions

1. *Heart* ACh hyperpolarizes the SA nodal cells and decreases their rate of diastolic depolarization. As a result, rate of impulse generation is reduced—*bradycardia* or even cardiac arrest may occur.

At the A-V node and His-Purkinje fibres refractory period (RP) is increased and *conduction is slowed*: P-R interval increases and partial to complete A-V block may be produced. The *force of atrial contraction is markedly reduced* and RP of atrial fibres is abbreviated. Due to nonuniform vagal innervation, the intensity of effect on RP and conductivity of different atrial fibres varies considerably, inducing inhomogeneity and predisposing to atrial fibrillation or flutter.

Ventricular contractility is also decreased but the effect is not marked.

2. *Blood vessels* All blood vessels are dilated, though only few (skin of face, neck) receive cholinergic innervation. As a result, fall in BP and flushing, especially in the blush area occurs. Muscarinic receptors (M_3) are present on vascular endothelial cells: vasodilatation is primarily mediated through the release of an *endothelium-dependent relaxing factor* (EDRF) which is nitric oxide (NO).

Stimulation of cholinergic nerves to the penis causes erection by releasing NO and dilating cavernosal vessels through M_3 receptors. However, this response is minimal with injected cholinomimetic drugs.

3. *Smooth muscle* The smooth muscle in most organs is contracted by ACh. Tone and peristalsis in the gastrointestinal tract is increased and sphincters relax. This may cause abdominal cramps and evacuation of bowel.

Peristalsis in ureter is increased. The detrusor muscle contracts while the bladder trigone and sphincter relaxes → voiding of bladder.

Bronchial muscles constrict producing bronchospasm and dyspnoea. Asthmatics are highly sensitive, in whom an attack of asthma may be precipitated.

4. *Glands* Secretion from all parasympathetically innervated glands is increased—sweating, salivation, lacrimation, tracheobronchial and gastric secretion. The effect on pancreatic and intestinal glands is not marked. Secretion of milk and bile is not affected.

5. *Eye* Contraction of circular muscle of iris produces miosis.

Contraction of ciliary muscle causes spasm of accommodation, increased aqueous outflow facility and reduction in intraocular tension (especially in glaucomatous patients).

B. Nicotinic actions

1. *Autonomic ganglia* Both sympathetic and parasympathetic ganglia are stimulated. This effect is manifested at higher doses.

High dose of ACh given after atropine causes tachycardia and rise in BP due to sympathetic ganglionic stimulation.

2. Skeletal muscles Iontophoretic application of ACh to muscle endplate causes contraction of the fibre. Intra-arterial injection of high dose can cause twitching and fasciculations, but i.v. injection is generally without any effect (due to rapid hydrolysis of ACh).

C. CNS actions

ACh injected i.v. does not penetrate blood-brain barrier and no central effects are seen. However, other cholinergic drugs which enter brain, produce complex behavioral and neurological effects.

The important features of other cholinesters are summarized in Table 5.3.

Uses Choline esters are practically not used now.

Cholinomimetic alkaloids

Pilocarpine It is obtained from the leaves of *Pilocarpus microphyllus* and other species. It has prominent muscarinic actions but stimulates ganglia as well.

Pilocarpine causes marked sweating, salivation and increase in other secretions. The cardiovascular effects of pilocarpine are complex. Applied to the eye, it penetrates cornea and promptly causes miosis, ciliary muscle contraction and fall in intraocular tension lasting 4–8 hours. Pilocarpine (0.5-4.0% eye drops) is used in the eye as second or third choice drug in glaucoma. It can be used orally for xerostomia, but is not available commercially for this purpose.

Muscarine It occurs in poisonous mushrooms *Amanita muscaria* and *Inocybe* species and has only muscarinic actions. It is not used therapeutically but is of toxicological importance in mushroom poisoning.

Arecoline It is found in betel nut *Areca catechu*. It has muscarinic as well as nicotinic actions including prominent CNS effects.

ANTICHOLINESTERASES

Anticholinesterases (anti-ChEs) are agents which inhibit ChE, protect ACh from hydrolysis—produce cholinergic effects *in vivo* and potentiate ACh both *in vivo* and *in vitro*. Some anti-ChEs like neostigmine have additional direct action on nicotinic cholinoceptors.

Anti-ChEs are mostly esters of carbamic acid or derivatives of phosphoric acid.

$$R_1-O-\overset{\overset{O}{\|}}{C}-N{<}{\overset{R_2}{R_3}} \qquad \overset{R_2}{\underset{R_3}{>}}\overset{\overset{O}{\|}}{P}-R_1$$

CARBAMATES   ORGANOPHOSPHATES

In carbamates R_1 may have a nonpolar tertiary amino N, e.g. in physostigmine, rendering the compound lipid soluble. In others, e.g. neostigmine, R_1 has a quaternary N^+—rendering it lipid insoluble. All organophosphates are highly lipid soluble except echothiophate which is water soluble.

The anti-ChEs react with the enzyme essentially in the same way as ACh. The carbamates and phosphates respectively carbamylate and phosphorylate the esteratic

Table 5.3: Properties of choline esters

Choline ester	Hydrolysis by		Actions		Selective action on
	AChE	BuChE	Musc	Nico.	
Acetylcholine	+++	++	++	+	Nonselective
Methacholine	+	–	++	±	CVS
Carbachol	–	–	+	++	g.i.t., bladder
Bethanechol	–	–	+	–	g.i.t., bladder

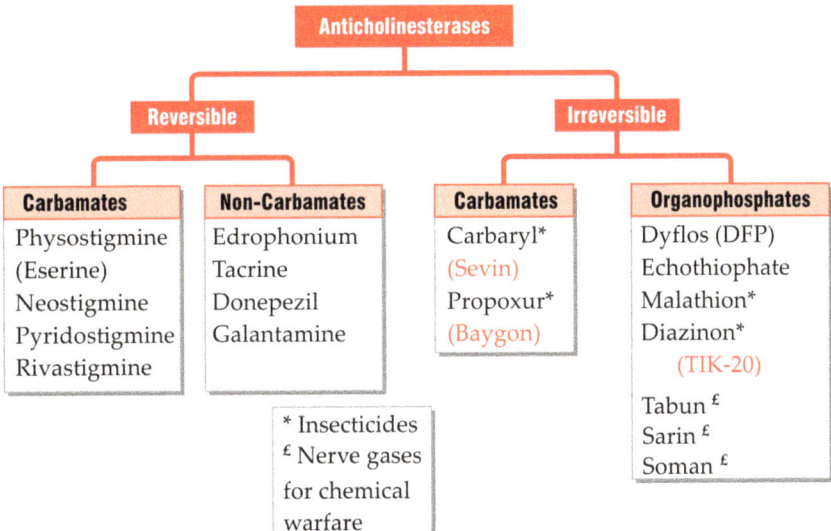

site of the enzyme. Whereas the acetylated enzyme (produced momentarily when ACh reacts with ChE) reacts with water extremely rapidly and the esteratic site is freed in a fraction of a millisecond, the carbamylated enzyme (reversible inhibitors) reacts slowly and the phosphorylated enzyme (irreversible inhibitors) reacts extremely slowly or not at all. The half-life of reactivation of carbamylated enzyme (30 min to 6 hrs) is less than that of synthesis of fresh enzyme protein, while that of phosphorylated enzyme (in days) is more than the regeneration time. Thus, apparently reversible and irreversible enzyme inhibition is obtained, though the basic pattern of inhibitor-enzyme interaction remains the same.

Pharmacological actions

The actions of anti-ChEs are qualitatively similar to that of directly acting cholinoceptor stimulants. However, relative intensity of action on muscarinic, ganglionic, skeletal muscle and CNS sites varies among the different agents.

Lipid-soluble agents (physostigmine and organophosphates) have more marked muscarinic and CNS effects. They stimulate ganglia but action on skeletal muscles is less prominent. The centrally acting anti-ChEs produce a generalized alerting response; cognitive function may improve in Alzheimer's disease.

Lipid-insoluble agents (neostigmine and other quaternary ammonium compounds) produce more marked effect on the skeletal muscles (direct action on muscle endplate cholinoceptors in addition to potentiation of ACh.), stimulate ganglia, but muscarinic effects are less prominent. They do not penetrate CNS and have no central effects.

After treatment with anti-ChEs, the ACh released by a single nerve impulse in skeletal muscle is not immediately destroyed—rebinds to the same receptor and diffuses to act on neighbouring receptors as well as on prejunctional fibres which may fire repetitively producing twitching and fasciculations. Force of contraction in partially curarized and myasthenic muscles is increased. Higher doses cause persistent depolarization of endplates resulting in blockade of neuromuscular transmission → weakness and paralysis.

The cardiovascular effects of anti-ChEs are complex: depend on the agent and its dose. Smooth muscles and glands of the gastrointestinal, respiratory and urinary tracts as well as in the eye are stimulated.

Pharmacokinetics

Physostigmine is rapidly absorbed from the g.i.t. and parenteral sites. Applied to the eye, it penetrates cornea freely. It crosses blood-brain barrier and is disposed after hydrolysis by ChE.

Neostigmine and congeners are poorly absorbed orally; oral dose is 20–30 times higher than parenteral dose. They do not effectively penetrate cornea or cross blood-brain barrier.

Organophosphates are absorbed from all sites including intact skin and lungs. They are hydrolyzed as well as oxidized in the body and little is excreted unchanged.

Uses

1. *Glaucoma:* Glaucoma is a progressive form of optic nerve damage associated with raised intraocular tension (i.o.t.). Miotics like pilocarpine and physostigmine lower i.o.t. by different mechanisms in the two principal types of glaucoma:

    Open angle (chronic simple) glaucoma: Miotics increase the tone of ciliary muscle which pulls on and improves the outflow facility of trabecular meshwork. However, they are now 3rd line drugs to latanoprost ($PGF_{2\alpha}$ analogue), ocular β blockers, brimonidine (α_2 agonist clonidine congener), dorzolamide (ocular carbonic anhydrase inhibitor) and dipivefrine (prodrug of adrenaline).

    Angle closure (narrow angle, acute congestive) glaucoma: Miotics contract sphincter pupillae muscle changing the direction of forces in the iris to lessen its contact with the lens → pupillary block is removed and iridocorneal angle is freed, aqueous outflow is restored.
2. *To reverse the effect of mydriatic:* After refraction testing.
3. *To prevent/break adhesions between iris and lens/cornea:* A miotic is alternated with a mydriatic.
4. *Myasthenia gravis:* It is an autoimmune disorder due to development of antibodies to the muscle endplate nicotinic receptors resulting in weakness and easy fatigability. Neostigmine and its congeners improve muscle contraction by preserving ACh as well as by directly depolarizing the endplate.
5. *Postoperative decurarization:* To reverse the effect of nondepolarizing muscle relaxants.
6. *Postoperative paralytic ileus/urinary retention.*
7. *Cobra bite:* To antagonize the curare-like action of cobra neurotoxin.
8. *Belladonna poisoning:* Physostigmine is the drug of choice for poisoning with atropine and other anticholinergic drugs.
9. *Alzheimer's disease:* This is a neurodegenerative disorder affecting primarily the cholinergic neurones in the brain. The relatively cerebroselective anti-ChEs, rivastigmine, donepezil and galantamine afford some symptomatic improvement.

Anticholinesterase poisoning

Anticholinesterases are easily available and extensively used as agricultural and household insecticides; accidental as well as suicidal and homicidal poisoning is common.

Local muscarinic manifestations at the site of exposure (skin, eye, g.i.t.) occur immediately and are followed by complex systemic effects due to muscarinic, nicotinic and central actions.

Treatment

1. Termination of further exposure to the poison—fresh air, wash the skin and mucous membranes with water, gastric lavage according to need.
2. Maintain patent airway, positive pressure respiration if it is failing.

3. Supportive measures—maintain BP, hydration, control of convulsions with judicious use of diazepam.
4. Specific antidotes—

(a) *Atropine* It is highly effective in counteracting the muscarinic symptoms, but higher doses are required to antagonize the central effects. It does not reverse peripheral muscular paralysis which is a nicotinic action.

(b) *Cholinesterase reactivators* Oximes are used to restore neuromuscular transmission in case of organophosphate anti-ChE poisoning. They provide more reactive OH groups which react with phosphorylated enzyme to form oxime phosphonate and release free cholinesterase. Pralidoxime is the most commonly used oxime.

ANTICHOLINERGIC DRUGS
(Muscarinic Receptor Antagonists, Atropinic, Parasympatholytic)

Conventionally the term 'anticholinergic drugs' is restricted to those which block actions of ACh on autonomic effectors and in the CNS exerted through muscarinic receptors. Though nicotinic receptor antagonists also block certain actions of ACh, they are generally referred to as 'ganglion blockers' and 'neuromuscular blockers'.

Atropine, the prototype drug of this class. It is highly selective for muscarinic receptors, but some of its synthetic substitutes do possess significant nicotinic blocking property in addition. All anticholinergic drugs are competitive antagonists.

In addition, many other classes of drugs, i.e. tricyclic antidepressants, phenothiazines, H_1 antihistamines, disopyramide possess significant antimuscarinic actions.

The natural alkaloids are found in plants of the solanaceae family: atropine in *Atropa belladonna* and *Datura stramonium*, hyoscine

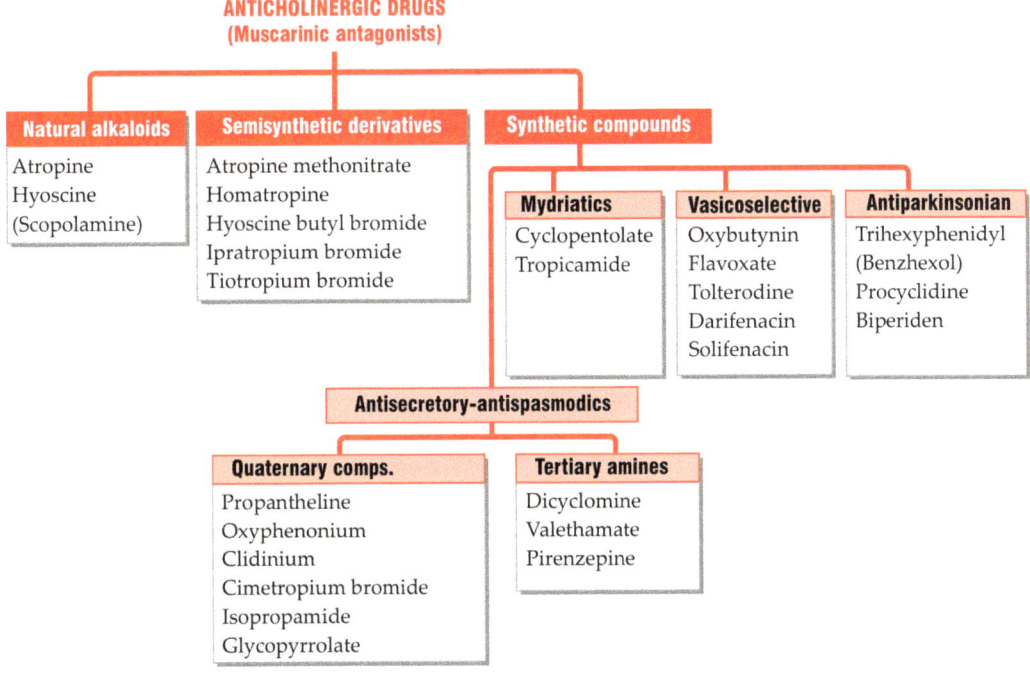

in *Hyoscyamus niger*. The levo-isomers are much more active than the dextro-isomers. Atropine is racemic while scopolamine is l-hyoscine.

PHARMACOLOGICAL ACTIONS
(Atropine as prototype)

The actions of atropine can be largely predicted from knowledge of parasympathetic responses. Prominent effects are seen in organs which normally receive strong parasympathetic tone. Atropine blocks all subtypes of muscarinic receptors.

1. CNS Atropine has an overall CNS stimulant action. However, these effects are not appreciable at low doses which mainly produce peripheral effects because of restricted entry of atropine into the brain.

- Atropine stimulates many medullary centres —vagal, respiratory, vasomotor.
- It depresses vestibular excitation and has antimotion sickness property.
- By blocking the relative cholinergic overactivity in basal ganglia, it suppresses tremor and rigidity of parkinsonism.
- High doses cause cortical excitation, restlessness, disorientation, hallucinations and delirium followed by respiratory depression and coma.

Hyoscine differs from atropine in producing depressant (drowsiness, amnesia, fatigue) effects at low doses.

2. CVS

Heart The most prominent effect of atropine is tachycardia. This is due to blockade of M_2 receptors on SA node through which vagal tone decreases HR. Higher the existing vagal tone—more marked is the tachycardia (maximum in young adults, less in children and elderly). On i.m./s.c. injection, transient initial bradycardia often occurs. Earlier believed to be due to vagal centre stimulation, it is now thought to be caused by blockade of muscarinic autoreceptors (M_1) on vagal nerve endings thereby augmenting ACh release. Atropine abbreviates refractory period of A-V node and facilitates A-V conduction, especially if it has been depressed by high vagal tone. P-R interval is shortened.

BP Since cholinergic impulses are not involved in maintenance of vascular tone, atropine does not have any consistent or marked effect on BP. Atropine blocks vasodepressor action of cholinergic agonists.

3. Eye The autonomic control of iris muscles and the action of mydriatics as well as miotics is illustrated in Fig. 5.5. Topical instillation of atropine causes mydriasis, abolition of light reflex and cycloplegia lasting 7–10 days. This results in photophobia and blurring of near vision. The ciliary muscles recover somewhat earlier than the sphincter pupillae. The intraocular tension tends to rise, especially in narrow angle glaucoma. However, conventional systemic doses produce minor ocular effects.

4. Smooth muscles All visceral smooth muscles that receive parasympathetic motor innervation are relaxed by atropine (M_3 blockade). Tone and amplitude of contractions of stomach and intestine are reduced; the passage of chyme is slowed—constipation may occur, spasm may be relieved. However, peristalsis is only incompletely suppressed because it is primarily regulated by local reflexes in the enteric plexus, and other neurotransmitters (5-HT, enkephalin, etc.) are involved.

Atropine causes bronchodilatation and reduces airway resistance, especially in COPD and asthma patients. Inflammatory mediators of asthma like histamine, PGs, leucotrienes and kinins increase vagal activity in addition to their direct stimulant action on bronchial muscle and glands. Atropine attenuates their action by antagonizing the indirect vagal component.

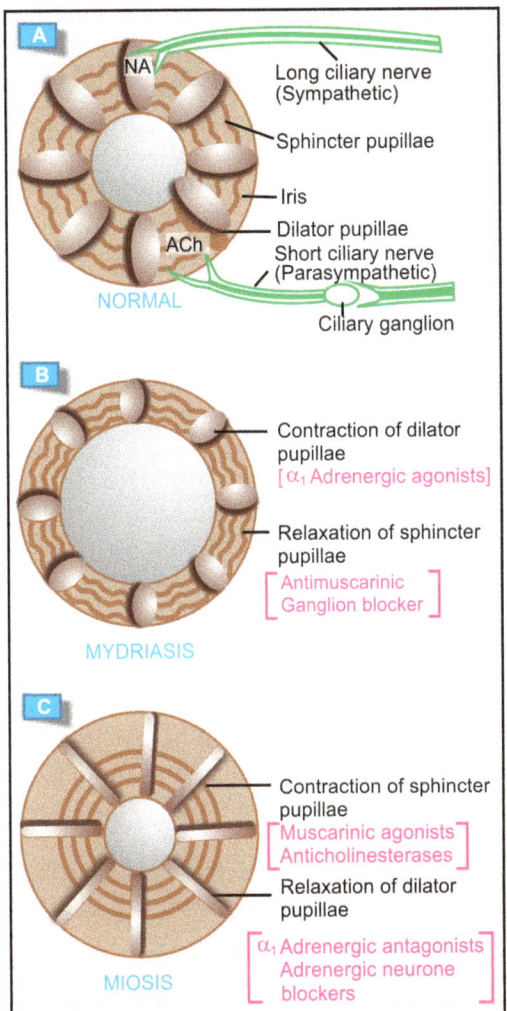

Fig. 5.5: Autonomic control of pupil (A); and site of action of mydriatics (B) and miotics (C)

Atropine has a relaxant action on ureter and urinary bladder; urinary retention can occur in older males with prostatic hypertrophy. However, this can be beneficial for increasing bladder capacity and controlling detrusor hyperreflexia in neurogenic bladder and enuresis. Relaxation of biliary tract is less marked and effect on uterus is minimal.

5. Glands Atropine markedly decreases sweat, salivary, tracheobronchial and lacrimal secretion (M3 blockade). Skin and eyes become dry, talking and swallowing may be difficult.

Atropine decreases secretion of acid, pepsin and mucus in the stomach, but the primary action is on volume of secretion so that pH of gastric contents may not be raised unless diluted by food. Relatively higher doses are needed and atropine is less efficacious than H_2 blockers in reducing acid secretion. Intestinal and pancreatic secretions are not significantly reduced. Bile production is not under cholinergic control, so not affected.

6. Body temperature Rise in body temperature occurs at higher doses. It is due to both inhibition of sweating as well as stimulation of temperature regulating centre in the hypothalamus. Children are highly susceptible to atropine fever.

The sensitivity of different organs and tissues to atropine varies and can be graded as—

Saliva, sweat, bronchial secretion > eye, bronchial muscle, heart > smooth muscle of intestine, bladder > gastric glands and smooth muscle.

PHARMACOKINETICS

Atropine and hyoscine are rapidly absorbed from g.i.t. Applied to eyes, they freely penetrate cornea. Passage across blood-brain barrier is somewhat restricted. About 50% of atropine is metabolized in liver and rest is excreted unchanged in urine. It has a t½ of 3–4 hours. Hyoscine is more completely metabolized and has better blood-brain barrier penetration.

ATROPINE SUBSTITUTES

Many semisynthetic derivatives of belladonna alkaloids and a large number of synthetic compounds have been introduced with the aim of producing more selective action on certain functions. Most of these differ only marginally from the natural alkaloids.

Hyoscine butyl bromide and *atropine methonitrate* are quaternary derivatives which do not produce CNS effects. They are used mainly for colics and functional g.i. disorders.

Ipratropium bromide is given by inhalation in bronchial asthma and chronic obstructive pulmonary disease (COPD). Unlike atropine, it does not depress mucociliary clearance by bronchial epithelium. *Tiotropium bromide* is a long acting and more broncho-selective congener of ipratropium.

Propantheline, oxyphenonium, clidinium, isopropamide are synthetic quaternary anticholinergics, mainly used as antisecretory-antispasmodic. *Cimetropium bromide* is another quaternary antispasmodic which is particularly promoted for irritable bowel syndrome (IBS).

Glycopyrrolate acts rapidly and is almost exclusively employed parenterally before and during anaesthesia.

Dicyclomine has additional direct smooth muscle relaxant and antiemetic properties. It has been used in morning sickness, motion sickness, IBS and in dysmenorrhoea.

Valethamate This antispasmodic-anticholinergic is mostly used to hasten dilatation of cervix during labour.

Oxybutynin, tolterodine, flavoxate, darifenacin and *solifenacin* are relatively vasicoselective anticholinergics with direct smooth muscle relaxant property. They are used for detrusor instability, urinary frequency and urge incontinence.

Pirenzepine is a selective M_1 antimuscarinic which inhibits gastric secretion with few atropinic side effects.

Homatropine, cyclopentolate, tropicamide are used exclusively as mydriatic and cycloplegic. They have quicker and briefer action than atropine.

Trihexyphenidyl, procyclidine and *biperiden* have more prominent central antimuscarinic action. They are used in parkinsonism.

USES (of atropine and its congeners)

1. Preanaesthetic medication: To check increased salivary and tracheobronchial secretions due to irritant general anaesthetics (which are infrequently used now), prevent reflex laryngospasm and to block vagal reflexes. Atropine and glycopyrrolate are occasionally employed *to prevent salivation during dental procedures and oral surgery.*

2. To afford symptomatic relief in abdominal cramps/colics, ureteric colic, dyspepsia and other functional g.i. disorders. Use of atropinic drugs in peptic ulcer is now obsolete.

3. The vasicoselective M_3 antimuscarinic drugs are used to relieve urinary frequency and urgency in overactive bladder, neurogenic disorders, enuresis in children.

4. Pulmonary embolism: Atropine benefits by reducing reflex respiratory secretions.

5. Bronchial asthma and COPD: Inhaled ipratropium bromide and tiotropium bromide are particularly useful in COPD and as adjuvant to inhaled $β_2$ agonists in severe/refractory bronchial asthma.

6. As mydriatic and cycloplegic for refraction testing and fundoscopy: tropicamide is preferred because of quickest and briefest action. The long-lasting mydriatic-cycloplegic action of atropine is very valuable for giving rest to intraocular muscles in iritis, iridocyclitis, choroiditis, keratitis and corneal ulcer.

7. To block vagal bradycardia in selected cases of myocardial infarction and digitalis toxicity.

8. Parkinsonism: Central anticholinergics reduce tremor and rigidity by counteracting unbalanced cholinergic activity in striatum, but are less effective than levodopa.

9. Motion sickness: Hyoscine is highly effective, especially valuable for vigorous motions. Dicyclomine is used in milder cases.

10. Atropine is the specific antidote for anticholinesterase poisoning and early mushroom poisoning (due to muscarine). It is also used to block the muscarinic side effects of neostigmine.

SIDE EFFECTS AND TOXICITY

Side effects are quite common with the use of atropine and its congeners. These are due to facets of its action other than for which it is being used. The side effects cause inconvenience but are rarely serious.

The dental implication is that xerostomia (due to reduced salivary flow) caused by regular use of atropinic drugs *can promote dental caries and oral candidiasis.*

Belladonna poisoning This may occur due to drug overdose or consumption of seeds and berries of belladonna/datura plant. Children are highly susceptible. Manifestations are due to exaggerated pharmacological actions.

Dry mouth, difficulty in swallowing and talking.

Dry, flushed and hot skin (especially over face and neck), fever, difficulty in micturition, a scarlet rash may appear.

Dilated pupil, photophobia, blurring of near vision, palpitation.

Excitement, psychotic behaviour, ataxia, delirium, hallucinations.

Hypotension, weak and rapid pulse, cardiovascular collapse with respiratory depression. Convulsions and coma occur only in severe poisoning.

Treatment If poison has been ingested, gastric lavage should be done with tannic acid ($KMnO_4$ is ineffective in oxidizing atropine). The patient should be kept in a dark quiet room. Cold sponging or ice bags are applied for reducing body temperature. Physostigmine 1–3 mg s.c. or i.v. antagonizes both central and peripheral effects. It may be repeated 4–6 hourly. Neostigmine is less satisfactory.

Other general measures (maintenance of blood volume, artificial respiration, diazepam to control convulsions) should be taken as appropriate.

Contraindications Atropinic drugs are absolutely contraindicated in individuals with a narrow iridocorneal angle—may precipitate acute congestive glaucoma. However, marked rise in intraocular tension is rare in patients with wide angle glaucoma.

Caution is advocated in elderly males with prostatic hypertrophy—urinary retention can occur.

Interactions

1. Absorption of most drugs is slowed because atropine delays gastric emptying. Extent of digoxin and tetracycline absorption may be increased due to longer transit time in the g.i.t.
2. Antihistaminics, tricyclic antidepressants, phenothiazines, disopyramide, pethidine have anticholinergic property—additive side effects occur with atropinic drugs.

Drugs acting on autonomic ganglia

Apart from *transdermal nicotine patches* and *nicotine chewing gum* which are used as aid in the treatment of smoking cessation, neither the ganglionic stimulants nor the ganglion blocking agents have any therapeutic value now. The above formulations of nicotine reduce craving for tobacco smoking/chewing and suppress the physical withdrawal symptoms of discontinuing tobacco use.

6
CHAPTER

Drugs Acting on Autonomic Nervous System-2
Adrenergic and Antiadrenergic Drugs

ADRENERGIC TRANSMISSION

Adrenergic (more precisely 'Noradrenergic') transmission is restricted to the sympathetic division of the ANS. There are three closely related endogenous catecholamines (CAs) which act as signal molecules.

Noradrenaline (NA) It acts as transmitter at postganglionic sympathetic sites (except at sweat glands, and some vasodilator fibres) and in certain areas of brain.

Adrenaline (Adr) It is secreted by adrenal medulla and may have a transmitter role in the brain, but not in periphery.

Dopamine (DA) It is a major transmitter in the basal ganglia, limbic system, CTZ, anterior pituitary, etc. and in a limited manner in the periphery (in renal blood vessels).

1. *Synthesis of CAs* Catecholamines are synthesized from the amino acid phenylalanine as depicted in Fig. 6.1. Synthesis of NA occurs in all adrenergic neurones, while that of Adr occurs only in the adrenal medullary cells and requires high concentration of glucocorticoids which reach there through intra-adrenal portal circulation for induction of the methylating enzyme.

2. *Storage of CAs* NA is stored in synaptic vesicles or 'granules' within the adrenergic nerve terminal (*see* Fig. 6.4). The vesicular membrane actively takes up DA from the cytoplasm and the final step of synthesis

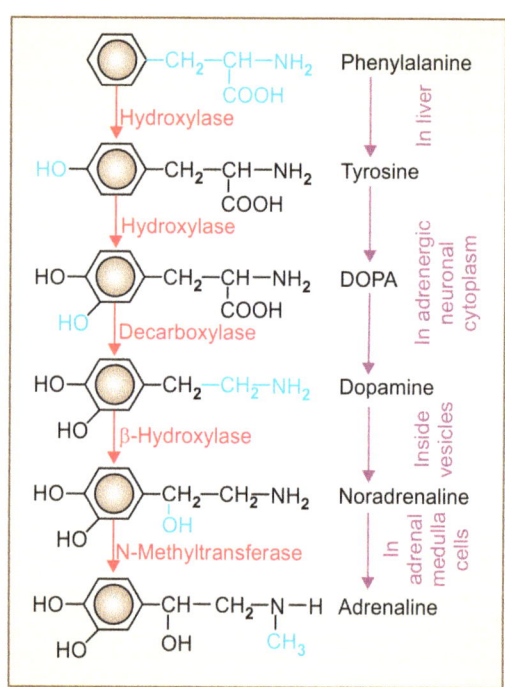

Fig. 6.1: Steps in the synthesis of catecholamines

of NA takes place inside the vesicle which contains dopamine β-hydroxylase. NA is then stored as a complex with ATP (in a ratio of 4:1) which is adsorbed on a protein *chromogranin*. The cytoplasmic pool of CAs is kept low by the enzyme monoamine oxidase (MAO) present on the outer surface of mitochondria.

3. Release of CAs The nerve impulse coupled release of CA takes place by exocytosis (*see* p. 81) and all the vesicular contents (NA or Adr, ATP, dopamine β hydroxylase, chromogranin) are poured out. The release is modulated by presynaptic receptors, of which α_2 inhibitory control is dominant.

Indirectly acting sympathomimetic amines (tyramine, etc.) also induce release of NA, but they do so by displacing NA from the nerve ending binding sites and by exchange diffusion utilizing norepinephrine transporter (NET) which is the carrier of uptake-1 (*see* below). This process is not exocytotic and does not require Ca^{2+}.

4. *Uptake of CAs* There is a very efficient mechanism by which NA released from the nerve terminal is recaptured. This occurs in two steps—

Axonal uptake An active amine pump (NET) is present at the neuronal membrane which transports NA at a higher rate than Adr (uptake-1). The indirectly acting sympathomimetic amines also utilize this pump for entering the neurone. This uptake is the most important mechanism for terminating the postjunctional action of NA and is inhibited by cocaine, desipramine and its congeners.

Vesicular uptake The membrane of intracellular vesicles has another amine pump the 'vesicular monoamine transporter' (VMAT-2) which transports CAs from the cytoplasm to the interior of vesicle. The vesicular NA is constantly leaking out into the axoplasm and is recaptured by this mechanism. This carrier also takes up DA formed in the axoplasm for further synthesis into NA. Thus, it is very important in maintaining the NA content of the neurone. This uptake is inhibited by reserpine resulting in depletion of CAs.

An extraneuronal uptake (uptake-2) of CAs involving a different transporter also occurs into nonneural cells. This is not inhibited by cocaine and is of minor importance.

5. *Metabolism of CAs* The pathways of metabolism of CAs are depicted in Fig. 6.2. Part of the NA leaking out from vesicles into cytoplasm as well as that taken up by axonal transport is first attacked by MAO, while that which diffuses into circulation is first acted upon by catechol-o-methyl transferase (COMT) in liver and other tissues. The alternative enzyme can subsequently act to produce vanillylmandelic acid (VMA) through intermediate steps shown in Fig. 6.2. The major metabolites excreted in urine are VMA and 3-methoxy-4-hydroxy phenyl glycol (a reduced product) along with some metanephrine, normetanephrine and 3,4 dihydroxy mandelic acid (DOMA). These metabolites are mostly conjugated with glucuronic acid or sulfate before excretion in urine. However, metabolism does not play an important role in terminating the action of neuronally released CAs. Action is terminated mainly by reuptake.

6. Adrenergic receptors Adrenergic receptors are membrane bound G-protein coupled receptors which function primarily by increasing or decreasing the intracellular production of second messengers cAMP or IP_3/DAG. In some cases, the activated G-protein itself operates K^+ or Ca^{2+} channels, or increases prostaglandin production.

On the basis of two distinct rank order of potencies of adrenergic agonists (Fig. 6.3), Ahlquist (1948) classified adrenergic receptors into two types α and β. This classification was confirmed later by the development of selective α and β adrenergic antagonists. Important features of α and β receptors are given in Table 6.1.

On the basis of relative organ specificity of selective agonists and antagonists, the β receptors were further subdivided into β_1 (cardiac) and β_2 (bronchial, vascular, uterine) subtypes. Later β_3 receptors were identified, which are located on adipocytes, mediate lipolysis and induce thermogenesis. The β_1 receptors are preferentially activated by dobutamine and blocked by metoprolol, while β_2 receptors are selectively activated by salbutamol and blocked by α-methyl propranolol.

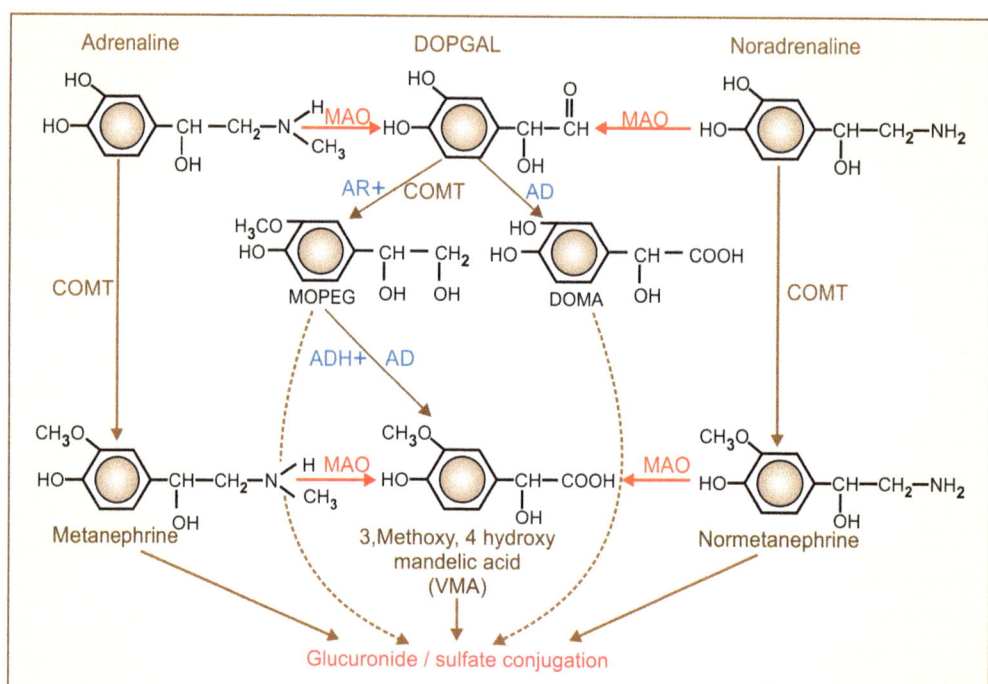

Fig. 6.2: Metabolism of catecholamines
MAO—Monoamine oxidase; COMT—Catechol-O-methyl transferase; AR—Aldehyde reductase; AD—Aldehyde dehydrogenase; ADH—Alcohol dehydrogenase; DOMA—3,4 dihydroxy mandelic acid; MOPEG—3-methoxy, 4-hydroxy phenyl glycol; VMA—vanillyl mandelic acid.

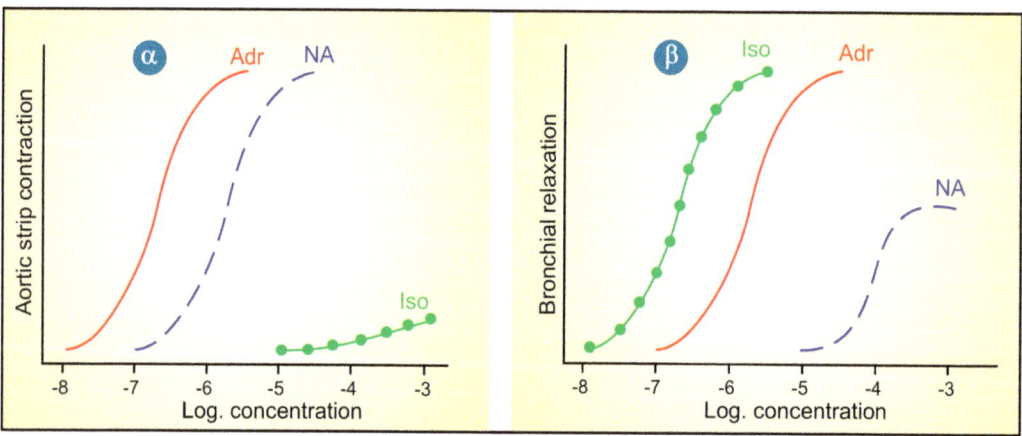

Fig. 6.3: Dose-response curves of 3 catecholamines adrenaline (Adr), noradrenaline (NA) and isoprenaline (Iso) on isolated aortic strip and isolated bronchial smooth muscle illustrating two distinct rank orders of potencies respectively for α and β adrenergic receptors

Adrenergic Transmission

Table 6.1: Differences between α and β adrenergic receptors

	α	β
1. Rank order of potency of agonists	Adr ≥ NA > Iso	Iso > Adr > NA
2. Antagonist	Phentolamine	Propranolol
3. Effector pathway	IP_3/DAG ↑, cAMP ↓, K^+ channel ↑	cAMP ↑, Ca^{2+} channel ↑

Similarly, subtypes of α adrenoceptor have also been identified. The $α_1$ subtype is located only postjunctionally. Phenylephrine and prazosin respectively are its selective agonist and antagonist. The $α_2$ subtype is present both pre- and postjuctionally. It is selectively activated by clonidine and blocked by yohimbine.

The adrenergic neuronal mechanisms and action of drugs which modify them are depicted in Fig. 6.4. A summary of drugs acting through adrenergic neuronal mechanisms is presented in Table 6.2.

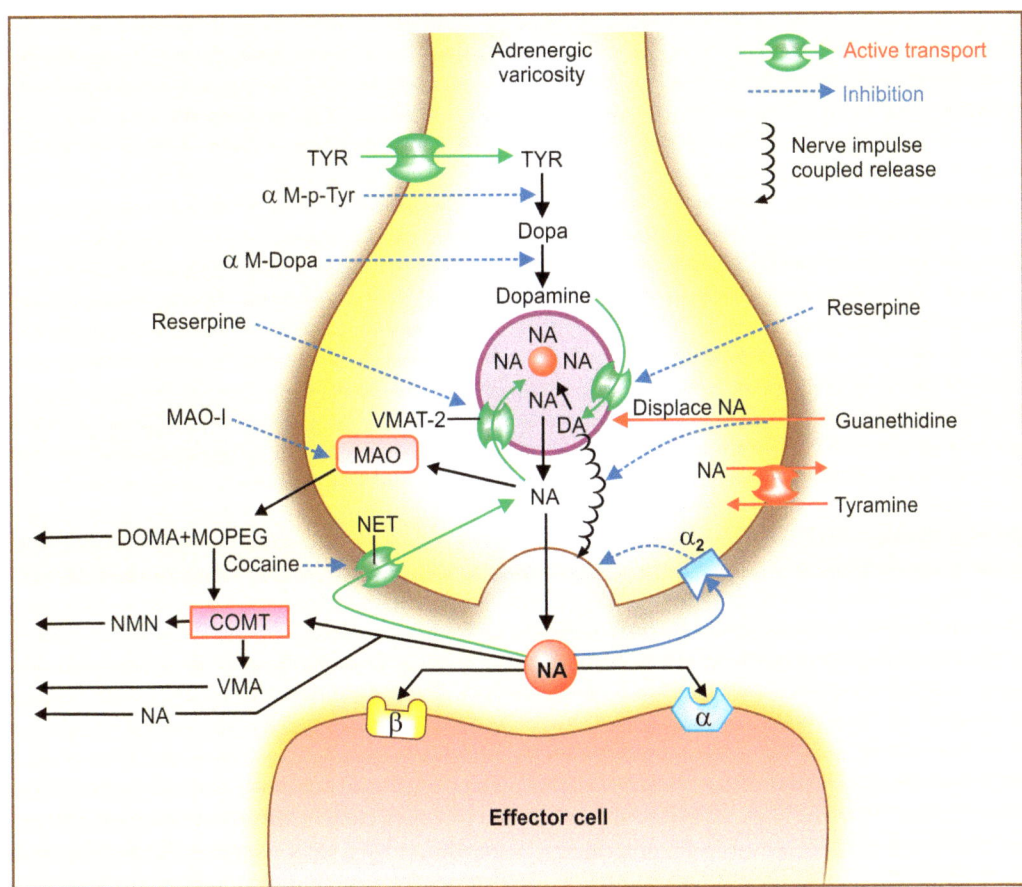

Fig. 6.4: Schematic representation of adrenergic neurotransmission and its modification by drugs
TYR—tyrosine; α M-p-Tyr—α methyl-p-tyrosine; α M-Dopa—α methyl dopa; MAO—monoamine oxidase; MAOI—monoamine oxidase inhibitor; COMT—catechol-o-methyl transferase; NMN—nor-metanephrine; VMA—vanillyl mandelic acid; NET—Norepinephrine transporter; VMAT-2—Vesicular monoamine transporter; DOMA—3,4 dihydroxy mandelic acid; MOPEG—3-Methoxy,4-hydroxy phenyl glycol.

Table 6.2: Summary of drug action through modification of adrenergic transmission

Step/site	Action	Drug	Response
1. Synthesis of NA	Inhibition Utilisation of same synthetic pathway	α-methyl-p-tyrosine α-methyl dopa	Depletion of NA Replacement of NA by α-methyl NA (false transmitter)
2. Axonal reuptake	Blockade	Cocaine, desipramine, guanethidine	Potentiation of NA (endo- and exogenous), inhibition of tyramine action
3. Vesicular uptake	Blockade	Reserpine	Depletion of NA (degraded by MAO)
4. Nerve impulse coupled release of NA	Inhibition	Guanethidine, bretylium	Loss of adrenergic transmission
5. Neuronal NA pool	Exchange diffusion	Tyramine, amphetamine	Indirect sympathomimetic
6. Metabolism	MAO inhibition	Nialamide tranylcypromine	Potentiation of NA (slight), of tyramine (marked)
	COMT inhibition	Tolcapone, entacapone	Potentiation of NA and DA (slight)
7. Receptors	Mimicking	Phenylephrine Clonidine	α_1 sympathomimetic α_2—inhibition of NA release, ↓ sympathetic outflow
		Isoprenaline	$\beta_1 + \beta_2$—sympathomimetic
		Salbutamol	β_2—sympathomimetic
	Blockade	Phentolamine	$\alpha_1 + \alpha_2$—blockade
		Prazosin	α_1—blockade
		Yohimbine	α_2—blockade
		Propranolol	$\beta_1 + \beta_2$—blockade
		Metoprolol	β_1—blockade

ADRENERGIC DRUGS (Sympathomimetics)

These are drugs with actions similar to that of Adr or that of sympathetic stimulation.

Direct sympathomimetics These drugs act directly as agonists on α and/or β adrenoceptors—Adr, NA, isoprenaline (Iso), phenylephrine, methoxamine, xylometazoline, salbutamol and many others.

Indirect sympathomimetics These drugs act on adrenergic neurone to release NA which then acts on the adrenoceptors, e.g. tyramine, amphetamine.

Mixed action sympathomimetics These drugs act directly as well as indirectly, e.g. ephedrine, mephentermine.

ACTIONS

The peripheral actions of Adr in most tissues have been clearly differentiated into those mediated by α or β receptors depending on the predominant receptor type present in a given tissue. These are tabulated in Table 6.3. The receptor subtype, wherever defined, has been mentioned in parenthesis. The actions of a particular sympathomimetic amine

Table 6.3: Adrenergic responses mediated through α and β receptors

α actions	β actions
1. Constriction of arterioles and veins → rise in BP ($\alpha_1 + \alpha_2$)	Dilatation of arterioles and veins → fall in BP (β_2)
2. Heart—no significant action	Cardiac stimulation (β_1), ↑ rate, force and conduction velocity
3. Bronchial muscle—no effect	Bronchodilatation (β_2)
4. Contraction of radial muscles of iris → mydriasis (α_1), decreased aqueous secretion	No effect on iris, slight relaxation ciliary muscle Enhanced aqueous secretion
5. Intestinal relaxation, contraction of sphincters	Intestinal relaxation (β_2)
6. Bladder trigone, prostate—contraction	Detrusor—relaxation (β_2, β_3)
7. Uterus—contraction (α_1)	Relaxation (β_2)
8. Splenic capsule—contraction	Mild relaxation (β_2)
9. Neuromuscular transmission facilitated, ↑ ACh release	Active state—prolonged in fast contracting muscle, abbreviated in slow contracting muscle; tremors (β_2)
10. Insulin secretion inhibited (α_2) (dominant)	Augmented insulin (mild) and glucagon secretion (β_2)
11. Liver —	Liver—glycogenolysis (β_2) → hyperglycaemia Muscle—glycogenolysis (β_2) → hyperlactacidaemia Fat—lipolysis ($\beta_1 + \beta_2 + \beta_3$) → increased blood FFA, calorigenesis
12. Renin release from kidney —	Renin release from kidney—augmented (β_1)
13. Male sex organs—ejaculation (α_1)	—
14. Salivary gland—K⁺ and water secretion (α_1)	Ptylin secretion
15. Adrenergic nerve terminals—inhibits NA release (α_2)	Facilitates NA release (weak action)

depend on its relative activity at different types of adrenergic receptors.

Adr: $\alpha_1 + \alpha_2 + \beta_1 + \beta_2$
NA: $\alpha_1 + \alpha_2 + \beta_1$ but no β_2 action
Iso: $\beta_1 + \beta_2$ but no α action

Important actions of Adr, NA and isoprenaline are compared in Table 6.4.
The overall actions are—

1. Heart Adr increases heart rate by increasing automaticity of SA node. It also activates latent pacemakers in A-V node and Purkinje fibres, cardiac arrhythmias can occur with high doses that raise BP markedly. Certain anaesthetics (chloroform, halothane) sensitize the heart to the arrhythmic action of Adr. Idioventricular rate is increased in patients with complete heart block.

Force of cardiac contraction is increased. Cardiac output and oxygen consumption of the heart are markedly enhanced.

Conduction velocity through A-V node, bundle of His, atrial and ventricular fibres is increased; partial A-V block may be overcome. Refractory period (RP) of all types of cardiac cells is reduced. All cardiac actions are predominantly β_1 receptor mediated.

When BP rises markedly, reflex bradycardia occurs due to stimulation of vagus. Bradycardia is the usual response seen when NA is injected i.v.

2. Blood vessels Both vasoconstriction (α) and vasodilatation (β_2) can occur depending on the drug, its dose and the vascular bed. Constriction predominates in cutaneous, mucous membrane and renal beds.

Table 6.4: Comparative effects of intravenous infusion of adrenaline, noradrenaline and isoprenaline

	Adr	NA	Iso
1. Heart rate	↑	↓	↑↑
2. Cardiac output	↑↑	—	↑↑
3. BP—Systolic	↑↑	↑↑	↑
Diastolic	↓↑	↑↑	↓↓
Mean	↑	↑↑	↓
4. Blood flow			
Skin and mm	↓	↓	—
Sk. muscle	↑↑	—,↓	↑
Kidney	↓	↓	—
Liver	↑↑	—	↑
Coronary	↑	↑	↑
5. Bronchial muscle	↓↓	—	↓↓
6. Intestinal muscle	↓↓	↓	↓
7. Blood sugar	↑↑	—,↑	↑

Vasoconstriction occurs through both α_1 and α_2 receptors. Vasodilatation predominates in skeletal muscles, liver and coronaries. The direct effect on cerebral vessels is not prominent—blood flow through this bed parallels change in BP.

Vasoconstrictor action is most marked on arterioles; larger arteries and veins are affected at higher doses.

3. BP The effect depends on the amine, its dose and rate of administration.

- NA causes rise in systolic, diastolic and mean BP; it does not cause vasodilatation (no β_2 action), peripheral resistance increases consistently due to α action.
- Isoprenaline causes rise in systolic but marked fall in diastolic BP (β_1—cardiac stimulation, β_2—vasodilatation). The mean BP generally falls.
- Adr given by slow i.v. infusion or s.c. injection causes rise in systolic but fall in diastolic BP; peripheral resistance decreases because vascular β_2 receptors are more sensitive than α receptors. Mean BP generally rises. Pulse pressure is increased.

When an α blocker has been given beforehand, only fall in BP is seen. This is called—*vasomotor reversal of Dale*.

4. Respiration Adr and Isoprenaline but not NA are potent bronchodilators (β_2). This action is more marked when the bronchi are constricted. Adr can directly stimulate respiratory centre (RC), but this action is seldom manifest at clinically used doses.

5. Eye Mydriasis occurs due to contraction of radial muscles of iris (α_1), but this is minimal after topical application because Adr penetrates cornea poorly. The intraocular tension tends to fall, especially in wide angle glaucoma, due to both reduction in aqueous formation as well as facilitation of outflow.

6. GIT In isolated preparations of gut activation of both α and β receptors causes relaxation. In intact animals and man, peristalsis is reduced and sphincters are constricted. However, the effects are brief and of no clinical import.

7. Bladder Detrusor is relaxed (β) and trigone is constricted (α): both actions tend to hinder micturition.

8. Uterus Adr can both contract or relax uterine muscle through respectively α and β receptors. The effect varies with hormonal and gestational status. Human uterus at term of pregnancy is relaxed by Adr; while at other times, its contractions are augmented.

9. Skeletal muscle Adr facilitates neuromuscular transmission. However, incomplete fusion of individual muscle fibre contractions along with enhanced firing of muscle spindles is responsible for the tremors produced by β_2 agonists.

10. CNS Adr, in clinically used doses, does not produce any marked CNS effects because of poor penetration in brain, but restlessness, apprehension and tremor may occur.

11. **Metabolic** Adr causes:
- Glycogenolysis → hyperglycaemia, hyperlactacidaemia (β_2)
- Lipolysis → rise in plasma free fatty acid (FFA) level
- Calorigenesis ($\beta_2 + \beta_3$)
- Transient hyperkalaemia followed by hypokalaemia due to initial release of K⁺ from liver followed by its uptake into muscles and liver.

In addition, metabolic effects result from reduction of insulin (α_2) and augmentation of glucagon (β_2) secretion.

Biochemical mediation of adrenergic responses

β actions The β actions are mediated through cAMP (*see* Fig. 3.5). Adr activates membrane bound enzyme *adenylyl cyclase* through a regulatory protein Gs → ATP is broken down to cAMP at the inner face. This in turn phosphorylates a number of intracellular cAMP-dependent protein kinases and initiates a series of reactions.

α actions The mediation of α actions is varied and less well defined. Vascular and other smooth muscle contractions are mediated through IP_3/DAG production and mobilization of intracellular Ca^{2+}. In other tissues, inhibition of cAMP production and hyperpolarization through K⁺ channel activation mediates the α adrenergic responses.

Administration CAs are absorbed from the intestine but are rapidly degraded by MAO and COMT present in the intestinal wall and liver. They are thus orally inactive.

For systemic effects *Adrenaline (epinephrine)* is administered by s.c. or i.m. injection in a dose of 0.2–0.5 mg. Its action lasts 0.5–2 hours. *In dental practice, Adr is used as a local vasoconstrictor added to lidocaine in a concentration of 1 in 200,000 to 80,000 for dental anaesthesia.*

ADRENALINE 1 mg/ml inj.;
in XYLOCAINE with ADRENALINE: Lidocaine 21.3 mg + Adrenaline 0.005 mg per ml inj, 30 ml vial; lidocaine 2% with adrenaline 1:80,000 in 1.5 ml cartridge for dental anaesthesia.

Noradrenaline (norepinephrine, levarterenol) is administered only by slow i.v. infusion at the rate of 2–4 µg/min, for raising BP in emergency situations.

Adverse effects and contraindications

- Transient restlessness, palpitation, anxiety, tremor, pallor may occur after s.c./i.m. injection of Adr.
- Marked rise in BP leading to cerebral haemorrhage, ventricular tachycardia/fibrillation, angina, myocardial infarction

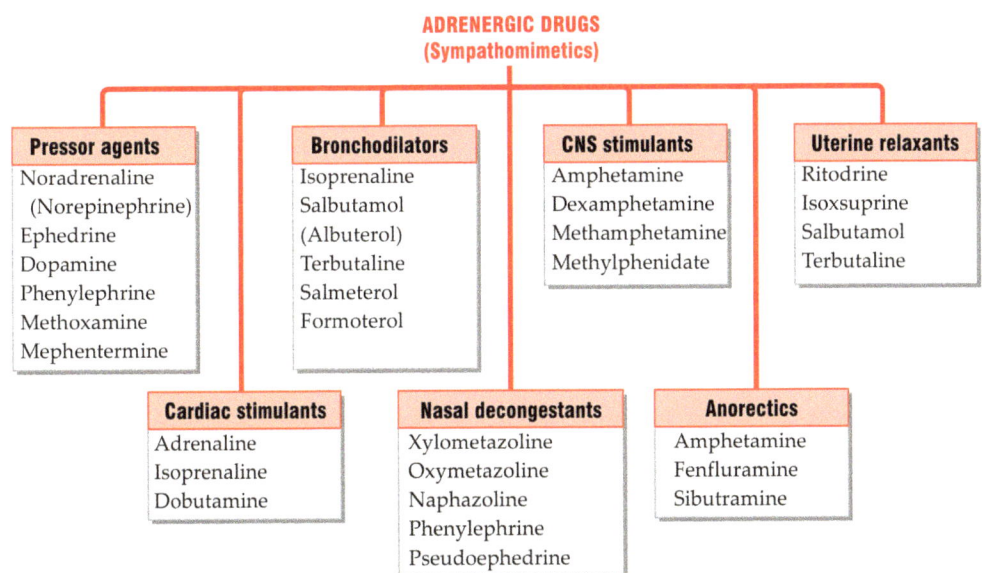

are the hazards of large doses or inadvertent i.v. injection of Adr.
- Adr is contraindicated in hypertensive, hyperthyroid and angina patients.
- *Adr mixed local anaesthetic should be used very cautiously for dental anaesthesia in patients with heart disease.*
- Adr should not be given during anaesthesia with halothane (risk of arrhythmias) and to patients receiving β blockers (marked rise in BP can occur).

Salient features of important adrenergic drugs are summarized below:

Dopamine (DA) It is a dopaminergic (D_1 and D_2 receptors) as well as weak adrenergic $β_1$ and very weak α agonist. The D_1 receptors in renal and mesenteric blood vessels are the most sensitive. Intravenous infusion of low dose of DA dilates these vessels increasing g.f.r. and Na^+ excretion. Moderately high doses produce a positive inotropic effect on the heart. Vasoconstriction ($α_1$ action) occurs only when large doses are infused. At doses normally infused i.v. (0.2–1 mg/min), it raises cardiac output and systolic BP with little effect on diastolic BP. This is useful in cardiogenic and septic shock.

Dobutamine A derivative of DA, but not a D_1 or D_2 receptor agonist. Dobutamine acts mainly on β adrenergic receptors, and is a weak α agonist. The only prominent action of clinically employed doses (2-8 μg/kg/min i.v. infusion) is increase in force of cardiac contraction and output. It is used as an inotropic agent in pump failure accompanying myocardial infarction, cardiac surgery, and for short-term management of severe congestive heart failure.

Ephedrine It is an alkaloid obtained from *Ephedra vulgaris* which mainly acts indirectly but has some direct action on α and β receptors as well. Repeated injections produce tachyphylaxis, primarily because the neuronal pool of NA available for displacement is small. Ephedrine is resistant to MAO, therefore, effective orally. It crosses to brain and causes stimulation.

Ephedrine is now infrequently used in mild chronic bronchial asthma and for hypotension during spinal anaesthesia.

Amphetamines These are synthetic compounds having the same pharmacological profile as ephedrine. They are orally active with long duration (4–6 hr). Amphetamines exert potent CNS stimulant and weak peripheral cardiovascular actions.

The central effects include alertness, increased concentration and attention span, euphoria, talkativeness, increased work capacity. Fatigue is allayed. Athletic performance is improved temporarily followed by deterioration. It is one of the drugs included in the 'dope test' for athletes. The reticular activating system is stimulated resulting in wakefulness and postponement of sleep deprivation induced physical disability. But this is short lived and may be accompanied by anxiety, restlessness, tremor, dysphoria and agitation.

Amphetamines stimulate respiratory centre, especially if it has been depressed. Hunger is suppressed as a result of inhibition of hypothalamic feeding centre. Peripheral effects on heart and BP are not significant at the usual doses, but tone of vesical sphincter is significantly increased.

Amphetamines are drugs of abuse and are capable of producing marked psychological but little or no physical dependence. Amphetamine abusers are generally teenagers seeking thrill or kick which is obtained on rapid i.v. injection. High doses produce euphoria, restlessness, panic, marked excitement which may progress to mental confusion, delirium, hallucinations and an acute psychotic state.

Repeated use is likely to produce long-lasting behavioural abnormalities; psychosis may be precipitated.

Adrenergic Drugs

Phenylephrine It is a selective α_1 agonist, with negligible β action. Phenylephrine raises BP by causing vasoconstriction. Topically, it is used as a nasal decongestant and for producing mydriasis when cycloplegia is not required. It is also a constituent of orally administered nasal decongestant preparations.

Methoxamine Another selective α_1 stimulant with no β actions; occasionally used as a pressor agent.

Mephentermine It produces both cardiac stimulation and vasoconstriction by directly activating α and β adrenergic receptors as well as by releasing NA. Administered orally or parenterally, it is used to prevent and treat hypotension due to spinal anaesthesia, shock and other hypotensive states.

SELECTIVE β_2 STIMULANTS

These include salbutamol, terbutaline, salmeterol, formoterol and ritodrine. They cause bronchodilatation, vasodilatation and uterine relaxation, without producing significant cardiac stimulation. However, β_2 selectivity is only relative. Salbutamol has β_2:β_1 action ratio of about 10. These drugs are primarily used in bronchial asthma (*see* Ch. 19). Occasionally ritodrine is employed to suppress uterine contractions and delay premature labour.

The most important side effect of β_2 agonists is muscle tremor.

NASAL DECONGESTANTS

These are α agonists which on topical application as dilute solution (0.05–0.1%) produce vasoconstriction in nasal mucosa. The imidazoline compounds—xylometazoline and oxymetazoline are relatively selective α_2 agonist (like clonidine). They have a longer duration of action (12 hr) than ephedrine. Rise in BP can occur in hypertensives after nasal instillation. Long-term use can produce anosmia and atrophic rhinitis.

ANORECTIC AGENTS

A number of drugs related to amphetamine have been developed which inhibit the feeding centre but have little/no CNS stimulant action or abuse liability. All of them act by releasing, NA/DA or 5-HT, or by inhibiting their reuptake, so as to enhance monoaminergic transmission in the brain.

Fenfluramine and its dextroisomer *dexfenfluramine* reduce food seeking behaviour by enhancing serotonergic transmission in the hypothalamus. They were extensively used by slimming centres, but are banned now.

Sibutramine which inhibits both NA and 5-HT reuptake was introduced subsequently. It is also banned now.

THERAPEUTIC USES

1. *Hypotensive states* (shock, spinal anaesthesia) One of the pressor agents can be infused along with volume replacement for neurogenic and haemorrhagic shock. In other hypotensive states, these drugs can be an expedient measure to maintain cerebral circulation. Slow i.v. infusion of dopamine is more appropriate, while NA is used only when potent vasoconstriction is required. Adr 0.5 mg injected promptly i.m. is the drug of choice for anaphylactic shock (*see* p. 72). It not only raises BP, but counteracts bronchospasm/laryngeal edema that may accompany. Because of the rapidity and profile of action, Adr is the only life-saving measure.

Postural or persistent hypotension due to autonomic neuropathy of diabetes, old age and hypotensive drugs may be treated with oral ephedrine or mephentermine, but these drugs cannot mimic the normal reflex vasoconstriction due to change of posture.

2. *Along with local anaesthetics* Adr 1 in 200,000 to 1 in 80,000 is often added to the local anaesthetic for infiltration, nerve block and spinal anaesthesia. Duration of anaesthesia is prolonged and systemic toxicity of the local anaesthetic is reduced. *Adr is routinely included in dental anaesthesia (unless contraindicated); serves to reduce bleeding as well (see* Ch. 24).

3. *Control of local bleeding* In cases of bleeding from skin, mucous membranes, tooth socket, epistaxis, etc: compresses or packs of Adr 1 in 10,000, soaked in cotton can control arteriolar and capillary bleeding.

4. *Nasal decongestant* In colds, rhinitis, sinusitis, blocked eustachian tube—one of the α-agonists is used as nasal drops.

5. *Cardiac arrest* (drowning, electrocution, Stokes-Adams syndrome and other causes) Adr injected i.v. along with external cardiac massage may be used to stimulate the heart.

6. *Partial or complete A-V block* Isoprenaline may be used as short-term measure to maintain sufficient ventricular rate.

7. *Congestive heart failure* Adrenergic inotropic drugs are not useful in the routine treatment of CHF. However, controlled short-term i.v. infusion of DA/dobutamine can tide over acute cardiac decompensation.

8. *Bronchial asthma* The β_2 adrenergic stimulants like salbutamol, terbutaline, salmeterol, etc. are the primary drugs for relief of reversible airway obstruction (see Ch. 19).

9. *Allergic disorders* Adr is life-saving in laryngeal edema and anaphylaxis, and can afford quick relief in urticaria, angioedema of mouth/face, etc., because it is a physiological antagonist of histamine.

10. *Ocular uses* Phenylephrine is used to facilitate fundus examination; cycloplegia is not required. It is also combined with tropicamide for refraction testing. Phenyephrine tends to reduce intraocular tension in wide angle glaucoma. The ester prodrug of Adr *dipivefrine* and selective α_2 agonist *brimonidine* are adjuvant drugs for open angle glaucoma.

11. *Attention deficit hyperkinetic disorder (ADHD)* Amphetamines have an apparently paradoxical effect to calm down hyperkinetic children. By increasing attention span, they improve the child's behaviour as well as performance in studies.

12. *Uterine relaxant* Selective β_2 stimulants, especially ritodrine, infused i.v. have been successfully used to postpone labour.

13. *Insulin hypoglycaemia* Adr may be used as an expedient measure to counteract hypoglycaemia, but glucose should be given as soon as possible.

ANTIADRENERGIC DRUGS (ADRENERGIC RECEPTOR ANTAGONISTS)

These are drugs which antagonize the action of adrenaline and related drugs on their receptors. They are competitive antagonists at α or β or both types of adrenergic receptors.

α ADRENERGIC BLOCKING DRUGS

These drugs inhibit adrenergic responses mediated through the α adrenergic receptors without affecting those mediated through β receptors.

GENERAL EFFECTS OF α BLOCKERS

1. Blockade of vasoconstrictor α_1 (also α_2) receptors reduces peripheral resistance and causes pooling of blood in capacitance vessels → venous return and cardiac output are reduced leading to fall in BP. Postural reflex is interfered with so that marked hypotension occurs on standing → dizziness and syncope. Hypovolemia accentuates the hypotension. Special care must be taken to ensure that *patients receiving an α blocker (e.g. prazosin or other α_1 adrenergic blocker for hypertension or benign prostatic hypertrophy) do not suddenly stand up after being supine on the dental chair*. These patients are also more prone to develop hypotension if they bleed during the dental procedure.

The α blockers abolish pressor action of Adr (injected i.v. in animals) which then produces only fall in BP due to β_2 mediated vasodilatation—*vasomotor reversal of Dale*.

α-Adrenergic Blocking Drugs

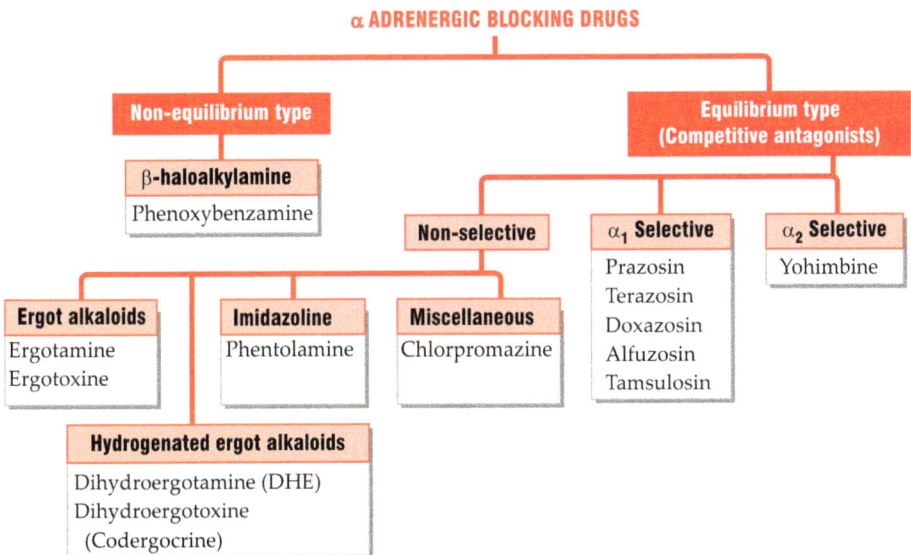

2. Reflex tachycardia occurs due to fall in mean arterial pressure and increased release of NA from cardiac sympathetic neurons due to blockade of presynaptic $α_2$ receptors.

3. Nasal stuffiness and miosis result from blockade of α receptors in nasal blood vessels and in radial muscles of iris respectively.

4. Hypotension due to α receptor blockage can reduce renal blood flow → g.f.r. is reduced and more complete reabsorption of Na^+ and water occurs in the tubules, resulting in Na^+ retention and expansion of blood volume. This is accentuated by reflex increase in renin release mediated through $β_1$ receptors.

5. Tone of smooth muscle in bladder trigone, sphincter and prostate is reduced by blockade of $α_1$ receptors (mostly of the $α_{1A}$ subtype) → urine flow in patients with benign hypertrophy of prostate (BHP) is improved.

6. Contractions of vas deferens and seminal vesicles which result in ejaculation are coordinated through α receptors. Therefore α blockers can inhibit ejaculation; this may manifest as impotence.

The α blockers have no effect on adrenergic cardiac stimulation, bronchodilatation, vasodilatation and most of the metabolic changes, because these are predominantly mediated through β receptors.

Apart from these common effects, most of which manifest as side effects, individual a blockers have some additional actions. Their pharmacological profile is governed by their central effects and by the relative activity on $α_1$ and $α_2$ receptor subtypes as well.

Side effects that may occur with any α blocker are—palpitation, postural hypotension, nasal blockage, fluid retention, inhibition of ejaculation and impotence.

Distinctive features of important α adrenergic blockers are outlined below:

Phenoxybenzamine This alkylamine cyclizes spontaneously in the body giving rise to a highly reactive ethyleniminium intermediate which reacts with α adrenoceptors and other biomolecules by forming strong covalent bonds. The α blockade is nonequilibrium (irreversible) and develops gradually. It lasts 3–4 days.

Phenoxybenzamine has been used primarily in pheochromocytoma; occasionally in secondary shock and peripheral vascular disease.

Natural and hydrogenated ergot alkaloids The amino acid alkaloids *ergotamine and ergotoxine* are partial agonists and antagonists at α adrenergic, serotonergic and dopaminergic receptors. The amine alkaloid ergometrine has no α blocking activity.

The natural ergot alkaloids produce long-lasting vasoconstriction which predominates over their α blocking action. This causes peripheral vascular insufficiency. Gangrene of toes and fingers occurs in ergotism.

The principal use of ergotamine is in migraine. Dihydroergotoxine has been used as a cognition enhancer.

Phentolamine It is a rapidly acting α blocker with short duration of action (in minutes) which has been utilized for diagnosis of pheochromocytoma, as well as for its intraoperative management. It can also be employed for control of hypertension due to clonidine withdrawal, cheese reaction, etc.

Prazosin It is first of the highly selective α_1 blockers having $\alpha_1 : \alpha_2$ selectivity ratio 1000:1. Prazosin blocks sympathetically mediated vasoconstriction and produces fall in BP which is attended by only mild tachycardia because NA release is not increased due to absence of α_2 blockade.

Prazosin dilates arterioles more than veins. Postural hypotension occurs, especially in the beginning—dizziness and fainting may be caused as 'first dose effect'. This can be minimized by starting with a low dose and taking it at bedtime.

Prazosin is primarily used as an antihypertensive. Other uses are—LVF, Raynaud's disease and prostatic hypertrophy. It blocks α_1 receptors in bladder trigone and prostate; thereby improves urine flow and reduces residual urine in bladder.

Terazosin and doxazosin are longer acting congeners of prazosin suitable for once daily dosing; particularly used in BHP.

Tamsulosin is relatively uroselective due to higher affinity for α_{1A} subtype of α_1 receptors which predominate in the bladder base and prostate. Thus, it does not cause significant changes in BP or HR at doses which relieve urinary symptoms of BHP. Dizziness and retrograde ejaculation are the only significant side effects. Its modified release (MR) capsule needs only once daily dosing.

Yohimbine An alkaloid from West African plant Yohimbehe. It is a relatively selective α_2 blocker with short duration of action. Yohimbine may cause congestion of genitals and has been claimed to be an aphrodisiac. This effect probably is only psychological. There are no valid indications for clinical use of yohimbine.

USES OF α BLOCKERS

1. *Pheochromocytoma* It is a tumour of adrenal medullary cells. Excess CAs are secreted which can cause intermittent or persistent hypertension. Estimation of urinary CA metabolites (VMA, normetanephrine) is diagnostic. In addition, a pharmacological test can be performed by injecting phentolamine 5 mg i.v. A fall in BP > 35 mmHg systolic or > 25 mmHg diastolic is indicative of pheochromocytoma.

Phenoxybenzamine can be used as definitive therapy for inoperable and malignant tumours. It is also employed before and during surgical removal of the tumour. Alternatively, phentolamine drip can be instituted during the operation.

2. *Hypertension* Prazosin and other selective α_1 blockers are useful antihypertensive drugs, but the nonselective $\alpha_1 + \alpha_2$ blockers have been a failure. However, phentolamine is of great value in controlling episodes of rise in BP during clonidine withdrawal and cheese reaction in patients on MAO inhibitors.

3. *Benign hypertrophy of prostate (BHP)* The urinary obstruction caused by BHP has a static component due to increased size of prostate and a dynamic component due to increased tone of smooth muscle in bladder neck and prostatic urethra. Since this increase in tone is mediated neurogenically through α_1 receptors, blockade of α_1 receptors relaxes these structures, reducing dynamic

obstruction, increasing urinary flow rate and causing more complete emptying of bladder in many patients of BHP.

Terazosin, doxazosin, alfuzosin and tamsulosin are the peferred blockers because of once daily dosing. Tamsulosin appears to cause fewer vascular side effects because of relative α_{1A} selectivity.

4. Peripheral vascular diseases The α blockers afford symptomatic relief when vasoconstriction is prominent, as in Raynaud's phenomenon, but not when vascular obstruction is organic as in Buerger's disease.

β ADRENERGIC BLOCKING DRUGS

These drugs inhibit adrenergic responses mediated through the β receptors. All β blockers are competitive antagonists.

The pharmacology of propranolol is described as prototype.

PROPRANOLOL

PHARMACOLOGICAL ACTIONS

1. CVS

(a) Heart Propranolol decreases heart rate, force of contraction (at relatively higher doses) and cardiac output (c.o.). The effects on a normal resting subject are not appreciable, but become prominent under sympathetic overactivity (exercise, emotion).

Cardiac work and oxygen consumption are reduced since the product of heart rate and aortic pressure decreases. Overall effect in angina patients is improvement of O_2 supply/demand status: exercise tolerance is increased.

Propranolol suppresses ectopic automaticity, especially if it has been augmented by adrenergic stimuli. The A-V conduction is slowed. At high doses, a direct depressant and membrane stabilizing (quinidine like) action is exerted, but this contributes little to the antiarrhythmic effect at usual doses. Propranolol blocks cardiac stimulant action of adrenergic drugs but not that of digoxin, methylxanthines or glucagon.

(b) Blood vessels Propranolol blocks vasodilatation and fall in BP evoked by isoprenaline and enhances the rise in BP caused by Adr; there is re-reversal of vasomotor reversal that is seen after α blockade. It has no direct effect on blood vessels and there is little acute change in BP. On prolonged administration, BP gradually falls in hypertensive subjects but not in

The β blockers are traditionally classified on the basis of their receptor subtype selectivity and other properties

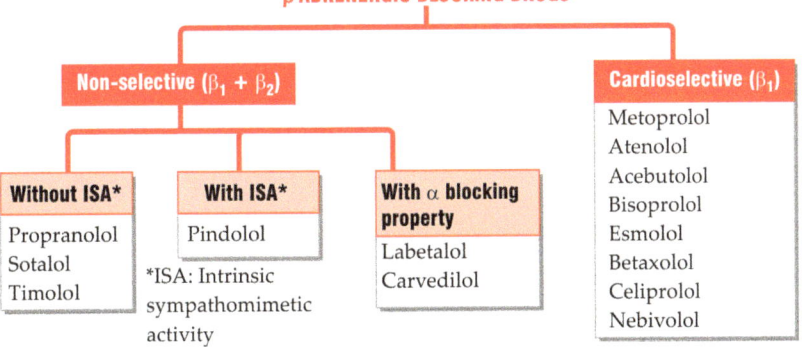

Another system classifies β blockers into 3 generations:

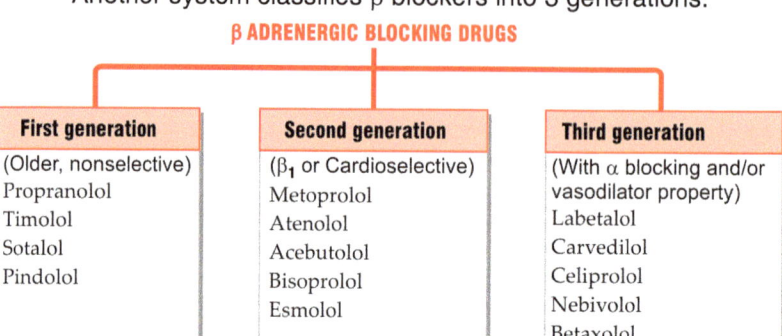

normotensives. Total peripheral resistance (t.p.r.) is increased initially (due to blockade of β mediated vasodilatation) and c.o. is reduced so that there is little change in BP. With continued treatment, resistance vessels gradually adapt to chronically reduced c.o.; t.p.r. decreases slowly—both systolic and diastolic BP fall. This is considered to be the most likely explanation of the antihypertensive action. Other mechanisms that may contribute are:
- Reduced NA release from sympathetic terminals.
- Decreased renin release from kidney (due to $β_1$ blockade).
- Central action reducing sympathetic outflow.

2. Respiratory tract Propranolol increases bronchial resistance by blocking the dilator $β_2$ receptors. The effect is hardly discernible in normal individuals because sympathetic bronchodilator tone is minimal. In asthmatics, however, the condition is consistently worsened and a severe attack may be precipitated.

3. CNS No overt central effects are produced by propranolol. However, subtle behavioural changes, forgetfulness, increased dreaming and nightmares have been reported with long-term use of relatively high doses.

4. Local anaesthetic Propranolol is a potent local anaesthetic, but is not clinically used for this purpose because of its irritant property.

5. Metabolic Propranolol blocks adrenergically induced lipolysis and consequent increase in plasma free fatty acid levels. Plasma triglyceride level and LDL/HDL-CH ratio is increased. It also inhibits glycogenolysis—recovery from insulin action is delayed. Though there is no effect on normal blood sugar level, prolonged propranolol therapy may reduce carbohydrate tolerance by decreasing insulin release.

6. Skeletal muscle Propranolol inhibits adrenergically provoked tremor. This is a peripheral action exerted directly on muscle fibre through $β_2$ receptors.

7. Eye Instillation of β blockers reduces secretion of aqueous humor. Consequently i.o.t. is lowered. There is no consistent effect on pupil size or accommodation.

PHARMACOKINETICS

Propranolol is well absorbed after oral administration, but has low bioavailability due to high first pass metabolism in liver. Oral: parenteral dose ratio of up to 40:1 has been found.

Metabolism of propranolol is dependent on hepatic blood flow. Chronic use of propranolol itself decreases hepatic blood flow, so that oral bioavailability is increased and its t½ is prolonged. Metabolites of propranolol, one of which is active, are excreted in urine.

INTERACTIONS

1. Additive depression of sinus node and A-V conduction occurs with digoxin and verapamil—cardiac arrest can occur.
2. Propranolol delays recovery from hypoglycaemia due to insulin and oral antidiabetics. Warning signs of hypoglycaemia mediated through sympathetic stimulation (tachycardia, tremor) are suppressed.
3. Phenylephrine, ephedrine and other α agonists present in cold remedies can cause marked rise in BP in β blocked subjects.
4. Though only low concentrations of *Adr are added to lidocaine for dental anaesthesia*, it may produce *some pressor* action in patients receiving nonselective β blockers.
5. Indomethacin and other NSAIDs attenuate the antihypertensive action of β blockers.
6. Propranolol retards lidocaine metabolism by reducing hepatic blood flow.

ADVERSE EFFECTS AND CONTRAINDICATIONS

Propranolol and other β blockers are generally well tolerated, but have the potential to produce many adverse effects.
1. Propranolol can accentuate myocardial insufficiency and worsen CHF. However, when compensation has been restored, careful addition of certain β_1 blockers (metoprolol, bisoprolol, nebivolol) is now established therapy to prolong survival.
2. Bradycardia: resting HR may be reduced to 60/min or less.
3. Propranolol worsens chronic obstructive lung disease, and can precipitate life-threatening attack of bronchial asthma; β blockers are contraindicated in asthmatics.
4. Propranolol exacerbates variant (vasospastic) angina due to unopposed α receptor mediated coronary constriction.
5. Carbohydrate tolerance may be impaired in prediabetics.
6. Plasma lipid profile may be altered on long-term use.
7. Withdrawal of propranolol after chronic use should be gradual, otherwise rebound hypertension, worsening of angina and even sudden death can occur.
8. Propranolol is contraindicated in partial or complete heart block: cardiac arrest may occur.
9. Tiredness and reduced exercise capacity may be felt.
10. Cold hands and feet may be noticed in winter due to blockade of vasodilator β_2 receptors.
11. Side effects not overtly due to β blockade are—g.i.t. upset, lack of drive, nightmares, forgetfulness, rarely hallucinations. Male patients on β blockers more frequently complain of sexual distress.

OTHER β BLOCKERS

A number of β blockers have been developed having some special features. The associated properties along with their significance can be summarized as:

Cardioselectivity (in metoprolol, atenolol, acebutolol, bisoprolol, nebivolol).

These drugs are more potent in blocking cardiac (β_1) than bronchial (β_2) receptors. Their features are:
1. Lower propensity to cause bronchoconstriction.
2. Less interference with carbohydrate metabolism.
3. Lower incidence of cold hands and feet.
4. No/less deleterious effect on blood lipid profile.
5. Ineffective in suppressing essential tremor.
6. Less liable to impair exercise capacity.

Partial agonistic (intrinsic sympathomimetic) action (in pindolol, acebutolol). These β blockers themselves activate β_1 and/or β_2 receptors submaximally.

1. Bradycardia and depression of contractility at rest are not prominent.
2. Withdrawal is less likely to exacerbate hypertension or angina.
3. Not effective in migraine prophylaxis—they dilate cerebral vessels.
4. Not suitable for secondary prophylaxis of MI.

Salient features of important β blockers are given below:

1. Sotalol Nonselective β blocker that has additional K^+ channel blocking and class III antiarrhythmic property.

2. Timolol Due to absence of local anaesthetic activity, this β blocker is used topically in the eye for glaucoma.

Betaxolol and Levobunolol are other β blockers employed topically for glaucoma.

3. Pindolol A potent β blocker with prominent intrinsic sympathomimetic activity.

4. Metoprolol It is the prototype of cardioselective ($β_1$) blockers. Its potency to block cardiac stimulation is similar to propranolol, but nearly 50 times higher dose is needed to block isoprenaline induced vasodilatation. Metoprolol has afforded prognostic benefit in CHF, and it is less likely to worsen asthma. It may be preferred in diabetics receiving insulin or oral hypoglycaemics.

5. Atenolol A relatively selective $β_1$ blocker having low lipid solubility. Oral absorption is incomplete, but first pass metabolism is not significant. Because of longer duration of action, once daily dose is often sufficient. It is one of the most commonly used β blockers for hypertension and angina.

6. Esmolol It is an ultrashort acting $β_1$ blocker devoid of partial agonist or membrane stabilizing actions. It is inactivated by esterases in blood; plasma t½ is < 10 min; action lasts 15–20 min after terminating i.v. infusion. Therefore, degree of β blockade can be titrated by regulating rate of infusion. Esmolol has been used to terminate supraventricular tachycardia, episodic atrial fibrillation or flutter, arrhythmia during anaesthesia, and to reduce HR and BP during and after cardiac surgery. It is also employed in early treatment of myocardial infarction.

7. Nebivolol This cardioselective β blocker also activates endothelial nitric oxide (NO) synthase. Increased NO production causes vasodilatation and has the potential to improve endothelial function.

USES

1. Hypertension β blockers are relatively mild antihypertensives. All agents, irrespective of associated properties, are nearly equally effective. β blockers are now generally used to suppliment other drugs, but are no longer first line antihypertensives (*see* Ch. 11).

2. Angina pectoris All β blockers benefit angina of effort, but the selective $β_1$ blockers are preferred. Taken on a regular schedule, they decrease frequency of attacks and increase exercise tolerance (*see* Ch. 11).

3. Cardiac arrhythmias β blockers suppress extrasystoles and tachycardias, especially those mediated adrenergically (during anaesthesia, digitalis induced). They may be used i.v. for this purpose. Esmolol is an alternative drug for paroxysmal supraventricular tachycardia (*see* Ch. 12).

4. Myocardial infarction (MI) In relation to MI, β blockers are used for two purposes:
(a) Secondary prophylaxis of MI: there is now firm evidence of benefit. Long-term therapy after recovery from MI has been found to decrease subsequent mortality by 20%.
(b) Myocardial salvage during evolution of MI: administered i.v. within 4–6 hours of an attack followed by continued oral therapy. β blockers—
  (i) May limit infarct size by reducing O_2 consumption.

(ii) May prevent arrhythmias including ventricular fibrillation.

However, β blockers can be given to only those patients not in shock or cardiac failure.

5. *Congestive heart failure* Although β blockers can worsen heart failure, several studies have reported beneficial haemodynamic effects of certain $β_1$ blockers in selected patients with dilated cardiomyopathy. Introduced gradually and maintained for long term, these drugs retard the progression of CHF and prolong life. The benefit may result from antagonism of deleterious effects of sympathetic overactivity on myocardium.

6. *Dissecting aortic aneurysm* β blockers help by reducing cardiac contractile force and aortic pulsation.

7. *Pheochromocytoma* β blockers may be added to α blockers to control tachycardia and arrhythmia, but should never be used alone.

8. *Thyrotoxicosis* Propranolol rapidly controls sympathetic symptoms (palpitation, nervousness, tremor, fixed stare, severe myopathy and sweating) without significantly affecting thyroid status. It is used before partial thyroidectomy, and while awaiting response to antithyroid drugs/radioactive iodine.

9. *Migraine* Propranolol is the most effective drug for chronic prophylaxis of migraine.

10. *Anxiety* Propranolol exerts an apparent antianxiety effect, especially under conditions which provoke nervousness and panic, e.g. examination, unaccustomed public appearance, etc. This is probably due to blockade of peripheral manifestations of anxiety (palpitation, tremor) which have a reinforcing effect on anxiety.

11. *Essential tremor* Nonselective β blockers have an established place in treating essential tremor.

12. *Glaucoma* Timolol and other ocular β blockers are commonly used for chronic simple (wide angle) glaucoma. They are also used as adjuvant in angle closure glaucoma.

13. *Hypertrophic obstructive cardiomyopathy* In this condition, the subaortic region is hypertrophic. β blockers improve c.o. in these patients during exercise, by reducing left ventricular outflow obstruction.

α + β ADRENERGIC BLOCKERS

Labetalol It is the first adrenergic antagonist capable of blocking both α and β receptors. The β blocking potency is about 1/3rd that of propranolol, while the α blocking potency is about 1/10th of phentolamine.

Labetalol is 3-5 times more potent in blocking β than α receptors. As such, effects of a low dose resemble those of propranolol alone; while at high doses, they are like a combination of propranolol and prazosin. It causes fall in BP which is attended by no change or slight decrease or increase in heart rate.

Labetalol is orally effective, but undergoes considerable first pass metabolism. It is a moderately potent hypotensive, and is especially useful in pheochromocytoma, pregnancy induced hypertension, and other hypertensive emergencies, as well as in essential hypertension. Most important side effect is postural hypotension, though other side effects of α and β blockers can also occur.

Carvedilol It is a $β_1 + β_2 + α_1$ adrenoceptor blocker which produces vasodilatation due to $α_1$ blockade as well as calcium channel blockade, and has antioxidant property. Carvedilol has been used in hypertension and is the β blocker especially employed as cardioprotective in CHF.

CHAPTER 7

Autacoids and Related Drugs

Autacoid This term is derived from Greek: *autos*—self, *akos*—healing substance or remedy. Autacoids are diverse substances produced by a *wide variety of cells* in the body, having intense biological activity, but generally *act locally* (e.g. within inflammatory pockets) at the site of synthesis and release.

They have also been called 'local hormones'. However, they differ from 'hormones' in two important ways—hormones are produced by *specific cells*, and are transported through circulation to act on *distant target tissues*.

Autacoids are involved in a number of physiological and pathological processes (especially inflammation and immunological reaction). Some autacoids, in addition, serve as transmitters or modulators in the nervous system. A number of useful drugs act by modifying their action or metabolism. The classical autacoids are—

Amine autacoids Histamine, 5-Hydroxytryptamine (Serotonin).

Lipid-derived autacoids Prostaglandins, Leukotrienes, Platelet activating factor.

Peptide autacoids Plasma kinins (Bradykinin, Kallidin), Angiotensin.

In addition, cytokines (interleukins, TNFα, GM-CSF, etc.) and several peptides like gastrin, somatostatin, vasoactive intestinal peptide, endothelins and many others may be considered as autacoids.

HISTAMINE

Histamine, meaning 'tissue amine' (*histos*—tissue) is almost ubiquitously present in animal tissues and in certain plants, e.g. stinging nettle.

Histamine is present primarily within storage granules of *mast cells*. Tissues rich in histamine are skin, gastric and intestinal mucosa, lungs, liver and placenta. Nonmast cell histamine occurs in brain, epidermis, gastric mucosa and at growing regions. Turnover of mast cell histamine is slow, while that of nonmast cell histamine is fast. Histamine is also present in blood, most body secretions, venoms and pathological fluids.

Synthesis, storage and destruction

Histamine is β imidazolylethylamine. It is synthesized locally from the amino acid histidine and degraded rapidly by oxidation and methylation (Fig. 7.1). Histamine is positively charged, and is held within mast cell granules by an acidic protein as well as heparin which are negatively charged. When the granules are extruded by exocytosis, Na^+ ions in e.c.f. exchange with histamine to release it in free form (Fig. 7.2). Increase in intracellular cAMP (caused by β adrenergic agonists and theophylline) inhibits histamine

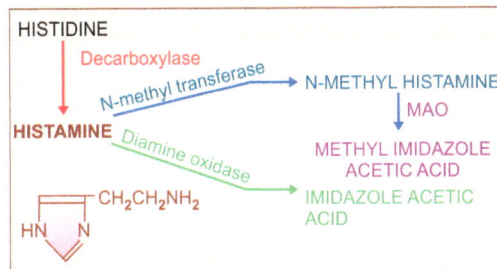

Fig. 7.1: Synthesis and degradation of histamine
MAO: Monoamine oxidase

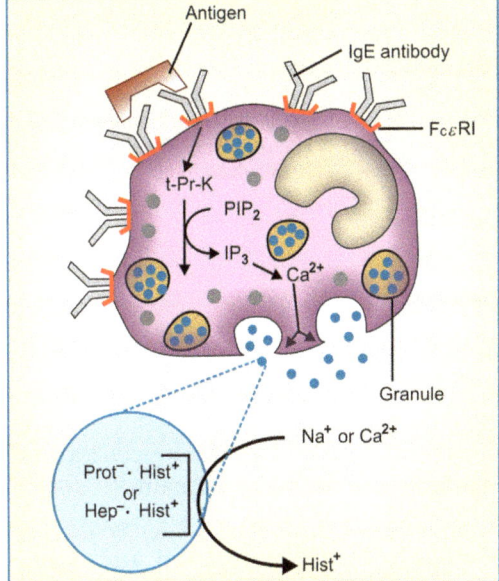

Fig. 7.2: Mechanism of antigen-antibody reaction induced release of histamine from mast cell

In sensitized atopic individual, specific reaginic (IgE) antibody is produced and gets bound to Fc epsilon receptor I (FcεRI) on the surface of mast cells. On challenge, the antigen bridges IgE molecules resulting in transmembrane activation of a tyrosine-protein kinase (t-Pr-K) which phosphorylates and activates phospholipase-Cγ. Phosphatidyl inositol bisphosphate (PIP_2) is hydrolysed and inositol trisphosphate (IP_3) is generated which triggers intracellular release of Ca^{2+}. The Ca^{2+} ions induce fusion of granule membrane with plasma membrane of the mast cell resulting in exocytotic release of granule contents. In the granule, positively charged histamine ($Hist^+$) is held complexed with negatively charged protein ($Prot^-$) and heparin (Hep^-) molecules. Cationic exchange with extracellular Na^+ (and Ca^{2+}) sets histamine free to act on the target cells.

release. Histamine is inactive orally because liver degrades all histamine that is absorbed from the intestines.

Histamine receptors Analogous to adrenergic α and β receptors, histaminergic receptors are classified into H_1 and H_2. Two more receptor subtypes (H_3 and H_4) have been identified and cloned subsequently, but have no clinical implication yet. The important features of H_1 and H_2 histamine receptors are given in Table 7.1.

PHARMACOLOGICAL ACTIONS

1. Blood vessels Histamine causes marked dilatation of smaller blood vessels, including arterioles, capillaries and venules. On s.c. injection flushing, heat, increased heart rate and cardiac output, with little or no fall in BP are produced. Rapid i.v. injection causes fall in BP which has an early short-lasting H_1 and a slow but more persistent H_2 component. Dilatation of cranial vessels causes pulsatile headache.

Like many other autacoids and ACh, vasodilatation caused by histamine is partly (H_1 component) indirect, mediated through release of 'endothelium-dependent relaxing factor' (EDRF) which is nitric oxide (NO); the H_1 receptor being located on the endothelial cells. H_2 receptors mediating vasodilatation are located directly on the vascular smooth muscle. Histamine also causes increased capillary permeability due to separation of endothelial cells, allowing exudation of plasma. This is primarily a H_1 response.

Injected intradermally, it elicits the *triple response* consisting of:

Red spot: due to intense capillary dilatation.
Wheal: due to exudation of fluid from capillaries and venules.
Flare: i.e. redness in the surrounding area due to arteriolar dilatation mediated by axon reflex.

Chapter 7: Autacoids and Related Drugs

Table 7.1: Distinctive features of H_1 and H_2 histaminergic receptors

	H_1	H_2
1. Selective agonists (relative selectivity $H_1 : H_2$)	2-Methyl histamine (8:1) 2-Pyridylethylamine (30:1) 2-Thiazolyl ethylamine (90:1)	Dimaprit (1:2000) Impromidine (1:10,000)
2. Selective antagonists (relative selectivity $H_1 : H_2$)	Mepyramine (6000:1) Chlorpheniramine (15000:1)	Cimetidine (1: 500) Ranitidine (I : >500)
3. Receptor type	G-protein coupled	G-protein coupled
4. Effector pathway	PIP_2 hydrolysis → IP_3/DAG : Release of Ca^{2+} from intracellular stores; Protein Kinase-C activation NO release → cGMP ↑	Adenylyl cyclase activation—cAMP ↑—phosphorylation of specific proteins

5. Distribution in body: actions mediated	a. Smooth muscle (intestine, airway, uterus)—contraction
	b. Blood vessels
	  i. Endothelium: Release of EDRF, PGI_2—vasodilatation. widening of gap junctions—increased capillary permeability
	  ii. Smooth muscle of large vessels— vasoconstriction.
	c. Afferent nerve endings— stimulation
	d. Ganglionic cell—stimulation.
	e. Adrenal medulla—release of CAs.
	f. Brain—transmitter.
		a. Gastric glands—acid secretion
		b. Blood vessels (smooth muscle) —dilatation
		c. Heart
		  Atria: +ive chronotropy
		  Ventricles: +ive inotropy
		d. Uterus (rat)—relaxation
		e. Brain—transmitter

PIP_2—Phosphatidyl inositol bisphosphate; IP_3—Inositol trisphosphate; DAG—Diacylglycerols; EDRF—Endothelium dependent relaxing factor: PGI_2—Prostacyclin; NO—Nitric oxide CAs—Catecholamines: cAMP—Cyclic 3', 5' adenosine monophosphate

2. Heart Direct effects of histamine on *in situ* heart are not prominent, but the isolated heart is stimulated.

3. Visceral smooth muscle Histamine causes bronchoconstriction; guinea pigs and patients of asthma are highly sensitive. Large doses cause abdominal cramps and colic by increasing intestinal contractions. Other visceral smooth muscles are not much affected.

4. Glands Histamine causes marked increase in gastric secretion—primarily of acid but also of pepsin (*see* Ch. 18). This is a direct action exerted on parietal cells through H_2 receptors and is mediated by increased cAMP generation, which in turn activates the membrane proton pump ($H^+ K^+$ ATPase).

5. Sensory nerve endings Itching occurs when histamine is injected i.v. or intracutaneously. Higher concentrations injected more deeply cause pain.

6. Autonomic ganglia and adrenal medulla Ganglia are stimulated and Adr is released, which can cause a secondary rise in BP.

PATHOPHYSIOLOGICAL ROLES

1. Gastric secretion Histamine has dominant physiological role in mediating secretion of HCl in the stomach (*see* Fig. 18.1). Histamine is released locally under the influence of all stimuli that evoke gastric secretion (feeding, vagal stimulation, cholinergic drugs and gastrin) and activates the proton pump (K^+H^+ATPase) through H_2 receptors to secrete HCl.

2. Allergic phenomena Released from mast cells following AG: AB reaction, histamine is causative in urticaria, angioedema, bronchoconstriction and anaphylactic shock. The H_1 antagonists are effective in controlling these manifestations to a considerable extent, except asthma and to a lesser extent anaphylactic fall in BP, in which leukotrienes (especially LTD_4) and PAF appear to be more important. Histamine is not involved in delayed or retarded type of allergic reactions.

3. *As transmitter* Histamine is believed to be the afferent transmitter which initiates the sensation of itch and pain at sensory nerve endings.

In the brain, it is involved in maintaining wakefulness; (H_1 antihistaminics owe their sedative action to blockade of this function) and appears to regulate many other functions.

4. *Inflammation* Histamine is implicated as a mediator of vasodilatation and other changes that occur during inflammation. It may also regulate microcirculation according to the local needs.

5. *Headache* Histamine has been implicated in certain vascular headaches, but there is no conclusive evidence.

Histamine has no therapeutic use. However, *beta histine,* an orally active histamine analogue, affords some relief of vertigo in Meniére's disease.

H_1 ANTAGONISTS
(Conventional antihistaminics)

These drugs competitively antagonize actions of histamine at the H_1 receptors.

Pharmacological actions

Qualitatively all H_1 antihistaminics have similar actions, but there are quantitative differences, especially in the sedative property.

1. *Antagonism of histamine* These drugs effectively block histamine induced bronchoconstriction, contraction of intestinal and other smooth muscle and triple response—especially wheal, flare and itch. Fall in BP produced by low doses of histamine is blocked, but additional H_2 antagonists are required for complete blockade of higher doses. Action of histamine on gastric secretion is singularly not affected by these drugs.

2. *Antiallergic action* Many manifestations of immediate hypersensitivity (type I reactions) are suppressed. Urticaria, itching and angioedema are well controlled. Anaphylactic fall in BP is only partially prevented. Asthma is practically unaffected in humans.

3. *CNS* The older antihistamines produce variable degree of CNS depression. This action appears to depend on the compound's ability to penetrate blood-brain barrier and its affinity for the central (compared to peripheral) H_1 receptors. Susceptibility of different individuals to sedative action of different antihistaminics varies considerably, but an overall grading is presented in Table 7.2. Some individuals also experience stimulant effects like restlessness and insomnia. Excitement and convulsions are frequently seen at toxic doses. The second generation antihistaminics are practically nonsedating.

Certain (*see* below) H_1 antihistamines are effective in preventing motion sickness. Promethazine controls vomiting of pregnancy and other causes as well.

Promethazine and a few other antihistaminics reduce tremor, rigidity and sialorrhoea of parkinsonism. Anticholinergic and sedative properties underlie the benefit. Some H_1 antihistamines are used as antitussives (*see* p. 315

Table 7.2: Clinical classification, doses and preparations of H_1 antihistaminics

Drug	Dose and route	Preparations
I. HIGHLY SEDATIVE		
Diphenhydramine	25–50 mg oral	BENADRYL 25 mg cap., 12.5 mg/5 ml syr
Dimenhydrinate	25–50 mg oral,	DRAMAMINE 16 mg/5 ml syr, 50 mg tab, GRAVOL 50 mg tab
Promethazine	25–50 mg oral, i.m. (1 mg/kg)	PHENERGAN 10, 25 mg tab., 5 mg/ml elixir, 25 mg/ml inj
Hydroxyzine	25–50 mg oral, i.m.	ATARAX 10, 25 mg tab, 10 mg/5 ml syr, 6 mg/ml drops, 25 mg/ml inj
II. MODERATELY SEDATIVE		
Pheniramine	20–50 mg oral, i.m.	AVIL 25 mg, 50 mg tab, 15 mg/5 ml syr, 22.5 mg/ml inj
Cyproheptadine	4 mg oral	PRACTIN, CIPLACTIN 4 mg tab, 2 mg/5 ml syrup,
Meclozine (Meclizine)	25–50 mg oral	In DILIGAN 12.5 mg + niacin 50 mg tab
Cinnarizine	25–50 mg oral	STUGERON, VERTIGON 25 mg and 75 mg tab
III. MILD SEDATIVE		
Chlorpheniramine	2–4 mg (0.1 mg/kg) oral, i.m.	PIRITON, CADISTIN 4 mg tab
Dexchlorpheniramine	2 mg oral	POLARAMINE 2 mg tab, 0.5 mg/5 ml syr
Triprolidine	2.5–5 mg oral	ACTIDIL 2.5 mg tab, .
Clemastine	1-2 mg oral	TAVEGYL 1 mg tab, 0.5 mg/5 ml syr
IV. SECOND GENERATION ANTIHISTAMINICS		
Fexofenadine	120–180 mg oral	ALLEGRA, ALTIVA, FEXO 120, 180 mg tab
Loratadine	10 mg oral	LORFAST, LORIDIN, LORMEG, 10 mg tab, 1 mg/ml susp
Desloratadine	5 mg oral	DESLOR, LORDAY, NEOLORIDIN 5 mg tab
Cetirizine	10 mg oral	ALERID, CETZINE, ZIRTIN, SIZON 10 mg tab, 5 mg/5ml syr
Levocetirizine	5-10 mg oral	LEVOSIZ, LEVORID, TECZINE 5, 10 mg tab. LEVOCET 5 mg tab, 2.5 mg/5ml syr
Azelastine	4 mg oral 0.28 mg intranasal	AZEP NASAL SPRAY 0.14 mg per puff nasal spray
Mizolastine	10 mg oral	ELINA 10 mg tab
Ebastine	10 mg oral	EBAST 10 mg tab
Rupatadine	10 mg oral	RUPAHIST 10 mg tab

4. *Anticholinergic action* Many H_1 blockers in addition antagonize muscarinic actions of ACh. The anticholinergic action can be graded as:

High	Low	Minimal/Absent
Promethazine	Chlorpheniramine	Fexofenadine
Diphenhydramine	Triprolidine	Loratadine
Dimenhydrinate	Cyproheptadine	Cetirizine
Pheniramine	Cinnarizine	Mizolastine

5. *Local anaesthetic* Some drugs have strong while others have weak membrane stabilizing property. However, antihistaminics are not used clinically as local anaesthetic because they cause irritation when injected s.c.

Membrane stabilizing activity also confers antiarrhythmic property to these compounds.

6. *BP* Most antihistaminics cause a fall in BP on i.v. injection due to direct smooth muscle

relaxation and weak α adrenergic blockade. However, fall in BP is not evident on oral administration.

Pharmacokinetics
The conventional H_1 antihistaminics are well absorbed from oral and parenteral routes, metabolized in the liver and excreted in urine. They are widely distributed in the body and enter brain. The newer compounds penetrate brain poorly, accounting largely for their mild/absent sedating action. Duration of action of most agents is 4–6 hours, except chlorpheniramine, loratadine, cetirizine and fexofenadine which act for 12–24 hours. On repeated use, many antihistamines induce their own metabolism.

Side effects and toxicity
Side effects with first generation H_1 antihistaminics are frequent, but are generally mild. Individuals show marked differences in susceptibility to the side effects with different drugs. Some degree of tolerance to the sedative side effects develops on repeated use.

Sedation, diminished alertness and concentration, light headedness, motor incoordination, fatigue and tendency to fall asleep are the most common. Objective testing shows impairment of psychomotor performance. Patients should be cautioned not to operate motor vehicles or machinery requiring constant attention. Alcohol synergises in producing these effects as do other CNS depressants. Few individuals, however, become restless, nervous and are unable to sleep. Second generation compounds are largely free of CNS effects.

Dryness of mouth, alteration of bowel movement, urinary hesitancy and blurring of vision can be ascribed to anticholinergic property.

Epigastric distress and headache may be felt. Local application can cause contact dermatitis.

SECOND GENERATION ANTIHISTAMINICS

The second generation antihistaminics (SGAs) may be defined as those H_1 receptor blockers marketed after 1980 which have one or more of the following properties:
- Absence of CNS depressant property.
- Higher H_1 selectivitiy: no anticholinergic side effects.
- Additional antiallergic mechanisms apart from histamine blockade; such as modification of release or action of leukotrienes, PAF and cytokines.

These newer drugs have the advantage of not impairing psychomotor performance (driving, etc. need not be contraindicated), produce no subjective effects, no sleepiness, do not potentiate alcohol or benzodiazepines. Some patients do complain of sedation, but incidence is similar to that with placebo. However, SGAs have a narrow spectrum of therapeutic usefulness which is limited by the extent of involvement of histamine (acting through H_1 receptors) in the disease state. The principal indications of SGAs are:
- Allergic rhinitis and conjunctivitis, hay fever, pollinosis; they control sneezing, runny but not blocked nose, and red, watering, itchy eyes.
- Urticaria, dermographism, atopic eczema.
- Acute allergic reactions to drugs and foods.

SGAs have poor antipruritic, antiemetic and antitussive actions.

A life-threatening adverse effect due to overdose or drug interaction occurred with some SGAs. Terfenadine, the first SGA introduced clinically, was found to cause polymorphic ventricular tachycardia (*Torsades de pointes*) in a few patients. The risk was markedly increased in liver disease or when erythromycin, clarithromycin, ketoconazole or itraconazole (inhibitors of CYP 3A4) were given concurrently. This adverse effect occurs due to blockade of cardiac K^+ channels by high concentrations of terfenadine (but not by its active metabolite). Similar incidences have been reported with astemizole and are possible with ebastine, but not with other SGAs. Terfenadine and astemizole are banned.

Fexofenadine It is the active metabolite of terfenadine which does not block delayed rectifier K⁺ channels in the heart—does not prolong QTc interval. Therefore, it has been introduced as a substitute of terfenadine which is largely free of arrhythmogenic potential. Sedative and atropinic side effects are minimal/absent.

Loratadine Another long-acting selective peripheral H_1 antagonist which lacks CNS depressant effects and is fast acting. Good efficacy has been reported in urticaria and atopic dermatitis.

Desloratadine is the major active metabolite of loratadine with similar properties and is effective at half the dose.

Cetirizine It has high affinity for peripheral H_1, receptors and penetrates brain poorly, but subjective somnolence and mild sedation is felt by many recipients. In addition to H_1 blockade, it inhibits release of histamine and cytotoxic mediators from platelets. Eosinophil chemotaxis during the secondary phase of the allergic response is also interfered. Thus, it may benefit allergic disorders by other actions as well. Cetirizine is indicated in upper respiratory allergies, pollinosis, urticaria and atopic dermatitis.

Its active R(–) enantiomer has been marketed as *Levocetirizine*, which is claimed to produce fewer side effects.

Azelastine This newer H_1 blocker has good topical activity. Given by nasal spray for seasonal and perennial allergic rhinitis, it provides quick symptomatic relief lasting 12 hr. Stinging in the nose and altered taste perception are the local side effects.

USES

The uses of H_1 antihistaminics are based on their ability to block certain effects of histamine released endogeneously, as well as on their sedative and anticholinergic properties.

1. *Allergic disorders* Antihistaminics do not suppress AG: AB reaction, but block the effects of released histamine—are only palliative. They effectively control certain immediate type of allergies, e.g. itching, urticaria, seasonal hay fever, allergic conjunctivitis and angioedema of lips, eyelids, etc. in which histamine is a major mediator. However, their action is slow; therefore, Adr alone is life saving in laryngeal angioedema. Similarly, they cannot be relied upon in anaphylactic shock and have a secondary place to Adr. Benefits are less marked in perennial vasomotor rhinitis, atopic dermatitis and chronic urticarias.

Certain newer compounds like cetirizine have adjuvant role in seasonal asthma.

Type I hypersensitivity reactions to drugs (except asthma and anaphylaxis) are suppressed. Some skin rashes also respond.

2. *Other conditions involving histamine* The H_1 blockers afford symptomatic relief in insect bite and ivy poisoning. Abnormal dermographism is suppressed. They have prophylactic value in blood/saline infusion induced rigor.

3. *Pruritides (Itching)* Though relief is often incomplete, older antihistaminics like chlorpheniramine, diphenhydramine remain the first choice drugs for itching.

4. *Common cold* Antihistaminics do not affect the course of the illness, but may afford symptomatic relief by anticholinergic (reduce rhinorrhoea) and sedative actions. The newer nonsedating antihistamines are less effective in this respect.

5. *Motion sickness* Promethazine, diphenhydramine, dimenhydrinate and meclozine have prophylactic value in motion sickness. They should be taken one hour before starting journey. Promethazine can also be used in morning sickness, drug induced and postoperative vomiting.

6. *Vertigo* Vertigo is primarily a vestibular disorder producing sense of rotation of

surroundings or movement when there is none. Cinnarizine is the H1 antihistaminic having additional anticholinergic, anti-5-HT, sedative and vasodilator properties which has been widely used in vertigo. It inhibits vestibular sensory nuclei in the inner ear, possibly by reducing stimulated influx of Ca2+ from endolymph into the vestibular sensory cells. Dimenhydrinate is also used for vertigo.

7. *Preanaesthetic medication* Promethazine has been used in preanaesthetic medication for its anticholinergic and sedative properties.

8. *Cough* Antihistaminics like chlorpheniramine, diphenhydramine, promethazine are constituents of many popular cough remedies. They have no selective cough suppressant action, but may afford symptomatic relief by sedative and anticholinergic action.

9. *Parkinsonism* Promethazine and some others afford mild symptomatic relief in early cases. This is based on their anticholinergic and sedative property.

10. *Acute muscle dystonia* Caused by antiemetic-antipsychotic drugs is promptly relieved by parenteral promethazine or hydroxyzine. This is again based on central anticholinergic action of the drugs.

11. *As sedative, hypnotic, anxiolytic* Antihistamines with CNS depressant action have been used as sedative and to induce sleep, but are not as dependable as benzodiazepines. Promethazine, commonly used to sedate children, has produced severe respiratory depression in some young children. It is contraindicated below 2 years age.

H_2 antagonists They are primarily used in peptic ulcer and other gastric hypersecretory states (*see* Ch. 18).

5-HYDROXYTRYPTAMINE (5-HT, Serotonin)

Serotonin was the name given to the vasoconstrictor substance which appeared in serum when blood clotted, and was shown to be *5-hydroxytryptamine* (5-HT). About 90% of body's content of 5-HT is localized in the intestines; most of the rest is in platelets and brain.

Synthesis, storage and destruction

5-HT is synthesized from the amino acid tryptophan and degraded primarily by MAO and to a small extent by a dehydrogenase (Fig. 7.3).

Like NA, 5-HT is actively taken up by an amine pump *serotonin transporter* (SERT) which operates at the membrane of platelets (therefore, 5-HT does not circulate in free form in plasma) and that of serotonergic nerve endings. This pump is inhibited by tricyclic antidepressants and selective serotonin reuptake inhibitors (SSRIs). Again, like CAs, 5-HT is stored within storage vesicles and its uptake at the vesicular membrane is inhibited by reserpine.

Serotonergic (5-HT) receptors

Four families of 5-HT receptors (5-HT$_1$, 5-HT$_2$, 5-HT$_3$, 5-HT$_{4-7}$) comprising of 14 receptor subtypes have so far been recognized. However, only some of these have been functionally correlated or their selective agonists/antagonists defined. Knowledge of subtypes of 5-HT receptors is important, because some newer drugs can only be described as 5-HT receptor subtype selective agonists or antagonists.

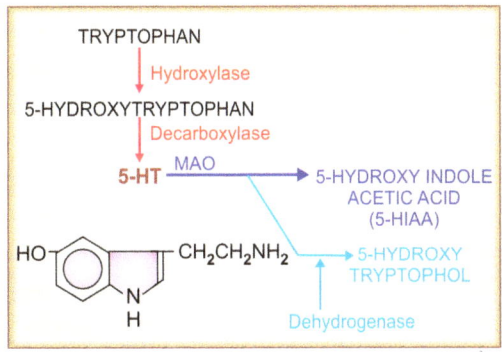

Fig. 7.3: Synthesis and degradation of 5-hydroxytryptamine (5-HT)

Important 5-HT receptor subtypes

5-HT$_1$: Autoreceptors; which inhibit serotonergic neural activity in brain.

    5-HT$_{1A}$—present in raphe nuclei and hippocampus; *buspirone* appears to exert antianxiety action through these receptors.

    5-HT$_{1B/1D}$—constricts cranial blood vessels and inhibits release of inflammatory neuropeptides in them; *sumatriptan* controls migraine through these receptors.

5-HT$_{2A}$: Most important postjunctional receptor mediating direct actions of 5-HT like vascular and visceral smooth muscle contraction, platelet aggregation, neuronal activation in brain; *ketanserin* blocks these receptors.

5-HT$_3$: Depolarizes neurones by gating cation channels; elicits reflex effects of 5-HT, such as emesis, gut peristalsis, bradycardia, transient hypotension, apnoea, pain, and itch. *Ondansetron* acts as antiemetic by blocking these receptors.

5-HT$_4$: Mediate intestinal secretion, augmentation of peristalsis. *Renzapride* is a selective 5-HT$_4$ agonist.

All 5-HT receptors (except 5-HT$_3$) are G protein coupled receptors, while the 5-HT$_3$ is a ligand gated cation (Na$^+$, K$^+$) channel which on activation elicits fast depolarization.

Actions

5-HT is a potent depolarizer of nerve endings. It thus exerts direct as well as reflex and indirect effects. Tachyphylaxis is common with repeated doses of 5-HT. The overall effects, therefore, are often variable; important ones are:

1. Constriction of larger arteries and veins, but dilatation of arterioles: variable and phasic effect on BP.
2. Isolated heart is stimulated, but in the intact animal bradycardia due to coronary chemoreflex predominates.
3. Enhanced peristalsis and secretion in gut causing diarrhoea.
4. Inhibition of gastric acid and pepsin secretion; augmentation of mucus production in stomach exerting ulceroprotective effect.
5. Activation of afferent nerve endings causing tingling or pricking sensation, pain; cardiovascular and respiratory reflexes are elicited.
6. Proaggregatory action on platelets.

Pathophysiological roles

The functions ascribed to 5-HT are:

1. Neurotransmitter in brain; involved in sleep, temperature regulation, cognitive function, behavior and mood, vomiting and pain perception.
2. Regulation of gut peristalsis.
3. Precursor of melatonin in pineal gland: regulation of biological clock.
4. Control of anterior pituitary hormone function by hypothalamus.
5. Nausea and vomiting, especially that evoked by cancer chemotherapy/radiotherapy.
6. Migraine: probably involved in initiating constriction of cranial vessels and inducing neurogenic inflammation of vessel wall.
7. Haemostasis: by promoting platelet aggregation and blood vessel retraction.
8. Vasospastic disorders like Raynaud's phenomenon and variant angina.
9. Carcinoid syndrome: 5-HT mediates bowel hypermotility and bronchoconstriction.

PROSTAGLANDINS AND LEUKOTRIENES
(Eicosanoids)

Prostaglandins (PGs) and Leukotrienes (LTs) are biologically active derivatives of 20 carbon atom polyunsaturated essential fatty acids that are released from cell membrane phospholipids. They are the major lipid-derived autacoids.

Chemistry, biosynthesis and degradation

Chemically, PGs may be considered to be derivatives of *prostanoic acid*, though prostanoic acid does not naturally occur in the body. Prostanoic acid has a five membered ring and two side chains projecting in opposite directions at right angle to the plane of the ring. There are many series of PGs designated A, B, C,..., I, and thromboxanes (TXs) depending on the ring structure and the substituents on it. Each series has members with subscript 1, 2, 3 indicating the number of double bonds in the side chains.

Leukotrienes are so named because they were first obtained from leukocytes (*leuko*) and have 3 conjugated double bonds (*triene*). They have also been similarly designated A, B, C,..., F and given subscripts 1, 2, 3, 4.

In the body PGs, TXs and LTs are all derived from 5,8,11,14 *eicosa tetraenoic acid (arachidonic acid)*. During PG, TX and prostacyclin (PGI) synthesis, 2 of the 4 double bonds of arachidonic acid get saturated in the process of cyclization, leaving 2 double bonds in the side chain. Thus, subscript 2 PGs are the most important in man, e.g. PGE_2, $PGF_{2\alpha}$, PGI_2, TXA_2. No cyclization or reduction of double bonds occurs during LT synthesis—the LTs of biological importance are LTB_4, LTC_4, LTD_4.

Eicosanoids are the most universally distributed autacoids in the body. Practically, every cell and tissue is capable of synthesizing one or more types of PGs or LTs. The pathways of biosynthesis of eicosanoids are summarized in Fig. 7.4.

There are no preformed stores of PGs and LTs. They are synthesized locally, and the rate of synthesis is governed by the rate of release of arachidonic acid from membrane lipids in response to appropriate stimuli. These stimuli activate hydrolases, including phospholipase A.

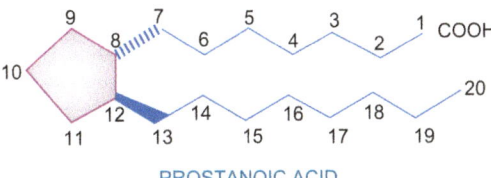

PROSTANOIC ACID

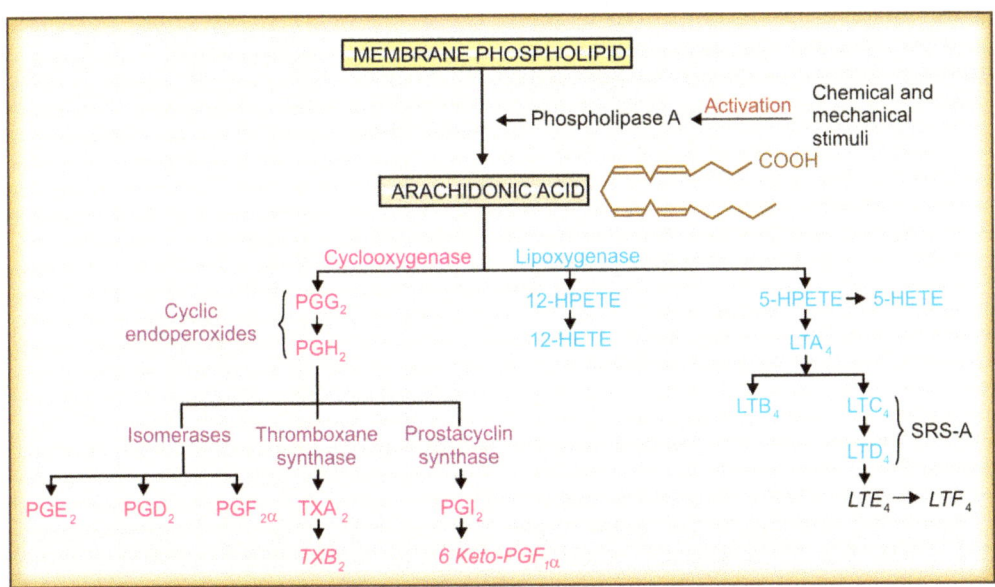

Fig. 7.4: Biosynthesis of prostaglandins (PG) and leukotrienes (LT). Less active metabolites are shown in italics

TX—Thromboxane, PGI—Prostacyclin; HPETE—Hydroperoxy eicosatetraenoic acid (Hydroperoxy arachidonic acid); HETE—Hydroxyeicosatetraenoic acid (Hydroxy arachidonic acid); SRS-A—Slow-reacting substance of anaphylaxis

Cyclooxygenase (COX) pathway It generates eicosanoids with a ring structure (PGs, TXs, prostacyclin) while *lipoxygenase* (LOX) produces open chain compounds (LTs). All tissues have COX—can form cyclic endoperoxides PGG_2 and PGH_2 which are unstable compounds. Further course in a particular tissue depends on the type of isomerases or other enzymes present in it. PGE_2 and $PGF_{2\alpha}$ are the major prostaglandins. Lung and spleen can synthesize the whole range of COX products. Platelets primarily synthesize TXA_2 which is chemically unstable, spontaneously changes to TXB_2. Endothelium mainly generates prostacyclin (PGI_2) that is also chemically unstable and rapidly converts to 6-keto $PGF_{1\alpha}$.

The cyclooxygenase enzyme is known to exist in two isoforms COX-1 and COX-2. While both isoforms catalyse the same reactions, COX-1 is a constitutive enzyme in most cells, i.e. it is synthesized even in the basal unstimulated state, and the level of COX-1 does not change much once the cell is fully grown. On the other hand, COX-2 normally present in insignificant amounts, is inducible by cytokines, growth factors and other stimuli during the inflammatory response. It is believed that eicosanoids produced by COX-1 participate in physiological (house keeping) functions such as secretion of mucus for protection of gastric mucosa, haemostasis and maintenance of renal function, while those produced by COX-2 lead to inflammatory and other pathological changes. However, certain sites in the kidney and brain constitutively express COX-2 which may play physiological role.

Lipoxygenase pathway It appears to operate mainly in the lung, WBC and platelets. Its most important products are the LTs, (generated by 5-LOX), particularly LTB_4 (potent chemotactic) and LTC_4, LTD_4 which together constitute the *'slow reacting substance of anaphylaxis'* (SRS-A).

Inhibition of synthesis

Synthesis of COX products can be inhibited by nonsteroidal anti-inflammatory drugs (NSAIDs). Aspirin acetylates COX at a serine residue and causes irreversible inhibition, while other NSAIDs are competitive and reversible inhibitors. Most NSAIDs are nonselective COX-1 and COX-2 inhibitors, but some later ones like celecoxib, etoricoxib are selective for COX-2.

NSAIDs do not inhibit the production of LTs. Rather, production of LTs may be increased since all the arachidonic acid becomes available to the LOX pathway.

Glucocorticosteroids inhibit the release of arachidonic acid from membrane lipids (by enhancing production of proteins called *annexins* which inhibit phospholipase A_2). Thus, they indirectly reduce production of all eicosanoids—PGs, TXs and LTs. Moreover, steroids inhibit the induction of COX-2 by cytokines at the site of inflammation.

Degradation

Biotransformation of arachidonates occurs rapidly in most tissues, but fastest in the lungs. Most PGs, TXA_2 and prostacyclin have plasma t½ of a few seconds to a few minutes. First a specific carrier mediated uptake into cells occurs, the side chains are then oxidized and double bonds are reduced in a stepwise manner to yield inactive metabolites. Metabolites are excreted in urine. PGI_2 is catabolized mainly in the kidney.

PROSTAGLANDINS, THROMBOXANES AND PROSTACYCLIN

Actions

The cyclic eicosanoids produce a wide variety of actions depending upon the particular PG (or TX or PGI), species on which tested, tissue, hormonal status and other factors. PGs differ in their potency to produce a given action and different PGs sometimes have opposite effects. Even the same PG may have opposite effects under different circumstances. The actions of biologically important PGs (PGE_2, $PGF_{2\alpha}$, PGI_2, TXA_2) are summarized in Table 7.3.

Table 7.3: A summary of the actions of major prostaglandins, prostacyclin and thromboxane

Organ	Prostaglandin E$_2$ (PGE$_2$)	Prostaglandin F$_{2\alpha}$ (PGF$_{2\alpha}$)	Prostacyclin (PGI$_2$)	Thromboxane A$_2$ (TXA$_2$)
1. Blood vessels	Vasodilatation, ↓ BP	Constricts larger veins and some arteries, little effect on BP	Vasodilatation (marked and widespread), ↓ BP	Vasoconstriction
2. Heart	Weak inotropic, reflex cardiac stimulation	Weak inotropic	—	—
3. Platelets	Variable effect	—	Antiaggregatory	Aggregation and release reaction
4. Uterus	Contraction (*in vivo*), softening of cervix	Contraction (*in vivo* and *in vitro*), softening of cervix	—	Contraction (*in vitro*)
5. Bronchi	Dilatation, inhibit histamine release	Constriction	Dilatation (mild), inhibit histamine release	Constriction
6. Stomach	↓ acid secretion, ↑ mucus production	—	↓ acid secretion (weak action), mucosal vasodilatation	—
7. Intestine	Contracts longitudinal & relaxes circular muscles, ↑ peristalsis, ↑ Cl⁻ & water secretion	Spasmogenic, ↑ fluid & electrolyte secretion (weak action)	Weak spasmogenic, inhibit toxin-induced fluid secretion	Weak spasmogenic
8. Kidney	Natriuresis, ↓ Cl⁻ reabsorption, inhibit ADH action, vasodilatation, renin release	—	Natriuresis, vasodilatation, renin release	Vasoconstriction
9. CNS	Pyrogenic	—	—	—
10. Afferent nerves	Sensitize to noxious stimuli → tenderness	—	Same as PGE$_2$	—
11. Endocrine system	Release of ant. pituitary hormones, steroids, insulin; TSH-like action	—	—	—
12. Metabolism	Antilipolytic, insulin-like action, mobilization of bone Ca^2	—	—	—

Patho-physiological roles

Since virtually all cells and tissues are capable of forming PGs, these autacoids have been implicated as mediators or modulators of a number of physiological processes and pathological states.

1. PGs have no role in regulating systemic BP, but PGI_2 generated by vascular endothelium is probably involved in the regulation of local vascular tone as a dilator.
2. PGE_2 is continuously produced locally in the ductus arteriosus during foetal life and keeps it patent. At birth its synthesis stops and closure occurs. Aspirin and indomethacin have been found to induce closure by inhibiting PG synthesis.
3. PGs, along with LTs and other autacoids may mediate vasodilatation and exudation at the site of inflammation.
4. TXA_2 (produced by platelets) and PGI_2 (produced by vascular endothelium) probably constitute a mutually antagonistic system: preventing aggregation of platelets while in circulation and inducing aggregation on injury, when plugging and thrombosis are needed.

    Aspirin interferes with haemostasis by inhibiting platelet aggregation. TXA_2 produced by platelet COX-1 amplifies platelet aggregation. Before it is deacetylated in the liver, aspirin acetylates COX-1 in platelets while they are in portal circulation. This action is long lasting, because platelets are unable to regenerate fresh COX-1 (lack nucleus: do not synthesize protein). On the other hand, vessel wall is able to regenerate fresh COX enzyme; inhibition of PGI_2 synthesis is brief. Therefore, in low doses, aspirin selectively inhibits TXA_2 production and has antithrombotic effect lasting > 3 days.
5. PGs produced by foetal tissues at term probably mediate initiation and progression of labour. Aspirin has been found to delay the initiation of labour and also prolongs its duration.
6. Dysmenorrhoea occurring in some women is due to uterine cramps and ischaemia induced by increased PG synthesis by endometrium. Aspirin group of drugs are highly effective in relieving dysmenorrhoea in most women.
7. PGs may be involved in mediating toxin induced increased fluid movement in secretory diarrhoeas. PGs appear to play a role in the growth of colonic polyps and colon cancer. Regular intake of low dose aspirin lowers incidence of colon cancer.
8. PGs (especially PGI_2) may be functioning as natural ulcer protectives by enhancing gastric mucus and bicarbonate production as well as by improving mucosal circulation. The ulcerogenic action of NSAIDs may be due to loss of this protective influence.
9. PGs appear to function as intrarenal regulators of blood flow as well as tubular reabsorption in kidney. Accordingly, the NSAIDs tend to retain salt and water. The diuretic action of furosemide is blunted by indomethacin. This indicates a facilitatory role of PGs by increasing renal blood flow and/or augmenting inhibition of tubular reabsorption.
10. PGE_2 may mediate bacterial or other pyrogen-induced fever and malaise at the level of hypothalamus. Aspirin and other inhibitors of PG synthesis are antipyretic.
11. PGs (especially E_2 and I_2) sensitize afferent nerve endings to pain inducing chemical and mechanical stimuli (Fig. 7.5). They irritate mucous membranes and produce long lasting dull pain on intradermal injection.

    PGs appear to serve as algesic agents during inflammation. They cause tenderness and amplify the action of other algesics. Inhibition of PG synthesis is a major anti-inflammatory mechanism.
12. $PGF_{2\alpha}$ lowers intraocular tension (i.o.t.) by enhancing uveoscleral and trabecular outflow of aqueous humor. Several nonirritating PG congeners like *latanoprost* are first line drugs for open angle glaucoma.

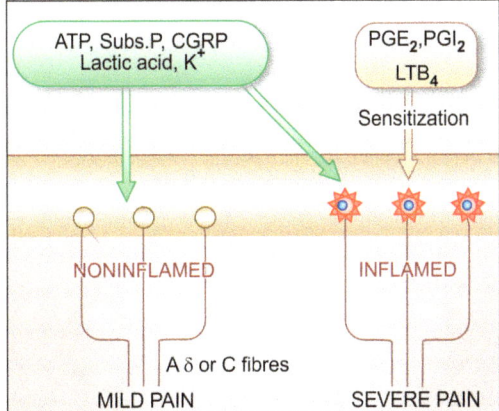

Fig. 7.5: Sensitization of nociceptors (pain receptors) to mediators of pain by prostaglandins at the inflammatory site

LEUKOTRIENES

The straight chain lipoxygenase products of arachidonic acid are produced by a limited number of tissues. The LTB_4 is produced mainly by neutrophils, while the LTC_4 and LTD_4 (the cysteinyl LTs) are produced primarily by macrophages. However, they are pathophysiologically as important as PGs.

1. CVS and blood LTC_4 and LTD_4 injected i.v. evoke a brief rise in BP followed by a more prolonged fall. The fall in BP is not due to vasodilatation, because no relaxant action has been seen on blood vessels. It is probably a result of coronary constriction induced decrease in cardiac output and reduction in circulating volume due to increased capillary permeability. These LTs markedly increase capillary permeability and are more potent than histamine in causing local edema formation.

The LTB_4 is highly chemotactic for T-lymphocytes, neutrophils and monocytes. Migration of neutrophils through capillaries and their clumping at sites of inflammation in tissues is also promoted by LTB_4. The LTC_4 and LTD_4 are chemotactic for eosinophils.

Role LTs are important mediators of inflammation. They are produced (along with PGs) locally at the site of injury. While LTC_4 and D_4 cause exudation of plasma, LTB_4 attracts the inflammatory cells which reinforce the reaction. These LTs play greater role in chronic inflammatory states.

2. Visceral smooth muscle LTC_4 and D_4 contract most smooth muscles. They are potent bronchoconstrictors and induce spastic contraction of g.i.t. at low concentrations.

They also increase mucus secretion in the airways.

Role The cysteinyl LTs (C_4 and D_4) are the most important mediators of human allergic asthma. They are released along with PGs and other autacoids during AG: AB reaction in the lungs. In comparison to other mediators, they are more potent and are metabolized slowly in the lungs, therefore exert a long lasting action. LTs may also be responsible for abdominal colics during systemic anaphylaxis.

3. Afferent nerves Like PGE_2 and I_2, the LTB_4 also sensitizes afferents carrying pain impulses, thereby contributes to pain and tenderness of inflammation.

PROSTANOID RECEPTORS

PGs, TX and prostacyclin act on their own specific receptors located on cell membrane. Five major types of prostanoid receptors have been designated, each after the natural PG for which it has the greatest affinity. Viz. DP (for PGD_2), EP (for PGE_2) FP (for $PGF_{2\alpha}$), IP (for prostacyclin or PGI_2) and TP (for TXA_2). All prostanoid receptors are G-protein coupled receptors which utilize the IP_3/DAG or cAMP transducer mechanisms. Prostanoid receptors have been categorized into three groups (Fig. 7.6).

- 'Contractile' group (EP_1, FP, TP): They cause smooth muscle contraction, platelet aggregation, etc.
- 'Relaxant' group (DP_1, EP_2, EP_4, IP): They cause smooth muscle relaxation, inhibition of platelet aggregation, etc.

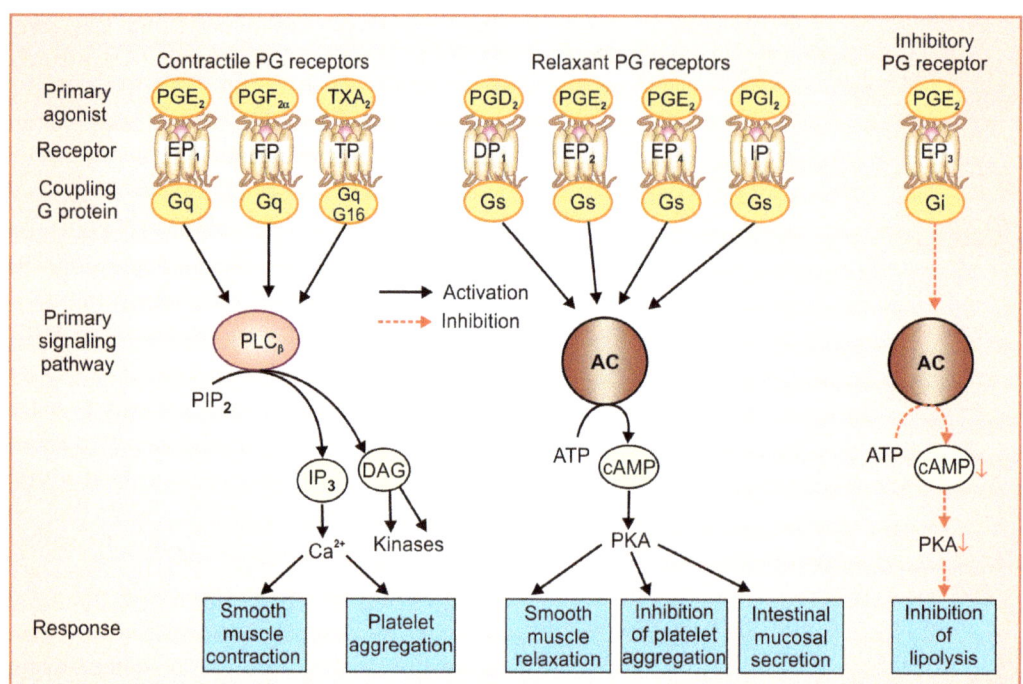

Fig. 7.6: Prostanoid receptors, their primary signaling pathways and major responses elicited through them. All prostanoid receptors are G-protein coupled receptors. On the basis of their functional characterization, prostanoid receptors have been grouped into contractile, relaxant and inhibitory groups.
PLC_β—Phospholipase Cβ; IP_3—Inositol trisphosphate; DAG—Diacyl glycerol; AC—Adenylyl cyclase; cAMP—Cyclic AMP; PKA—Protein kinase A.

- 'Inhibitory' group (EP_3): It causes inhibition of lipolysis.

LEUKOTRIENE RECEPTORS

Separate receptors for LTB_4 (designated BLT), and for the cysteinyl LTs (designated *cys* LT_1 and *cys* LT_2 for LTC_4, LTD_4) have been defined. All LT receptors function through the IP_3/DAG transducer mechanism. The *cys* LT_1 receptor is expressed in bronchial and intestinal muscle. Few *cys* LT_1 receptor antagonists, *viz.* Montelukast, Zafirlukast, are now valuable drugs for bronchial asthma (*see* Ch. 19).

USES

The clinically useful natural and synthetic prostaglandins are listed in the chart below.

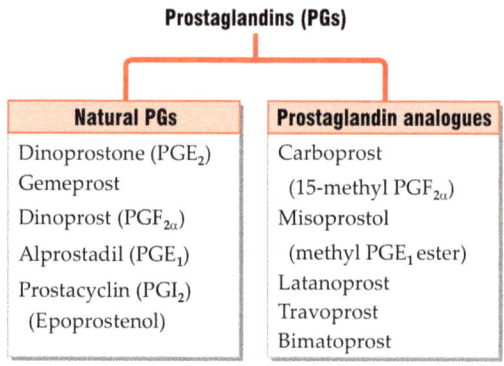

Prostaglandins (PGs)

Natural PGs	Prostaglandin analogues
Dinoprostone (PGE_2)	Carboprost
Gemeprost	(15-methyl $PGF_{2\alpha}$)
Dinoprost ($PGF_{2\alpha}$)	Misoprostol
Alprostadil (PGE_1)	(methyl PGE_1 ester)
Prostacyclin (PGI_2)	Latanoprost
(Epoprostenol)	Travoprost
	Bimatoprost

Clinical use of PGs and their analogues is rather restricted because of short lasting action, cost, side effects and other practical considerations. Their approved indications are:

1. **Abortion:** Single oral dose of misoprostol after 2 days of mifepristone (antiprogestin)

priming is used to terminate pregnancy of up to 7 weeks duration. Extra- or intra- amniotic injection of PGE_2 or $PGF_{2\alpha}$ can be used for 2nd trimester abortion.

2. Induction/augmentation of labour: Intravaginal PGE_2 or $PGF_{2\alpha}$ are alternative to i.v. oxytocin, but are less reliable.

3. Cervical priming (ripening): Low doses of PGE_2 applied in cervical canal/vagina make the cervix soft and more compliant for abortion/delivery.

4. Postpartum haemorrhage: Carboprost (15-methyl $PGF_{2\alpha}$) i.v. is an alternative drug to ergometrine/oxytocin to stop bleeding.

5. Peptic ulcer: Misoprostol (PGE_1 analogue) can be used to heal NSAID-associated peptic ulcer.

6. Glaucoma: Topical latanoprost/travoprost/bimatoprost that are FP receptor agonists, are first line drugs to lower i.o.t.

CHAPTER 8

General Anaesthetics and Skeletal Muscle Relaxants

GENERAL ANAESTHETICS

General anaesthetics (GAs) are drugs which produce reversible loss of all sensation and consciousness. The cardinal features of general anaesthesia are:
- Loss of all sensation, especially pain
- Sleep (unconsciousness) and amnesia
- Immobility and muscle relaxation
- Abolition of somatic and autonomic reflexes.

In the modern practice of balanced anaesthesia, these modalities are achieved by using a combination of inhaled and i.v. drugs, each drug for a specific purpose. Anaesthesia has developed as a highly specialized science in itself. *In dental practice, general anaesthesia is employed only in few cases. It is administered and managed by a qualified anaesthetist, and not by the dental surgeon himself.*

Mechanism of general anaesthesia

The mechanism of action of GAs is not precisely known. A wide variety of chemical agents produce general anaesthesia. Therefore, GA action had been related to some common physicochemical property of the drugs. Mayer and Overton (1901) pointed out a direct parallelism between lipid/water partition coefficient of the GAs and their anaesthetic potency.

Minimal alveolar concentration (MAC) It is the lowest concentration of the anaesthetic in pulmonary alveoli needed to produce immobility in response to a painful stimulus (surgical incision) in 50% individuals. It is accepted as a valid measure of potency of inhalational GAs, because it remains fairly constant for most young adults.

The MAC of a number of GAs shows excellent correlation with their oil/gas partition coefficient. However, this only reflects capacity of the anaesthetic to enter into CNS and attain sufficient concentration in the neuronal membrane, but not the mechanism by which anaesthesia is produced.

It is now clear that different anaesthetics may be acting through different molecular mechanisms and various components of the anaesthetic state involve action at discrete loci in the cerebrospinal axis. The principal locus of causation of unconsciousness appears to be in the thalamus or the reticular activating system, amnesia may result from action in cerebral cortex and hippocampus, while spinal cord is the likely seat of immobility on surgical stimulation.

Recent findings show that ligand gated ion channels (but not voltage sensitive ion channels) are the major targets of anaesthetic action. The $GABA_A$ receptor gated Cl^- channel is the most important of these. Many inhalational anaesthetics, barbiturates, benzodiazepines and propofol potentiate the action of inhibitory transmitter GABA to open Cl^- channels. Each of the above anaesthetics appears to interact with its own specific binding site on the $GABA_A$ receptor-Cl^- channel complex, but none binds to the GABA binding site as such. Action of glycine (another inhibitory transmitter which also activates Cl⁻ channels) in the spinal cord and medulla is augmented by barbiturates, propofol and many inhalational anaesthetics. This action may block responsiveness to painful stimuli resulting in immobility of the anaesthetic state. Certain fluorinated anaesthetics and barbiturates, in addition, inhibit neuronal cation channel gated by nicotinic cholinergic receptor which may mediate analgesia and amnesia.

On the other hand, N_2O and ketamine do not affect GABA or glycine gated Cl⁻ channels. Rather they selectively inhibit the excitatory NMDA type of glutamate receptor. This receptor gates mainly Ca^{2+} selective cation channels in the neurones and their inhibition appears to be the primary mechanism of anaesthetic action of ketamine as well as N_2O. The volatile anaesthetics have little action on this receptor.

Unlike local anaesthetics which act primarily by blocking axonal conduction, the GAs appear to act by depressing synaptic transmission.

Stages of anaesthesia

GAs cause an irregularly descending depression of the CNS, i.e. the higher functions are lost first and progressively lower areas of the brain are involved, but in the spinal cord lower segments are affected somewhat earlier than the higher segments. The vital centres located in the medulla are paralysed the last as the depth of anaesthesia increases.

Guedel (1920) described four stages with *ether* anaesthesia.

I. *Stage of analgesia* From beginning of anaesthetic inhalation to loss of consciousness; pain is progressively abolished; some minor procedures can be performed, but it is difficult to maintain.

II. *Stage of delirium* From loss of consciousness to beginning of regular respiration; excitement, struggling, breath-holding, jerky breathing, sympathetic stimulation occur. No procedure can be carried out. This stage is inconspicuous in modern anaesthesia.

III. *Surgical anaesthesia* From onset of regular respiration to cessation of spontaneous breathing. Most dental/surgical procedures are carried out at lighter planes of this stage.

IV. *Medullary paralysis* From cessation of breathing to failure of circulation and death. It is never attempted.

These clear-cut stages are not seen now-a-days with the use of faster acting GAs, premedication and employment of many drugs together. The precise sequence of events differs somewhat with different anaesthetics.

The modern anaesthetist has to depend on several other observations to gauge the depth of anaesthesia.
- If eyelash reflex is present and patient is making swallowing movements—Stage II has not been reached.
- Loss of response to a painful stimulus like pressure on the upper nasal border of the orbit—indicates that stage III has been reached.
- If incision of the skin causes reflex increase in respiration, BP rise or other effects; insertion of endotracheal tube is resisted and induces coughing, vomiting, laryngospasm; tears appear in the eye; passive inflation of lungs is resisted—anaesthesia is light.
- Fall in BP, cardiac and respiratory depression are signs of deep anaesthesia.

In the present-day practice, anaesthesia is generally kept light; adequate analgesia, amnesia and muscle relaxation are produced by the use of intravenous drugs. Concentrations of inhalational anaesthetics exceeding 1.5 MAC are infrequently used. Some effects common to most inhalational anaesthetics are:
- The EEG initially shows activation, but increasing concentrations of potent GAs cause progressive EEG suppression culminating in electrical silence at >2 MAC.
- Decrease in cerebral metabolic rate which indirectly reduces cerebral blood flow

(CBF). However, at higher concentrations, their direct vasodilatory action predominates and CBF may actually increase. These higher concentrations should be avoided in patients with raised intracranial pressure.
- All fluorinated anaesthetics depress cardiac contractility and lower BP.
- Respiratory depression, bronchodilatation and reduced airway mucociliary function occurs; so that prolonged anaesthesia predisposes to respiratory complications.
- Limited and reversible lowering of GFR and urine flow.
- Reduced gastrointestinal motility.

Pharmacokinetics of inhalational anaesthetics

Inhalational anaesthetics are gases or vapours that diffuse rapidly across pulmonary alveoli and tissue barriers. The depth of anaesthesia depends on the potency of the agent (MAC is an index of potency) and its partial pressure (PP) in the brain, while induction and recovery depend on the rate of change of PP in the brain. Transfer of the anaesthetic between lung and brain depends on a series of tension gradients which may be summarized as—

$$\text{Alveoli} \rightleftharpoons \text{Blood} \rightleftharpoons \text{Brain}$$

Factors affecting the PP of anaesthetic attained in the brain are—

1. *PP of anaesthetic in the inspired gas* Higher the inspired tension more anaesthetic will be transferred to the blood hastening induction.

2. *Pulmonary ventilation* It governs delivery of the GA to the alveoli. Hyperventilation will bring in more anaesthetic per minute and quicken induction.

3. *Alveolar exchange* The GAs diffuse freely across alveoli, but if alveolar ventilation and perfusion are mismatched (as occurs in emphysema and other lung diseases) the attainment of equilibrium between alveoli and blood will be delayed. Induction and recovery both are slowed.

4. *Solubility of anaesthetic in blood* This is the most important property determining induction and recovery. Both induction and recovery are slow with an anaesthetic that is highly soluble in blood (e.g. ether). On the other hand, drugs with low blood solubility, e.g. N_2O, sevoflurane, desflurane induce quickly.

5. *Solubility of anaesthetic in tissues* Majority of GAs are equally soluble in lean tissues as in blood but more soluble in fatty tissue. Anaesthetics with greater lipid solubility (halothane) continue to enter adipose tissue for hours and also leave it slowly prolonging residual sedation.

6. *Cerebral blood flow* Brain is a highly perfused organ; as such GAs are quickly delivered to it. This can be hastened by CO_2 inhalation which causes cerebral vasodilatation—induction and recovery are accelerated.

Elimination When anaesthetic inhalation is discontinued, gradients are reversed and the channel of absorption (pulmonary epithelium) becomes the channel of elimination. Same factors which govern induction also govern recovery. Anaesthetics, in general, persist for long periods in adipose tissue because of their high lipid solubility and low blood flow through fatty tissues. Most GAs are eliminated unchanged. Metabolism is significant only for halothane which is about 20% metabolized in liver.

Second gas effect and diffusion hypoxia
In the initial part of induction, diffusion gradient from alveoli to blood is high and larger quantity of anaesthetic is entering blood. If the inhaled concentration of anaesthetic is high, substantial loss of alveolar gas volume will occur and the gas mixture will be sucked in, independent of ventilatory exchange—gas flow will be higher than the tidal volume. This is significant only with N_2O, since it is given at 70–80% concentration. Though it has low solubility in blood, about 1 litre/min of N_2O enters blood in the first few minutes. As such, gas flow is 1 litre/min greater than the minute volume. If another potent anaesthetic, e.g. halothane (given at 1–2% concentration) is being administered at the same time, it also will be delivered to blood at a rate 1 litre/min higher than minute volume and induction will be faster. This is called *second gas effect*.

The reverse occurs when N_2O is discontinued after prolonged anaesthesia; N_2O having low blood solubility rapidly diffuses into alveoli and dilutes the alveolar air. Consequently, PP of oxygen in alveoli is reduced. The resulting hypoxia, called *diffusion hypoxia*, is not of much consequence if cardiopulmonary reserve is normal, but may be dangerous if it is low. This can be prevented by continuing 100% O_2 inhalation for a few minutes after discontinuing N_2O, instead of straight away switching over to air. Diffusion hypoxia is not significant with other anaesthetics because they are administered at low concentrations (0.2–4%) and cannot dilute alveolar air by more than 1–2%.

Properties of an ideal anaesthetic

A. *For the patient* The anaesthetic should be pleasant, nonirritating, should not cause nausea or vomiting. Induction and recovery should be fast with no after effects.

B. *For the surgeon* It should provide adequate analgesia, immobility and muscle relaxation. It should be noninflammable and nonexplosive so that cautery may be used.

C. *For the anaesthetist* Its administration should be easy, controllable and versatile.
- Margin of safety should be wide—no fall in BP. Heart, liver and other organs should not be affected.
- It should be potent so that low concentrations are needed and oxygenation of the patient does not suffer.
- Rapid adjustments in depth of anaesthesia should be possible.
- It should be cheap, stable and easily stored.
- It should not react with rubber tubing or soda lime.

The inhalational anaesthetics have a steep concentration-response relationship: increasing the concentration only by 10% over MAC immobilizes>90 individuals (at MAC only 50% are immobilized), and 2–3 MAC is often lethal.

The important physical and anaesthetic properties of inhalational anaesthetics are presented in Table 8.1.

Table 8.1: Physical and anaesthetic properties of inhalational anaesthetics

Anaesthetic	Boiling point (°C)	Inflammability	Irritancy (odour)	Oil: Gas partition coefficient*	Blood: Gas partition coefficient*	MAC (%)	Induction	Muscle relaxation
1. Ether	35	Infl. + Explo.	+++ (Pungent)	65	12.1	1.9	Slow	V. good
2. Halothane	50	Noninfl.	– (Pleasant)	224	2.3	0.75	Interm.	Fair
3. Isoflurane	48	Noninfl.	± (Unpleasant)	99	1.4	1.2	Interm.	Good
4. Desflurane	24	Noninfl.	+ (Unpleasant)	19	0.42	6.0	Fast	Good
5. Sevoflurane	59	Noninfl.	– (Pleasant)	50	0.68	2.0	Fast	Good
6. Nitrous oxide	Gas	Noninfl.	–	1.4	0.47	105	Fast	Poor

* At 37°C
MAC—Minimal alveolar concentration; Infl.—Inflammable; Explo.—Explosive; Interm.—Intermediate

CLASSIFICATION

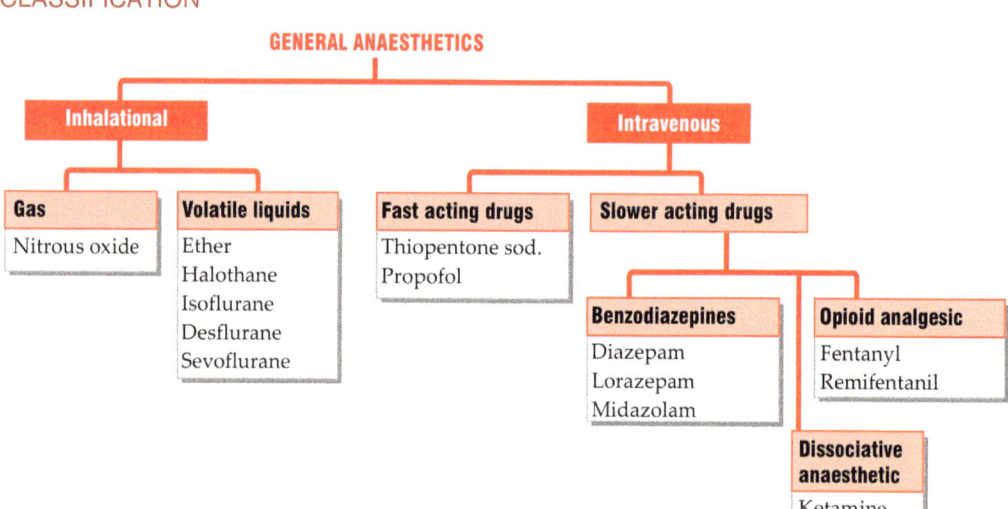

INHALATIONAL ANAESTHETICS

1. Nitrous oxide (N₂O) It is a colourless, odourless, heavier than air, noninflammable gas supplied under pressure in steel cylinders. It is a nonirritating but low potency anaesthetic; unconsciousness cannot be produced in all individuals without concomittent hypoxia: MAC is 105% implying that even pure N₂O cannot produce adequate anaesthesia at 1 atmosphere pressure.

Nitrous oxide is a good analgesic (even 20% produces moderate analgesia) but weak muscle relaxant. Onset of N₂O action is quick and smooth (but thiopentone is often used for induction), recovery is rapid. Second gas effect and diffusion hypoxia are possible only with N₂O. Post-anaesthetic nausea is not marked.

Nitrous oxide is generally used as a carrier and as adjuvant to other anaesthetics. A mixture of 70% N₂O + 25–30% O₂ + 0.2–2% another potent anaesthetic is employed for most surgical procedures.

In dental practice N₂O is now used to provide 'conscious sedation' for allaying anxiety and apprehension (*see* p. 136). It is nontoxic to liver, kidney and brain. It is cheap and very commonly used.

2. Ether (Diethyl ether) It is a highly volatile liquid, produces irritating vapours which are inflammable and explosive. Though ether is a potent anaesthetic, produces good analgesia and marked muscle relaxation, it has gone out of use, because it is unpleasant and inflammable.

3. Halothane (FLUOTHANE) It is a volatile liquid with sweet odour, nonirritant and noninflammable. Solubility in blood is moderate, therefore induction is reasonably quick and pleasant.

Halothane is a potent anaesthetic. For induction 2–4% and for maintenance 0.5–1% is delivered by the use of a special vaporizer. It is not a good analgesic or muscle relaxant, but it potentiates competitive neuromuscular blockers.

Halothane causes direct depression of myocardial contractility. Cardiac output is reduced with deepening anaesthesia. BP starts falling early and parallels the depth. Heart rate is often reduced by direct depression of SA nodal automaticity and absence of reflex of baroreceptor activation even when BP falls. Halothane causes relatively greater depression of respiration;

breathing is shallow and rapid. Ventilatory support with added oxygen is frequently required.

Pharyngeal and laryngeal reflexes are abolished early and coughing is suppressed while bronchi dilate making it the preferred anaesthetic for asthmatics. It inhibits intestinal and uterine contractions.

Hepatitis occurs rarely in susceptible individuals, especially after repeated use. A genetically determined reaction *malignant hyperthermia* occurs rarely. This is due to intracellular release of Ca^{2+} from sarcoplasmic reticulum through an abnormal RyR calcium channel causing persistent muscle contraction and increased heat production.

About 20% of halothane that enters blood is metabolized in the liver, the rest is exhaled out. Recovery from halothane anaesthesia is smooth and reasonably quick; shivering may occur but nausea and vomiting are rare. Psychomotor performance and mental ability remain depressed for several hours after regaining consciousness.

Halothane is still used because it is cheap. However, in affluent countries it has been replaced by the newer and costlier congeners.

4. Isoflurane (SOFANE) This potent fluorinated anaesthetic has properties similar to halothane, but is less soluble in blood. Therefore, induction and recovery are relatively fast. Fall in BP is like halothane, but isoflurane tends to increase heart rate. It does not sensitize the heart to adrenergic arrhythmias.

Respiratory depression is prominent because of which assistance is usually needed to avoid hypercarbia. Secretions are slightly increased. Renal and hepatic toxicity has not been encountered. Postanaesthetic nausea and vomiting is mild.

Though somewhat pungent, isoflurane has many advantages, i.e. better adjustment of depth of anaesthesia and low toxicity. It does not provoke seizures and is preferred for neurosurgery. In many hospitals it has become the routine anaesthetic.

5. Desflurane This newer all fluorinated congener of isoflurane has gained popularity as an anaesthetic for out-patient surgery. Its distinctive properties are high volatility, lower lipid solubility and very low solubility in blood as well as in tissues, because of which induction and recovery are very fast. Depth of anaesthesia changes rapidly with change in inhaled concentration. Postanaesthetic cognitive and motor impairment is shortlived. Therefore, patient can be discharged a few hours after surgery.

Desflurane is less potent than isoflurane; higher concentration has to be used for induction. Because of somewhat pungent odour, this higher concentration irritates air passages and can induce coughing, breath-holding, and laryngospasm, making it difficult to use for induction. Degree of respiratory depression, muscle relaxation, vasodilatation and fall in BP, as well as maintained cardiac contractility and coronary circulation are similar to isoflurane. In addition to its suitability for outpatient surgery, desflurane can serve as a good alternative to isoflurane for routine surgery as well, especially for prolonged operations.

6. Sevoflurane It is the latest polyfluorinated anaesthetic with properties intermediate between isoflurane and desflurane. Solubility in blood and tissues as well as potency are less than isoflurane but higher than desflurane. Induction and emergence from anaesthesia are fast. Consequently, rapid changes in depth can be achieved. Absence of pungency makes it pleasant and administrable through face mask. Unlike desflurane, it poses no problem in induction. Acceptability is good, even by pediatric patients. Recovery is smooth; orientation, cognitive and motor functions are regained almost as quickly as with desflurane. Sevoflurane is suitable for both outpatient as well as inpatient surgery, but its high cost and need for high flow open system makes it very expensive to use.

INTRAVENOUS ANAESTHETICS

FAST ACTING DRUGS

These are drugs which on i.v. injection produce loss of consciousness in one arm-brain circulation time (~11 sec); are generally used for induction because of rapidity of onset of action. Anaesthesia is then usually maintained by an inhalational agent. They also serve to reduce the amount of maintenance anaesthetic. Supplemented with analgesics and muscle relaxants, they can also be used as the sole anaesthetic.

1. Thiopentone sod It is an ultrashort acting thiobarbiturate, highly soluble in water yielding a strongly alkaline solution, which must be prepared freshly before injection. Extravasation of the solution or inadvertent intraarterial injection produces intense pain. Subsequently, necrosis and gangrene may occur.

Injected i.v. (3–5 mg/kg) it produces unconsciousness in 15–20 sec. The undissociated form of thiopentone has high lipid solubility—enters brain almost instantaneously. Initial distribution depends on organ blood flow—brain gets large amounts. However, as other less vascular tissues (muscle, fat) gradually take up the drug, blood concentration falls and it back diffuses from the brain; consciousness is regained in 6–10 min (t½ of distribution phase is 3 min).

On repeated injection, the extracerebral sites are gradually filled up, so that lower doses produce anaesthesia which lasts longer. Its ultimate disposal occurs mainly by hepatic metabolism (elimination t½ is 7–12 hr). Residual CNS depression may persist for > 12 hr. The patient should not be allowed to leave the hospital without an attendant before this time.

Thiopentone is a poor analgesic. Painful procedures should not be carried out under its influence unless an opioid or N_2O has been given; otherwise, the patient may struggle, shout and show reflex changes in BP and respiration. Laryngospasm can also occur. Shivering and delirium may complicate recovery, but post-anaesthetic vomiting is uncommon.

It is a weak muscle relaxant. BP falls immediately after injection mainly due to vasodilatation, but recovers rapidly.

Thiopentone has now been largely replaced by propofol. It is seldom employed in dentistry.

2. Propofol It is an oily liquid employed as a 1% emulsion for i.v. induction and short duration anaesthesia. Unconsciousness after propofol injection occurs in 15–45 sec and lasts 5–10 min. Propofol distributes rapidly (distribution t½ 2–4 min). Due to rapid metabolism, elimination t½ (100 min) is much shorter than that of thiopentone. As such, propofol has largely superseded thiopentone.

Intermittent injection or continuous infusion of propofol has been used for total i.v. anaesthesia when supplemented by fentanyl. It lacks airway irritancy and is not likely to induce laryngospasm. Propofol is particularly suited for outpatient surgery because residual impairment is less marked and incidence of post-operative nausea and vomiting is low. Excitatory effects and involuntary movements are noted in few patients. Induction apnoea lasting ~1 min is common. Fall in BP, due primarily to vasodilatation occurs consistently and is occasionally marked, but short lasting. Bradycardia is also frequent.

In subanaesthetic doses it has been used for sedating intubated patients in intensive care units.

SLOWER ACTING DRUGS

1. Benzodiazepines (BZDs) In addition to their use in preanaesthetic medication, BZDs are now frequently employed for inducing, maintaining and supplementing anaesthesia as well as for conscious sedation. Relatively higher doses (diazepam 0.2–0.5 mg/kg or equivalent) injected i.v. produce sedation, amnesia and then unconsciousness in 5–10 min. If no other anaesthetic or opioid is given, the patient becomes responsive in about 1 hr due to redistribution of the drug (distribution t½ of diazepam is 15 min), but amnesia persists for 2–3 hr and sedation for 6 hr or more. BZDs are poor analgesics: an opioid or N_2O is usually added if the procedure is painful.

By themselves, BZDs do not markedly depress respiration, cardiac contractility or BP; but when opioids are also given, these functions are considerably compromised. They do not provoke postoperative nausea or vomiting. Involuntary movements are not stimulated.

BZDs are now the preferred drugs for endoscopies, cardiac catheterization, angiographies, conscious sedation during local/regional anaesthesia for dental procedures, fracture setting, etc. They are a frequent component of balanced anaesthesia employing several drugs. The anaesthetic action of BZDs can be rapidly reversed by flumazenil 0.5–2 mg i.v.

Diazepam 0.2–0.5 mg/kg by slow undiluted injection in a running i.v. drip: this technique reduces the burning sensation in the vein and incidence of thrombophlebitis. Diazepam is less popular as i.v. anaesthetic now, due to irritant action on veins.

Lorazepam It is 3 times more potent, slower acting and less irritating than diazepam. It distributes more gradually—awakening may be delayed. Amnesia is more profound.

Midazolam Water soluble, nonirritating to veins, faster and shorter acting and 3 times more potent than diazepam. It is being preferred over diazepam for anaesthetic use and for sedation of dental patients, as well as intubated and mechanically ventilated patients.

2. Ketamine It induces the so-called '*dissociative anaesthesia*' which is characterized by profound analgesia, immobility, amnesia with light sleep. The patient appears to be conscious, but is unable to process sensory stimuli and does not react to them. Thus, the patient appears to be dissociated from his own body and the surroundings. The primary site of action of ketamine is in the cortex and subcortical areas; not in the reticular activating system.

Respiration is not depressed, airway reflexes are maintained and muscle tone increases. Heart rate, cardiac output and BP are elevated due to sympathetic stimulation. The above effects are produced within a min and recovery starts after 10–15 min, but the patient remains amnesic for 1–2 hr. Emergence delirium, hallucinations and involuntary movements occur in up to 50% patients. Ketamine injection is not painful. Children tolerate the drug better. Its elimination t½ is 3–4 hr.

Ketamine has been employed for dental and other operations on the head and neck, in patients who have bled, in asthmatics (because it relieves bronchospasm), in those who do not want to lose consciousness and for short operations. It may be dangerous for hypertensives and in ischaemic heart disease, but is good for hypovolemic patients.

3. Fentanyl This short acting (30–50 min) potent opioid analgesic related to pethidine is generally given i.v. at the beginning of painful surgical procedures. Fentanyl is frequently used as supplement in balanced anaesthesia. This permits use of lower anaesthetic concentrations with better haemodynamic stability. Combined with benzodiazepines, it can obviate the need for inhaled anaesthetics for diagnostic, endoscopic, angiographic, dental and other minor procedures in poor risk patients, as well as for burn dressing.

After i.v. fentanyl (2–4 µg/kg) the patient remains drowsy but conscious and his cooperation can be commanded. Respiratory depression is marked, but predictable; the patient may be encouraged to breathe and assistance may be provided. Heart rate decreases, because fentanyl stimulates vagus. Fall in BP is slight. Spasm of masseter and chest muscles may occur if fentanyl is injected rapidly.

Nausea, vomiting and itching often occur during recovery. The opioid antagonist naloxone can be used to counteract persisting respiratory depression and mental clouding.

4. Remifentanil It is a faster acting congener of fentanyl with a still shorter and more predictable duration of action. After i.v. injection it produces profound analgesia within 1–2 min which fades in 10–15 min. The very brief action is due to rapid metabolism by plasma and tissue esterases yielding a plasma t½ of 10–15 min. Administered by bolus i.v. injection followed by continuous i.v. infusion, remifentanil is mainly used to provide strong and titratable analgesia to cover short and painful procedures.

COMPLICATIONS OF GENERAL ANAESTHESIA

A. During anaesthesia
1. Respiratory depression and hypercarbia; can be overcome by providing respiratory assistance.
2. Salivation, respiratory secretions; this is less problematic now as nonirritant anaesthetics are mostly used.
3. Cardiac arrhythmias, asystole.
4. Fall in BP.
5. Aspiration of gastric contents: acid pneumonitis.
6. Laryngospasm and asphyxia.
7. Awareness: dreadful perception and recall of events during surgery; this is likely when light anaesthesia + analgesics and muscle relaxants are used.
8. Delirium, convulsions, excitatory effects.

B. After anaesthesia
1. Nausea and vomiting.
2. Persisting sedation: impaired psychomotor function.
3. Mucus plugging of airways, atelectasis and pneumonia.
4. Organ toxicities: liver, kidney damage.
5. Emergence delirium.
6. Cognitive defects: prolonged excess cognitive decline has been observed in some patients, especially the elderly.

DRUG INTERACTIONS

1. Patients on antihypertensives given general anaesthetics—BP may fall markedly.
2. Neuroleptics, opioids and clonidine potentiate anaesthetics.
3. Halothane sensitizes heart to Adr.
4. If a patient on corticosteroids is to be anaesthetized, give 100 mg i.v. hydrocortisone intraoperatively because anaesthesia is a stress—can precipitate adrenal insufficiency.
5. Insulin need of a diabetic is increased during GA: switch over to plain insulin even if the patient is on oral hypoglycaemics.

CONSCIOUS SEDATION

'Conscious sedation' is a monitored state of altered consciousness that can be employed along with local anaesthesia, to carry out dental procedures/surgery or other diagnostic/therapeutic interventions in apprehensive children (or adults) and in medically compromised patients. It allows operative procedure to be performed with minimal physiologic and psychologic stress. *Conscious sedation* is a technique in which drugs are used to produce a state of CNS depression (but not unconsciousness) sufficient to withstand the trespass of the procedure, while maintaining communication with the patient, who is able to respond to commands and maintain a patent airway throughout. The difference between conscious sedation and anaesthesia is one of degree. The protective airway and other reflexes are not lost during conscious sedation; therefore, it is safer. However, by itself, conscious sedation is not able to suppress the pain of dental procedure; local anaesthetic must be injected in addition. Drugs used for conscious sedation are diazepam, midazolam, propofol, nitrous oxide and fentanyl.

SKELETAL MUSCLE RELAXANTS

Skeletal muscle relaxants are drugs that act peripherally at neuromuscular junction/muscle fibre itself or centrally in the cerebrospinal axis to cause paralysis or to reduce muscle tone.

The neuromuscular blocking agents are used in conjunction with general anaesthetics to provide muscle relaxation for surgery, while centrally acting muscle relaxants are used primarily for painful muscle spasms and spastic neurological diseases.

NEUROMUSCULAR BLOCKING AGENTS

Curare It is the generic name for certain plant extracts used by south American tribals as arrow poison for game hunting. The animals got paralysed even if not killed by the arrow. Natural sources of curare are *Strychnos toxifera, Chondrodendron tomentosum* and related plants. The muscle paralysing active principles of these are tubocurarine, toxiferins, etc.

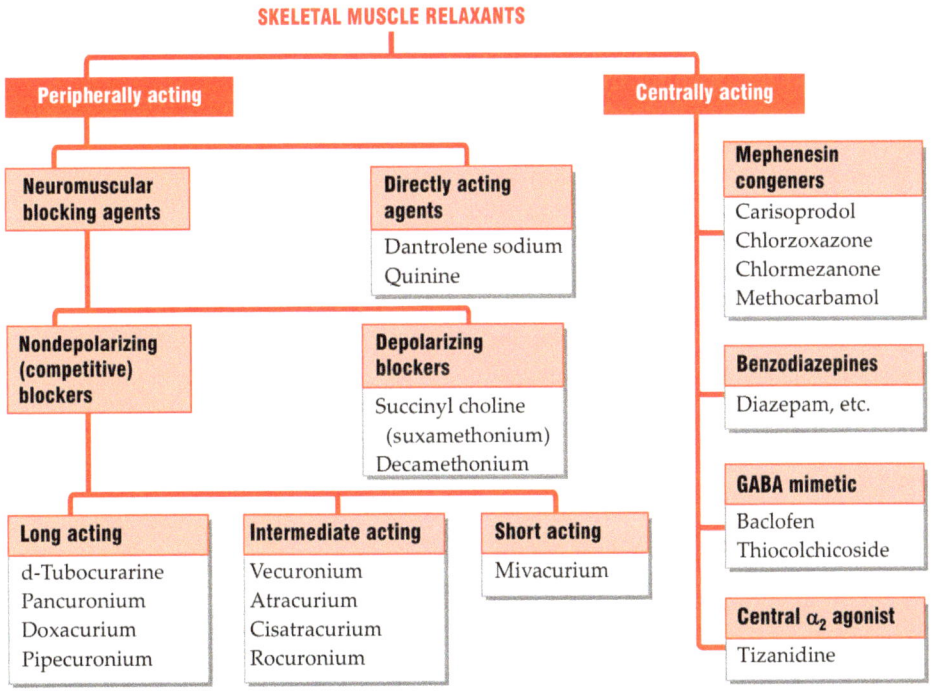

MECHANISM OF ACTION

The site of action of both competitive and depolarizing blockers is the endplate of skeletal muscle fibres.

Competitive block (Nondepolarizing block)

This is produced by curare and related drugs.

The competitive blockers have affinity for the nicotinic (N_M) cholinergic receptors at the muscle endplate but have no intrinsic activity. The N_M receptor has been isolated and studied in detail. It is a protein with 5 subunits (α2 β ε or γ and δ) which are arranged like a rosette surrounding the Na^+ channel (see Fig. 3.3). The two α subunits carry 2 ACh binding sites; these sites have negatively charged groups which combine with the cationic head of ACh and trigger opening of the Na^+ channel. Most of the competitive blockers have two or more quaternary N^+ atoms which provide the necessary attraction to the same site, but the bulk of the antagonist molecule does not allow conformational changes in the subunits needed for opening the channel. The ACh released from motor nerve endings is not able to combine with its receptors to generate endplate potential (EPP) and the muscle fails to contract in response to nerve impulse. The antagonism is surmountable by increasing the concentration of ACh *in vitro* and by anticholinesterases *in vivo*.

The competitive blockers also block the prejunctional nicotinic receptors located on motor nerve endings and supplement the post junctional block.

Depolarizing block
Decamethonium and SCh have affinity as well as submaximal intrinsic activity at the N_M cholinoceptors. They depolarize muscle endplates by opening Na^+ channels (just as ACh does) and initially produce twitching and fasciculations. These drugs do not dissociate rapidly from the receptor, thereby induce prolonged partial depolarization of the region around the muscle endplate. As a result, Na^+ channels get inactivated (because transmembrane potential drops to about –50 mV) → ACh released from motor nerve endings is unable to generate a propagated muscle action potential (MAP) producing flaccid paralysis. In other words, a zone of inexcitability is created around the end-plate preventing activation of muscle fibre.

Depolarizing blockers also have 2 quaternary N^+ atoms but the molecule is long, slender and flexible. The features of classical depolarizing block differ markedly from that of nondepolarizing block (Fig. 8.1 and Table 8.2).

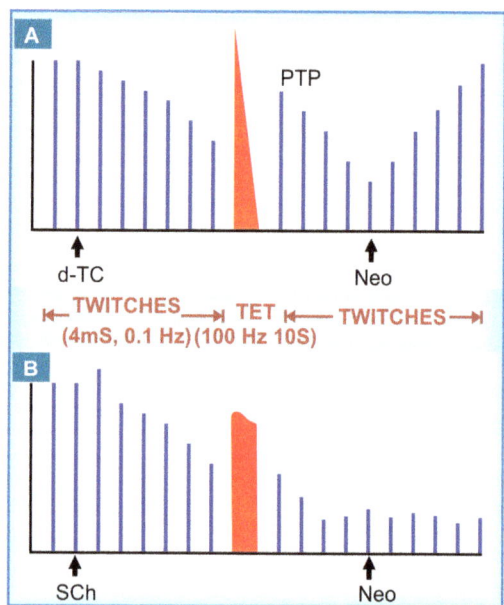

Fig. 8.1: Illustration of characteristics of competitive (A) and depolarizing (B) neuromuscular blockade in sciatic nerve-gastrocnemius muscle of cat;
A. Tubocurarine (d-TC) produces progressive decrease in twitch tension; tetanic stimulation (TET) produces poorly sustained contracture, which is followed by post-tetanic potentiation (PTP); Neostigmine (Neo) restores the twitch contractions.
B. Succinylcholine (SCh) produces initial augmentation of twitches followed by progressive block; tetanus is well sustained, but there is no PTP; block is not reversed (rather worsened) by neostigmine.

Table 8.2: Features of competitive and typical depolarizing block

	Competitive block (d-tubocurarine)	Depolarizing block (Succinyl cholile)
1. Paralysis in man	Flaccid	Fasciculations → flaccid
2. Paralysis in chick	Flaccid	Spastic
3. Effect on isolated frog's rectus muscle	No contraction, Antagonism of ACh	Contraction
4. Tetanic stimulation during partial block	Poorly sustained contraction	Well-sustained contraction
5. Neostigmine	Antagonises block	No effect
6. Ether anaesthesia	Synergistic	No effect
7. Order of paralysis	Fingers, eyes → limbs → neck, face → trunk → respiratory	Neck, limbs → face, jaw, eyes, pharynx → trunk → respiratory
8. Effect of lowering temperature	Reduces block	Intensifies block
9. Effect of cathodal current to endplate	Lessens block	Enhances block

In many species, e.g. dog, rabbit, rat, monkey, in slow contracting soleus muscle of cat, and under certain conditions in man the classical depolarizing block described above (phase I block) is followed by a phase II block, which is due to desensitization of the N_M receptor to ACh. This block superficially resembles nondepolarizing block in features. SCh readily produces phase II block in patients with atypical or deficient pseudocholinesterase.

ACTIONS

1. *Skeletal muscles* Intravenous injection of nondepolarizing blockers rapidly produces muscle weakness followed by flaccid paralysis. Small fast response muscles (fingers, extraocular) are affected first; paralysis spreads to hands, feet—arm, leg, neck, face—trunk—finally intercostal muscles—diaphragm: respiration stops. Recovery occurs in the reverse sequence; diaphragmatic contractions resume first.

Depolarizing blockers typically produce fasciculations lasting a few seconds before inducing flaccid paralysis, but fasciculations are not prominent in well-anaesthetized patients. Though the sequence in which muscles are involved is somewhat different from the competitive blockers (Table 8.2), the action of SCh develops with such rapidity that this is often not perceived. Apnoea generally occurs within 45–90 sec, but lasts only 2–5 min followed by rapid recovery.

2. *Autonomic ganglia* Because the cholinergic receptors in autonomic ganglia are also nicotinic (though of a different subclass N_N), competitive neuromuscular blockers produce some degree of ganglionic blockade. SCh may cause brief ganglionic stimulation by agonistic action on ganglionic nicotinic receptors.

3. *Histamine release* d-TC releases histamine from mast cells resulting in hypotension, flushing, bronchospasm and increased respiratory secretions. Histamine releasing potential of other neuromuscular blockers is graded in Table 8.3.

4. *C.V.S.*
d-Tubocurarine produces a significant fall in BP. This is due to—
(a) ganglionic blockade,
(b) histamine release, and
(c) reduced venous return—a result of paralysis of limb and respiratory muscles.

Table 8.3: Comparative properties of neuromuscular blocking drugs

Drug	Dose£ (mg/kg)	Onset* (min)	Duration@ (min)	Hist. release	Gang. block	Vagal block
LONG ACTING						
1. d-Tubocurarine	0.2–0.4	4–6	40–60	+++	++	±
2. Pancuronium	0.04–0.1	4–6	60–120	±	±	+
3. Doxacurium	0.03–0.08	4–8	60–120	+	–	–
4. Pipecuronium	0.05–0.08	2–4	50–100	±	–	–
INTERMEDIATE ACTING						
5. Vecuronium	0.08–0.1	2–4	30–50	±	–	±
6. Atracurium	0.3–0.6	2–4	20–40	+	–	–
7. Rocuronium	0.6–0.9	1–2	25–40	–	–	±
SHORT ACTING						
8. Mivacurium	0.15–0.2	2–4	15–30	+	–	–
9. Succinylcholine	0.5–0.8	1–1.5	5–8	++	St.	St.

£ Initial paralysing dose during opioid/nitrous oxide-oxygen anaesthesia. In patients anaesthetised with ether/halothane/isoflurane, the dose may be 1/3–1/2 of the figure given.
* Time to maximal block after i.v. injection.
@ Duration of surgical grade relaxation after usual clinical doses; time to 95% recovery of muscle twitch is nearly double of the figure given (especially for long-acting drugs). Duration is also dose dependent.
St. — Stimulation

Heart rate may increase due to vagal ganglionic blockade. All newer nondepolarizing drugs have much less effects on BP and HR.

Cardiovascular effects of SCh are variable. BP occasionally falls on account of its muscarinic action causing vasodilatation.

5. *G.I.T.* The ganglion blocking activity of competitive blockers may enhance postoperative paralytic ileus after abdominal operations.

6. *C.N.S.* All neuromuscular blockers are quaternary compounds—do not cross blood-brain barrier—no CNS effects.

PHARMACOKINETICS

All neuromuscular blockers are quaternary compounds. They are highly ionized, therefore not absorbed orally. They are practically always given i.v. Muscles with higher blood flow receive more drug and are affected earlier. Redistribution to non-muscular tissues plays a significant role in the termination of action of a single dose. They do not cross placenta or penetrate brain. Pancuronium, doxacurium and pipecuronium are partly metabolized while vecuronium, atracurium, rocuronium and mivacurium are largely metabolized in the body. Atracurium is inactivated in plasma by spontaneous nonenzymatic degradation (Hofmann elimination) in addition to that by cholinesterases. The unchanged drug is excreted in urine as well as in bile.

SCh is rapidly hydrolysed by plasma pseudocholinesterase. Its action lasts for 3 to 5 min. Some patients have genetically determined abnormality of pseudocholinesterase (low affinity for SCh) or deficiency of pseudocholinesterase. In them, SCh causes dominant phase II blockade resulting in muscle paralysis and apnoea lasting for hours.

INTERACTIONS

1. *Thiopentone sod* and SCh solutions should not be mixed in the same syringe; they react chemically.
2. *General anaesthetics* potentiate competitive blockers.
3. *Anticholinesterases* reverse the action of competitive blockers. Neostigmine 0.5–2 mg i.v. is almost routinely used after pancuronium and other long acting blockers to hasten recovery at the end of operation.
4. *Antibiotics* Aminoglycoside antibiotics reduce ACh release from prejunctional nerve endings and have a weak stabilizing action on the postjunctional membrane. In clinically used doses aminoglycoside antibiotics do not by themselves produce muscle relaxation but potentiate competitive blockers. Tetracyclines (by chelating Ca^{2+}), polypeptide antibiotics, clindamycin and lincomycin also synergise with competitive blockers.
5. *Calcium channel blockers* Verapamil and others potentiate both competitive and depolarizing neuromuscular blockers.
6. *Diuretics* produce hypokalaemia which enhances competitive block.
7. *Diazepam, propranolol* and *quinidine* intensify competitive block, while high dose of corticosteroids reduce it.

TOXICITY

1. Respiratory paralysis and prolonged apnoea is the most important complication of neuromuscular blockers.
2. Flushing due to histamine release can occasionally occur with atracurium and mivacurium.
3. Fall in BP and cardiovascular collapse can occur, especially in hypovolemic patients.
4. Cardiac arrhythmias and even arrest have occurred, especially with SCh.
5. An attack of asthma may be precipitated by histamine releasing neuromuscular blockers.
6. Postoperative muscle soreness is often felt after SCh.

USES

1. The most important use of neuromuscular blockers is as adjuvants to general anaesthesia; adequate muscle relaxation can be achieved at lighter planes. They are specially valuable in abdominal and thoracic surgery. In *dentistry they may be needed for setting of mandibular fractures.*

Vecuronium, atracurium and rocuronium are the most frequently employed non-depolarizing blockers for surgical procedures. Succinylcholine is employed for brief procedures, e.g. endotracheal intubation, laryngoscopy, bronchoscopy, oesophagoscopy, reduction of fractures and to counteract laryngospasm.

2. Assisted ventilation of critically ill patients in intensive care units can be facilitated by continuous infusion of a competitive neuromuscular blocker by reducing chest wall resistance to inflation. Vecuronium is generally selected for this purpose.
3. Convulsions and trauma from electroconvulsive therapy can be avoided by the use of muscle relaxants.
4. Severe cases of tetanus and status epilepticus may be paralysed by a neuromuscular blocker, and then maintained on intermittent positive pressure respiration.

DIRECTLY ACTING MUSCLE RELAXANTS

Dantrolene This muscle relaxant is chemically and pharmacologically entirely different from neuromuscular blockers. It does not affect neuromuscular transmission or MAP, but uncouples contraction from depolarization of the muscle membrane. Depolarization triggered release of Ca^{2+} from sarcoplasmic reticulum is reduced by dantrolene.

Dantrolene reduces spasticity in upper motor neurone disorders, hemiplegia, paraplegia, cerebral palsy and multiple sclerosis. It is administered orally for this purpose.

Used i.v. it is the drug of choice for malignant hyperthermia which is due to persistent release of Ca^{2+} from sarcoplasmic reticulum (induced by fluorinated anaesthetics and SCh in genetically susceptible individuals having an abnormal RyR1 calcium channel).

Muscular weakness is the dose limiting side effect. Troublesome diarrhoea is another problem. Long-term use can cause serious liver toxicity.

Quinine This antimalarial drug increases refractory period and decreases excitability of motor endplates. Muscle tone in myotonia congenita is reduced. Taken at bed time it may abolish nocturnal leg cramps in some patients.

CENTRALLY ACTING MUSCLE RELAXANTS

These are drugs which reduce skeletal muscle tone and lessen muscle spasm by a selective action in the cerebrospinal axis, without altering consciousness. They selectively depress spinal and supraspinal polysynaptic reflexes involved in the regulation of muscle tone, without significantly affecting monosynaptically mediated stretch reflex. Polysynaptic pathways in the ascending reticular formation which are involved in the maintenance of wakefullness are also depressed, though to a lesser extent. Therefore, all centrally acting muscle relaxants do have some sedative property and they overlap with antianxiety drugs. They have no effect on neuromuscular transmission and on the muscle fibres, but reduce decerebrate rigidity, upper motor neurone spasticity and hyperreflexia. Prominent differences between centrally and peripherally acting muscle relaxants are listed in Table 8.4.

Mephenesin was the first drug found to reduce muscle tone by depressing spinal internuncial neurones, which modulate polysynaptic reflexes that maintain muscle tone. It is not used clinically because of toxicity. Congeners of mephenesin, *viz.* *carisoprodol, chlorzoxazone, chlormezanone* and *methocarbamol* have low toxicity and are used for musculoskeletal disorders associated with muscle spasm. They are often combined with NSAIDs. However, clinical efficacy of none of the above drugs as muscle relaxant is impressive. Gastric irritation and sedation are the most important side effects.

Table 8.4: Comparative features of centrally acting and peripherally acting muscle relaxants

Centrally acting	Peripherally acting
1. Decrease muscle tone without reducing voluntary power	Cause muscle paralysis, voluntary movements lost
2. Selectively inhibit polysynaptic reflexes in CNS	Block neuromuscular transmission
3. Cause some CNS depression	No effect on CNS
4. Given orally, sometimes parenterally	Practically always given i.v.
5. Used in chronic spastic conditions, acute muscle spasms, tetanus	Used for short-term purposes (surgical operations)

Diazepam (see Ch. 9) is the prototype of benzodiazepines (BZDs) which act in the brain on specific BZD receptors enhancing GABAergic transmission. Diazepam reduces muscle tone by supraspinal rather than spinal action. Sedation limits the dose which can be used for reducing muscle tone, but gastric tolerance is very good. It is particularly valuable in spinal injuries and tetanus. Combined with analgesics, it is popular for rheumatic disorders associated with muscle spasm.

Baclofen It is an analogue of the inhibitory transmitter GABA, and acts as selective $GABA_B$ receptor agonist.

The GABA receptors have been divided into:

$GABA_A$ receptor It is an intrinsic ion channel receptor (see Fig. 9.2), which increases Cl⁻ conductance, and is blocked by bicuculline. This receptor is facilitated by BZDs.

$GABA_B$ receptor It is a G-protein coupled receptor which hyperpolarizes neurones by increasing K^+ conductance and altering Ca^{2+} flux. The $GABA_B$ receptor is bicuculline insensitive.

Baclofen does not affect Cl⁻ transport and its actions are not antagonized by bicuculline.

Skeletal Muscle Relaxants

The primary site of action of baclofen is in the spinal cord where it depresses both polysynaptic and monosynaptic reflexes. As such, it does produce muscle weakness. Baclofen reduces spasticity in many neurological disorders like multiple sclerosis, amyotropic lateral sclerosis, spinal injuries and flexor spasms, but is relatively ineffective in stroke, cerebral palsy, rheumatic and traumatic muscle spasms and in parkinsonism.

Thiocolchicoside It is believed to be a GABA mimetic and glycinergic muscle relaxant. Combined with NSAIDs, it is being used for painful muscle spasms, e.g. sprains, torticollis, backache, etc.

Tizanidine This clonidine congener is a central α_2 adrenergic agonist—inhibits release of excitatory amino acids in spinal interneurones. Facilitation of inhibitory transmitter glycine has also been demonstrated. Tizanidine inhibits polysynaptic reflexes; reduces muscle tone and frequency of muscle spasms without reducing muscle strength.

Tizanidine is indicated in spasticity due to neurological disorders and in painful muscle spasms of spinal origin. Side effects are drymouth, drowsiness, night-time insomnia and hallucinations. Dose-dependent elevation of liver test values has been noted.

Uses of Centrally Acting Muscle Relaxants

1. *Acute muscle spasms* Overstretching of a muscle, sprain, tearing of ligaments and tendons, dislocation, fibrositis, bursitis, etc. cause painful spasm of muscles. The mephenesin-like and BZD muscle relaxants are often combined with analgesics. *They may help to relieve trismus occurring after a dental procedure.* However, efficacy of these drugs is modest or uncertain.

2. *Torticollis, lumbago, backache, neuralgias* respond in the same way as acute muscle spasms.

3. *Anxiety and tension* is often associated with increased tone of muscles and *bruxism* (involuntary grinding of teeth during sleep; mostly stress related). Diazepam like drugs may afford some relief.

4. *Spastic neurological diseases* like hemiplegia, paraplegia, spinal injuries, multiple sclerosis, and cerebral palsy are somewhat benefited by baclofen, diazepam, tizanidine and dantrolene.

5. *Tetanus* Most commonly diazepam is infused i.v. and the dose is titrated by the response. Methocarbamol is an alternative.

6. *Electroconvulsive therapy* Diazepam may be used to suppress convulsions.

7. *Orthopaedic manipulations* may be performed under the influence of diazepam or methocarbamol given i.v.

CHAPTER 9

Drugs Acting on Central Nervous System-1
Sedative-Hypnotics, Ethyl Alcohol, Antiepileptics and Antiparkinsonian Drugs

SEDATIVE-HYPNOTICS

Sedative A drug that subdues excitement and calms the subject without inducing sleep, though drowsiness may be produced. Sedation refers to decreased responsiveness to stimulation. It is associated with some decrease in alertness, motor activity and ideation.

Hypnotic A drug that induces and/or maintains sleep, similar to normal arousable sleep. This is not to be confused with 'hypnosis' meaning a trans like state in which the subject becomes passive and highly suggestible.

The sedatives and hypnotics are CNS depressants with somewhat differing time-action and dose-action relationships. Those with quicker onset, shorter duration and steeper dose-response relationships are prefered as *hypnotics*, while more slowly acting drugs with flatter dose-response curves are employed as *sedatives*. However, there is considerable overlap; a hypnotic at lower dose may act as sedative. Hypnotics given in high doses can produce general anaesthesia. Thus, sedation—hypnosis—general anaesthesia may be regarded as increasing grades of CNS depression. However, benzodiazepines (BZDs) cannot be considered non-selective or global CNS depressants like barbiturates.

Treatment of insomnia is the most important use of this class of drugs.

Sleep

The duration and pattern of sleep varies considerably among individuals. Age has an important effect on quantity and depth of sleep. It has been recognized that sleep is an architectured cyclic process in which the

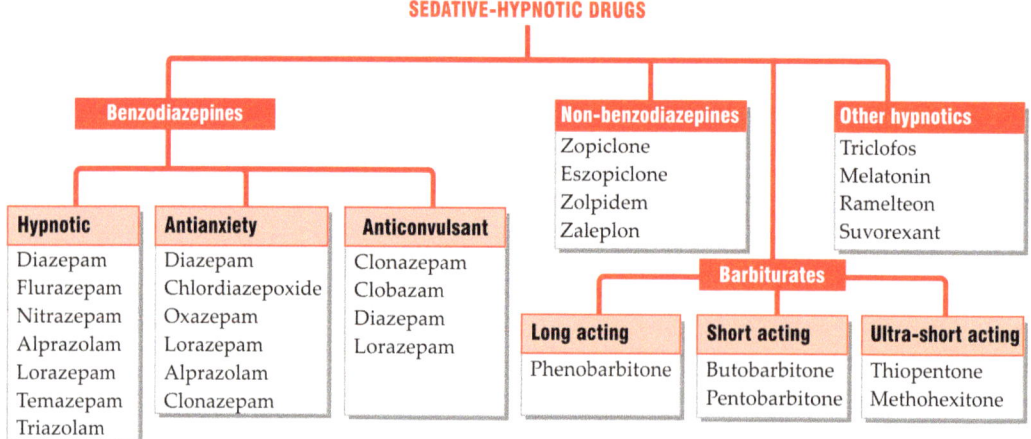

Sedative-Hypnotics

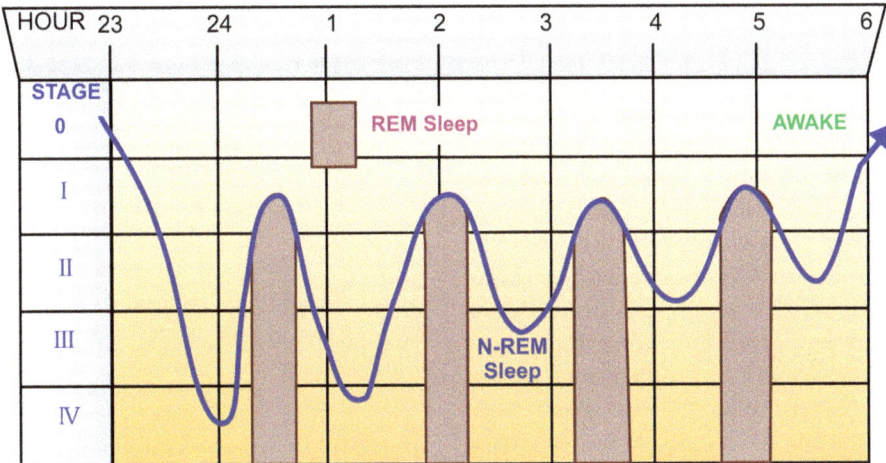

Fig. 9.1: A normal sleep cycle
REM—Rapid eye movement

subject passes from stage 0 (awake) to stage 4 (cerebral sleep) through stage 1 (dozing), stage 2 (unequivocal sleep) and stage 3 (deep sleep transition) of non-rapid eye movement (N-REM) sleep interspersed with REM (paradoxical) sleep (Fig. 9.1). About 20–30% of sleep time is spent in REM, while stage 2 occupies the major part of NREM sleep. Dreams and nightmares occur during REM sleep. The cyclic pattern of sleep stages, particularly REM, is considered to be essential for sleep to be refreshing.

BARBITURATES

Barbiturates have been popular hypnotics and sedatives of the last century up to 1960s but are not used now. However, they are described first as they are the prototype of CNS depressants.

Barbiturates are substituted derivatives of barbituric acid (malonyl urea). Lipid solubility of different members differs; the more lipid soluble ones are more potent and shorter acting. Barbiturates are insoluble in water but their sodium salts dissolve yielding highly alkaline solution.

Pharmacological actions

Barbiturates are general depressants for all excitable cells, more so for the CNS.

1. CNS Barbiturates produce dose-dependent effects:

sedation → sleep → anaesthesia → coma. Hypnotic dose shortens the time taken to fall asleep and increases sleep duration. REM and stage 3, 4 sleep are decreased; REM-NREM sleep cycle is disrupted. The effects on sleep become progressively less marked if the drug is taken every night consecutively. A rebound increase in REM sleep and nightmares is often noted when the drug is discontinued after a few nights of use. Hangover (dizziness, distortions of mood, irritability and lethargy) may occur in the morning after a nightly dose.

Sedative dose (smaller dose of a longer acting barbiturate) given at daytime can produce drowsiness, reduction in anxiety and excitability. However, barbiturates do not have selective antianxiety action. They can impair learning, short-term memory and judgement. Euphoria may be experienced by addicts.

Barbiturates have anticonvulsant property. Phenobarbitone has higher anticonvulsant: sedative ratio, i.e. it has specific anticonvulsant action.

Barbiturates depress all areas of the CNS, but reticular activating system is the most sensitive; its depression is primarily responsible for inability to maintain wakefulness.

Mechanism of action Barbiturates appear to act primarily at the GABA : BZD receptor–Cl⁻

channel complex (*see* Fig. 9.2) and potentiate GABAergic inhibition by increasing the lifetime of Cl⁻ channel opening induced by GABA. They do not bind to the BZD receptor, but bind to another site on the same macromolecular complex to exert the GABA-facilitatory action. At high concentrations, barbiturates directly increase Cl⁻ conductance (GABA-mimetic action). This is in contrast to BZDs which have only GABA-facilitatory property. Moreover, at high doses barbiturates inhibit Ca^{2+} dependent release of neurotransmitters, depress glutamate-induced neuronal depolarization through AMPA receptors (a type of excitatory amino acid receptors), and depress voltage sensitive Na^+ and K^+ channels. A dose dependent effect on multiple neuronal targets appears to confer barbiturates the ability to produce any grade of CNS depression.

2. Other actions
At relatively higher doses, barbiturates depress respiration, lower BP, decrease cardiac contractility and heart rate, but reflex tachycardia can occur due to fall in BP. Muscle tone, bowel motility and urine output are also reduced. Toxic doses cause respiratory failure and cardiovascular collapse.

Pharmacokinetics
Barbiturates are well absorbed from the g.i. tract. They are widely distributed in the body. The rate of entry into CNS is dependent on lipid solubility: highly lipid soluble thiopentone has practically instantaneous entry while less lipid soluble ones (pentobarbitone) take longer; phenobarbitone enters very slowly. Plasma protein binding varies with the compound, e.g. thiopentone 75%, phenobarbitone 20%.

Three processes are involved in termination of action of barbiturates: the relative importance of each varies with the compound.

(a) *Redistribution* This is important in the case of highly lipid soluble thiopentone and other ultrashort acting barbiturates. After their i.v. injection, consciousness is regained in 6–10 min due to redistribution (*see* Ch. 2), while the ultimate disposal occurs by metabolism (t½ of elimination phase is 9 hours).

(b) *Metabolism* Drugs with intermediate lipid solubility (short acting barbiturates) are primarily metabolized in liver by oxidation, dealkylation and conjugation. Their plasma t½ ranges from 12–40 hours.

(c) *Excretion* Barbiturates with low lipid solubility (long acting agents) are significantly excreted unchanged in urine. The t½ of phenobarbitone is 80–120 hours. Alkalinization of urine increases ionization and excretion.

Barbiturates induce hepatic microsomal enzymes and increase the rate of their own metabolism as well as that of many other drugs.

Uses
Except for phenobarbitone in epilepsy and thiopentone in anaesthesia, barbiturates are not used now.

Adverse effects
Side effects Hangover, mental confusion, impaired performance and traffic accidents.

Hypersensitivity Rashes, swelling of eyelids, lips, etc.

Tolerance and dependence Both cellular and pharmacokinetic tolerance develops on repeated use.

Addiction as well as physical dependence occurs, and barbiturates have considerable abuse liability. This is one of their major disadvantages. Withdrawal symptoms are—excitement, hallucinations, delirium, convulsions; even deaths have occurred.

Acute barbiturate poisoning
Manifestations are due to excessive CNS depression. The patient is flabby and comatose with shallow and failing respiration, fall in BP and cardiovascular collapse, renal shut down, pulmonary complications, bullous eruptions.

Lethal dose of a barbiturate depends on its lipid solubility. It is 2–3 g for the more lipid soluble agents (short acting barbiturates) and 5–10 g for less lipid soluble phenobarbitone.

Treatment
Gastric lavage; supportive measures such as patent airway, assisted respiration, oxygen, maintenance of blood volume by fluid infusion and use of vasopressors. Alkaline diuresis: with mannitol and sodium bicarbonate is indicated in the case of long acting barbiturates only. Haemodialysis is highly effective in removing long acting as well as short acting barbiturates.

There is no specific antidote for barbiturates. The approach is to keep the patient alive till the poison has been eliminated.

Interactions

1. Barbiturates induce several CYP iso-enzymes and enhance the metabolism of warfarin, steroids (including contraceptives),

tolbutamide, griseofulvin, chloramphenicol, theophylline and many other drugs, reducing their effectiveness.

2. Additive action with other CNS depressants such as alcohol, antihistamines, opioids, etc.

BENZODIAZEPINES (BZDs)

Benzodiazepines (BZDs) are selective CNS depressants which produce sedation, relieve anxiety, facilitate sleep, suppress seizures and reduce muscle tone.

Chlordiazepoxide and diazepam were introduced around 1960 as antianxiety drugs. Since then, this class has proliferated and has replaced barbiturates as hypnotic and sedative, because—

1. BZDs have a high therapeutic index. Ingestion of even 20 hypnotic doses does not usually endanger life.
2. Hypnotic doses do not affect respiration or cardiovascular functions.
3. BZDs have practically no action on other body systems. Only on i.v. injection the BP falls and cardiac contractility decreases.
4. BZDs cause less distortion of sleep architecture.
5. BZDs do not alter disposition of other drugs by microsomal enzyme induction.
6. They have lower abuse liability than barbiturates; tolerance is mild, dependence and withdrawal syndrome are less marked.
7. A specific BZD antagonist *flumazenil* is available, which can be used in case of poisoning.

CNS actions The overall action of all BZDs is qualitatively similar, but there are prominent differences in selectivity and time course of action. Different members are preferred for use as hypnotic, anxiolytic, anticonvulsant and muscle relaxant.

BZDs hasten onset of *sleep,* reduce intermittent awakening and increase total sleep time. Time spent in stage 2 is increased while that in stage 3 and 4 is decreased. They tend to shorten REM phase, but effect is less marked than with barbiturates. Most subjects wake up with a feeling of refreshing sleep. Some degree of tolerance develops to the sleep promoting action of BZDs after repeated nightly use.

Given i.v., diazepam causes analgesia. In contrast to barbiturates, BZDs do not produce hyperalgesia. They also produce centrally mediated skeletal muscle relaxation and exert anticonvulsant activity (*see* p. 142, 158).

Other actions Diazepam decreases nocturnal gastric secretion and prevents stress ulcers. BZDs do not significantly affect bowel movement.

Site and mechanism of action

Benzodiazepines act preferentially on midbrain ascending reticular formation (which maintains wakefulness) and on limbic system (thought and mental functions). Muscle relaxation is produced by a primary medullary site of action and ataxia is due to action on cerebellum.

BZDs act by enhancing presynaptic/postsynaptic inhibition through a specific BZD receptor which is an integral part of the $GABA_A$ receptor–Cl^- channel complex. The subunits of this complex form a pentameric transmembrane anion channel (Fig. 9.2) gated by the primary ligand (GABA), and modulated by secondary ligands which include BZDs. The modulatory BZD receptor increases the frequency of Cl^- channel opening induced by submaximal concentrations of GABA. The $GABA_A$ antagonist bicuculline antagonizes BZD action in a noncompetitive manner. It is noteworthy that the BZDs do not themselves increase Cl^- conductance; have only GABA facilitatory but no GABA mimetic action. This probably explains the lower ceiling CNS depressant effect of BZDs.

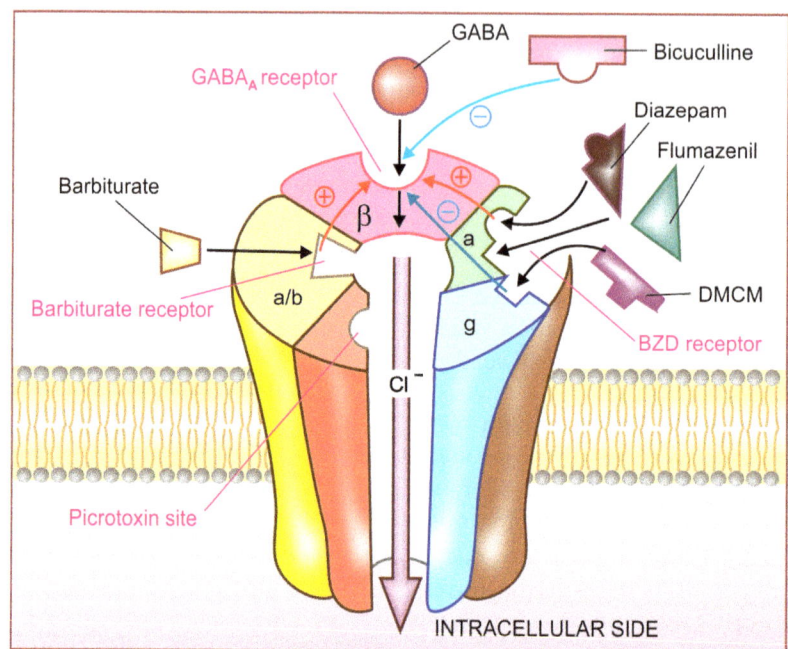

Fig. 9.2: Schematic depiction of $GABA_A$-benzodiazepine receptor-chloride channel complex
The chloride channel is gated by the primary ligand GABA. The benzodiazepine (BZD) receptor modulates $GABA_A$ receptor in either direction: agonists like diazepam facilitate, while inverse agonists like DMCM hinder GABA mediated Cl^- channel opening, and BZD antagonist flumazenil blocks the action of both. The barbiturate receptor, located elsewhere, also facilitates GABA and is capable of opening Cl^- channel directly as well. Bicuculline blocks $GABA_A$ receptor, while picrotoxin blocks the Cl^- channel directly

The BZD receptor exhibits a considerable degree of constitutive activation. As such, it is capable of fine tuning GABA action in either direction. While the BZD-agonists enhance GABA induced hyperpolarization (due to influx of Cl^- ions), and decrease firing rate of neurones, other compounds called *BZD-inverse agonists* like dimethoxyethyl-carbomethoxy-β-carboline (DMCM) inhibit GABA action and are convulsants. The competitive BZD-antagonist flumazenil blocks the sedative action of BZDs as well as the convulsant action of DMCM.

Lately, several subtypes of the BZD receptor have been described which may explain the differing pharmacological profile of individual BZD compounds.

Pharmacokinetics

There are marked pharmacokinetic differences among BZDs, because they differ in lipid solubility by > 50-fold. Oral absorption of some is rapid while that of others is slow. Absorption from i.m. sites is irregular except for lorazepam. Plasma protein binding also varies markedly (flurazepam 10% to diazepam 99%). BZDs are widely distributed in the body. The more lipid soluble members enter brain rapidly and have a two phase plasma concentration decay curve; first due to distribution and later due to elimination. A relatively short duration of action is obtained with single dose of a drug that is rapidly redistributed, even though it may have a long elimination t½. Using the elimination t½ alone to predict duration of action may be misleading. However, elimination t½ determines duration of action in case of BZDs whose elimination is by far the dominant feature or when the drug is given repeatedly.

Benzodiazepines are metabolized in the liver by dealkylation and hydroxylation to many metabolites, some of which may be active. The biological effect half-life of these drugs may be longer than the plasma t½ of the administered compound. Some BZDs (e.g. diazepam) undergo enterohepatic circulation. BZDs and their phase I metabolites are excreted in urine as glucuronide conjugates. BZDs cross placenta and are secreted in milk.

Benzodiazepines with a long t½ or those which generate active metabolites cumulate on nightly use; their action may then extend into the next day. Some features of BZDs used as hypnotic are given in Table 9.1.

Adverse effects

Benzodiazepines are relatively safe drugs. Side effects of hypnotic doses are dizziness, ataxia, disorientation, amnesia, prolongation of reaction time—impairment of psychomotor skills (the subject should not drive). Hangover is less common. Weakness, blurring of vision, dry mouth and urinary incontinence are occasional side effects. Like any hypnotic, BZDs can aggravate sleep apnoea.

Tolerance to the sedative effects develops gradually, but there is little tendency to increase the dose. Cross tolerance to alcohol and other CNS depressants occurs.

The dependence producing liability of BZDs is low. They are weak reinforcers (less pleasurable) and seldom abused alone. Drug abusers find them rather bland and prefer other CNS depressants. Withdrawal syndrome is generally mild. Drug seeking behaviour is not prominent. Anxiety, insomnia, restlessness, malaise, loss of appetite, bad dreams is all that occurs on withdrawal in most cases. Agitation, panic reaction, tremors and delirium are occasional; convulsions are rare.

Interactions

BZDs synergise with alcohol and other CNS depressants leading to excessive impairment. Concurrent use with sod. valproate has provoked psychotic symptoms.

Drug interactions due to microsomal enzyme induction are not significant.

Action of BZDs can be prolonged by CYP 3A4 inhibitors like ketoconazole, erythromycin and others. Cimetidine, isoniazid and oral contraceptives also retard BZD metabolism.

NON-BENZODIAZEPINE HYPNOTICS

This newer group of hypnotics is chemically different from BZDs, but acts as agonist on a subset of BZD receptors, producing hypnotic-amnesic action with minimal antianxiety and anticonvulsant effects. Their duration of action is relatively short, because of which they are being preferred for treatment of insomnia.

Table 9.1: Some pharmacokinetic and clinical features of benzodiazepines used as hypnotics

Drug	t½ (hr)*	Redistribution$	Hypnotic dose (mg)	Clinical indications
I. Long acting				
Flurazepam	50–100	–	15–30	Chronic insomnia, short-term insomnia
Diazepam	30–60	+	5–10	with anxiety; Frequent nocturnal awakening;
Nitrazepam	30	±	5–10	Night before operation or dental procedure
Lorazepam	10–20	–	1–2	
II. Short acting				
Alprazolam	12	+	0.25-0.5	Individuals who react unfavourably to
Temazepam	8–12	+	10–20	unfamiliar surroundings or unusual timings
Triazolam	1–3	–	0.125–0.25	of sleep. Sleep onset difficulties.

* t½ of elimination phase, including that of active metabolite
$ + indicates that redistribution contributes to termination of action of single dose

Zopiclone The effect of zopiclone on sleep resembles that of BZDs, but it does not alter REM sleep and tends to prolong stages 3 and 4. It is reported not to disturb sleep architecture; but some degree of next morning impairment can occur. Zopiclone has been used to wean-off insomniacs taking regular BZD medication. Its t½ is 5-6 hours.

Zopiclone is indicated for short-term (<2 weeks) treatment of insomnia.

Eszopiclone This is the active (S) enantiomer of zopiclone which is needed at ½ the dose. It is claimed to produce little tolerance or dependence, and can be used in chronic insomniacs as well.

Zolpidem Hypnotic effect of zolpidem is pronounced, but anticonvulsant, muscle relaxant and antianxiety effects are not evident. Its advantages are: relative lack of effect on sleep stages; minimal residual daytime sedation and fading of hypnotic action on repeated nightly use; no/little rebound insomnia on discontinuation; near absence of tolerance or physical dependence and low abuse potential combined with safety in overdose like BZDs. The t½ is short (2 hr).

Zaleplon This is the shortest acting of the newer non-BZD hypnotics. Zaleplon is rapidly absorbed and rapidly cleared by hepatic metabolism with a t½ of 1 hour. As such, it is effective only in sleep-onset insomnia; does not prolong total sleep time or reduce the number of awakenings. Because of brevity of action, it can be taken late at night without causing morning sedation. No tolerance or dependence has been reported and hypnotic effect does not fade on nightly use. However, its use should be limited to 1-2 weeks.

Uses

Currently, BZDs are one of the most frequently prescribed drugs. They have also been combined with many other categories of drugs with a view to improve efficacy by relieving attendant anxiety.

1. As hypnotic When indicated, BZDs are the hypnotic of choice and the newer non-BZD compounds zopiclone, zolpidem or zaleplon are being increasingly preferred.

Insomnia arises under a variety of circumstances. It could be a long term (months-years), short term (weeks) or transient (a day or two, mostly situational) problem.

Dentists are likely to need to prescribe a hypnotic either to ensure sleep night before the dental procedure in an apprehensive patient, or to supplement analgesics before and after dental surgery. A longer acting BZD, like diazepam, is mostly preferred for such use.

2. Other uses
- As anxiolytic and for daytime sedation.
- As anticonvulsant, especially emergency control of status epilepticus, febrile convulsions, tetanus, etc.
- As centrally acting muscle relaxant for muscular spasms and spasticity.
- For preanaesthetic medication, i.v. anaesthesia or conscious sedation.
- Alcohol withdrawal in dependent subjects.
- Along with analgesics, NSAIDs, spasmolytics, antiulcer and many other drugs.

BENZODIAZEPINE ANTAGONIST

Flumazenil It is a BZD analogue which has little intrinsic activity (practically no effect on normal subjects), but competes with BZD agonists as well as inverse agonists for the BZD receptor and reverses their depressant or stimulant effects respectively.

Flumazenil abolishes the hypnogenic, psychomotor, cognitive and EEG effects of BZDs. On i.v. injection, the action of flumazenil starts in seconds and lasts for 1–2 hr; elimination t½ is 1 hr. It has been used to reverse the effect of BZD employed for i.v.

anaesthesia or for conscious sedation, and as an antidote for BZD overdose/poisoning.

OTHER HYPNOTICS

Triclofos It is similar to the very old hypnotic chloral hydrate, but lacks the acrid odour, burning taste and gastric irritancy of the latter. Triclofos is rapidly hydrolysed to the active metabolite trichloroethanol which acts in 30 min, and the action lasts 6–8 hours. Though obsolete, triclofos is occasionally employed to sedate children, and to induce sleep in adults.

Melatonin It is the principal hormone of the pineal gland which is secreted at night, and plays an important role in entraining the sleep-wake cycle with the circadian rhythm. Started before intercontinental flight, melatonin has been shown to reduce jet-lag symptoms and to hasten reentrainment with the day-night cycle of the new place. Shift workers may also be benefited by melatonin.

Ramelteon This melatonin receptor agonist has been recently introduced as a hypnotic for sleep-onset insomnia, that is free of BZD-like side effects. Taken ½ hr, before going to bed, ramelteon has been shown to hasten sleep-onset and to increase sleep duration, without causing next-morning impairment. However, the efficacy of ramelteon as hypnotic remains to be established.

Suvorexant This novel hypnotic is a 'dual orexin receptor antagonist'. Orexins are neuropeptides which promote wakefulness by acting upon 2 types of orexin receptors in the brain. Orexin levels are high during daytime and low at night. Moreover, narcolepsy (episodes of sudden sleep) is associated with loss of orexin neurones. Suvorexant blocks both types of orexin receptors, and has been found to hasten sleep onset, as well as increase total sleep time. However, day-time somnolence may occur. The value of suvorexant as hypnotic compared to BZDs needs to be worked out.

ETHYL ALCOHOL (Ethanol)

When unqualified, 'alcohol' refers to *ethyl alcohol* or *ethanol*. Pharmacology of alcohol is important for its presence in beverages (which have been used since recorded history) and for alcohol intoxication, rather than as a drug.

Pharmacological actions

Local actions Ethanol is a mild rubefacient and counterirritant when rubbed on skin. By evaporation it produces cooling. Applied to delicate skin (scrotum) or mucous membranes (oral mucosa) it produces irritation and burning sensation. Alcohol should not be applied in the mouth.

Alcohol is an astringent—precipitates surface proteins and hardens skin. By precipitating bacterial proteins it acts as an antiseptic. The antiseptic action increases with concentration from 20 to 70%, remains constant from 70 to 90% and decreases above that.

CNS Alcohol is a neuronal depressant. Since the highest areas are most easily deranged and these are primarily inhibitory—apparent excitation and euphoria are experienced at lower plasma concentrations (30–100 mg/dl). Hesitation, caution, self-criticism and restraint are lost first. Mood and feelings are altered; anxiety may be allayed. Some individuals experience what is labelled as 'high'. With increasing concentration (100–150 mg/dl) mental clouding, disorganization of thought, impairment of memory and other faculties, alteration of perception and drowsiness supervene. At 150–200 mg/dl the person is sloppy, ataxic and drunk; 200–300 mg/dl result in stupor and above this unconsciousness prevails, medullary centres are paralysed and death may occur.

Any measurable concentration of alcohol produces a measurable slowing of reflexes: driving is dangerous. Performance is impaired, fine discrimination and precise movements are obliterated; errors increase.

Alcohol can induce sleep but is not a dependable hypnotic. Some individuals report poor quality of sleep and early morning awakening. Sleep architecture may be disorganized and sleep apnoea aggravated. Alcohol, when present in the brain, exerts anticonvulsant action, but this is followed by lowering of seizure threshold. Seizures may be precipitated in epileptics when alcohol level falls. Chronic alcohol abuse damages brain neurones.

Other actions Alcohol affects many body functions in a dose-dependent manner.
1. Vasodilatation, flushing, tachycardia, mild rise in BP at low doses (due to sympathetic stimulation), but fall in BP at high levels (due to vasodilatation, cardiac and vasomotor centre depression).
2. Respiratory centre is depressed at high concentrations.
3. Though alcohol is reputed to combat cold because it produces a sense of warmth due to cutaneous vasodilatation, heat loss is actually greater in cold surroundings.
4. Dilute alcohol (10%) stimulates gastric secretion, but higher concentrations inhibit it and cause mucosal congestion progressing to gastritis. Gastroesophageal reflux is worsened due to decrease in the tone of lower esophageal sphincter. Bowel movement may be altered.
5. Moderate amounts of alcohol do not cause liver damage in well-nourished individuals, but chronic alcoholism along with nutritional deficiencies may cause alcoholic cirrhosis of liver.
6. Regular intake of small to moderate amounts of alcohol raises HDL-cholesterol level: risk of coronary artery disease is reduced by 15–35%.
7. Urine flow may increase due to inhibition of ADH secretion.
8. Though reputed as an aphrodisiac, alcohol actually impairs performance of sexual act.
9. Hyperglycaemia (due to Adr release) occurs initially, but high levels deplete hepatic glycogen and cause hypoglycaemia.

Pharmacokinetics

Though some alcohol is absorbed from stomach, very rapid absorption occurs when it reaches duodenum and small intestine. Limited first pass metabolism takes place in stomach wall and in liver. Alcohol gets distributed widely in the body (vol of distribution 0.7 L/kg), crosses blood-brain barrier efficiently: concentration in brain is very near blood concentration. It also crosses placenta freely. Alcohol is oxidized in liver to the extent of 98%. Even with high doses, not more than 10% escapes metabolism.

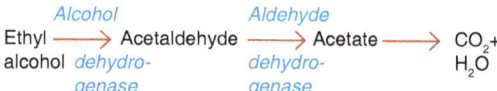

Metabolism of alcohol follows *zero order* kinetics, i.e. a constant amount (8–12 ml of absolute alcohol/hour) is degraded in unit time, irrespective of blood concentration. Thus, rate of consuming drinks governs whether a person will get drunk.

Excretion occurs though kidney and lungs, but neither is quantitatively significant. Concentration in exhaled air is about 0.05% of blood concentration. This is utilized for medicolegal determination of drunken state by using portable hand-held breath-analyser which measures alcohol content of exhaled air.

Interactions

1. Alcohol synergises with tranquilizers, antidepressants, antihistaminics, hypnotics, opioids. As a result marked CNS depression with motor impairment can occur. Chances of accidents increase.
2. Individuals taking sulfonylureas, certain *cephalosporins* (cefoperazone) or *metronidazole* have experienced *bizarre reactions when they consume alcohol*.
3. Acute alcohol ingestion inhibits, while chronic intake induces tolbutamide, phenytoin (and many other drugs) metabolism.
4. Alcohol enhances hypoglycaemia produced by insulin and sulfonylureas.

5. *Aspirin and other NSAIDs cause more gastric bleeding when taken with alcohol.*
6. Alcoholics are more prone to paracetamol toxicity due to enhanced generation of its toxic metabolite, N-acetyl-p-benzozuinone imine (NABQI).

Food value

Alcohol requires no digestion and is metabolized rapidly. It is an energy yielding substrate: 7 Cal/g, but these calories cannot be stored. It also does not supply body building and other essential constituents of food. Those who consume substantial part of their caloric intake as alcohol, often suffer from nutritional deficiencies. Thus, alcohol is an imperfect and expensive food.

Toxicity

A. Side effects of moderate drinking Nausea, vomiting, flushing, hangover, traffic accidents.

B. Acute alcoholic intoxication Hypotension, gastritis, hypoglycaemia, collapse, respiratory depression, coma and death.

C. Chronic alcoholism On chronic intake, low degree tolerance develops to the subjective and behavioral effects of alcohol. Addiction may develop even with moderate drinking, depending on the individual's likings and attitudes.

Physical dependence occurs only on heavy and round-the-clock drinking, when alcohol is present in the body continuously. Heavy drinking is often associated with nutritional deficiencies, because food is neglected and malabsorption may occur. In addition to impaired mental and physical performance, neurological afflictions are common in alcoholics. They often suffer from polyneuritis, pellagra, tremors, seizures, loss of brain mass, Wernicke's encephalopathy, Korsakoff's psychosis and megaloblastic anaemia.

Alcoholic cirrhosis of liver, hypertension, cardiomyopathy, CHF, arrhythmias, stroke, acute pancreatitis, impotence, gynaecomastia, infertility and skeletal myopathy are the other complications. Incidence of oropharyngeal, esophageal and hepatic malignancy, and respiratory infections is high; immune function is depressed.

Dental implications Alcoholics have higher incidence of heavy dental plaque, calculus deposits, chronic periodontitis and tooth loss due to poor oral hygiene. *While prescribing metronidazole or certain cephalosporins for periodontal infections, dentists should warn patients about the possibility of bizarre reactions, if they drink. Concurrent ingestion of NSAIDs and alcohol should be prohibited.*

Clinical uses

Medicinal uses of ethanol are primarily restricted to external application, and as a vehicle for liquid preparations used internally.

1. As antiseptic and disinfectant: because of good cleansing property and that it evaporates without leaving any residue, *alcohol is used to disinfect working surfaces in dentistry.* Being irritant, it is not suitable for application to oral mucosa.
2. Rubefacient and counterirritant for sprains, joint pains, etc.
3. Rubbed into the skin to prevent (but not to treat) bedsores. Astringent action of alcohol is utilized in antiperspirant and aftershave lotions.
4. Low concentrations of alcohol may be used as appetite stimulant and carminative.
5. Ethyl alcohol can be used to treat methanol poisoning.

ANTIEPILEPTIC DRUGS

Epilepsies These are a group of disorders of the CNS characterized by paroxysmal cerebral dysrhythmia, manifesting as brief episodes (seizures) of loss or disturbance of consciousness, with or without characteristic body movements (convulsions), sensory or psychiatric phenomena. Epilepsy has a focal origin in the brain, manifestations depend on the site of the focus, regions into which the discharges spread and postictal depression of these regions. Epilepsies have been classified variously; major types are:

1. Generalised seizures

1. Generalised tonic-clonic seizures (GTCS, major epilepsy, grand mal): lasts 1–2 min.
The usual sequence is aura—cry—unconsciousness—the patient falls—tonic spasm of all body muscles—clonic jerking followed by prolonged sleep and depression of all CNS functions.

2. Absence seizures (minor epilepsy, petit mal): prevalent in children, lasts about 1/2 min.
No or only momentary loss of consciousness, patient apparently freezes and stares in one direction, no muscular component or little bilateral jerking. EEG shows characteristic 3 cycles per second spike and wave pattern.

3. Atonic seizures (Akinetic epilepsy): Brief loss of consciousness with relaxation of all muscles due to excessive inhibitory discharges. Patient may fall.

4. Myoclonic seizures Shock-like momentary contraction of muscles of a limb or the whole body.

II. Partial seizures

1. Simple partial seizures (SPS) There is sudden onset unilateral jerking of a group of muscles or a limb lasting 30–90 sec., or localized sensory disturbances such as pinpricks, auditory/visual hallucinations, etc. The patient remains conscious and aware of the attack.

2. Complex partial seizures (CPS, temporal lobe epilepsy, psychomotor): attacks of bizarre and confused behaviour, dream-like state, and purposeless movements or emotional changes lasting 1–2 min along with impairment of consciousness. An aura often precedes. The seizure focus is located in the temporal lobe.

3. Simple partial or complex partial seizures secondarily generalized The partial seizure occurs first and evolves into generalized tonic-clonic seizures with loss of consciousness.

Most of the cases of epilepsy are primary (idiopathic), some may be secondary to trauma/surgery on the head, intracranial tumour, tuberculoma, cysticercosis, cerebral ischaemia, etc. Treatment is symptomatic and depends primarily on the seizure type.

Phenobarbitone

Phenobarbitone is the first efficacious antiepileptic drug introduced in 1912. Enhancement of $GABA_A$ receptor mediated synaptic inhibition appears to be its most

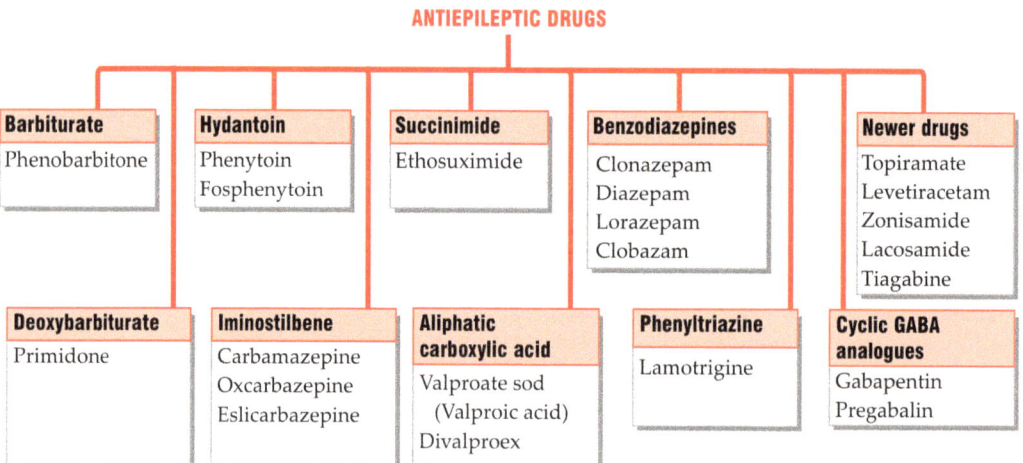

important mechanism of sedative as well as anticonvulsant action. Phenobarbitone has specific anticonvulsant activity which is not entirely dependent on general CNS depression. With continued use of phenobarbitone sedation wanes off but not the anticonvulsant action.

The major drawback of phenobarbitone as an antiepileptic is its sedative action. Long-term administration (as needed in epilepsy) may produce additional side effects like—behavioral abnormalities, diminution of intelligence, impairment of learning and memory, hyperactivity in children, mental confusion in older people.

Uses Phenobarbitone has broad-spectrum efficacy in generalized tonic-clonic (GTC), simple partial (SP) and complex partial (CP) seizures: but is infrequently used now.

Status epilepticus: Phenobarbitone may be injected i.m. or i.v. but response is slow to develop.

It is not effective in absence seizures.

Primidone It is a deoxybarbiturate which is converted by liver to phenobarbitone and phenylethyl malonamide (PEMA). Activity is mainly due to these active metabolites. Antiepileptic efficacy and side effects are similar to phenobarbitone.

Phenytoin (Diphenylhydantoin)

Phenytoin is not a global CNS depressant. Only mild sedation occurs at therapeutic doses. Tonic-clonic epilepsy is suppressed but paroxysmal focal EEG discharge and 'aura' persist.

Mechanism of action Phenytoin prevents repetitive detonation of normal brain cells. This is achieved by prolonging the inactivated state of voltage sensitive neuronal Na$^+$ channel (Fig. 9.3) that governs the refractory period of the neurone. As a result, high frequency discharges are inhibited with little effect on normal low frequency discharges. Intracellular accumulation of Na$^+$ that occurs during repetitive firing is prevented.

Ability of phenytoin to selectively inhibit high frequency firing confers efficacy in trigeminal neuralgia as well.

Pharmacokinetics Absorption of phenytoin by oral route is slow, and it is 80–90% bound to plasma proteins.

Phenytoin is metabolized in liver by hydroxylation and glucuronide conjugation. The kinetics of metabolism is *capacity limited*; changes from first order to zero order over the therapeutic range—small increments in dose produce disproportionately high plasma concentrations. The t½ (normally 12–24 hr) progressively increases (up to 60 hr) when plasma concentration rises.

Adverse effects Phenytoin produces numerous side effects; some occur at therapeutic plasma concentration after prolonged use:

Gum hypertrophy: Commonest side effect (20% incidence), more in younger patients. It is due to overgrowth of gingival collagen fibres. It can be minimized by maintaining good oral hygiene.

- Hirsutism, coarsening of facial features (especially troublesome in young girls), acne.
- Hypersensitivity reactions are—rashes, DLE, lymphadenopathy; neutropenia is rare, but requires discontinuation of therapy.
- Megaloblastic anaemia: phenytoin decreases folate absorption.
- Osteomalacia: phenytoin interferes with vit D activation.
- Given during pregnancy, phenytoin can produce foetal hydantoin syndrome (hypoplastic phalanges, cleft palate, hare lip, microcephaly).

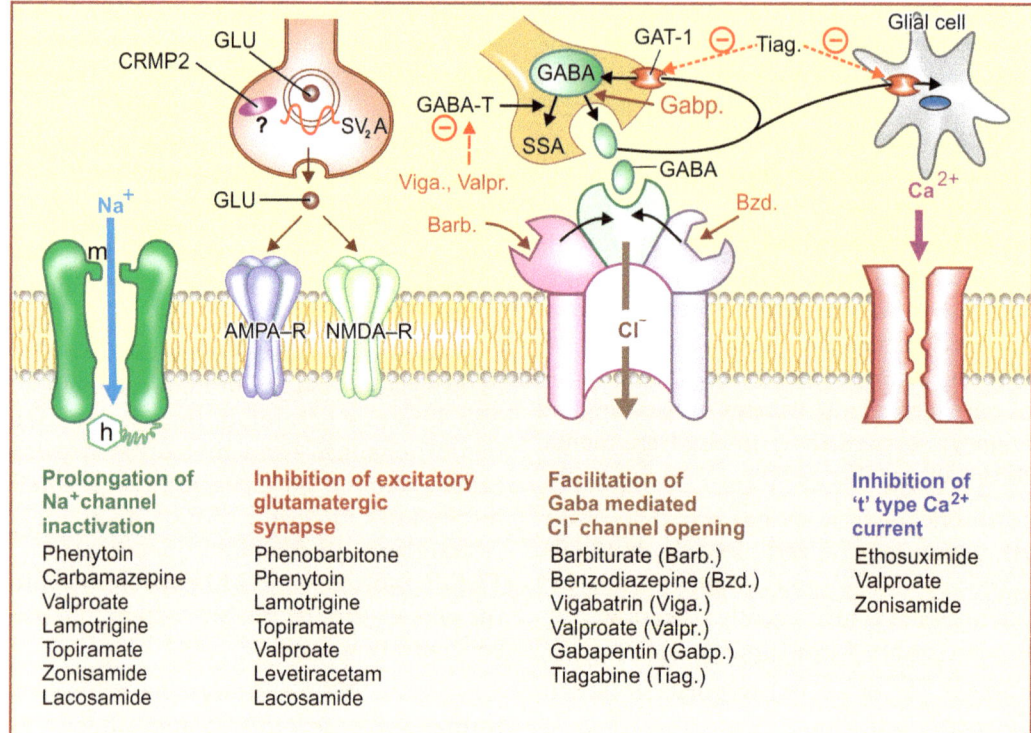

Fig. 9.3: Major mechanisms of anticonvulsant action
m—Activation gate; h—Inactivation gate; GABA-T—GABA transaminase; SSA—Succinic semialdehyde; GAT-1—GABA transporter; GLU—Glutamate; SV$_2$A—Synaptic vesicular protein 2A; CRMP2—collapsin-response mediator protein; NMDA-R—N-methyl D-aspartate receptor; AMPA-R—α aminohydroxy methyl isoxazole propionic acid receptor

Overdose toxicity due to high plasma concentration of phenitoin produces:
(a) Cerebellar and vestibular manifestations: ataxia, vertigo, diplopia and nystagmus.
(b) Drowsiness, behavioral alterations, mental confusion and hallucinations.
(c) Epigastric pain, nausea and vomiting.

Interactions Phenobarbitone competitively inhibits phenytoin metabolism, while by enzyme induction both enhance each other's degradation—unpredictable overall interaction.
- Carbamazepine and phenytoin induce each other's metabolism.
- Valproate displaces protein bound phenytoin and decreases its metabolism: plasma level of unbound phenytoin increases.
- Chloramphenicol, isoniazid, cimetidine, dicumarol, and warfarin inhibit phenytoin metabolism, and can precipitate its toxicity.
- Phenytoin induces microsomal enzymes and increases degradation of steroids (failure of oral contraceptives), doxycycline, theophylline and many other drugs.

Uses Phenytoin is one of the first line antiepileptic drugs for—
1. Generalized tonic-clonic, simple and complex partial seizures. It is ineffective in absence seizures.
2. Trigeminal neuralgia: second choice drug to carbamazepine.

Fosphenytoin
This water soluble prodrug of phenytoin has replaced phenytoin for i.v. use in status epilepticus, because it is less damaging to the intima of the vein.

Carbamazepine

Chemically related to imipramine, it was introduced in the 1960s for trigeminal neuralgia; but soon became a first line drug for partial seizures as well as for GTCS. The action of carbamazepine on Na$^+$ channels (prolongation of inactivated state) is similar to that of phenytoin. High frequency neuronal discharges are inhibited, and its presynaptic action may decrease transmitter release.

Carbamazepine has a therapeutic effect in mood disorders, and an antidiuretic action by enhancing ADH action on renal tubules.

Oral absorption of carbamazepine is slow and variable. It is 75% bound to plasma proteins and metabolized in liver by oxidation to an active metabolite (10-11 epoxy carbamazepine) as well as by hydroxylation and conjugation to inactive ones. Initially, its plasma t½ is 20–40 hours but decreases to 10–20 hr on chronic medication due to autoinduction of metabolism.

Adverse effects Carbamazepine produces dose-related neurotoxicity—sedation, dizziness, vertigo, diplopia and ataxia. Vomiting, diarrhoea, worsening of seizures are also seen with higher doses.
Hypersensitivity reactions are rashes, photosensitivity, hepatitis, lupus like syndrome and rarely agranulocytosis, aplastic anaemia. Increased incidence of minor foetal malformations has been reported. Its combination with valproate doubles teratogenic frequency.

Interactions Carbamazepine is an enzyme inducer. It can reduce efficacy of haloperidol and oral contraceptives. Metabolism of carbamazepine is induced by phenobarbitone, phenytoin, valproate and vice versa.

Erythromycin, fluoxetine, isoniazid inhibit metabolism of carbamazepine.

Uses Carbamazepine is the most effective drug for CPS, and shares first choice drug status for GTCS and SPS as well.

Trigeminal and related neuralgias: Carbamazepine is the drug of choice. These neuralgias are characterized by attacks of high intensity electric shock-like or stabbing pain set off by even trivial stimulation of certain trigger zones in the mouth or on the face. Drugs benefit by interrupting temporal summation of afferent impulses (by a selective action on high frequency neuronal discharges). Carbamazepine is not an analgesic but has a specific action (almost diagnostic) in these neuralgias. About 60% patients of trigeminal neuralgia respond well. Phenytoin and baclofen are less efficacious alternatives.

Manic depressive illness and acute mania: as an alternative to lithium.

Oxcarbazepine
This congener of carbamazepine does not generate the epoxide metabolite, so that toxic effects and drug interactions due to this metabolite are avoided. Indications are similar to carbamazepine, but doses required are 1½ times larger.

Eslicarbazepine
This (s)+ enantiomer prodrug is rapidly converted to the same active metabolite as is oxcarbazepine. As such, therapeutic utility and toxic effects of eslicarbazepine are similar to those of oxcarbazepine, but it is suitable for once daily dosing. It is an add-on drug for partial seizures.

Ethosuximide
It has an entirely different profile of anticonvulsant action than phenytoin and is clinically effective only in absence seizures. However, ethosuximide has been superseded by sod. valproate.

Valproic acid (Sodium valproate)

It is a broad-spectrum anticonvulsant effective in several experimental models of epilepsy. Remarkably, valproate produces little sedation or other central effects. It is effective in partial seizures, GTCS as well as in absence, myoclonic and atonic seizures.

Valproate appears to act by multiple mechanisms:
(i) A phenytoin-like frequency dependent prolongation of Na^+ channel inactivation.
(ii) Attenuation of Ca^{2+} mediated 'T' current (ethosuximide like).
(iii) Enhanced release of inhibitory transmitter GABA by inhibiting its degradation (by GABA-transaminase).
(iv) Blockade of excitatory NMDA type of glutamate receptor.

Valproate is well absorbed, 90% plasma protein bound, completely metabolized and then excreted in urine. Plasma t½ is 10–15 hours.

Adverse effects Toxicity of valproate is low. Anorexia, vomiting, drowsiness, ataxia and tremor are dose-related side effects. However, cognitive and behavioral effects are not prominent.
Alopecia, curling of hair, and increased bleeding tendency have been observed. *The dentist may face excess bleeding while executing a dental procedure.*
A rare but serious adverse effect is fulminant hepatitis, which occurs only in children (especially below 3 yr age).
Administered during pregnancy, it has produced neural tube defects (spina bifida) in the offspring.

Uses Valproic acid is the drug of choice for absence seizures, and one of the 1st line drugs for GTCS, SPS and CPS. Though, control is often incomplete, valproate is the most effective drug for myoclonic and atonic seizures.
Mania and bipolar illness: Valproate is now extensively used.

Interactions

- Valproate increases plasma levels of phenobarbitone and lamotriazine by inhibiting their metabolism.
- It displaces phenytoin from protein binding site and decreases its metabolism; phenytoin toxicity may occur.
- Valproate inhibits hydrolysis of active epoxide metabolite of carbamazepine.
- Concurrent administration of clonazepam and valproate is contraindicated because absence status may be precipitated.
- Foetal abnormalities are more common if valproate and carbamazepine are given concurrently.

Divalproex This coordination compound of valproic acid with sodium valproate has better gastric tolerance, but is absorbed more slowly. Its indications are similar to those of valproate.

Clonazepam

It is a benzodiazepine with prominent anticonvulsant properties, but is singularly ineffective in GTCS.
Benzodiazepines potentiate GABA induced Cl⁻ influx to produce sedation and the same mechanism has been held responsible for the anticonvulsant property. At large doses, high frequency discharges are inhibited akin to phenytoin.
The most important side effect of clonazepam is sedation and dullness. Motor disturbances and ataxia are dose-related adverse effects.
Clonazepam has been primarily employed in absence seizures. It is also useful in myoclonic and akinetic epilepsy. However, its value is limited by development of tolerance.

Clobazam This BZD analogue is generally used as adjuvant to other antiepileptic drugs in refractory epilepsy.

Diazepam

Diazepam has anticonvulsant activity but is not used for long-term therapy of epilepsy because of prominent sedative action and rapid development of tolerance to the antiepileptic effect. However, administered i.v., it is one of the drugs for emergency control of convulsions, e.g. status epilepticus, tetanus, eclampsia, convulsant drug poisoning, etc.
Rectal instillation of diazepam is the preferred therapy for febrile convulsions in children.

Lorazepam Injected i.v., it is better suited than diazepam for emergency control of seizures with the advantage of more sustained effect.

Lamotrigine A newer anticonvulsant having carbamazepine-like action profile. Prolongation of Na$^+$ channel inactivation and suppression of high frequency firing has been demonstrated. In addition, it may directly block voltage sensitive Na$^+$ channels, thus stabilizing the presynaptic membrane and preventing release of excitatory neurotransmitters, mainly glutamate and aspartate.

Lamotrigine is a broad-spectrum antiepileptic found useful in refractory cases of partial seizures and GTCS, both as add-on drug as well as monotherapy. Absence, myoclonic and akinetic epilepsy cases have also been successfully treated.

Side effects are sleepiness, dizziness, diplopia, ataxia and vomiting.

Gabapentin This lipophilic GABA derivative crosses to the brain and enhances GABA release, but does not act as agonist at GABA$_A$ receptor. Added to a first line drug, it reduces seizure frequency in refractory partial seizures with or without generalization. Gabapentin and its newer congener *pregabalin* exert a specific analgesic effect in neuropathic pain. They are now considered to be first line drugs for pain due to diabetic neuropathy, postherpetic and other neuralgias. Some prophylactic effect in migraine has been noted. Side effects are sedation, dizziness and unsteadiness.

Pregabalin This newer congener of gabapentin has been particularly used for neuropathic pain, but has similar antiseizure property as well. It appears to cause less sedation than gabapentin.

Topiramate This weak carbonic anhydrase inhibitor has broad-spectrum anticonvulsant activity. It appears to act by multiple mechanisms, *viz* phenytoin-like prolongation of Na$^+$ channel inactivation, GABA potentiation, antagonism of certain glutamate receptors and neuronal hyperpolarization.

Topiramate is indicated as monotherapy, as well as for supplementing primary antiepileptic drug in refractory SPS, CPS and GTCS. Promising results have been obtained in myoclonic epilepsy also.

Zonisamide Another newer weak carbonic anhydrase inhibitor with multiple anticonvulsant actions. It is indicated mainly as 'add-on' therapy for refractory partial seizures.

Levetiracetam A unique anticonvulsant which does not appear to act by any of the major anticonvulsant mechanisms of action, but by altering release of glutamate and/or GABA across the synapse. It is used as adjuvant medication for refractory partial seizures with or without generalization. It produces few side effects. Drug interactions are unlikely.

Lacosamide This newer antiepileptic drug acts by enhancing Na$^+$ channel inactivation and suppressing repetitive firing of neurones. It is used as add-on therapy of partial seizures with or without generalization. Side effects are ataxia, vertigo, depression and cardiac arrhythmia.

TREATMENT OF EPILEPSIES

Antiepileptic drugs suppress seizures but do not cure the disorder; the disease may fade out though after years of successful control. The aim of drugs is to control and totally prevent all seizure activity at an acceptable level of side effects. The cause of epilepsy should be searched in the patient; if found and treatable, an attempt to remove it should be made. Some general principles of symptomatic treatment with antiepileptic drugs are:

1. Choice of drug (Table 9.2) and dose is according to the seizure type(s) and need of the individual patient.

Table 9.2: Choice of antiseizure drugs

Type of seizure	First line drugs	Alternative/Add-on drugs	Reserve/Add-on drugs
1. Partial seizures (SPS, CPS) with or without generalization	Carbamazepine, Lamotrigine, Valproate, Oxcarbazepine	Levetiracetam, Clobazam, Phenytoin, Gabapentin, Topiramate	Lacosamide, Phenobarbitone, Zonisamide, Tiagabine
2. Generalized seizures • Tonic-clonic	Valproate, Lamotrigine, Carbamazepine	Clobazam, Oxcarbazepine, Phenytoin	Levetiracetam, Topiramate, Phenobarbitone
• Absence	Valproate, Ethosuximide	Lamotrigine, Clobazam, Clonazepam	Levetiracetam, Topiramate, Zonisamide
• Myoclonic	Valproate	Topiramate, Levetiracetaim	Clobazam, Clonazepam
• Atonic	Valproate	Lamotrigine	Topiramate, Clonazepam
3. Febrile seizures	Diazepam (rectal)	—	—
4. Status epilepticus	Lorazepam (i.v.) Diazepam (i.v.)	Fosphenytoin (i.v.)	Phenobarbitone (i.m.)

2. Initiate treatment early, because each seizure episode increases the propensity to further attacks. Start with a single drug, gradually increase dose till full control of seizures or side effects appear. Use combinations when all reasonable monotherapy fails.
3. Therapy should be as simple as possible. A seizure diary should be maintained.
4. All drug withdrawals should be gradual (except in case of toxicity). Prolonged therapy (may be life long, or at least 3 years after the last seizure) is needed. Withdrawal may be attempted in selected cases.
5. Dose regulation may be facilitated by monitoring of steady-state plasma drug levels.
6. When women on antiepileptic therapy conceive, antiepileptic drugs should not be stopped. Though most antiseizure drugs have been shown to increase the incidence of birth defects, discontinuation of therapy carries a high risk of status epilepticus. It may be advisable to substitute valproate by another antiepileptic drug, and to give folic acid supplementation.

Dental implications

1. Dentists have to recognise and manage phenytoin induced gum hypertrophy.
2. *In an epileptic patient dental procedure should be carried out only after ensuring that the patient is under adequate anticonvulsant drug cover and has taken his/her medication.*
3. *In the event of a patient developing an attack of tonic-clonic seizures during dental procedure, the first priority is to prevent injuries due to biting or fall. Ensure that the patient is secure on the flat dental chair or on the floor. Any denture or instrument should be immediately removed from the mouth. The head should be turned to the side to prevent the tongue from falling back and obstructing the airway. Give oxygen through a face mask to support respiration if any sign of cyanosis is seen. Do not attempt to stop convulsive movements by restraining the patient.*

The seizure usually passes off in a few minutes, but the patient may be confused or dazed. He/She should be allowed to rest and recover for some time. Continuation or postponement of the procedure after the fit is over depends on the circumstances.

The patient must be sent back home with an escort. *In case the seizures do not stop or recur within 10–20 minutes, management is as for status epilepticus.*

Status epilepticus When seizure activity occurs for >30 min, or two or more seizures occur in quick succession, the condition is labelled 'status epilepticus'. Recurrent tonic-clonic convulsions without recovery of consciousness is an emergency; fits have to be controlled as quickly as possible to prevent death and permanent brain damage.

- The first priority is to maintain patent airway. Dextrose (20–50 ml of 50% solution) is injected i.v. to correct hypoglycaemia, if that is responsible for the seizure.
- *Lorazepam* 4 mg injected i.v. over 2 min, repeated once if required, is the first choice drug now. It produces more sustained anticonvulsant effect than diazepam.
- *Diazepam* 10 mg injected i.v. at 2 mg/min is an alternative.
- *Fosphenytoin* 100–150 mg/min i.v. infusion to a maximum of 15 mg/kg, under continuous ECG monitoring is a slower acting drug which may be given to suppress seizures that have not responded, and to pave the way for long-term seizure treatment.
- *Phenobarbitone sod.* 50–100 mg i.v. is another slower acting drug to be used as alternative.
- Refractory cases may be treated with i.v. midazolam/propofol/thiopentone anaesthesia, with or without curarization.
- General measures, including maintenance of airway (intubation if required), oxygenation, fluid and electrolyte balance, BP, normal cardiac rhythm, euglycaemia and care of the unconscious must be taken.

ANTIPARKINSONIAN DRUGS

These are drugs that have a therapeutic effect in parkinsonism.

Parkinsonism It is an extrapyramidal motor disorder characterized by *rigidity, tremor* and *hypokinesia* with secondary manifestations like defective posture and gait, mask-like face and sialorrhoea; dementia may accompany. If untreated, the symptoms progress over several years to end-stage disease in which the patient is rigid, unable to move, unable to breathe properly; succumbs mostly to chest infections/embolism.

Parkinson's disease (PD) is a progressive degenerative disorder, mostly affecting older people, first described

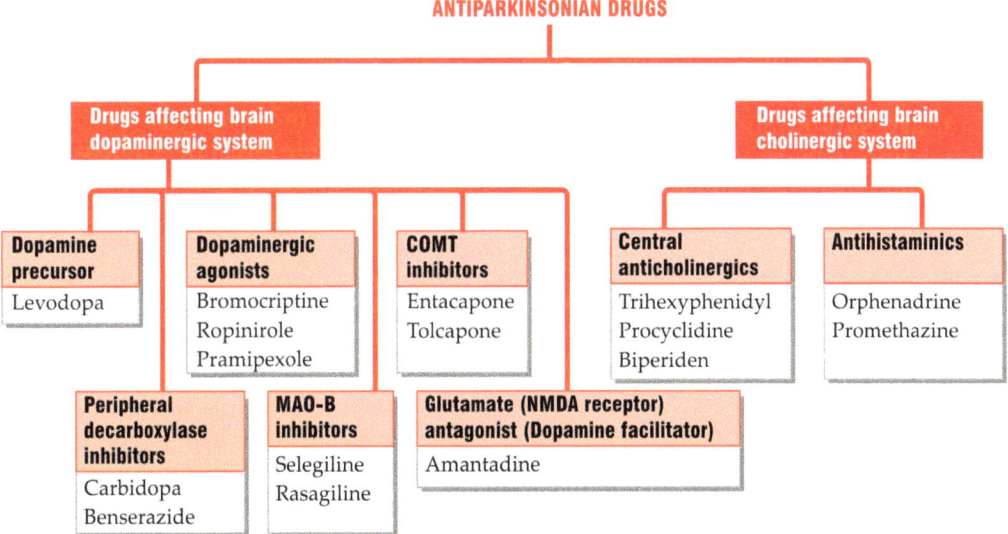

by James Parkinson in 1817. The most consistent lesion in PD is degeneration of neurones in substantia nigra pars compacta and the nigrostriatal (dopaminergic) tract. This results in deficiency of dopamine (DA) in the striatum which controls muscle tone and coordinates movements. An imbalance between dopaminergic (inhibitory) and cholinergic (excitatory) system in the striatum occurs giving rise to the motor defect.

Drug-induced reversible parkinsonism due to neuroleptics, metoclopramide (dopaminergic blockers) is now fairly common.

Levodopa

Levodopa, the precursor of the transmitter dopamine (DA), has a specific salutary effect in PD: efficacy exceeding that of any other drug used alone. More than 95% of an oral dose of levodopa is decarboxylated in the peripheral tissues (mainly gut and liver). DA thus formed acts on heart, blood vessels, other peripheral organs and on CTZ (though located in the brain, i.e. floor of IV ventricle, it is not bound by blood-brain barrier). About 1–2% of the administered levodopa crosses to the brain, is taken up by the surviving dopaminergic neurones, converted to DA which is stored and released as a transmitter.

Actions

1. **CNS** Levodopa hardly produces any effect in normal individuals, but marked symptomatic improvement occurs in parkinsonian patients. Hypokinesia and rigidity resolve first, later tremor as well. Secondary symptoms of posture, gait, handwriting, speech, facial expression, mood, self-care and interest in life are gradually normalized.

2. **CVS** The DA formed in the periphery can cause tachycardia by acting on cardiac β adrenergic receptors. Postural hypotension due to central and ganglionic action of DA is quite common.

3. **CTZ** The peripherally formed DA gains access to the CTZ without hindrance—elicits nausea and vomiting by stimulating dopaminergic D2 receptors.

4. **Endocrine** DA acts on pituitary mammotropes to inhibit prolactin release → blood prolactin level falls.

Pharmacokinetics

Levodopa is metabolized, both in the periphery as well as in the brain by two principal enzymes, *viz.* monoamine oxidase-B (MAO-B) and catechol-o-methyltransferase (COMT), which act sequentially producing homovanillic acid (HVA). This is excreted in urine, mostly after conjugation. The plasma t½ of levodopa is 1–2 hours.

Adverse effects Side effects of levodopa therapy are frequent and often troublesome. Some are prominent in the beginning of therapy while others appear late.

1. Nausea and vomiting: This is due to activation of D2 receptors in the CTZ. Tolerance gradually develops and then the dose can be progressively increased.
2. Postural hypotension: It occurs in about 1/3rd of patients, but is mostly asymptomatic; some patients experience dizziness, few have fainting attacks. *Care should be taken by the dentist that patients on levodopa therapy do not sit up and leave the dental chair abruptly from a reclining position.*
3. Cardiac arrhythmias
4. Exacerbation of angina
5. Alteration in taste sensation
6. Abnormal movements: Facial tics, grimacing, tongue thrusting, choreoathetoid movements of limbs, etc. start appearing after a few months of use of levodopa. These symptoms may become as disabling as the original disease itself. *Orofacial dyskinesias may make brushing difficult—damage teeth and pose difficulty in wearing dentures.*
7. Behavioural effects: Range from mild anxiety, nightmares, etc. to severe depression, mania, hallucinations, mental confusion or frank psychosis.
8. Fluctuation in motor performance: After 2–5 years of therapy, the level of

control of parkinsonian symptomatology starts showing fluctuation. 'End of dose' deterioration, develops into rapid 'switches' or 'on-off' effect. With time 'all or none' response develops, i.e. the patient is alternately well and disabled.

Interactions

1. Pyridoxine: Abolishes the therapeutic effect by enhancing peripheral decarboxylation of levodopa.
2. Phenothiazines, butyrophenones, metoclopramide reverse the therapeutic effect of levodopa by blocking DA receptors.
3. Antihypertensives: postural hypotension is accentuated.

PERIPHERAL DECARBOXYLASE INHIBITORS

Carbidopa and *benserazide* are extracerebral dopa decarboxylase inhibitors. They do not penetrate blood-brain barrier and do not inhibit conversion of levodopa to DA in the brain. Administered along with levodopa, they increase its t½ in the periphery and make more of it available to cross blood-brain barrier to reach its site of action.

Benefits obtained on combining with levodopa are—
1. The plasma t½ of levodopa is prolonged and its dose is reduced to approximately 1/4th.
2. Systemic concentration of DA is reduced, nausea and vomiting are minimized.
3. Cardiac complications are minimized.
4. Pyridoxine reversal of levodopa effect does not occur.
5. 'On-off' effect is minimized due to more sestained DA levels.
6. Degree of improvement may be higher.

Problems not resolved or accentuated are—
1. Involuntary movements
2. Behavioral abnormalities
3. Postural hypotension.

Currently, levodopa is practically always used along with a decarboxylase inhibitor

DOPAMINERGIC AGONISTS

The DA agonists can act on striatal DA receptors even in advanced patients who have largely lost the capacity to synthesize, store and release DA from the administered levodopa. Moreover, they can be longer acting, exert subtype selective activation of DA receptors involved in parkinsonism, and not share the concern expressed about levodopa of contributing to dopaminergic neuronal damage by oxidative metabolism.

Bromocriptine It is an ergot derivative which acts as potent agonist on D2, but as partial agonist or antagonist on D1 receptors. Bromocriptin improves parkinsonian symptoms, but has been replaced by the newer DA agonists ropinirole and pramipexole.

Ropinirole and Pramipexole These are two nonergoline, selective D2/D3 receptor agonists with negligible affinity for D1 and nondopaminergic receptors. They have therapeutic effect in PD comparable to levodopa and bromocriptin, but are better tolerated. Side effects are nausea, dizziness, hallucinations, postural hypotension and episodes of day time sleep.

Ropinirole and pramipexole are used for monotherapy as well as to supplement levodopa, with the advantage of lower incidence of dyskinesias and motor fluctuations.

MAO-B INHIBITOR

Selegiline (Deprenyl) It is a selective and irreversible MAO-B inhibitor which retards intracerebral metabolism of DA; has mild antiparkinsonian action in early cases and prolongs levodopa action when given along with the latter. Two isoenzyme forms of MAO, termed MAO-A and MAO-B are recognized. Both are present in peripheral adrenergic structures and intestinal mucosa, while the latter predominates in brain and blood platelets. Unlike nonselective MAO inhibitors, selegiline in low doses (10 mg/day) does not interfere with peripheral metabolism of dietary amines;

CA accumulation and hypertensive reaction does not develop.

Selegiline interacts with pethidine causing excitement, rigidity, hyperthermia, respiratory depression. It may interact with tricyclic antidepressants and selective serotonin reuptake inhibitors as well.

Rasagiline This newer selective MAO-B inhibitor is more potent, longer acting and better tolerated. It is being preferred over selegiline for prolonging the action of levodopa.

COMT INHIBITORS

Two selective and reversible COMT inhibitors *Entacapone* and *Tolcapone* were introduced as adjuvants to levodopa-carbidopa for advanced PD. Because of hepatotoxicity, tolcapone is practically not used now. When peripheral decarboxylation of levodopa is blocked by carbidopa/benserazide, it is mainly metabolized by COMT to 3-O-methyldopa. Blockade of this pathway by entacapone prolongs the t½ of levodopa and allows a larger fraction of the administered dose to cross to brain. Entacapone acts only in the periphery.

Entacapone may be used to smoothen 'wearing off' effect, or to increase 'on' time with levodopa-carbidopa.

GLUTAMATE ANTAGONIST (DOPAMINE FACILITATOR)

Amantadine Developed as an antiviral drug for prophylaxis of influenza A_2, amantadine was found serendipitiously to benefit parkinsonism. It acts rapidly, but has lower efficacy than levodopa. Though, up to 2/3rd patients derive some benefit, tolerance develops over few months and the efficacy is lost. Amantadine acts primarily by exerting an antagonistic action on NMDA type of glutamate receptors, through which striatal dopaminergic system controls motor function. It also promotes presynaptic synthesis and release of DA in the brain.

Amantadine is occasionally used to supplement levodopa.

CENTRAL ANTICHOLINERGICS

These are drugs having a higher central: peripheral anticholinergic action ratio than atropine, but the pharmacological profile is similar to it. In addition, certain H_1 antihistaminics have significant central anticholinergic property. There is little to choose clinically among these drugs, though trihexyphenidyl is most commonly used.

These drugs act by reducing the unbalanced cholinergic activity in the striatum of parkinsonian patients. Sialorrhoea is controlled by their peripheral action. The overall efficacy is much lower than levodopa, and they may be used alone in mild cases. In others, they can be combined with levodopa-carbidopa.

Anticholinergics are the only drugs effective in neuroleptic drug induced parkinsonism. *Xerostomia caused by antiparkinsonian anticholinergics may aggravate dental caries.*

Chapter 10

Drugs Acting on Central Nervous System-2
Psychopharmacological Agents

The psychopharmacological agents or psychotropic drugs are medicines having primary effects on *psyche* (mental processes) and are used for treatment of psychiatric disorders.

In order to understand the categorization of psychotropic drugs and their actions, it is necessary to know the broad features of various types of psychiatric illnesses, which are outlined below.

Psychoses These are severe psychiatric illness with serious distortion of thought, behaviour, capacity to recognise reality and of perception (delusions and hallucinations). There is inexplicable misperception and misevaluation; the patient is unable to meet the ordinary demands of life.

(a) *Acute and chronic organic brain syndromes (cognitive disorders)* Such as delirium and dementia; some toxic or pathological basis can often be defined; prominent features are confusion, disorientation, defective memory and disorganized thought and behaviour.

(b) *Functional disorders* No underlying cause can be defined; memory and orientation are mostly retained but emotion, thought, reasoning and behaviour are seriously altered.

(i) *Schizophrenia* (split mind), i.e. splitting of perception and interpretation from reality, characterized by hallucinations, inability to think coherently with little impairment of alertness and intellect.

(ii) *Paranoid states* with marked persecutory or other kinds of fixed delusions (false beliefs) and loss of insight into the abnormality.

(iii) *Mood (affective) disorders* The primary symptom is change in mood state; may manifest as:

Mania—elation, hyperactivity, uncontrollable thought and speech, may be associated with violent behaviour, or

Depression—sadness, loss of interest and pleasure, worthlessness, guilt, physical and mental slowing, melancholia, self destructive ideation.

A common form of mood disorder is *bipolar disorder* with cyclically alternating manic and depressive phases. The relapsing mood disorder may also be *unipolar* (mania or depression) with waxing and waning course.

Neuroses These are less serious; the ability to comprehend reality is not lost, though the patient may undergo extreme suffering. Depending on the predominant feature, it may be labelled as:

(a) *Anxiety* An unpleasant emotional state associated with uneasiness, worry, tension and concern for the future.

(b) *Phobic states* Fear of the unknown or of some specific objects, person or situations.

(c) *Obsessive compulsive disorder* (OCD) Limited abnormality of thought or behaviour (ritual like) which the patient is not able to overcome even on voluntary effort.

(d) *Reactive depression* due to physical illness, loss, blow to self-esteem or bereavement, but is excessive or disproportionate.

(e) *Post-traumatic stress disorder* (PTSD) Varied symptoms following distressing experiences like war, riots, earthquakes, etc.

(f) *Hysterical* Dramatic symptoms resembling serious physical illness, but situational, and always in the presence of others. The patient does not feign but actually undergoes the symptoms, though the basis is only psychic and not physical.

Pathophysiology of mental illness is not clear, though some ideas have been formed, e.g. dopaminergic overactivity in the limbic system may be involved in schizophrenia and mania; monoaminergic (NA, 5-HT) deficit may underlie depression. Treatment is empirical, symptom oriented and not disease specific. However, it is highly effective in many situations.

Depending on the primary use, the psychotropic drugs may be grouped into:

1. *Antipsychotic* (neuroleptic, ataractic, major tranquilliser) useful in all types of functional psychosis, especially schizophrenia.

2. *Antimanic* (mood stabiliser) used to control mania and to break into cyclic affective disorders (bipolar disorder).

3. *Antidepressants* used for minor as well as major depressive illness, phobic states, obsessive- compulsive behaviour, and certain anxiety disorders.

4. *Antianxiety* (anxiolytic-sedative, minor tranquilliser) used for anxiety and phobic states.

5. *Psychotomimetic* (psychedelic, psychodysleptic, hallucinogen). These drugs are seldom used therapeutically but produce psychosis like states. Most of them are drugs of abuse like LSD, cannabis.

Tranquillizer It is an old term meaning "a drug which reduces mental tension and produces calmness without inducing sleep or depressing mental faculties." It has been interpreted differently by different people; some extend it to cover both chlorpromazine-like and antianxiety drugs, others feel that it should be restricted to the antianxiety drugs only. The term 'tranquillizer' is therefore best avoided.

ANTIPSYCHOTIC DRUGS (Neuroleptics)

These are drugs having a salutary therapeutic effect in psychoses.

Pharmacology of chlorpromazine (CPZ) is described as the prototype of 'typical antipsychotics' which have potent dopamine D2 receptor blocking action and produce extrapyramidal motor side effects. These drugs are also called neuroleptic drugs. In addition, several atypical antipsychotic drugs are available which have weak D2 blocking action and produce fewer side effects. Comparative features of various antipsychotic drugs are presented in Table 10.1.

PHARMACOLOGICAL ACTIONS

1. CNS Effects differ in normal and psychotic individuals.

In nonpsychotic individuals CPZ produces indifference to surroundings, paucity of thought, psychomotor slowing, emotional

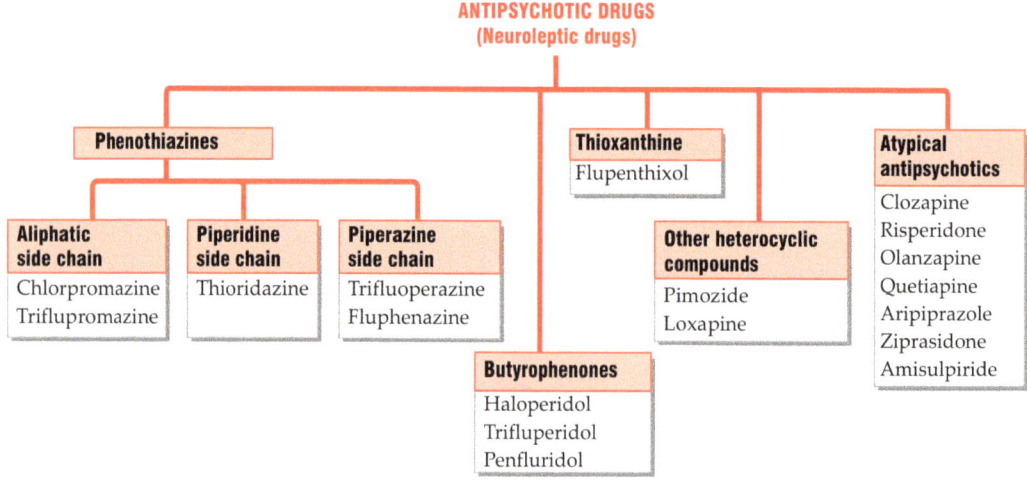

Table 10.1: Comparative properties of antipsychotic drugs

Drug	Antipsychotic dose (mg/day)	Relative activity Extrapyramidal	Sedative	Hypotensive	Antiemetic	Trade name
1. Chlorpromazine	100–800	++	+++	+++	++	LARGACTIL
2. Triflupromazine	50–200	++±	+++	++	+++	SIQUIL
3. Thioridazine	100–400	+	+++	+++	±	MELLERIL, THIORIL
4. Trifluoperazine	2–20	+++	+	+	+++	TRINICALM
5. Fluphenazine	1–10	+++	+	+	+++	ANATENSOL
6. Haloperidol	2–20	+++	+	+	+++	SERENACE, HALOPIDOL
7. Trifluperidol	1–8	+++	+	+	+++	TRIPERIDOL
8. Flupenthixol	3–15	+++	+	+	+	FLUANXOL
9. Pimozide	2–6	+++	+	+	+	ORAP, NEURAP
10. Loxapine	20–50	++	+	++	+	LOXAPAC
11. Clozapine	100–300	–	++	++	–	LOZAPIN, SIZOPIN
12. Risperidone	2–8	++	+	+	–	RESPIDON, SIZODON
13. Olanzapine	2.5–20	±	++	+	–	OLACE, OLZAP
14. Quetiapine	50-400	±	+++	++	–	QUEL, SOCALM
15. Aripiprazole	5-30	±	±	±	–	ARIPRA, BILIEF
16. Ziprasidone	40-160	±	+	±	–	AZONA, ZIPSYDON

+ to +++ increasing intensity of action; – absence of an action

quietening, reduction in initiative and tendency to go off to sleep from which the subject is easily arousable. Spontaneous movements are minimized, but slurring of speech, ataxia or motor incoordination does not occur. Most normal individuals perceive these effects as 'neutral' or 'unpleasant'.

In a psychotic CPZ reduces irrational behaviour, agitation and aggressiveness and controls psychotic symptomatology. Disturbed thought and behaviour are gradually normalised, anxiety is relieved. Hyperactivity, hallucinations and delusions are suppressed.

All phenothiazines, thioxanthenes and butyrophenones have the same antipsychotic efficacy, but potency differs in terms of equieffective doses. The aliphatic and piperidine side chain phenothiazines (CPZ, triflupromazine, thioridazine) have low potency, produce more sedation and cause greater potentiation of hypnotics, opioids, etc. The sedative effect is produced immediately while antipsychotic effect takes weeks to develop. Moreover, tolerance develops to the sedative but not to the antipsychotic effect. Thus, the two appear to be independent actions.

Performance and intelligence are relatively unaffected but vigilance is impaired. Extrapyramidal motor disturbances (*see* adverse effects) are intimately linked to the antipsychotic effect but are more prominent in the high potency compounds and least in thioridazine, clozapine and other atypical antipsychotics. No consistent effect on sleep architecture has been noted.

Chlorpromazine lowers seizure threshold, and can precipitate fits in untreated epileptics. Temperature control is knocked off at relatively higher doses—body temperature falls if surroundings are cold. The medullary respiratory and other vital centres are not affected, except at very high doses. It is very difficult to produce coma with these drugs. Phenothiazines and butyrophenones, except thioridazine, have potent antiemetic action exerted through the CTZ. However, they are ineffective in motion sickness.

Mechanism of action The typical antipsychotic drugs have potent dopamine D2 receptor blocking action; antipsychotic potency has shown good correlation with their capacity to bind to D2 receptor. Blockade of dopaminergic projections to the temporal and prefrontal areas constituting the 'limbic system' and in mesocortical areas is probably responsible for the antipsychotic action.

The '*dopaminergic theory of schizophrenia*' envisages that dopaminergic overactivity in limbic areas of brain is responsible for the disorder. Accordingly, blockade of this overactivity by the antipsychotic drugs is responsible for the therapeutic effect.

The atypical antipsychotics like clozapine have weak D2 blocking action. However, clozapine has additional 5-HT$_2$ and α_1 adrenergic blocking action, and is relatively selective for D4 receptors. Thus, antipsychotic property may depend on a specific profile of action of the drugs on several neurotransmitter receptors.

Dopaminergic blockade in the basal ganglia appears to cause the extrapyramidal symptoms, while that in CTZ is responsible for antiemetic action.

2. ANS Neuroleptics have varying degrees of α adrenergic blocking activity which may be graded as:

CPZ = triflupromazine > thioridazine > fluphenazine > haloperidol > trifluoperazine > clozapine > pimozide, i.e. more potent compounds have lesser α blocking activity.

Anticholinergic property of neuroleptics is weak and may be graded as:

thioridazine > chlorpromazine > triflupromazine > trifluoperazine = haloperidol.

The phenothiazines have weak H_1-antihistaminic and anti-5-HT actions as well.

3. Local anaesthetic Chlorpromazine is a potent local anaesthetic. Other antipsychotics have weaker membrane stabilizing action.

4. CVS Neuroleptics produce hypotension (primarily postural) by a central as well as peripheral action on sympathetic tone. The hypotensive action is more marked after parenteral administration and roughly parallels the α adrenergic blocking potency. Reflex tachycardia accompanies hypotension.

High doses of CPZ directly depress the heart and produce ECG changes (Q-T prolongation and suppression of T wave). CPZ exerts some antiarrhythmic action, probably due to membrane stabilization. Arrhythmia may occur in overdose, especially with thioridazine.

5. Endocrine Neuroleptics consistently increase prolactin release by blocking the inhibitory action of DA on pituitary lactotropes. This may result in galactorrhoea and gynaecomastia. Secretion of several pituitary hormones is reduced, but clinically significant consequences are infrequent.

On long-term use, certain antipsychotic drugs impair glucose tolerance, aggravate diabetes and elevate serum triglycerides.

Tolerance and dependence Tolerance to the sedative and hypotensive actions develops within days or weeks of CPZ therapy, but the antipsychotic, extrapyramidal and other actions based on DA antagonism do not display tolerance.

Neuroleptics are hedonically (pertaining to pleasure) bland drugs. No drug seeking behaviour is evident. Physical dependence is probably absent.

PHARMACOKINETICS

Oral absorption of CPZ is somewhat unpredictable and bioavailability is low. More consistent effects are produced after i.m. or i.v. administration. It is highly bound to plasma as well as tissue proteins. Volume of distribution is large (20 L/kg). CPZ is metabolized by liver into a number of metabolites. The acute effects of a single dose generally last for 6–8 hours. The elimination t½ is variable, but mostly is in the range of 18–30 hours.

Atypical (second generation) antipsychotics Lately some antipsychotic drugs like *clozapine, risperidone, olanzapine, quetiapine, aripiprazole, ziprasidone,* etc. have been introduced which have a pharmacological profile distinct from CPZ. They produce few extrapyramidal symptoms and no/mild hyperprolactinaemia. Tardive dyskinesia is rare. These atypical antipsychotics tend to suppress both positive and negative symptoms of schizophrenia, while the older drugs have little effect on negative symptoms. Many patients refractory to the typical antipsychotics respond to these drugs. The atypical antipsychotics have only weak D2 blocking, but potent 5-HT_2 antagonistic activity alongwith variable α adrenergic, muscarinic and H_1 histaminergic blocking property. These features may account for the above differences. Quetiapine is short acting with prominent sedative property, while aripiprazole is not sedating and long acting.

The major limitation of clozapine is higher incidence of agranulocytosis and other blood dyscrasias. This is not the case with olanzapine, risperidone and others. Another limitation of clozapine and olanzapine is weight gain, precipitation of diabetes and dyslipidaemia. Currently, atypical antipsychotics are being increasingly prescribed. Though, there is no convincing evidence of higher efficacy, they produce fewer side effects and neurological complications. Some atypical antipsychotics are effective in mania and bipolar disorder as well.

ADVERSE EFFECTS

Antipsychotics are safe drugs in single or infrequent doses, but side effects are common.

I. Based on pharmacological actions (dose related)

1. **CNS** Drowsiness, lethargy, mental confusion: more with low potency agents; increased appetite and weight gain; aggravation of seizures in epileptics.

2. **α Adrenergic blockade** *Postural hypotension*, palpitation, inhibition of ejaculation (especially with thioridazine) are more common with low potency phenothiazenes. *Dentists should instruct patients to get up slowly from a reclining dental chair.*

3. **Anticholinergic** Dry mouth (may promote caries tooth), blurring of vision, constipation, urinary hesitancy in elderly males (thioridazine has the highest propensity). High potency agents lack anticholinergic property.

4. **Endocrine** Amenorrhoea, infertility, gynaecomastia, galactorrhoea—due to hyperprolactinaemia. Impaired glucose tolerance, precipitation of diabetes, raised serum triglyceride levels.

5. **Extrapyramidal disturbances** These are the major dose limiting side effects; more prominent with high potency drugs like fluphenazine, haloperidol, pimozide, etc., least with thioridazine and atypical antipsychotics. Extrapyramidal syndromes are of following types.

(a) *Parkinsonism* with typical manifestations—rigidity, tremor, hypokinesia, mask like facies, shuffling gait. Anticholinergic antiparkinsonian drugs may counteract these symptoms.

A rare form of extrapyramidal side effect is *perioral tremors 'rabbit syndrome'* that generally occurs after few years of therapy.

(b) *Acute muscular dystonias* Bizarre muscle spasms, mostly involving linguo-facial muscles—grimacing, tongue thrusting, torticollis, locked jaw; occurs within a few hours of a single dose or at the most in the first week of therapy. It is more common in children below 10 years and in girls, particularly after parenteral administration. These dystonias last for one to few hours and then resolve spontaneously. One of the central anticholinergics, promethazine or hydroxyzine injected i.m. clears the reaction within 10–15 minutes.

(c) *Akathisia Restlessness,* feeling of discomfort, apparent agitation manifested as a compelling desire to move about, but without anxiety, is seen in some patients.

(d) *Malignant neuroleptic syndrome* It occurs rarely with high doses of potent agents; the patient develops marked rigidity, immobility, tremor, fever, semiconsciousness, fluctuating BP and heart rate; lasts for 5–10 days after drug withdrawal and may be fatal.

(e) *Tardive dyskinesia* It occurs late in therapy, sometimes even after withdrawal of the neuroleptic drug; manifests as purposeless involuntary facial and limb movements like constant chewing, pouting, puffing of cheeks, lip licking, choreoathetoid movements. *Dental problems may arise because of involvement of orofacial muscles. Attrition of teeth may result from grinding.* There is no satisfactory solution of the problem.

6. **Miscellaneous** Weight gain, blue pigmentation of exposed skin, corneal and lenticular opacities, retinal degeneration, cardiac arrhythmia are rare complications.

II. Hypersensitivity reactions These are not dose related.

1. Cholestatic jaundice.
2. Skin rashes, urticaria, contact dermatitis, photosensitivity.
3. Agranulocytosis is rare; more common with clozapine.

INTERACTIONS

1. Neuroleptics *potentiate all CNS depressants*—hypnotics, anxiolytics, alcohol, opioids and antihistaminics. *Dentists should be careful while prescribing any of the above drugs* to patients receiving neuroleptics.
2. Neuroleptics block the actions of levodopa and direct DA agonists in parkinsonism.
3. CPZ and few others abolish the antihypertensive action of clonidine and methyldopa, probably because they block central α_2 adrenergic receptors.

USES

1. Schizophrenia The antipsychotic drugs are used primarily in functional psychoses. They have indefinable but definite therapeutic effect: produce a wide range of symptom relief. Both typical and atypical antipsychotics control positive symptoms (hallucinations, delusions, disorganized thought, restlessness, insomnia, anxiety, fighting, aggression), but for negative symptoms (apathy, loss of insight and volition, affective flattening, poverty of speech, social withdrawal) the atypical ones are more effective. Some patients do not respond, and virtually none responds completely. Antipsychotics are only symptomatic treatment, do not remove the cause of illness.

2. Mania Antipsychotics are required for rapid control of acute mania; may be given i.m. Lithium or valproate may be started simultaneously or added after the acute phase is controlled.

3. Bipolar disorder Some atypical antipsychotics, *viz.* olanzapine, aripiprazole, quetiapine, are useful in bipolar disorder as well.

4. Organic brain syndromes Neuroleptics are not very effective. May be used on a short-term basis.

5. Anxiety Antipsychotics should not be used for simple anxiety. Patients not responding to BZDs, or those having a psychotic basis for anxiety may be treated with a neuroleptic.

6. As antiemetic Neuroleptics are potent antiemetics—control a wide range of drug and disease induced vomiting at doses much lower than those needed in psychosis. They are ineffective in motion sickness: probably because dopaminergic pathway through the CTZ is not involved in this condition.

DRUGS FOR MANIA AND BIPOLAR DISORDER

These are drugs which control mania and stabilize mood in bipolar disorder.

DRUGS FOR MANIA AND BIPOLAR DISORDER

- Lithium carbonate
- **Anticonvulsants**
  - Sodium valproate
  - Carbamazepine
  - Lamotrigine
- **Atypical antipsychotics**
  - Olanzapine
  - Risperidone
  - Quetiapine
  - Aripiprazole

Lithium carbonate

Lithium is a small monovalent cation. In 1949, it was found to exert beneficial effects in manic patients.

Actions and mechanism

Lithium has practically no acute effects in normal individuals as well as in patients of bipolar disorder. It is neither sedative nor euphorient; but on prolonged administration, it acts as a mood stabiliser in bipolar disorder. Given to patients in acute mania, it gradually suppresses the episode taking 1–2 weeks. Continued treatment prevents cyclic mood changes. The markedly reduced sleep time in manic patients is normalized.

The mechanism of antimanic and mood stabilizing action of lithium is not known. It has been proposed that:

(a) Li^+ partly replaces body Na^+ and is nearly equally distributed inside and outside the cells; this may affect ionic fluxes of Na^+ and K^+ across brain cells.

(b) Li^+ may correct imbalance in the turnover of brain monoamines.

(c) The above hypothesis cannot explain why Li^+ has no effect on people not suffering from mania. An attractive hypothesis has been put forward based on the finding that lithium inhibits hydrolysis of inositol-1-phosphate. As a result, the supply of free inositol for regeneration of membrane phosphatidyl-inositides, which are the source of IP_3 and DAG, is reduced (Fig. 10.1). The hyperactive neurones involved in the manic state may be preferentially affected, because supply

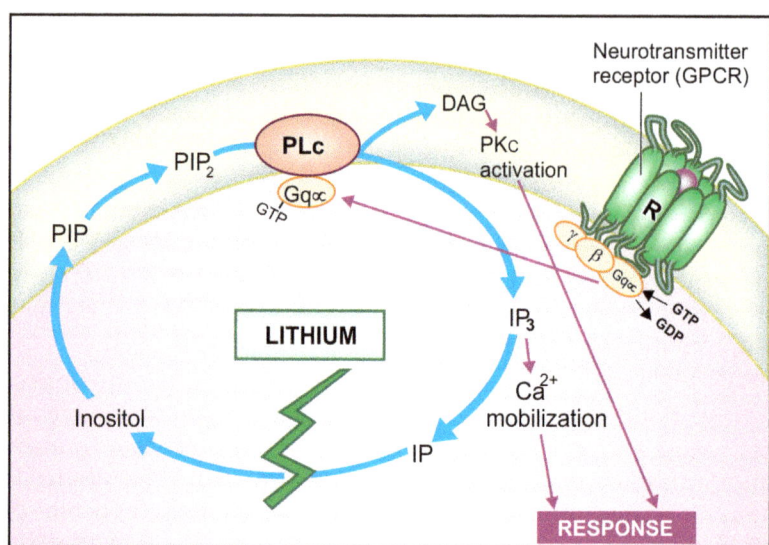

Fig. 10.1: Proposed mechanism of antimanic action of lithium
PIP-Phosphatidyl inositol phosphate; PIP_2-Phosphatidyl inositol bisphosphate; IP3-Inositol trisphosphate; IP-Inositol-1-phosphate; PLc-Phospholipase C; DAG-Diacyl glycerol; PKc-Protein kinase C; Gq-Coupling Gq protein; R- Neurotransmitter receptor

of inositol from extracellular sources is meagre. Thus, lithium may ignore normally operating receptors, but 'search out' and selectively, though indirectly, dampen signal transduction in the overactive ones.

Other actions of lithium are:
It inhibits the action of ADH on distal tubules and causes a diabetes insipidus like state.
It has some insulin-like action on glucose metabolism.
Leukocyte count is increased by lithium therapy.
Lithium reduces thyroxine synthesis by interfering with iodination of tyrosine.

Pharmacokinetics and control of therapy

Lithium is well absorbed orally. It first distributes in the extracellular water and then gradually enters cells and slowly penetrates into the CNS, ultimately attaining a rather uniform distribution in total body water.

Lithium is handled by the kidney in much the same way as Na^+. Most of the filtered Li^+ is reabsorbed in the proximal convoluted tubule. After a single dose of Li^+, urinary excretion is rapid for 10–12 hours followed by a much slower phase lasting several days. The t½ of the latter phase is 16–30 hours.

There is marked individual variation in the rate of lithium excretion. Since the margin of safety is narrow, monitoring of serum lithium concentration is essential for optimal therapy. Serum lithium level 0.5–0.8 mEq/L is considered optimum for maintenance therapy in bipolar disorder, while 0.8–1.1 mEq/L is required for episodes of mania. Toxicity symptoms occur frequently when serum levels exceed 1.5 mEq/L.

Adverse effects Side effects are common but are mostly tolerable. Toxicity occurs at levels only marginally higher than therapeutic levels.
1. Nausea, vomiting and mild diarrhoea.
2. Thirst and polyuria are experienced by most patients.
3. Fine tremors and rarely seizures.

4. CNS toxicity manifests when plasma concentration rises further—coarse tremors, giddiness, ataxia, motor incoordination, nystagmus, mental confusion, slurred speech, hyper-reflexia. In acute intoxication, these symptoms progress to muscle twitchings, drowsiness, delirium, coma and convulsions. Vomiting, severe diarrhoea, albuminuria, hypotension and cardiac arrhythmias are the other features.

There is no specific antidote to lithium.
5. On long-term use, some patients develop renal diabetes insipidus and goiter.
6. Lithium is contraindicated during pregnancy; foetal goiter and other congenital abnormalities can occur.

Interactions
1. Diuretics (thiazide, furosemide) raise plasma levels of lithium.
2. NSAIDs also cause Li$^+$ retention (along with Na$^+$ retention). *Dentists should refer patients for monitoring and adjusting Li$^+$ therapy when they prescribe NSAIDs.* Tetracyclines and ACE inhibitors are other drugs capable of producing Li$^+$ retention.
3. Lithium tends to enhance insulin/sulfonylurea induced hypoglycaemia.

Use

1. *Acute manic episode* (inappropriate cheerfulness, motor restlessness, nonstop talking, racing thoughts, flight of ideas and progressive loss of contact with reality; sometimes violent behaviour). Though lithium is effective in controlling acute mania, response is slow. Most psychiatrists prefer to use an atypical antipsychotic generally by i.m. route, with or without diazepam, and start lithium after the episode is under control. Maintenance lithium therapy is generally given to prevent recurrences.

2. *Bipolar disorder* Lithium has proven efficacy in bipolar disorder. It lengthens the interval between cycles of mood swings: episodes of mania as well as depression are attenuated, if not totally prevented.

Recurrent *unipolar depression* also responds to lithium therapy.
3. Lithium is sporadically used in many other *recurrent neuropsychiatric illness*, cluster headache, etc.

Anticonvulsants

Over the last two decades, several anticonvulsants and atypical antipsychotics have emerged as effective and better tolerated alternatives to lithium for mania and bipolar disorder. Moreover, about 30% cases of mania/bipolar disorder do not respond to lithium, and many do not tolerate it, necessitating use of other drugs.

1. Sodium valproate
In acute mania, high dose valproate acts faster than lithium and is an alternative to antipsychotic medication. It is also an effective prophylactic in bipolar disorder. Valproate and its compound *divalproex* have a favourable tolerability profile. Their use to prevent cyclic mood changes in bipolar illness has now exceeded that of lithium. A combination of valproate and lithium may succeed in resistant cases of bipolar disorder.

2. Carbamazepine
Carbamazepine is another anticonvulsant which prolongs remission in bipolar disorder, but its efficacy is lower than that of valproate or lithium. Moreover, side effects of carbamazepine are more pronounced. As such, its use in psychiatry has declined.

3. Lamotrigine
This newer anticonvulsant has been found to afford prophylaxis of depression in bipolar disorder, but is not effective either for treatment or for prevention of mania. It is being used as maintenance therapy in bipolar patients who suffer recurrent episodes of major depression alternating with hypomania. The tolerability profile of lamotrigine is favourable.

Atypical antipsychotics

Atypical antipsychotic drugs like olanzapine, risperidone, aripiprazole and quetiapine ± a benzodiazepine are now first line drugs for mania, but severe cases are better treated with a parenteral neuroleptic like haloperidol. Given as maintenance therapy, aripiprazole prevents episodes of mania, while quetiapine has good efficacy in bipolar depression. Olanzapine suppresses both manic and depressive phases.

ANTIDEPRESSANT DRUGS

These are drugs which can elevate mood in depressive illness. Practically all antidepressants affect monoaminergic transmission in the brain in one way or the other, and many of them have other associated properties. While the earliest antidepressants were introduced in the 1950s, over the past three decades, a large number of compounds with an assortment of effects on reuptake/metabolism of biogenic amines and on pre/post-junctional aminergic/cholinergic receptors have become available.

REVERSIBLE INHIBITORS OF MAO-A (RIMAs)

Monoamine oxidase (MAO) is a mitochondrial enzyme involved in the oxidative deamination of biogenic amines (Adr, NA, DA, 5-HT). Two isoenzyme forms of MAO have been identified.

MAO-A: Preferentially deaminates 5-HT and NA, and is inhibited by clorgyline, moclobemide.

MAO-B: Preferentially deaminates phenylethylamine and is inhibited by selegiline.

Dopamine is degraded equally by both isoenzymes.

Their distribution also differs. Peripheral adrenergic nerve endings, intestinal mucosa and human placenta contain predominantly MAO-A, while

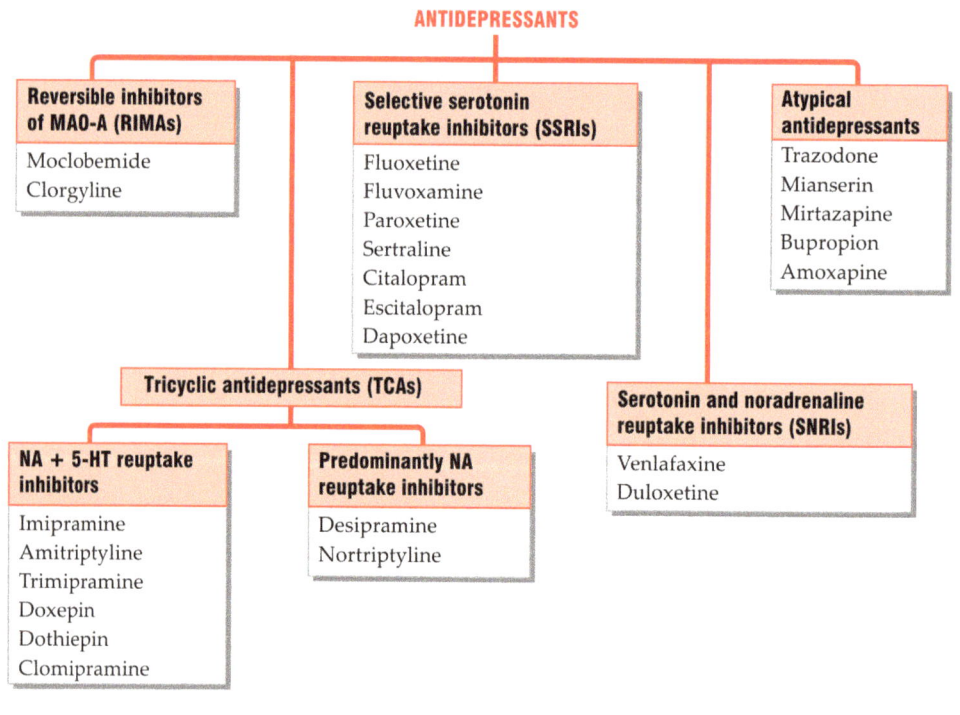

MAO-B predominates in certain areas of brain and in platelets. Liver contains both isoenzymes.

In the 1950s, iproniazid and related drugs that were nonselective and irreversible MAO inhibitors were used briefly as antidepressants, but were abandoned because of high toxicity and interaction with several foods and drugs. The most important interaction known as *cheese reaction* occurs when the subject receiving MAO inhibitor ingests tyramine rich foods including certain cheese, beer, wines, etc. The ingested tyramine escapes degradation in the intestinal wall and liver → reaches systemic circulation in high concentration and displaces large amounts of NA from transmitter loaded sympathetic nerve endings → hypertensive crisis, cerebrovascular accident and other complications. Similar hypertensive reaction can occur with cold remedies, levodopa, tricyclic antidepressants as well.

Lately, some MAO-A selective and reversible inhibitors have been introduced which have useful antidepressant property coupled with low toxicity and freedom from dangerous interactions in the recommended dose range.

Moclobemide It is a reversible and selective MAO-A inhibitor with short duration of action; full MAO activity is restored within 1–2 days of stopping the drug. Because of competitive inhibition of MAO-A, tyramine is able to displace moclobemide from the enzyme so that potentiation of pressor response to ingested amines is weak and dietary restrictions are not required. Clinical trials have shown moclobemide to be an efficacious antidepressant, comparable to tricyclic antidepressants (TCAs), except in severe cases. Moclobemide is free of the anticholinergic, sedative and cardiovascular adverse effects of typical TCAs and is safer in overdose. This makes it a particularly good option in elderly patients and in those with heart disease.

Adverse effects of moclobemide are nausea, dizziness, headache, insomnia, rarely excitement and liver damage. Caution is advised while coprescribing pethidine, SSRIs and TCAs.

TRICYCLIC ANTIDEPRESSANTS (TCAs)

Imipramine, an analogue of CPZ, was found during clinical trials in the 1950s to selectively benefit depressed but not agitated psychotics. In contrast to CPZ, it inhibited NA and 5-HT reuptake into neurones. A large number of congeners were soon added and are called *tricyclic antidepressants (TCAs)*.

Pharmacological actions

The TCAs inhibit monoamine reuptake by inhibiting norepinephrine transporter (NET) and serotonin transporter (SERT) located in the neuronal and platelet membrane. In addition, they interact with a variety of receptors *viz.* muscarinic, α adrenergic, histamine H_1, $5-HT_1$, $5-HT_2$ and occasionally dopamine D2. However, relative potencies at these sites differ among different compounds. The actions of imipramine are described as prototype.

1. CNS Effects differ in normal individuals and in the depressed.

In normal individuals Imipramine induces a peculiar clumsy feeling, tiredness, light-headedness, sleepiness, difficulty in concentrating and thinking, unsteady gait. These effects tend to provoke anxiety. There is no mood elevation or euphoria; effects are rather unpleasant.

In depressed patients little acute effects are produced, except sedation. After 2–3 weeks of continuous treatment, the mood is gradually elevated, patients become more communicative and start taking interest in self and surroundings. Thus, TCAs are not euphoriants but only antidepressants. The sedative property varies among different compounds (*see* Table 10.2). The more sedative ones are suitable for depressed patients showing anxiety and agitation. The less sedative or stimulant ones are better for withdrawn and retarded patients.

Chapter 10: Drugs Acting on Central Nervous System-2

Table 10.2: Comparative properties and trade names of tricyclic and related antidepressants

Drug	Sedation	Antimuscarinic	Hypotension	Cardiac arrhythmia	Seizure precipitation	Daily dose (mg)	Trade name
Tricyclic antidepressants (TCAs)							
1. Imipramine	+	++	++	+++	++	50–200	DEPSONIL, ANTIDEP
2. Amitriptyline	+++	+++	+++	+++	++	50–200	AMLINE, TRYPTOMER
3. Trimipramine	+++	++	++	+++	++	50–150	SURMONTIL
4. Doxepin	+++	++	++	+++	++	50–150	SPECTRA, DOXIN
5. Clomipramine	++	++	+	+++	+++	50–150	CLOFRANIL, CLONIL
6. Dothiepin	++	++	++	++	++	50–150	PROTHIADEN
7. Nortriptyline	+	++	+	++	+	50–150	SENSIVAL
Selective serotonin reuptake inhibitors (SSRIs)							
1. Fluoxetine	±	–	–	–	±	20–40	FLUDAC, FLUNIL
2. Fluvoxamine	±	–	–	–	–	50–200	FLUVOXIN
3. Paroxetine	+	+	–	–	–	20–50	XET
4. Sertraline	–	–	–	–	–	50–150	SERENATA
5. Citalopram	–	±	–	+	–	20–40	CELICA
6. Escitalopram	–	±	–	–	–	10-20	ESDEP, FELIZ-S
Serotonin and noradrenaline reuptake inhibitors (SNRIs)							
1. Venlafaxine	±	–	–	±	–	75–150	VENLOR
2. Duloxetine	+	++	–	–	–	30-80	DELOK
Atypical antidepressants							
1. Trazodone	+++	–	+	±	–	50–200	TRAZODAC
2. Mianserin	++	+	++	+	++	30–100	TETRADEP
3. Bupropion	–, ↑	–	–	–	+++	150–300	SMOQUIT
4. Amoxapine	+	+	++	++	++	100–300	DEMOLOX
5. Mirtazapine	+++	+	±	–	–	15–45	MIRT, MIRTAZ

+ to +++ increasing intensity of action; – absence of an action

The TCAs lower seizure threshold and produce convulsions in overdose. Clomipramine and bupropion have the highest seizure precipitating potential. Amitriptyline and imipramine depress respiration in overdose only.

Mechanism of antidepressant action The TCAs and related drugs inhibit NET and SERT, the transporters which mediate active reuptake of biogenic amines NA and 5-HT into their respective neurones and thus potentiate them. Antidepressants, however, differ markedly in their selectivity and potency for different amines (*see* classification above). Most of the compounds do not inhibit DA uptake, except bupropion. Tentative conclusions drawn are:

- Inhibition of NA and 5-HT uptake is associated with antidepressant action.
- Inhibition of DA uptake correlates with stimulant action; but is not primarily involved in antidepressant action.

Uptake blockade appears to initiate a series of time-dependent changes in the number and sensitivity of aminergic receptors that culminate in antidepressant effect after a few weeks.

None of these compounds, except amoxapine, block DA receptors or possess antipsychotic activity.

2. ANS Most TCAs are potent anticholinergics—cause dry mouth, blurring of vision, constipation and urinary hesitancy as side effect. The anticholinergic potency is graded in Table 10.2. They potentiate exogenous and endogenous NA by blocking uptake.

3. CVS Effects on cardiovascular function are prominent, and may be dangerous in overdose.

Tachycardia: due to anticholinergic and NA potentiating actions.

Postural hypotension: due to inhibition of cardiovascular reflexes and α_1 blockade.

ECG changes and cardiac arrhythmias: T wave suppression or inversion is the most consistent change. Arrhythmias occur in overdose due to interference with intraventricular conduction. The NA potentiating + ACh blocking actions along with direct myocardial depression compound the proarrhythmic potential. Older patients are more susceptible. The SSRIs, SNRIs and atypical antidepressants are safer in this regard.

Tolerance and dependence

Tolerance to the anticholinergic and hypotensive effects of imipramine-like drugs develops gradually, though antidepressant action is sustained. Addiction is rare because their acute effects are not pleasant.

There is some evidence of physical dependence occurring when high doses are given for long periods, but TCAs do not carry abuse potential.

Pharmacokinetics

The oral absorption of TCAs is good, though often slow. They are highly bound to plasma and tissue proteins—have large volumes of distribution (~20 L/kg). They are extensively metabolized in liver; the major route for imipramine and amitriptyline is demethylation whereby active metabolites—desipramine and nortriptyline respectively are formed. Metabolites are excreted in urine over 1–2 weeks. The plasma t½ of amitriptyline, imipramine and doxepin range between 16–24 hours.

Adverse effects

Side effects are common with tricyclic antidepressants.

1. Anticholinergic: dry mouth, bad taste, constipation, epigastric distress, urinary retention (especially in males with enlarged prostate), blurred vision, palpitation. Decreased salivation *increases risk of dental caries, oral thrush, etc.*
2. Sedation, mental confusion and weakness, especially with amitriptyline and more sedative congeners.
3. Increased appetite and weight gain is noted with most TCAs and trazodone, but not with SSRIs and bupropion.
4. Some patients may switch to hypomania or mania. Probably, this reflects a basic

bipolar illness, the other pole being unmasked by the antidepressant.
5. Sweating and fine tremors are relatively common.
6. Seizure threshold is lowered—fits may be precipitated, especially in children.
7. Postural hypotension, especially in older patients. This is less severe with desipramine like drugs and insignificant with SSRIs. *Patients should not abruptly sit up or stand from a reclining position on the dental chair.*
8. Cardiac arrhythmias, especially in patients with ischaemic heart disease. This may be responsible for sudden death in these patients.

Acute poisoning Antidepressant poisoning is frequent; usually self-attempted by the depressed patients, and may endanger life. Manifestations are:
Excitement, delirium and other anticholinergic symptoms followed by muscle spasms, convulsions and coma. Respiration is depressed, body temperature may fall, BP is low, tachycardia is prominent. ECG changes and ventricular arrhythmias are common.

Treatment is primarily supportive with gastric lavage, respiratory support, fluid infusion, maintenance of BP and body temperature. Acidosis must be corrected by bicarbonate infusion.

Diazepam may be injected i.v. to control convulsions and delirium. Most important is treatment of cardiac arrhythmias, for which propranolol/lidocaine may be used.

Interactions

1. TCAs potentiate directly acting *sympathomimetic amines* that may be present in cold/asthma remedies. *Adrenaline containing local anaesthetic should be avoided for dental anaesthesia due to risk of potentiation and precipitation of cardiac arrhythmia.*
2. TCAs potentiate *CNS depressants*, including alcohol and antihistaminics.
3. Carbamazepine and other enzyme inducers enhance metabolism of TCAs.
4. SSRIs inhibit metabolism of many drugs including TCAs—dangerous toxicity can occur if the two are given concurrently.
5. When used together, the anticholinergic action of neuroleptics and TCAs may add up.

SELECTIVE SEROTONIN REUPTAKE INHIBITORS (SSRIs)

The major limitations of TCAs (first generation antidepressants) are:
- Frequent anticholinergic, cardiovascular and neurological side effects.
- Relatively low safety margin; they are hazardous in overdose; fatalities are likely.
- Significant number of patients respond incompletely and some do not respond.

To overcome these shortcomings, a large number of newer (second generation) antidepressants have been produced since 1980s. The SSRIs selectively inhibit SERT, SNRIs inhibit both SERT and NET, while uptake blockade is weak/absent in the atypical antidepressants. Antidepressant efficacy of some of these drugs is now rated higher than the older TCAs. In fact, some patients not responding to one type of drug may respond to the other. More importantly, the newer drugs have improved tolerability and safety in therapeutic dose as well as in overdose.

The relative safety and better acceptability of SSRIs has made them 1st line drugs in depression and allowed their extensive use in anxiety, phobias, OCD and related disorders. The SSRIs, produce little or no sedation, do not interfere with cognitive and psychomotor function or produce anticholinergic side effects. They are devoid of α adrenergic blocking action, so that postural hypotension does not occur, making them suitable for elderly patients. They have practically no seizure precipitating propensity and do not inhibit cardiac conduction. As such, overdose arrhythmias are not a problem. However, they frequently produce nausea. Weight gain is not a problem with SSRIs, but they more commonly interfere with ejaculation or orgasm. A new constellation of mild side effects, *viz.* nervousness, restlessness, insomnia, anorexia, dyskinesia, headache and diarrhoea is associated with them, but patient acceptability is good. Increased incidence of epistaxis and ecchymosis has been reported, probably due to impairment of platelet function. *Gastric blood loss due to NSAIDs may be increased by SSRIs.*

The SSRIs inhibit drug metabolizing isoenzymes CYP2D6 and CYP3A4: elevate plasma levels of TCAs, haloperidol, clozapine, warfarin, β blockers, some BZDs and carbamazepine. *Use of tramadol to relieve dental pain should be avoided in patients receiving SSRIs* due to risk of 'Serotonin syndrome' manifesting as agitation, muscle rigidity, twitchings, convulsions and hyperthermia.

Other uses of SSRIs The SSRIs are now 1st choice drugs for OCD, panic disorder, social phobia, eating disorders and post-traumatic stress disorder (PTSD). They are also being increasingly used for many anxiety disorders, body dysmorphic disorder, compulsive buying, kleptomania and premature ejaculation. Elevation of mood and increased work capacity has been reported in postmyocardial infarction and other chronic somatic illness patients.

SEROTONIN AND NORADRENALINE REUPTAKE INHIBITORS (SNRIs)

1. Venlafaxine It is a novel antidepressant which inhibits uptake of both NA and 5-HT, but, in contrast to older TCAs, does not interact with cholinergic, adrenergic or histaminergic receptors or have sedative property. Venlafaxine does not produce the usual side effects of TCAs; tends to raise rather than depress BP and is safer in overdose. *Desvenlafaxine* is an active metabolite of venlafaxine with similar actions, uses and side effects.

2. Duloxetine This is another SNRI similar in properties to venlafaxine. In addition to depression, duloxetine is useful in panic attacks, diabetic neuropathic pain, fibromyalgia and stress urinary incontinence in women. Mild sedation and antimuscarinic effects occur.

ATYPICAL ANTIDEPRESSANTS

Rather than primarily blocking amine reuptake, these antidepressants appear to act by other mechanisms, and have their own distinctive features.

1. Trazodone It is the first atypical antidepressant which selectively but less efficiently blocks 5-HT uptake, and has prominent α adrenergic as well as weak 5-HT$_2$ antagonistic actions. It is sedative but not anticholinergic, causes bradycardia rather than tachycardia, does not interfere with intracardiac conduction—less prone to cause arrhythmia. Inappropriate, prolonged and painful penile erection (priapism) occurs in a few recipients as does postural hypotension. Antidepressant action is rather modest.

2. Mianserin It is unique in not inhibiting either NA or 5-HT uptake; but blocks presynaptic α$_2$ receptors, thereby increases release and turnover of NA in brain. This may be responsible for the antidepressant effect. Blood dyscrasias and liver dysfunction have restricted its use.

3. Mirtazapine It acts by a novel mechanism *viz.* blocks α$_2$ auto- (on NA neurones) and hetero- (on 5-HT neurones) receptors enhancing both NA and 5-HT release. Selective enhancement of antidepressive

5-HT_1 receptor action is claimed to be exerted by concurrent blockade of 5-HT_2 receptors. Accordingly, it has been labelled as *"noradrenergic and specific serotonergic antidepressant"* (NaSSA). It is a H_1 blocker and quite sedative, but not anticholinergic or antidopaminergic. Efficacy in depression is reported to be comparable to TCAs.

4. Bupropion This inhibitor of DA and NA uptake has excitant rather than sedative property. It is metabolized into an amphetamine like compound. It is marketed in a sustained release formulation as an aid to smoking cessation. Side effects are insomnia, agitation, dry mouth and nausea. Seizures occur in overdose.

5. Amoxapine This tetracyclic compound is unusual in that it blocks dopamine D2 receptors in addition to inhibiting NA reuptake. It has mixed antidepressant + neuroleptic properties; may be used for patients with psychotic depression unresponsive to other antidepressants.

Uses

1. Endogenous (major) depression: The aim of drug therapy is to relieve symptoms of depression and restore normal social behaviour. The tricyclic and related antidepressants are of proven value. Response takes at least 2–3 weeks to appear, full benefits take still longer. The SSRIs, SNRIs and atypical antidepressants are currently used as first choice for their good tolerability, safety in overdose, and possibly higher efficacy. The order TCAs are mostly used as alternatives in nonresponsive/nontolerant patients. After a depressive episode has been controlled, continued treatment at maintenance doses for months is recommended to prevent relapse. Therapy is generally not continued beyond one year.

2. Obsessive-compulsive disorder (OCD): The SSRIs are the drugs of choice due to better patient acceptability. TCAs, especially clomipramine, are highly effective in OCD and panic disorders. SSRIs and TCAs also reduce compulsive eating in *bulimia*, and help patients with *body dysmorphic disorder, compulsive buying* and *kleptomania*, though these habits may not completely die.

3. Anxiety disorders: Antidepressants, especially SSRIs and SNRIs exert a slow onset but sustained beneficial effect in many patients of generalized anxiety disorder and phobic states. They may be used along with a short course of BZDs to cover exacerbations. SSRIs have also proven helpful in *post-traumatic stress disorder*.

4. Neuropathic pain: Amitriptyline and other TCAs afford considerable relief in post-herpetic neuralgia, diabetic and some other types of chronic pain. Duloxetin, a SNRI, is now a first line drug for diabetic neuropathy, fibromyalgia, etc.

5. Attention deficit-hyperactivity disorder (ADHD) in children: TCAs with less depressant properties like imipramine and amoxapine are now first line drugs in this disorder.

6. Premature ejaculation This refers to repeated occasions of ejaculation before or shortly after penetration. Most SSRIs and some TCAs like clomipramine delay/inhibit ejaculation as a side effect, which can be utilized in premature ejaculation cases as the desired effect. Dapoxetine, a SSRI drug has been especially used for this purpose, because it acts rapidly and more predictively.

7. Enuresis: Imipramine 25 mg at bedtime reduces bedwetting in children above 5 years.

8. Smoking cessation: The atypical antidepressant bupropion is approved as an aid to smoking cessation. It reduces craving and is comparable in efficacy to nicotine gum.

9. Pruritus: Some tricyclics have antipruritic property.

ANTIANXIETY DRUGS

Anxiety Some degree of anxiety is a part of normal life. Treatment is needed when it is disproportionate to the situation and excessive. Some psychotics and depressed patients also exhibit pathological anxiety.

Antianxiety drugs These are an ill-defined group of drugs, mostly mild CNS depressants which are aimed to control the symptoms of anxiety, produce a restful state of mind without interfering with normal mental or physical functions. *In dentistry, the most important application of antianxiety drugs is for premedication of apprehensive patients and as adjuncts to local anaesthesia.* Antianxiety BZDs also counteract the CNS toxicity of local anaesthetics injected for dental anaesthesia. The anxiolytic-sedative drugs differ markedly from antipsychotics, and more closely resemble sedative-hypnotics. They:

1. Have no therapeutic effect to control thought disorder of schizophrenia.
2. Do not produce extrapyramidal side effects.
3. Have anticonvulsant property.
4. Produce dependence and carry abuse liability.

In addition to the above drugs, antidepressants, especially the SSRIs and SNRIs are effective in obsessive-compulsive disorder (OCD), phobias, panic and many types of severe generalized anxiety disorders.

Benzodiazepines

The pharmacology of benzodiazepines (BZDs) as a class is described in Ch. 9. Some members have a slow and prolonged action, relieve anxiety at low doses without producing significant CNS depression. In contrast to barbiturates, they are more selective for the limbic system and have proven clinically better in both quality and quantity of improvement in anxiety and stress-related symptoms. At antianxiety doses, cardiovascular and respiratory depression is minor.

Because anxiety is a common complaint and is a part of most physical as well as mental illness, and because BZDs:

(i) have little effect on other body systems,
(ii) have lower dependence producing liability,
(iii) are relatively safe even in gross overdosage,

they are presently one of the most widely used class of drugs. Potent BZDs like lorazepam and clonazepam injected i.m. have adjuvant role in the management of acutely psychotic and manic patients. Higher doses induce sleep and impair performance.

Adverse effects of BZDs produced in their use as hypnotics are described in Ch. 9. *Side effects* that occur in their use to relieve anxiety are—sedation, light-headedness, psychomotor and cognitive impairment, vertigo, confusional

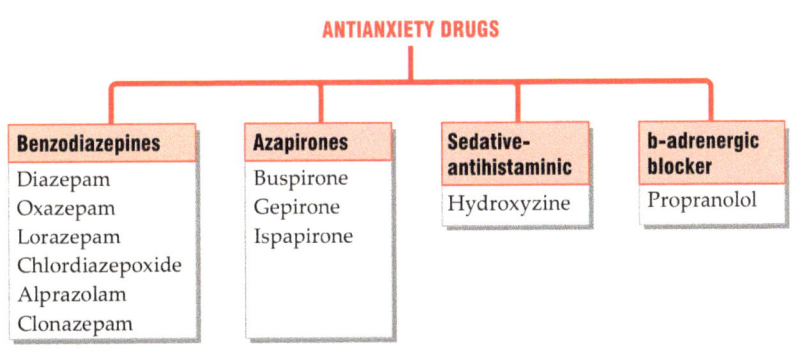

state (especially in the elderly), increased appetite and weight gain, alterations in sexual function. The major constraint in their long-term use for anxiety disorders is their potential to impair mental functions, and to produce dependence.

Differences between individual BZDs recommended for anxiety are primarily pharmacokinetic: choice of one over the other is largely empirical.

Buspirone

It is the first azapirone, a class of selective antianxiety drugs, distinctly different from BZDs. Buspirone:

- Does not produce significant sedation or cognitive/functional impairment.
- Does not interact with BZD receptor or modify GABAergic transmission.
- Does not produce tolerance or physical dependence.
- Does not suppress BZD or barbiturate withdrawal syndrome.
- Has no muscle relaxant or anticonvulsant activity.

Buspirone relieves generalized anxiety of mild to moderate intensity, but is ineffective in severe cases, in those showing panic reaction and in OCD. The therapeutic effect develops slowly; maximum benefit may be delayed up to 2 weeks. The mechanism of anxiolytic action is not clearly known, but may be dependent on its selective partial agonistic action on 5-HT_{1A} receptors. By stimulating presynaptic 5-HT_{1A} autoreceptors, it reduces activity of dorsal raphe serotonergic neurones.

Side effects of buspirone are minor: dizziness, nausea, headache, light-headedness, rarely excitement. It does not potentiate alcohol and other CNS depressants. Though most patients on buspirone remain alert, those operating machinery/motor vehicles should be cautioned.

Hydroxyzine It is a H_1 antihistaminic with sedative, antiemetic, antimuscarinic and spasmolytic properties. It may be used in reactive anxiety or that associated with marked autonomic symptoms.

β Blockers (see Ch. 6)

Many symptoms of anxiety (palpitation, rise in BP, shaking, tremor, gastrointestinal hurrying, etc.) are due to sympathetic overactivity, and these symptoms reinforce anxiety. Propranolol and other nonselective β blockers benefit anxious patients troubled by these symptoms, by breaking the vicious cycle and provide symptomatic relief. They do not affect the psychological symptoms such as worry, tension and fear, but are valuable in acutely stressful situations (examination fear, unaccustomed public appearance, etc.). β blockers may be used for performance/situational anxiety or as adjuvant to BZDs.

Cardiovascular Drugs-1
Drugs Affecting Renin-Angiotensin System, Calcium Channel Blockers, Drugs for Hypertension, Angina Pectoris and Myocardial Infarction

Drugs having their major action on the heart or blood vessels, or those used primarily for cardiovascular disorders are designated 'Cardiovascular drugs'. They can act directly on the cardiovascular structures or through the autonomic/central nervous system, kidney, autacoids or hormones which regulate cardiovascular function.

DRUGS AFFECTING RENIN-ANGIOTENSIN SYSTEM

Renin-angiotensin system (RAS)

Angiotensin II (Ang II) is an octapeptide generated in the plasma from a precursor plasma α_2 globulin. It is involved in electrolyte, blood volume and pressure homeostasis. Drugs that interfere with the generation or action of Ang II have assumed great importance in the treatment of cardiovascular diseases.

The generation and metabolism of Ang II in circulation is depicted in Fig. 11.1. The enzyme *renin* secreted by kidney splits off a decapeptide *Angiotensin I* (Ang I) from angiotensinogen. Ang I is largely inactive but is rapidly converted to Ang II by *angiotensin-converting enzyme* (ACE) which removes 2 amino acids from the carboxy terminus of the decapeptide. The ACE is located primarily on the luminal surface of vascular endothelial cells (especially in lungs). Circulating Ang II has a very short t½ (1 min); due to serial degradation by peptidases termed *angiotensinases*.

Local renin-angiotensin systems: Many tissues, especially heart, blood vessels, brain, kidneys, adrenals generate Ang II on the surface of their cells or inside their cells. Thus, local renin-angiotensin systems appear to operate in several organs in addition to the circulating one.

Actions of Angiotensin II

1. The most prominent action of Ang II is vasoconstriction, which is produced directly as well as by enhancing Adr/NA release from adrenal medulla/adrenergic nerve endings and by increasing central sympathetic outflow. As a result, BP rises acutely. Ang II is much more potent pressor agent than NA.

2. Ang II increases force of myocardial contraction, but reflex bradycardia predominates due to rise in BP. Cardiac output is often reduced, while cardiac work is increased (due to rise in peripheral resistance).

3. Acting on a chronic basis Ang II induces hypertrophy and hyperplasia in the myocardium and vascular smooth muscle by direct cellular effects. Indirectly, volume overload and increased t.p.r. caused by Ang II contributes to the hypertrophy and remodeling (abnormal redistribution of muscle mass) in heart and blood vessels. Fibrosis and dilatation of infarcted area with hypertrophy of the noninfarcted ventricular wall is seen after myocardial infarction.

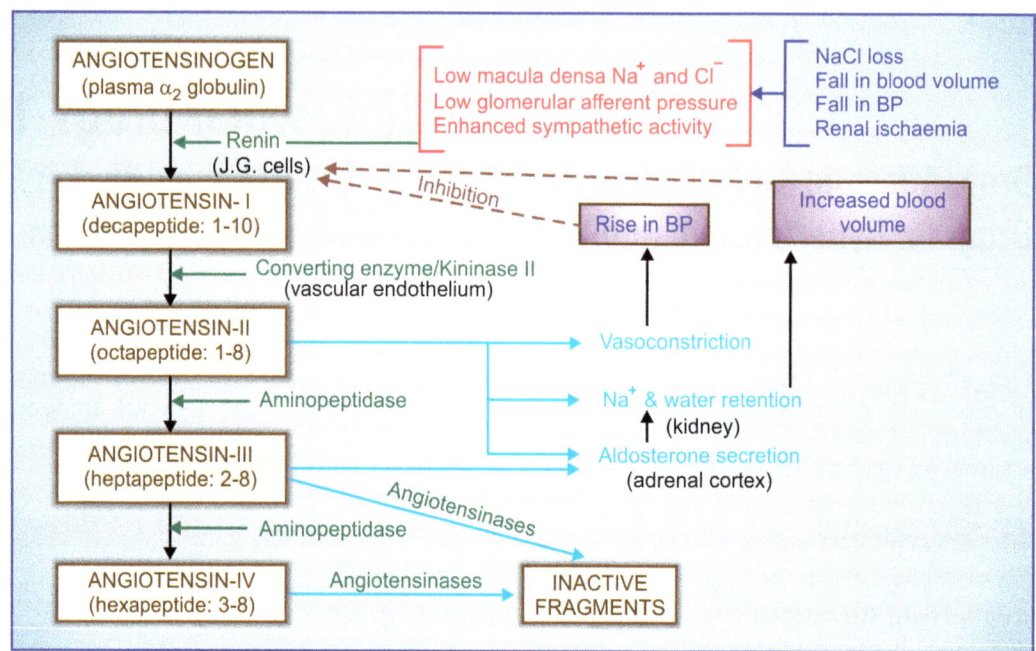

Fig. 11.1: Physiological regulation of electrolyte balance, plasma volume and blood pressure by the renin-angiotensin system
J.G. cells—Juxtaglomerular cells

Progressive cardiac myocyte death and fibrotic transformation occurs in CHF. Ang II plays a pivotal role in the causation of vascular and ventricular hypertrophy, apoptosis and remodeling. Accordingly, ACE inhibitor therapy retards/reverses many of these changes which are important risk factors for cardiovascular mortality and morbidity.

4. Ang II contracts many visceral smooth muscles *in vitro*, but *in vivo* effects are insignificant.

5. Ang II and Ang III are trophic to zona glomerulosa of the adrenal cortex—enhance synthesis and release of aldosterone. This acts on distal tubule to promote Na$^+$ reabsorption and K$^+$/H$^+$ excretion. These effects are exerted at concentrations lower than those required to cause vasoconstriction.

6. Ang II promotes Na$^+$/H$^+$ exchange in proximal tubule leading to increased Na$^+$, Cl$^-$ and HCO$_3^-$ reabsorption.

Angiotensin receptors Specific Ang II receptors are expressed on the surface of target cells. Two subtypes (AT$_1$ and AT$_2$) have been differentiated pharmacologically: *Losartan* is a selective AT$_1$ antagonist, while PD 123177 is a selective AT$_2$ antagonist. Both subtypes are G-protein coupled receptors. However, all major actions of Ang II are mediated by AT$_1$ receptor.

Pathophysiological Roles of RAS

1. *Mineralocorticoid secretion* Ang II (also Ang III) is the physiological stimulus for aldosterone secretion from adrenal cortex.

2. *Electrolyte, blood volume and pressure homeostasis* The RAS plays an important role in maintaining electrolyte composition and volume of extracellular fluid (see Fig. 11.1). Changes that lower blood volume or pressure, or decrease Na$^+$ content induce renin release.

Increased renin is translated into increased plasma Ang II which produces acute rise in BP by vasoconstriction, and more long-lasting effects by directly as well as indirectly increasing Na^+ and water reabsorption in the kidney. Rise in BP, in turn, inhibits renin release.

3. *Development of hypertension* The RAS is directly involved in renovascular hypertension. In essential hypertension and in pregnancy-induced hypertension it appears to have a permissive role.

4. *Secondary hyperaldosteronism* The RAS is instrumental in the development of secondary hyperaldosteronism.

5. *CNS* Ang II can be formed locally in the brain and may function as transmitter or modulator. Regulation of thirst, hormone release and sympathetic outflow may be the responses mediated.

Inhibition of Renin-angiotensin System

This can be achieved by:
1. Sympathetic blockers (β blockers, central sympatholytics)—decrease renin release.
2. Direct renin inhibitors (DRIs, e.g. aliskiren) block renin action—interfere with generation of Ang I from angiotensinogen (rate limiting step).
3. Angiotensin converting enzyme (ACE) inhibitors (e.g. captopril) prevent generation of the active principle Ang II.
4. Angiotensin receptor (AT_1) blockers (ARBs, e.g. losartan) antagonise the action of Ang II on target cells.
5. Aldosterone antagonists (e.g. spironolactone) block mineralocorticoid receptors.

ANGIOTENSIN CONVERTING ENZYME INHIBITORS

Captopril, an orally active dipeptide analogue ACE inhibitor, was introduced in 1977 and quickly gained wide usage. A multitude of ACE inhibitors like *enalapril, lisinopril, benazepril, ramipril, perindopril, trandolapril,* and *fosinopril,* etc. are now available. The pharmacology of captopril is described as prototype since most of its effects are class effects common to all ACE inhibitors.

Captopril

It is a sulfhydryl containing dipeptide surrogate of proline which inhibits ACE and abolishes the pressor action of Ang I without affecting that of Ang II. It does not block angiotensin receptors.

By inhibiting their degradation it can also increase plasma kinin levels and potentiate the hypotensive action of exogenously administered bradykinin. Elevated kinins (and PGs whose synthesis is enhanced by kinins) may be responsible for the cough and angioedema induced by ACE inhibitors in susceptible individuals. However, kinins do not appear to be important for the hypotensive action of these drugs in the long term.

Captopril lowers BP. This effect is more marked in Na^+ depleted subjects and in those with overactive RAS. Captopril-induced hypotension is a result of decrease in total peripheral resistance. Both systolic and diastolic BP fall. It has no effect on cardiac output. Cardiovascular reflexes are not interfered, and there is little dilatation of capacitance vessels. Because of these features, postural hypotension is not a problem.

Reflex (postural) changes in plasma aldosterone are abolished and its basal levels are decreased as a consequence of loss of regulation by Ang II. However, physiologically sufficient mineralocorticoid is still secreted under the influence of ACTH and plasma K^+.

Pharmacokinetics About 70% of orally administered captopril is absorbed. Presence of food in stomach reduces its bioavailability. Penetration in brain is poor. It is partly metabolized and partly excreted unchanged in urine. The plasma t½ is ~2 hours, but actions last for 6–12 hours.

Adverse effects The adverse effect profile of all ACE inhibitors is similar. Captopril is well tolerated by most patients; adverse effects are:
1. *Hypotension.*
2. *Hyperkalemia:* This is more likely in patients with impaired renal function and in those taking K⁺ sparing diuretics, NSAIDs or β blockers.
3. *Cough:* A persistent brassy cough occurs in 4-16% patients within 1–8 weeks. This is not dose related and appears to be caused by inhibition of bradykinin/substance P breakdown in the lungs of susceptible individuals.
4. *Rashes, urticaria.*
5. *Angioedema*: Resulting in swelling of lips, mouth, nose, larynx may develop within hours to a few days.
6. *Dysguesia:* Reversible loss or alteration of taste sensation.
7. *Foetopathic:* Foetal growth retardation, hypoplasia of organs and foetal death may occur if ACE inhibitors are given during later half of pregnancy.
8. *Headache, dizziness, nausea and bowel upset.*
9. *Acute renal failure:* This may be precipitated by ACE inhibitors in patients with bilateral renal artery stenosis.

Interactions Indomethacin (and other NSAIDs) attenuate the hypotensive action of ACE inhibitors, while diuretics synergise with them. Hyperkalemia can occur if K^+ supplements/K^+ sparing diuretics are given along with captopril. Antacids reduce bioavailability of captopril, while ACE inhibitors reduce Li^+ clearance and predispose to its toxicity.

Other ACE inhibitors Differences among ACE inhibitors are primarily pharmacokinetic, reflected in time course of their action; no single drug is superior to others. Their important features are listed in Table 11.1. Enalapril is a prodrug: has to be converted in the body to the active form *enaprilat*. Therefore, it acts slowly; is less likely to cause sudden hypotension and is longer acting. Other ACE inhibitors are also slow and longer acting and more potent than captopril. Ramipril is claimed to cause greater inhibition of tissue RAS because of extensive tissue distribution.

USES

1. Hypertension ACE inhibitors are first line drugs in all grades of hypertension. About 50% patients respond to monotherapy with ACE inhibitors, and majority of the rest to their combination with diuretics or β blockers or both. ACE inhibitors offer many advantages:

Table 11.1: Comparative features of ACE inhibitors

	Captopril	Enalapril	Lisinopril	Perindopril	Ramipril
1. Chemical nature	Sulfhydryl	Carboxyl	Carboxyl	Carboxyl	Carboxyl
2. Activity status	Active	Prodrug	Active	Prodrug	Prodrug
3. Bioavailability (as active form)	70%	50%	25%	20%	60%
4. Time to peak action	1 hr	4–6 hr	6–8 hr	6 hr	3–6 hr
5. Elimination t½	2 hr	11 hr	12 hr	25–30 hr	8–48 hr
6. Mode of excretion	Renal	Renal	Renal	Renal	Renal
7. Duration of action	6–12 hr	24 hr	> 24 hr	> 24 hr	>24 hr
8. Daily dose (mg)	25–150	2.5–40	5–40	2–8	1.25–10

- Freedom from postural hypotension, electrolyte disturbances, feeling of weakness and CNS effects.
- Safety in asthmatics, diabetics and peripheral vascular disease patients.
- Left ventricular hypertrophy and increased wall-to-lumen ratio of blood vessels that occurs in hypertensive patients is reversed.
- No hyperuricaemia, no deleterious effect on plasma lipid profile.
- No rebound hypertension on withdrawal.
- Minimum worsening of quality of life parameters like general wellbeing, work performance, sleep, sexual performance, etc.

2. CHF ACE inhibitors cause both arteriolar and venodilatation in CHF patients: reduce afterload as well as preload. Considerable symptomatic relief is obtained in nearly all grades of CHF.

ACE inhibitors also retard the progression of left ventricular systolic dysfunction and prolong survival of CHF patients. Long-term benefits of ACE inhibitors may also accrue from withdrawal of Ang II mediated ventricular hypertrophy, remodeling, accelerated myocyte apoptosis and fibrosis.

As such, ACE inhibitors are the first line drugs in CHF.

3. Myocardial infarction (MI) ACE inhibitors administered while MI is evolving (within 24 hr of an attack) and continued for 6 weeks reduce early as well as long-term mortality.

4. Prophylaxis in high cardiovascular risk subjects ACE inhibitors are protective in high cardiovascular risk subjects even when there is no associated hypertension or left ventricular dysfunction. Protective effect is exerted both on myocardium as well as on vasculature, and is independent of the hypotensive action.

5. Diabetic nephropathy Prolonged ACE inhibitor therapy has been found to prevent or delay end-stage renal disease in type I as well as type II diabetics.

Chronic renal failure due to nondiabetic causes may also be improved by ACE inhibitors.

6. Scleroderma crisis ACE inhibitors produce dramatic improvement and are life saving.

ANGIOTENSIN RECEPTOR BLOCKERS (ARBs)

Over the past 3 decades, several nonpeptide orally active AT_1 receptor antagonists have been developed as alternatives to ACE inhibitors. These include *losartan, candesartan, irbesartan, valsartan, telmisartan, valsartan* and *olmesartan*. The ARBs are now more commonly used than ACE inhibitors. Losartan is described as the prototype.

Losartan It is a competitive antagonist and inverse agonist of Ang II, 10,000 times more selective for AT_1 than for AT_2 receptor. It does not block any other receptor or ion channel. All overt actions of Ang II, *viz.* vasoconstriction, central and peripheral sympathetic stimulation, release of aldosterone and Adr from adrenals, renal actions promoting salt and water reabsorption, central actions like thirst, vasopressin release and growth-promoting actions on heart and blood vessels are blocked. No inhibition of ACE has been noted.

Pharmacologically, ARBs differ from ACE inhibitors in that they do not interfere with degradation of bradykinin and other ACE substrates: no rise in level or potentiation of bradykinin occurs. Consequently, many patients who develop cough with ACE inhibitors, tolerate an ARB nicely.

Losartan causes fall in BP in hypertensive patients which lasts for 24 hours, while HR remains unchanged and cardiovascular reflexes are not interfered. No significant effect on plasma lipid profile, carbohydrate tolerance or insulin sensitivity has been noted. Losartan has the same potential for regressing hypertensive left ventricular hypertrophy as ACE inhibitors.

Pharmacokinetics Oral bioavailability of losartan is only 33% due to first pass metabolism. It is partially carboxylated in liver to an active metabolite (E3174) which is a 10–30 times more potent and noncompetitive AT_1 antagonist. Both compounds are 98% plasma protein bound, do not enter brain and are excreted by the kidney. The plasma t½ of losartan is 2 hours, but that of E3174 is 6–9 hours.

Adverse effects Losartan is well tolerated; has side effect profile similar to placebo. Like ACE inhibitors, it can cause hypotension and hyperkalemia, but first dose hypotension is uncommon. Losartan is largely free of cough and dysguesia inducing potential. Headache, dizziness, weakness and upper g.i. side effects are mild and occasional.

Candesartan is dose to dose more potent, *valsartan* and *telmisartan* nearly equipotent, while *Irbesartan* is less potent than losartan, but their pharmacological profile and uses are similar.

Uses of angiotensin receptor blockers
Losartan and other ARBs are now first line antihypertensive drugs as alternative to ACE inhibitors, comparable in efficacy and other desirable features, with the advantage of not inducing cough and a low incidence of angioedema, rash and dysguesia. They are also as effective as ACE inhibitors in CHF, MI and in diabetic nephropathy.

DIRECT RENIN INHIBITOR
Aliskiren
A nonpeptide orally active drug aliskiren, which binds to the catalytic site of renin and competitively inhibits the generation of Ang I, is now available. It has antihypertensive effect similar to ACE inhibitors and ARBs. Though, it offers no specific advantage over ACE inhibitors and ARBs, it can be used as an alternative to them, or added to them for more complete RAS blockade.

CALCIUM CHANNEL BLOCKERS

These are an important class of cardiovascular drugs which act by inhibiting L-type of voltage sensitive calcium channels in the smooth muscles and heart. There are 3 pharmacologically distinct subclasses of calcium channel blockers (CCBs); *see* chart.

The two most important actions of CCBs are:
1. Smooth muscle (especially vascular) relaxation.
2. Negative chronotropic, inotropic and dromotropic action on the heart.

Smooth muscle Smooth muscles depolarise primarily by inward Ca^{2+} movement through a voltage sensitive L-type channel. These Ca^{2+} ions trigger release of more Ca^{2+} ions from the intracellular stores, and together bring about excitation-contraction coupling (*see* Fig. 11.5). The CCBs cause relaxation by decreasing intracellular availability of Ca^{2+}.

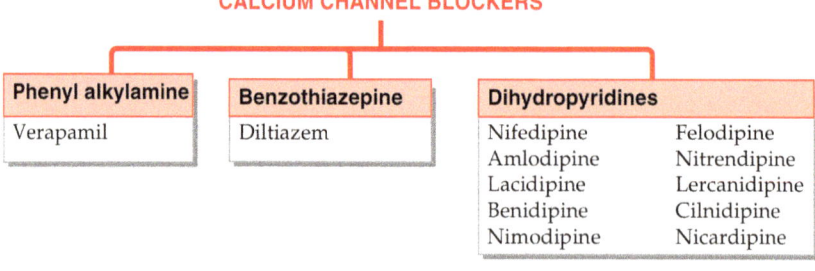

They markedly relax arterioles, but have mild effect on veins. Extravascular smooth muscle (bronchial, biliary, intestinal, vesical, uterine) is also relaxed. Among the CCBs, the dihydropyridines (DHPs) have the most marked smooth muscle relaxant and vasodilator action.

Heart In the working atrial and ventricular fibres, Ca^{2+} moves in during the plateau phase of AP and elicits contraction through binding to troponin. The CCBs would thus have negative inotropic action by reducing Ca^{2+} availability.

The 0 phase depolarization in SA and A-V nodes is largely Ca^{2+} mediated. Automaticity and conductivity of these cells appear to be dependent on the rate of recovery of the Ca^{2+} channel (Fig. 11.2).

The L-type Ca^{2+} channels activate as well as inactivate at a slow rate. Consequently, Ca^{2+} depolarized cells (SA and A-V nodal) have a considerably less steep 0 phase depolarization and longer refractory period. The recovery process which restores the channel to the state from which it can again be activated is delayed by verapamil and to a lesser extent by diltiazem (resulting in depression of pacemaker activity and conduction) but not by DHPs (they have no negative chronotropic/dromotropic action). Moreover, channel blockade by verapamil is enhanced at higher rates of stimulation, that by nifedipine is independent of frequency, while diltiazem is intermediate.

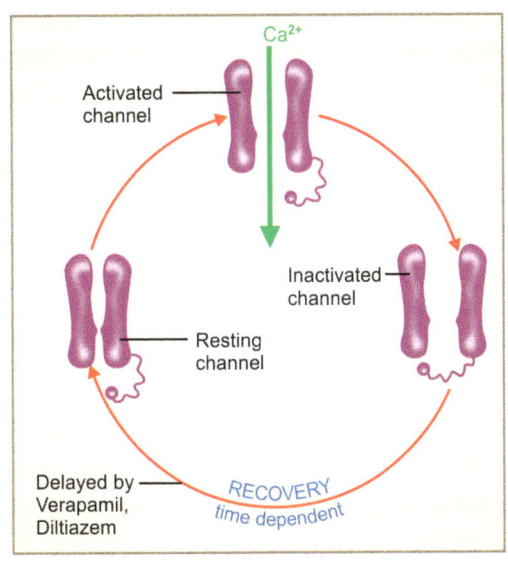

Fig. 11.2: Activation–inactivation–recovery cycle of cardiac Ca^{2+} channels

Thus, verapamil slows sinus rate and A-V conduction, but nifedipine does not. Effect of diltiazem on sinus node automaticity and A-V conduction is similar to that of verapamil.

The relative potencies to block slow channels in the smooth muscle do not parallel those in the heart. The DHPs are more selective for smooth muscle L channels. At concentrations which cause vasodilatation they have negligible negative inotropic action. Diltiazem causes less depression of contractility than verapamil. Important differences between the three representative CCBs are summarized in Table 11.2.

Table 11.2: Comparative properties of representative calcium channel blockers

	Verapamil	Nifedipine	Diltiazem
1. Channel blocking potency	++	+++	+
2. Frequency dependence of channel blockade	++	–	+
3. Channel recovery rate	Much delayed	No effect	Delayed
4. Cardiac effects (In vivo at usual clinical doses)			
Heart rate	↓	↑	↓, –
A-V conduction velocity	↓↓	–	↓↓
Contractility	–, ↓	↑	↓, ↑
Output	–, ↓	↑	–, ↑
5. Vascular smooth muscle relaxation	++	+++	+

Verapamil causes vasodilatation as well as cardiac depression. Along with lowering of BP, it produces bradycardia, slowing of A-V conduction and may worsen heart failure. It should not be used concurrently with β blockers or other cardiac depressants.

Diltiazem has less marked cardiodepressant activity. The fall in BP is attended by little change or decrease in the HR. Though it produces milder side effects, drug interactions and contraindications of diltiazem remain the same as for verapamil.

Nifedipine is a rapidly acting dihydropyridine (DHP) with short duration of action. It frequently produces flushing, palpitation, headache and ankle edema. Direct depression of heart is minimal, and is overshadowed by reflex sympathetic stimulation. Nifedipine has paradoxically worsened angina pectoris in some patients and has been associated with higher mortality among postmyocardial infarct subjects. The slow onset and long-acting DHPs have replaced nifedipine.

Amlodipine is pharmacokinetically the most distinct DHP. It is absorbed very slowly (peak after 6–9 hours) and acts for > 24 hours. The early vasodilator side effects like flushing, palpitation, headache, postural dizziness are largely avoided. A single daily dose is sufficient.

Felodipine, nitrendipine, lercanidipine, benidipine and lacidipine are the other highly vasoselective long-acting DHPs.

Nicardipine It is a highly vasoselective short-acting DHP with pronounced action on coronary and cerebral vessels. Nicardipine is one of the few DHPs that is water soluble, and available for i.v. use. It has a rapid onset and offset of hypotensive effect which can be controlled by adjusting the rate of i.v. infusion. As such, it has become popular for a variety of hypertensive emergencies. The t½ of i.v. nicardipine is 45 min, and its action lasts for 3–4 hours.

An infrequent adverse effect of prolonged CCB therapy having implications in dentistry is *gum hyperplasia*.

USES

1. *Angina pectoris* All CCBs are effective in reducing frequency and severity of classical as well as variant angina. Benefit in classical angina appears to be primarily due to reduction in cardiac work as a consequence of reduced afterload. Though, they can increase coronary flow in normal individuals, this is unlikely to be significant in patients with fixed arterial obstruction. Exercise tolerance is increased.

On the other hand, myocardial ischaemia may be aggravated by short-acting DHPs. This may be due to decreased coronary flow secondary to fall in mean arterial pressure, reflex tachycardia and coronary steal. Trials using high dose regular short-acting nifedipine formulation have reported increased mortality among MI patients. The sudden rush of sympathetic activity evoked by each dose of these preparations has been held responsible for the deleterious effect. The long-acting DHPs (e.g. amlodipine) do not aggravate ischaemia, and are extensively used. The direct cardiac effect of verapamil and diltiazem to reduce O_2 requirement as well as less marked reflex sympathetic stimulation makes these drugs less likely to accentuate ischaemia.

The capacity of CCBs to prevent arterial spasm is undoubtedly responsible for the beneficial effect in variant angina.

2. *Hypertension* The CCBs are one of the first line antihypertensive drugs. Though all 3 subgroups of CCBs are efficacious, the long-acting DHPs (e.g. amlodipine) are most commonly used followed by diltiazem. The CCBs lower BP by reducing peripheral resistance without compromising cardiac output. Their advantages are:

1. Do not compromise haemodynamics: no impairment of physical and mental work capacity, no sedation.
2. Can be used in asthma, angina and peripheral vascular disease patients.

3. Do not affect male sexual function.
4. No deleterious effect on plasma lipid profile, uric acid level or electrolyte balance.
5. Do not impair renal perfusion.
6. No impairment of quality of life.
7. No adverse foetal effects when given during pregnancy.

Verapamil and diltiazem are not suitable for patients with CHF or cardiac conduction defects, because of their negative inotropic and dromotropic actions. On the other hand, DHPs may accentuate bladder voiding difficulty in elderly males and gastroesophageal reflux.

3. *Cardiac arrhythmias* Verapamil and diltiazem are highly effective in PSVT, and for control of ventricular rate in supraventricular arrhythmias.

4. *Hypertrophic cardiomyopathy* The negative inotropic action of verapamil can be salutary in this condition.

ANTIHYPERTENSIVE DRUGS

These are drugs used to lower BP in hypertension.

Hypertension is a very common disorder, particularly past middle age. *As such, many patients presenting for dental treatment are likely to be on long-term antihypertensive drug therapy.*

Hypertension is not a disease in itself but is an important risk factor for cardiovascular morbidity and mortality. Almost all hypertension management guidelines including WHO-ISH (2003), NICE (2011), JNC 8 (2014) and European Society of Hypertension (2007, 2013) define the cutoff level between normotensives and hypertensives to be 140 mm Hg (systolic) and 80 mm Hg (diastolic).

Majority of cases are of essential (primary) hypertension, i.e. the cause is not known. Sympathetic and renin-angiotensin systems may or may not be overactive, but they do contribute to tone of blood vessels and c.o. in hypertensives, as they do in normotensives. Many antihypertensive drugs interfere with these regulatory systems at one level or the other (*see* chart on next page).

The ACE inhibitors, angiotensin antagonists, direct renin inhibitor and CCBs have already been described.

DIURETICS

Diuretics have been a first line antihypertensive drugs over the past 4 decades, but they do not lower BP in normotensives. Their pharmacology is described in Ch. 13.

Thiazides Hydrochlorothiazide (HCZ) and chlorthalidone are the diuretic of choice for uncomplicated hypertension. Both have similar efficacy and are dose to dose equivalent. Their proposed mechanism of antihypertensive action is:

1. Initially, the diuresis reduces plasma and e.c.f. volume by about 10% and this decreases c.o.
2. Subsequently, compensatory mechanisms operate to almost regain Na^+ balance and plasma volume; c.o. is restored, but the fall in BP is maintained by a slowly developing reduction in t.p.r.
3. The reduction in t.p.r. is most probably an indirect consequence of a small (~5%) persisting Na^+ and volume deficit. Decrease in intracellular Na^+ concentration in the vascular smooth muscle may reduce stiffness of vessel wall, increase their compliance and dampen responsiveness to constrictor

WHO-ISH: World Health Organization and International Society of Hypertension.
JNC 8: Evidence-based guidelines for the management of high blood pressure in adults; report from the panel members appointed to the Joint National Committee (USA).
NICE: National Institute for Health Care Excellence (UK); Hypertension in adults: diagnosis and management (CG 127).

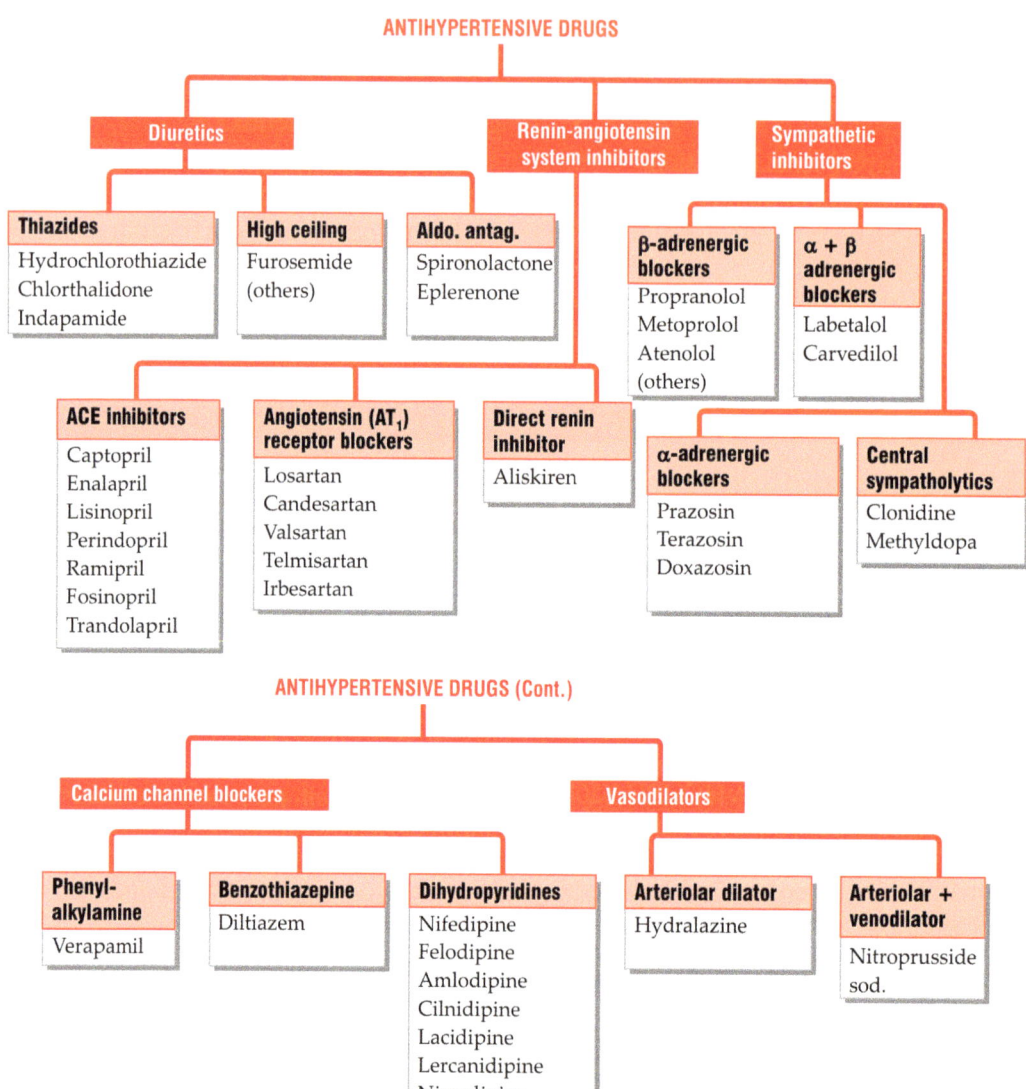

stimuli (NA, Ang II). Similar effects are produced by salt restriction.

The fall in BP is mild (~10 mm Hg) and develops gradually over 2–4 weeks. During long-term treatment with thiazides, the heart rate and c.o. remain unaffected, while t.p.r. is reduced. Thiazides have no effect on capacitance vessels, sympathetic reflexes are not impaired: postural hypotension is rare. They potentiate all other antihypertensives (except DHPs) and prevent development of tolerance to these drugs by not allowing expansion of plasma volume. Maximal antihypertensive efficacy is reached at doses equivalent to 25 mg of HCZ which has minimal diuretic effect. At 12.5–25 mg/day doses, complications of diuretic therapy like hypokalaemia, fatigue, loss of energy, impotence, carbohydrate intolerance, dyslipidemia, hyperuricaemia are absent or mild. As such, thiazides are a first choice antihypertensive, alone or in combination.

Indapamide It is a mild diuretic, chemically related to chlorthalidone; reduces BP at doses which cause little diuresis or K^+ loss.

High ceiling diuretics Furosemide is a strong diuretic, but a weaker antihypertensive than thiazides. The explanation of this paradox may lie in its brief duration of action. The natriuretic action lasting only for 4–6 hours after the conventional morning dose may not maintain Na^+ deficient state in vascular smooth muscle round the clock. High ceiling diuretics are indicated in hypertension only when it is complicated by:
(a) Chronic renal failure: thiazides are ineffective in renal failure patients.
(b) Coexisting refractory CHF.
(c) Resistance to combination regimens containing a thiazide, or marked fluid retention due to use of potent vasodilators.

Aldosterone antagonists Spironolactone and eplerenone themselves lower BP slightly. Accordingly, they are used only in conjunction with a thiazide diuretic to prevent K^+ loss and to augment the antihypertensive action. The aldosterone antagonists (spironolactone, eplerenone) may, in addition, afford prognostic benefit by counteracting the deleterious cardic and vascular effects of aldosterone. The current NICE and JNC 8 guidelines recommend adding one of these drugs to the regimen if the target BP level is not attained.

β-ADRENERGIC BLOCKERS

The pharmacology and mechanism of antihypertensive action of β blockers is described in Ch. 6. β-lockers are mild antihypertensives, and do not significantly lower BP in normotensives. Used alone they suffice in only 30–40% patients—mostly mild-to-moderate cases. Additional BP lowering may be obtained by combining with other drugs.

The BP lowering develops over 1–3 weeks and is well sustained. Despite short and differing plasma half-lives, the antihypertensive action of most β blockers is maintained over 24 hours with single daily dose.

All β blockers, irrespective of associated properties, exert similar antihypertensive effect.

There are several contraindications to β blockers, including cardiac, pulmonary and peripheral vascular disease and diabetes. The nonselective β blockers have an unfavourable effect on lipid profile (raise triglyceride level and LDL/HDL ratio). They have also fared less well on quality of life parameters like decreased work capacity, fatigue, loss of libido and subtle cognitive effects (forgetfulness, low drive). The patients acceptability of a $β_1$ selective hydrophilic drug like atenolol is better than that of propranolol.

Mainly due to inferior efficacy in primary prevention of MI and stroke, as well as other drawbacks pointed out above, β blockers are no longer considered first-line antihypertensive drugs for monotherapy, except in patients with other compelling indications.

β + α ADRENERGIC BLOCKERS

Labetalol It is a combined α and β blocker; reduces t.p.r. and acts faster than pure β blockers. It has been used i.v. for rapid BP reduction in hyperadrenergic states. Oral labetalol therapy is restricted to moderately severe hypertension not responding to pure β blocker.

Carvedilol This nonselective β + weak selective $α_1$ blocker produces vasodilatation and has additional antioxidant/free radical scavenging properties. It is approved for use in hypertension as well as in CHF.

α-ADRENERGIC BLOCKERS

The non-selective ($α_1 + α_2$) adrenergic blockers are not useful antihypertensive drugs; only the selective $α_1$ blockers are employed to supplement the 1st line antihypertensive drugs in selected cases.

Prazosin (See Ch. 6)

It is the prototype of selective α_1 antagonists which dilates both resistance and capacitance vessels; effect on the former predominating. The haemodynamic effects are reduction in t.p.r. and mean BP accompanied by only slight decrease in venous return and c.o. There is little reflex cardiac stimulation and renin release during long-term therapy. Tachycardia does not compensate for the fall in BP, because α_2 (presynaptic) receptors which normally inhibit NA release are not blocked. Thus, autoregulation of NA release remains intact.

Renal blood flow and g.f.r. are maintained but fluid retention may attend fall in BP. Cardiovascular reflexes are not appreciably impaired by chronic therapy, but postural hypotension and fainting may occur in the beginning—called 'first dose effect'. However, it may persist in the elderly patients. Dentists must be careful when patients made to recline on the dental chair sit up.

Prazosin does not impair carbohydrate tolerance, and may have a small favourable effect on lipid profile. Symptomatic improvement may occur in males with prostatic hypertrophy.

Though, prazosin is a moderately potent antihypertensive, it is not used as a first choice drug because fluid retention and tolerance gradually develops, and risk of CHF is increased.

Terazosin, Doxazosin

These are long-acting congeners of prazosin with similar properties and are suitable for once daily dosing.

CENTRAL SYMPATHOLYTICS

Clonidine

It is an imidazoline derivative having complex actions. Clonidine is a partial agonist with high affinity and high intrinsic activity at α_2 receptors. The major haemodynamic effects result from stimulation of α_{2A} receptors present in medulla (vasomotor centre) causing reduction in sympathetic outflow → fall in BP and bradycardia.

Clonidine is a moderately potent antihypertensive.

Clonidine is active orally; metabolized as well as excreted unchanged in urine with a t½ of 8-12 hours. Effect of a single dose lasts for 6–24 hours.

Adverse effects Side effects with clonidine are relatively common and disturbing.
- Sedation, mental depression, disturbed sleep; dryness of mouth, nose and eyes, constipation.
- Impotence, salt and water retention, bradycardia.
- Postural hypotension occurs, but is mild.
- Rebound hypertension with tachycardia, restlessness, headache, sweating occurs on sudden stoppage of clonidine therapy due to:
  a. Sudden removal of central sympathetic inhibition resulting in release of large quantities of stored CAs.
  b. Supersensitivity of peripheral adrenergic structures to CAs.

Regular schedule of drug administration must be maintained to prevent rebound phenomena.

Interactions Tricyclic antidepressants and chlorpromazine abolish the antihypertensive action of clonidine, probably by blocking α receptors on which clonidine acts.

Use Because of relatively higher incidence of side effects, impairment of quality of life and risk of withdrawal hypertension, clonidine is now infrequently used in hypertension; only to supplement the 1st line drugs in selected cases.

Other possible uses of clonidine are opioid withdrawal syndrome, postoperative epidural analgesia and menopausal syndrome.

Methyldopa

It is the α-methyl analogue of dopa, the precursor of dopamine (DA) and NA. The α methyl-NA (a selective α_2 agonist) formed in the brain from methyldopa acts on central α_2 receptors to decrease efferent sympathetic activity. In large doses it inhibits the enzyme dopa decarboxylase and reduces NA synthesis, but the primary site of action is central, as outlined above.

Methyldopa is a moderate efficacy antihypertensive. Circulating levels of NA and renin tend to fall due to reduction in sympathetic tone.

Adverse effects Sedation, lethargy and reduced mental capacity are common side effects. Cognitive impairment may develop. Dryness of mouth, nasal stuffiness, headache, fluid retention, weight gain, impotence and postural hypotension are the other side effects.

Hypersensitivity phenomena such as positive Coombs' test, haemolytic anaemia, fever, rash, hepatitis, 'flu' like illness can also occur with methyldopa.

Use Methyldopa was widely used for mild-to-moderate hypertension, but use has declined now because of the availability of better tolerated agents. It is safe during pregnancy.

VASODILATORS

Hydralazine/Dihydralazine It is a directly acting arteriolar vasodilator with little action on venous capacitance vessels; reduces t.p.r. and causes greater reduction of diastolic than systolic BP. Reflex compensatory mechanisms are evoked which cause tachycardia, increase in c.o. and renin release → increased aldosterone → Na^+ and water retention. Angina may be precipitated due to increased cardiac work as well as steal phenomenon. Tolerance to the hypotensive action develops unless diuretics or β blockers or both are given together to block the compensatory mechanisms. The mechanism of vascular smooth muscle relaxant action is not clearly known; may involve interference with Ca^{2+} release, K^+ channel opening and/or NO generation.

Hydralazine is well absorbed orally. The chief metabolic pathway is acetylation, and there are slow or fast acetylators.

The hypotensive effect lasts for 12 hours.

Adverse effects are frequent and mainly due to vasodilatation.
1. Facial flushing, conjunctival injection, throbbing headache, dizziness, palpitation, nasal stuffiness, fluid retention, edema, CHF.
2. Angina and MI may be precipitated in patients with coronary artery disease.
3. Paresthesias, tremor, muscle cramps, edema, rarely peripheral neuritis.
4. Lupus erythematosus or rheumatoid arthritis like symptoms develop on prolonged use of doses above 100 mg/day.

Use Hydralazine is rarely used now in moderate-to-severe hypertension not controlled by the first line drugs. Usually, low doses are added to diuretics and β blockers.

It is one of the preferred antihypertensives during pregnancy.

Sodium nitroprusside It is a rapidly (within seconds) and consistently acting vasodilator with brief duration of action (2–5 min), so that vascular tone can be titrated with the rate of i.v. infusion. Nitroprusside relaxes both resistance and capacitance vessels: reduces t.p.r. as well as c.o. (by decreasing venous return). Myocardial work is reduced. In contrast to hydralazine, ischaemia is not accentuated.

Endothelial cells, RBCs (and may be other cells) split nitroprusside to generate NO which relaxes vascular smooth muscle. The enzymes involved are different from those that produce NO from glyceryl trinitrate. In addition, nitroprusside generates NO (and CN) nonenzymatically with the help of glutathione. This may be responsible for the different pattern of vasodilator action compared to nitrates, as well as for the fact that no nitrate like tolerance develops to nitroprusside action.

Nitroprusside is a second line drug for hypertensive emergencies with aortic dissection or acute heart failure.

Side effects due to the vasodilator action of nitroprusside are—palpitation, nervousness, vomiting, perspiration, pain in abdomen, weakness, disorientation, and lactic acidosis.

TREATMENT OF HYPERTENSION

The aim of antihypertensive therapy is to prevent morbidity and mortality associated with persistently raised BP by lowering it to the target level, with minimum inconvenience to the patient. Both systolic and diastolic BP predict the likelihood of target organ damage (TOD) and complications such as:
- Cerebrovascular disease, transient ischaemic attacks, stroke.
- Hypertensive heart disease—left ventricular hypertrophy, heart failure.
- Coronary artery disease, angina, myocardial infarction (MI), sudden cardiac death.
- Arteriosclerotic peripheral vascular disease, retinopathy.
- Dissecting aneurysm of aorta.
- Glomerulopathy, renal failure.

Nonpharmacological measures (life style modification—diet, exercise, weight reduction, mental relaxation, etc.) should be tried first and concurrently with drugs.

Hypertension has been graded (NICE 2011 guidelines) as given in the Box:

Hypertension	BP (mm Hg)	
	Systolic	Diastolic
Stage I	140–159	90–99
Stage II	160–179	100–109
Severe	≥180	≥110

Till recently, four groups, *viz.* thiazide diuretics, β blockers, ACE inhibitors/ARBs and CCBs have been regarded as 1st line antihypertensive drugs. However, the recent JNC 8 (2014) and NICE (2011) hypertension treatment guidelines have excluded the β blockers from the list of 1st line drugs due to their lower efficacy in primary prevention of MI and stroke, as well as other drawbacks (see p. 193).

A *stepped care approach*, initially using a single drug and progressively adding one or more drugs from different groups according to need, is recommended.

Step I The drug to initiate therapy is selected on the basis of age and race of the patient. For young (<55 years) non-black subjects an ACE inhibitor/ARB is considered to be the most appropriate drug, because these subjects have higher plasma renin activity and respond better to ACE inhibitors/ARBs. For older non-blacks and blacks of all ages, a CCB or a thiazide diuretic is the preferred option for initiating therapy. The β blockers may be used to initiate therapy in young patients, only if they are pregnant or have any other contraindication to ACE inhibitors/ARBs.

Step II When the target BP is not achieved by a single drug, or when systolic BP is >20 mm Hg higher and/or diastolic BP is >10 mm Hg higher than the target BP, a combination of two drugs, i.e. ACE inhibitor/ARB + a CCB or diuretic (if CCB not suitable), is recommended irrespective of age or race of the patient.

Step III If lowering of BP to target level is still not achieved, all 3 first line drugs, *viz.* ACE inhibitor/ARB + CCB + diuretic are used together. Titration of dose of each drug within its therapeutic range may also be tried for optimal BP lowering.

Step IV Even the 3 drug combination (as above) may be inadequate in few patients with resistant hypertension. An aldosterone antagonist (e.g. eplerenone) or higher dose (≥50 mg) thiazide or a β blocker or selective α_1 blocker may be added as the 4th drug in such cases.

Hypertensive emergencies and urgencies

Markedly raised BP (> 220 mm Hg systolic or > 120 mm Hg diastolic, or both) is termed hypertensive 'emergency' when accompanied with target organ damage (TOD), and 'urgency' without target organ damage. This requires controlled reduction of BP over minutes (in emergencies) or hours (in urgencies) to counter threat to organ function and life.

Though unlikely to be encountered in dental practice, sudden rise in BP may occur when the patient suffers a stroke or MI. Pheochromocytoma, hypertensive encephalopathy, acute LVF or dissecting aortic aneurysm may also trigger hypertensive emergency.

Parenteral drugs

Hypertensive emergencies require use of drugs with controllable action infused i.v. to lower BP by about 25% over a period of 1–2 hours and then gradually to not lower than 160/100 mm Hg. Drugs employed are:

1. *Nicardipine* It is a dihydropyridine CCB available for i.v. use. Nicardipine has rapid onset and offset of hypotensive action, and is now the preferred drug for most hypertensive emergencies, because it is equally effective and less toxic than sodium nitroprusside.

2. *Sodium nitroprusside* This is another potent and rapidly acting hypotensive drug that was commonly used in the

past, but is now mostly restricted to cases with aortic dissection (combine with i.v. esmolol) or acute heart failure (combine with furosemide).

3. *Glyceryl trinitrate (GTN)* Though not a potent hypotensive, GTN infused i.v. is suitable (due to its venodilator action) for cases of MI or acute heart failure accompanied by rise in BP. However, infusion of GTN beyond 12 hours leads to development of tolerance. It also needs to be avoided in cases of stroke.

4. *Labetalol* This combined β + α adrenergic blocker is an efficacious hypotensive when injected i.v. Labetalol is particularly useful for lowering raised BP due to pheochromocytoma and other hyperadrenergic states. It is also indicated for severe hypertension complicating aortic dissection, MI, stroke, and in preeclampsia.

5. *Esmolol* It is a short-acting selective β_1 adrenergic blocker used by bolus i.v. injection, followed by slow i.v. infusion. Its action starts in 1–2 min, and lasts for 10–20 min after termination of infusion. Esmolol is suitable for cases with aortic dissection, because it reduces cardiac contractility and cardiac work. Combined with nicardipine or GTN, it is also indicated in MI associated with raised BP and tachycardia.

Oral drugs

Oral drugs that act slowly and decrease BP over 2–48 hours may be safer and more appropriate in hypertensive urgencies when there is no immediate threat to life or of organ damage. The preferred oral drugs are:

1. *Amlodipine* This slow and long acting oral DHP (see p. 190) is most commonly employed in a dose of 10 mg repeated after 12 hours and then once daily. It starts acting in 6–8 hours and may take 2–3 days to lower BP to the target level, but is safer. Amlodipine is particularly suitable for elderly patients and those prone to postural hypotension.

2. *Labetalol* In a dose of 100–200 mg oral twice daily, this combined β + α blocker starts acting in 2–4 hours and is satisfactory in many cases of severe hypertension without target organ damage. It is the 1st line drug in pheochromocytoma, preeclampsia and in those with ischaemic heart disease.

ANTIANGINAL DRUGS

Antianginal drugs are those that prevent, abort or terminate attacks of angina pectoris. Since a patient may develop an attack of angina during dental procedure, dentists should be familiar with its management.

Angina pectoris It is a pain syndrome due to induction of an adverse oxygen supply/demand situation in a portion of the myocardium. Metabolites that accumulate due to myocardial ischaemia elicit the pain. Two principal forms are recognized:

(a) *Classical angina* (common form) Attacks are predictably (stable angina) provoked by exercise, anxiety, eating or coitus and subside when the increased energy demand is withdrawn. The underlying pathology is—severe arteriosclerotic affliction of larger coronary arteries (conducting vessels) which run epicardially and send perforating branches to supply the deeper tissue (Fig. 11.3). The coronary obstruction is 'fixed'; blood flow fails to increase during increased demand despite local factors mediated dilatation of resistance vessels (Fig. 11.4) and ischaemic pain is felt. Due to inadequacy of

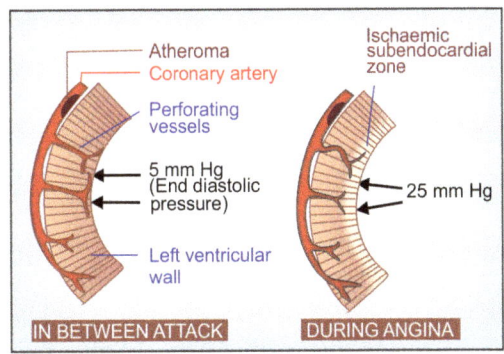

Fig. 11.3: Diagrammatic representation of subendocardial 'crunch' during an attack of angina

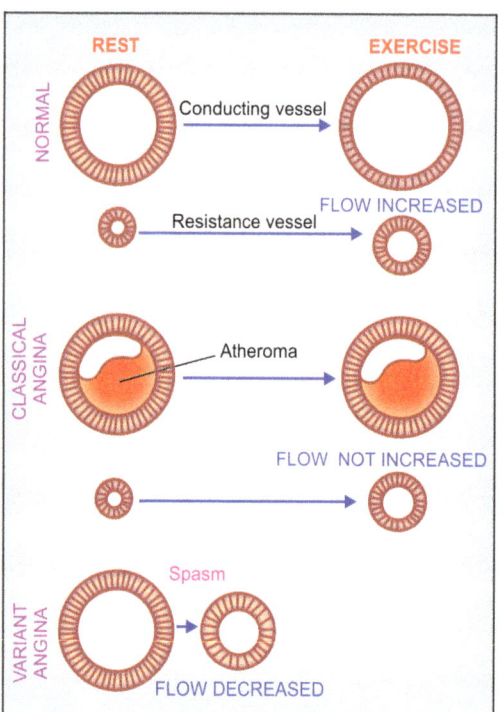

Fig. 11.4: Diagrammatic representation of coronary artery calibre changes in classical and variant angina

ischaemic left ventricle, the end diastolic left ventricular pressure rises from 5 to about 25 mm Hg—produces subendocardial 'crunch' during diastole (blood flow to the subendocardial region occurs only during diastole) and aggravates ischaemia in this region.

Drugs that are useful, primarily reduce cardiac work (directly by acting on heart or indirectly by reducing preload, hence end diastolic pressure, and afterload). They may also cause favourable redistribution of blood flow to the ischaemic areas.

(b) *Variant/Prinzmetal's/Vasospastic angina* (uncommon form) Attacks occur at rest or during sleep and are unpredictable. They are due to recurrent localized (occasionally diffuse) coronary vasospasm (Fig. 11.4) which may be superimposed on arteriosclerotic coronary artery disease. Abnormally reactive and hypertrophied segments in the coronary arteries have been demonstrated. Drugs are aimed at preventing and relieving the coronary vasospasm.

Unstable angina (UA) with rapid increase in duration and severity of attacks is mostly due to rupture of an atheromatous plaque attracting platelet deposition and incomplete occlusion of the coronary artery; occasionally with associated coronary vasospasm. However, myocardial necrosis is absent, but patients are at high risk of developing MI.

Antianginal drugs relieve cardiac ischaemia but do not alter the course of coronary artery pathology: no permanent benefit is afforded by these drugs.

The antianginal drugs are classified in the chart.

Clinical Classification

A. **Used to abort or terminate attack** Glyceryl trinitrate (GTN), Isosorbide dinitrate (sublingually).

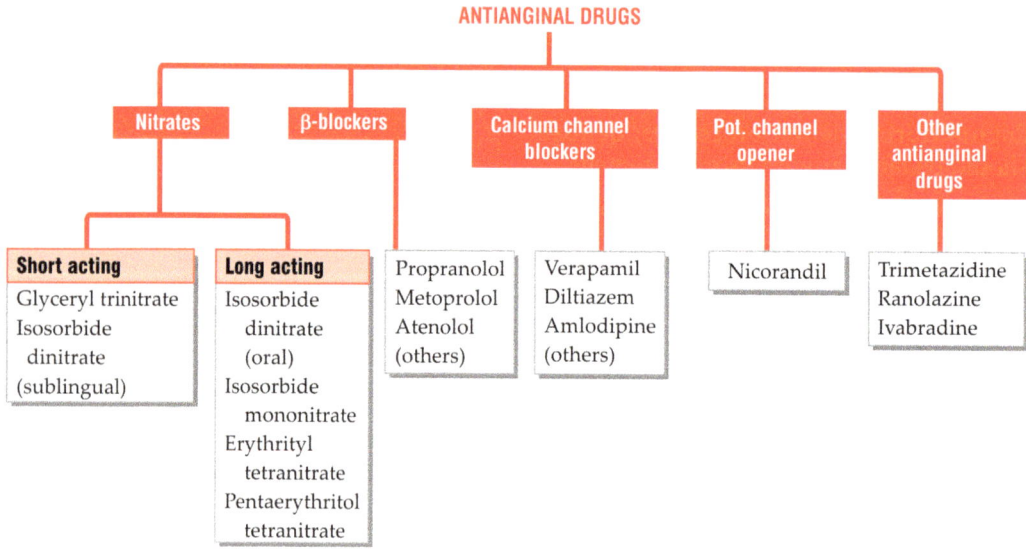

B. Used for chronic prophylaxis All other drugs.

NITRATES (GTN as prototype)

All organic nitrates share the same action; differ only in time course. The only major action is direct nonspecific smooth muscle relaxation.

Preload reduction Nitrates dilate veins more than arteries → peripheral pooling of blood → decreased venous return, i.e. preload on heart is reduced → end diastolic size and pressure are reduced → decreased cardiac work.

The decrease in end diastolic pressure abolishes the subendocardial crunch by restoring the pressure gradient across ventricular wall due to which subendocardial perfusion occurs during diastole. It is through their action on peripheral veins that nitrates exert major beneficial effects in classical angina.

After load reduction Nitrates also produce mild arteriolar dilatation → slightly decrease total peripheral resistance (t.p.r.) or afterload on heart; BP falls somewhat; systolic more than diastolic (reflex sympathetic activity tends to maintain diastolic BP). This action contributes to the reduction of cardiac work which is directly proportional to aortic impedance.

Redistribution of coronary flow In the arterial tree, nitrates preferentially relax bigger conducting (angiographically visible) coronary arteries than arterioles or resistance vessels. This pattern of action may cause favourable redistribution of blood flow to ischaemic areas in angina patients. Dilatation of conducting vessels all over by the nitrate along with ischaemia induced dilatation of autoregulatory resistance vessels only in the ischaemic zone increases blood flow to this area; while in the non-ischaemic zones, resistance vessels maintain their tone, and flow does not increase, or may decrease to compensate for increased flow to ischaemic zone. In fact, nitrates do not appreciably increase total coronary flow in angina patients.

Mechanism of relief of angina The relaxant effect on larger coronary vessels is the principal action of nitrates benefiting variant angina by counteracting coronary spasm. In classical angina, the primary action is to reduce cardiac work by action on peripheral vasculature, though increased blood supply to the ischaemic area may contribute. Exercise tolerance of angina patients is increased because the same amount of exercise causes lesser augmentation of cardiac work.

Heart and peripheral blood flow Nitrates have no direct stimulant or depressant action on the heart. They dilate cutaneous vessels (especially over face and neck → flushing) and meningeal vessels causing headache. Splanchnic and renal blood flow decreases to compensate for vasodilatation in other areas. Nitrates tend to decongest lungs by shifting blood to systemic circulation.

Other smooth muscles Bronchi, biliary tract and esophagus are relaxed; effect on intestine, ureter and uterus is variable and insignificant.

Mechanism of action Organic nitrates are rapidly denitrated enzymatically in the smooth muscle cell to release the reactive free radical *nitric oxide (NO)* which activates cytosolic soluble guanylyl cyclase → increased cGMP → causes dephosphorylation of myosin light chain kinase (MLCK) through a cGMP-dependent protein kinase (Fig. 11.5). Reduced availability of phosphorylated (active) MLCK interferes with activation of myosin → it fails to interact with actin to cause contraction. Consequently, relaxation occurs. Raised intracellular cGMP may also reduce Ca^{2+} entry—contributing to relaxation.

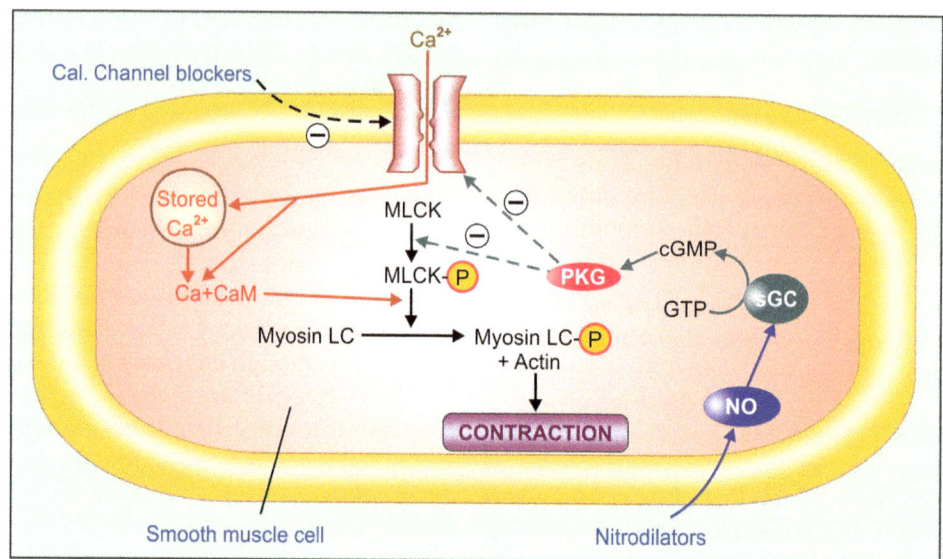

Fig. 11.5: Mechanism of vascular smooth muscle relaxant action of nitrodilators like glyceryl trinitrate and calcium channel blockers; (- - -→) Inhibition
CaM—Calmodulin; NO—Nitric oxide; MLCK—Myosin light chain kinase; MLCK-P—Phosphorylated MLCK; GTP—Guanosine triphosphate; cGMP—Cyclic guanosine monophosphate; Myosin LC—Myosic light chain; sGC—Soluble guanylyl cyclase; PKG—Protein kinase G

Pharmacokinetics Organic nitrates are lipid soluble: therefore well absorbed from buccal mucosa, intestines and skin. Ingested orally, all except isosorbide mononitrate undergo extensive and variable first pass metabolism in liver. They are rapidly denitrated by a glutathione reductase enzyme.

Adverse effects These are mostly due to vasodilatation.
1. Fullness in head, throbbing headache; some degree of tolerance develops on continued use.
2. Flushing, weakness, sweating, palpitation, dizziness and fainting; these symptoms are mitigated by lying down.
3. Rashes are rare.

Tolerance Attenuation of haemodynamic and anti-ischaemic effect of nitrates occurs if they are continuously present in the body. This tolerance weans off rapidly (within hours) when the body is free of the drug. Clinically, no significant tolerance develops on intermittent use of sublingual GTN for attacks of angina. However, it may become important when GTN is used orally, transdermally or by continuous i.v. infusion round the clock.

The most practical way to prevent nitrate tolerance is to provide nitrate free intervals every day.

Dependence on organic nitrates can also develop, so that sudden stoppage of nitrate after prolonged use may precipitate spasm of coronary and peripheral vessels. Angina may worsen; MI and sudden deaths are reported.

Interactions Sildenafil (a drug used for erectile dysfunction) causes dangerous potentiation of nitrate action: severe hypotension, MI and deaths are on record. Additive hypotension is also possible when nitrate is given to a patient receiving other vasodilators.

1. Glyceryl trinitrate (GTN, Nitroglycerine) It is a volatile liquid which is formulated by adsorbing on the inert matrix of the tablet.

The sublingual route is used when terminating an attack or aborting an imminent one is the aim. It acts within 1–2 min (peak blood level in 3–6 min) because of direct absorption into systemic circulation (bypassing liver where almost 90% is metabolized).

Plasma t½ of GTN is 2 min, duration of action depends on the period it remains available for absorption from buccal mucosa. The remaining part of the tablet may be spit or swallowed when no longer needed. A sublingual spray formulation of GTN is also available, which may act faster than the s.l. tablet. Sustained release oral capsules containing much larger amounts of GTN can be used for chronic prophylaxis.

Nitroglycerine is readily absorbed from the skin. A transdermal patch in which the drug is incorporated into a polymer bonded to adhesive plaster (see p. 11) has been developed which provides steady delivery of GTN for 24 hours. However, development of tolerance and dependence may jeopardise its value. It is advised that the patch be taken off for 8 hours daily.

Intravenous infusion of GTN has been successfully used for unstable angina, coronary vasospasm, LVF accompanying MI, hypertension during cardiac surgery, etc.

2. Isosorbide dinitrate It can be used sublingually at the time of attack (slightly slower in action than GTN, peak in 5–8 min) as well as orally for chronic prophylaxis. The t½ is 40 min, but sustained release formulation may afford protection for 6–10 hours.

3. Isosorbide mononitrate This is an active metabolite of isosorbide dinitrate. When administered orally, it undergoes little first pass metabolism: bioavailability is high, interindividual differences are minimal and it is longer acting (t½ 4–6 hr).

4. Erythrityl tetranitrate and pentaerythritol tetranitrate These are longer acting nitrates used only for chronic prophylaxis.

Uses

1. *Angina pectoris* Nitrates are effective in classical as well as variant angina. For aborting or terminating an attack, sublingual GTN tablet or isosorbide dinitrate is taken on 'as and when required' basis. Since dental procedures often provoke anxiety, an anginal attack may be precipitated. *Sublingual GTN tablet or spray should be readily available to abort/terminate such an attack on the dental chair.* Longer acting formulations (oral, transdermal) of GTN or other long-acting nitrates used on regular schedule increase exercise tolerance and postpone ECG changes of angina. Nitrates are useful in unstable angina as well. However, antiplatelet drugs are the primary measure in unstable angina.

2. *Myocardial infarction* Carefully titrated i.v. infusion of GTN to avoid tachycardia and started soon after the arterial occlusion, can relieve pulmonary congestion and limit the area of necrosis by favourably altering O_2 balance in the marginal partially ischaemic zone by reducing cardiac work.

3. *CHF and acute LVF* Nitrates afford relief in acute left ventricular failure by venous pooling of blood → reduced venous return → decreased end diastolic volume → improvement in failing left ventricular function. Intravenous GTN is the preparation of choice for emergency use.

4. *Biliary colic* Biliary colic due to gallstone and that caused by morphine responds to sublingual GTN or isosorbide dinitrate.

5. *Esophageal spasm* Sublingual GTN promptly relieves pain.

6. *Cyanide poisoning* Nitrates react with haemoglobin to generate methaemoglobin which has high affinity for cyanide radical. In cyanide poisoning, sod. nitrite injected i.v. produces methaemoglobin which then reacts with cyanide and forms

cyanomethaemoglobin. Cytochrome and other oxidative enzymes are thus protected from the cyanide.

β BLOCKERS

The β blockers do not dilate coronaries or other blood vessels; total coronary flow is rather reduced due to blockade of dilator $β_2$ receptors. However, flow to the ischaemic subendocardial region is not reduced because of favourable redistribution and decrease in ventricular wall tension. The β blockers act by preventing increase in cardiac work and O_2 consumption that occurs during exercise or anxiety.

The cardioselective β blockers (e.g. atenolol, metoprolol) are preferred over nonselective $β_1 + β_2$ blockers (e.g. propranolol) in classical angina. They decrease frequency and severity of attacks, and increase exercise tolerance. On the other hand, β blockers can worsen variant angina. Long-term β blocker therapy lowers risk of sudden cardiac death among ischaemic heart disease patients. The β blockers are to be taken on a regular schedule; not on 'as and when required' basis.

The β blockers are routinely used in unstable angina, provided there are no contraindications.

CALCIUM CHANNEL BLOCKERS

Described earlier (see p. 190).

POTASSIUM CHANNEL OPENERS

Since intracellular concentration of K^+ is much higher (150 mM) compared to extracellular (4–5 mM), K^+ channel opening results in outflow of K^+ ions and hyperpolarization. There are multiple types of K^+ channels, which serve diverse functions and exhibit different sensitivities to drugs. As such, K^+ channel openers exhibit considerable diversity in action.

Nicorandil It activates ATP sensitive K^+ channels and hyperpolarizes vascular smooth muscle. Like nitrates, nicorandil also acts as a NO donor—relaxes blood vessels by increasing cGMP. Thus, arterial dilatation is coupled with venodilatation. Coronary flow is increased; dilatation of both epicardial conducting vessels and deeper resistance vessels has been demonstrated. No significant effect on cardiac contractility and conduction has been noted.

Beneficial effects on angina frequency and exercise tolerance that are comparable to nitrates, β blockers and CCBs have been obtained with nicorandil.

Side effects are flushing, palpitation, weakness, headache, dizziness, nausea and vomiting. Mouth ulcers are frequent.

Nicorandil is sporadically used as an alternative to nitrates or CCBs for angina pectoris.

OTHER ANTIANGINAL DRUGS

1. Trimetazidine This antianginal drug acts by nonhaemodynamic mechanisms. There is no effect on determinants of myocardial O_2 consumption, such as HR and BP, both at rest as well as during exercise, but angina frequency is reduced and exercise capacity is increased. In patients not fully controlled by long-acting nitrate/β blocker/CCB, addition of trimetazidine further reduced anginal attacks and increased exercise duration. The mechanism of action of trimetazidine is uncertain, but it may improve cellular tolerance to ischaemia by inhibiting a key enzyme LC 3-KAT of fatty acid oxidation, thus shifting back ischaemic myocardial metabolism to utilize glucose and save O_2.

Trimetazidine is generally well tolerated; side effects are—gastric burning, dizziness, fatigue and muscle cramps. It is mostly used as additional medication to conventional therapy in angina and post-MI patients.

2. Ranolazine This novel antianginal drug acts primarily by reducing Ca^{2+} overload in the myocardium that occurs during ischaemia. Ranolazine is an inhibitor of a late Na⁺ current (late I_{Na}) in the myocardium, and this indirectly reduces Na^+/Ca^{2+} exchange to exert cardioprotective effect. A secondary action of ranolazine is to inhibit LC3-KAT, and thus shift back ATP production in ischaemic myocardium from fatty acid oxidation to more O_2 efficient carbohydrate oxidation.

Ranolazine decreases frequency of anginal attacks and improves exercise tolerance. It is mainly used in combination with one or more conventional antianginal drugs.

3. Ivabradine This pure heart rate lowering antianginal drug has been introduced as an alternative to β blockers. The only significant action of ivabradine is to block cardiac pacemaker (sinoatrial) cell 'f' or *'funny'* cation channels which open during early part of slow diastolic (phase 4) depolarization. This inward current (I_f) determines rate of phase 4 depolarization and thereby heart rate. Thus, ivabradine causes bradycardia without any other electrophysiological or inotropic effect. Reduction in heart rate decreases cardiac O_2 consumption and allows more time for myocardial perfusion which occurs during diastole. Ivabradine has been found to decrease angina frequency and to improve exercise tolerance. It can also be used to control inappropriate sinus tachycardia and in selected patients of grade II to grade IV heart failure.

DRUG THERAPY IN MYOCARDIAL INFARCTION

Myocardial infarction (MI) is ischaemic necrosis of a portion of the myocardium due to sudden occlusion of a branch of coronary artery. An acute thrombus at the site of atherosclerotic obstruction is the usual cause. Since an attack of MI can occur at any time, dental practitioners should be prepared to provide first hand treatment in their clinic. About 1/4th patients suffer cardiac arrest or ventricular fibrillation and die before therapy can be instituted. The remaining are best treated in specialized coronary care units with continuous monitoring of the haemodynamic parameters and ECG to guide the selection of drugs and dosage. Those who receive such facility can be greatly benefitted by drug therapy, which according to individual needs is directed to:

1. *Pain, anxiety and apprehension* When the chest pain is not relieved by 3 doses of s.l. GTN given 5 min. apart, MI is suspected and an opioid analgesic (morphine) or diazepam should be given parenterally.

2. *Oxygenation* By O_2 inhalation and assisted ventilation, if needed.

3. *Maintenance of blood volume, tissue perfusion and microcirculation* Slow i.v. infusion of saline/dextrose may be instituted if the BP falls.

4. *Correction of acidosis* Acidosis occurs due to lactic acid production; can be corrected by sod. bicarbonate i.v. infusion.

5. *Prevention and treatment of arrhythmias* Prophylactic i.v. infusion of a β blocker (unless contraindicated due to fall in BP/bradycardia, etc.) is recommended. Its continuation orally for a few days reduces the incidence of arrhythmias and mortality. β blockers used early in evolving MI can reduce the infarct size (myocardial salvage) and subsequent complications.

Tachyarrhythmias may be treated with lidocaine, procainamide or amiodarone. Bradycardia and heart block may be managed with atropine or electrical pacing.

6. *Pump failure* The objective is to increase c.o. and/or decrease filling pressure without unduly increasing cardiac work or lowering BP. Drugs used for this purpose are:

(a) *Furosemide*: It is indicated if pulmonary

wedge pressure is > 20 mm Hg. Furosemide acts by decreasing cardiac preload.

(b) *Vasodilators*: Slow i.v. infusion of GTN is mostly used to cause venodilation. This may be supplemented by i.v. esmolol or labetalol.

(c) *Inotropic agents*: dopamine or dobutamine i.v. infusion may be needed to augment the pumping action of heart and tide over crisis.

7. *Prevention of thrombus extension, embolism, venous thrombosis* All patients of MI should be immediately given aspirin (150–300 mg) for chewing and swallowing. This may be supplemented by other antiplatelet drugs (clopidogrel or prasugrel or ticagrelor). Anticoagulants (heparin or fondaparinux, followed by oral anticoagulants) are used primarily to prevent deep vein thrombosis/pulmonary embolism. Their value in checking coronary artery thrombus extension is uncertain.

8. *Thrombolysis* Fibrinolytic agents, i.e. plasminogen activators—alteplase/tenecteplase to achieve reperfusion of the infarcted area, are indicated only in ST segment elevation MI (STEMI). This is beneficial only when started within 1–2 hours of symptom onset. Primary percutaneous coronary intervention (PCI) with stent placement is the preferred revascularization procedure now.

9. *Prevention of remodeling and subsequent CHF* ACE inhibitors/ARBs have proven efficacy and afford long-term survival benefit. One of these drugs is started as soon as the patient is haemodynamically stable.

10. *Prevention of future attacks*

(a) Platelet function inhibitors—aspirin alone or combined with clopidogrel given on long-term basis is routinely prescribed.

(b) β blockers—these drugs reduce risk of reinfarction, CHF and mortality. All patients not having any contraindication are put on a $β_1$ blocker for at least 2 years.

(c) Control of hyperlipidaemia—dietary substitution with unsaturated fats, along with a statin hypolipidaemic drug is recommended irrespective of blood cholesterol level. Long-term statin therapy reduces risk of cardiovascular events.

CHAPTER 12

Cardiovascular Drugs
Drugs for Heart Failure and Cardiac Arrhythmia

CARDIAC GLYCOSIDES

These are glycosidic drugs having *cardiac inotropic* property. They increase myocardial contractility and output in a hypodynamic heart without a proportionate increase in O_2 consumption.

The cardiac glycosides are found in several plants and one is present in toad skin as well. Only one cardiac glycoside *digoxin* is currently in clinical use. It is obtained from the plant *Digitalis lanata*, and the term 'digitalis' refers to any cardiac glycoside. The cardiac glycosides consist of an aglycone moiety made of cyclopentanoperhydrophenanthrene (steroid) ring with attached 5 or 6 membered unsaturated lactone ring and a sugar moiety.

Pharmacological actions

Heart Digoxin has direct effects on myocardial contractility and electrophysiological properties. In addition, it has vagomimetic action, reflex effects due to alteration in haemodynamics and direct CNS effects altering sympathetic activity.

1. Digoxin causes a dose dependent increase in force of contraction of heart—a positive inotropic action. This is more prominent in the failing heart. When a normal heart is subjected to increased impedance to outflow, it generates greater tension so that stroke volume is maintained up to considerably higher values of impedance (Fig. 12.1), while the failing heart is not able to do so and the stroke volume progressively decreases. The digitalized failing heart regains some of its capacity to contract more forcefully when subjected to increased resistance to ejection. There is more complete emptying of the failing and dilated ventricles—cardiac output is increased.

2. The heart rate is decreased by digoxin. It produces bradycardia by increasing vagal tone as well as by a direct extravagal action exerted on SA and A-V nodes. In CHF patients improved circulation (due to positive inotropic action) restores the diminished vagal tone and abolishes sympathetic overactivity. Consequently, lowering of heart rate is more marked.

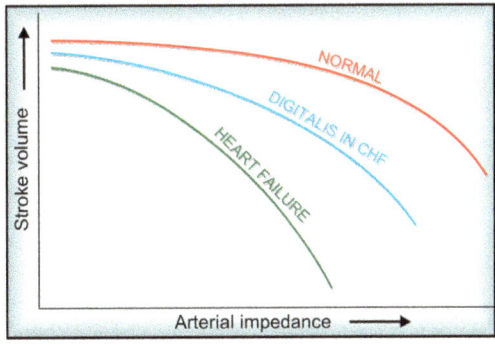

Fig. 12.1: Relationship between peripheral resistance and stroke output in normal and failing heart, and the action of digitalis on failing heart

3. The electrophysiological properties of different types of cardiac fibres are affected differently by digoxin:
- SA and A-V nodal automaticity is depressed while that in Purkinje fibres (PFs) and ectopic pacemakers is enhanced: arrhythmias may be produced.
- Effective refractory period (ERP) of A-V node and bundle of His is prolonged: the maximal rate at which impulses can be transmitted from atrium to ventricle is reduced.
- A-V conduction is slowed. Partial to complete A-V block can occur.
- Atrial ERP is abbreviated and made more inhomogeneous: atria become more prone to fibrillation. Ventricular ERP is also reduced.
- Myocardial excitability is enhanced, but may be depressed at toxic doses.

Mechanism of action Digoxin increases force of cardiac contraction by inhibiting membrane associated Na^+K^+ ATPase of myocardial fibres (Fig. 12.2). Inhibition of this cation pump results in progressive accumulation of Na^+ intracellularly. This indirectly results in intracellular Ca^{2+} accumulation by $Na^+ : Ca^{2+}$ exchange (for details *see* legend to Fig. 12.2).

The excess Ca^{2+} remaining in cytosol is taken up into sarcoplasmic reticulum (SR) which progressively get loaded with more Ca^{2+} → subsequent calcium transients (brief bursts of Ca^{2+} release attending action potentials) are augmented → better

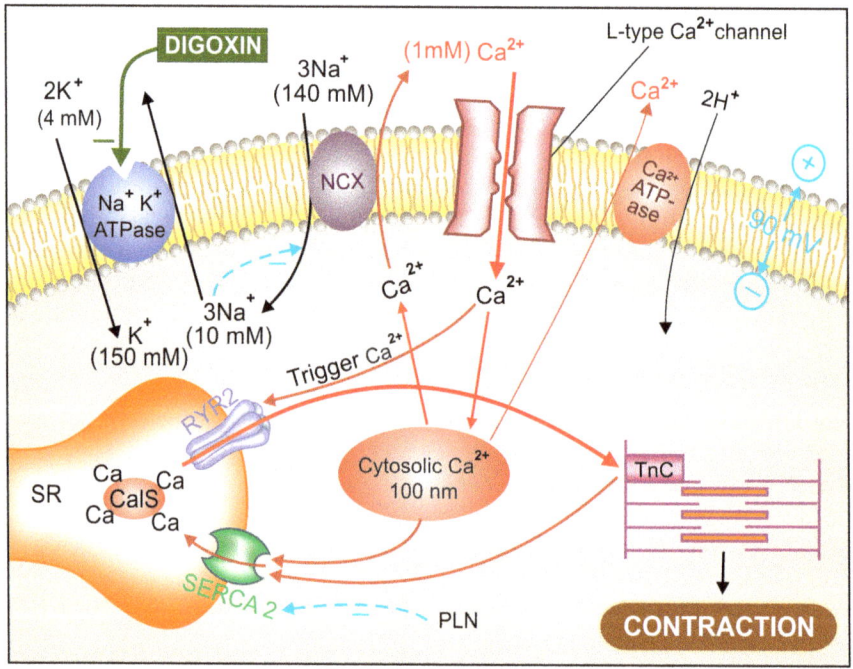

Fig. 12.2: Mechanism of positive inotropic action of digoxin.
During depolarization Ca^{2+} ions enter the cell driven by the steep Ca^{2+} gradient (>1 mM extracellular to < 100 nM cytosolic during diastole) through voltage sensitive L type Ca^{2+} channels. This triggers release of larger amount of Ca^{2+} stored in sarcoplasmic reticulum (SR) through Ryanodine calcium channel 2 (RYR2) → cytosolic Ca^{2+} increases transiently to about 500 nM (calcium transients) → triggers contraction by activating troponin C (TnC) on myofibrils. The sarcoplasmic-endoplasmic reticular Cal. ATPase 2 (SERCA 2) is then activated which pumps Ca^{2+} back into the SR where it is stored loosely bound to calsequestrin (CalS). In the resting state SERCA remains inhibited by a protein phospholamban (PLN). A fraction of cytosolic Ca^{2+} is extruded mainly by $3Na^+/1Ca^{2+}$ exchange transporter (NCX). Inhibition of $Na^+ K^+$ ATPase by digoxin reduces transmembrane gradient of Na^+ which drives extrusion of Ca^{2+}, raising cytosolic Ca^{2+} concentration

excitation-contraction coupling → increased force of contraction.

Binding of glycoside to $Na^+K^+ATPase$ is slow. Moreover, after $Na^+K^+ATPase$ inhibition, Ca^{2+} loading occurs gradually. As such, inotropic effect of digoxin takes hours to develop, even after i.v. administration.

At toxic doses of digoxin, excessive inhibition of Na^+ K^+ ATPase results in depletion of intracellular K^+ in the myocardium; toxicity is partially reversed by infusing K^+. Excessive Ca^{2+} loading of SR results in spontaneous cycles of Ca^{2+} release and uptake producing oscillatory after-depolarizations and after-contractions (arrhythmias).

Blood vessels Digoxin has weak direct vasoconstrictor action—peripheral resistance is increased in normal individuals. However, in CHF patients this is more than compensated by the indirect effect of improvement in circulation whereby reflex sympathetic overactivity is withdrawn and a net decrease in peripheral resistance occurs. Digoxin has no prominent effect on BP or on coronary circulation.

Kidney Digoxin promptly causes diuresis in CHF patients, secondary to improvement in circulation and renal perfusion. The retained salt and water is gradually excreted. No diuresis occurs in normal individuals or in patients with edema due to other causes.

CNS Digoxin has little apparent CNS effect in therapeutic dose. Higher doses cause CTZ activation → nausea and vomiting. Still higher doses produce hyperapnoea, central sympathetic stimulation, mental confusion, disorientation and visual disturbances.

Pharmacokinetics

The pharmacokinetic properties of digoxin are presented in Table 12.1. Bioavailability of digoxin tablets from different manufacturers differs considerably.

Table 12.1: Pharmacokinetic features of digoxin

	DIGOXIN
1. Oral absorption	60–80%
2. Plasma protein binding	25%
3. Duration of action	2–6 days
4. Plasma t½	40 hr
5. Daily maintenance dose	0.125–0.5 mg
6. Route of elimination (predominant)	Renal excretion
7. Administration	Oral, i.v.

Digoxin is concentrated in the heart (~20 times than plasma), skeletal muscle, liver and kidney. It is primarily excreted unchanged by the kidney: mainly by glomerular filtration; rate of excretion is altered parallel to creatinine clearance.

Cardiac glycosides are cumulative drugs. When maintenance doses are given from the beginning, steady-state levels and full therapeutic effect are attained after 4 t½, i.e. 6–7 days for digoxin.

Adverse effects

Toxicity of digoxin is high, margin of safety is low (therapeutic index 1.5–3) and fatalities have occurred occasionally. Hypokalaemia enhances digoxin toxicity. The manifestations of toxicity are:

Extracardiac Anorexia, nausea, vomiting and abdominal pain are usually reported first: are due to gastric irritation, mesenteric vasoconstriction and CTZ stimulation. Fatigue, malaise, headache, mental confusion, restlessness, hyperapnoea, disorientation, psychosis and visual disturbances are the other complaints.

Cardiac Almost every type of arrhythmia can be produced by digoxin: pulsus bigeminus, nodal and ventricular extrasystoles, ventricular tachycardia and terminally ventricular fibrillation. Partial to complete A-V block may be the sole cardiac toxicity or it may accompany other arrhythmias. Severe bradycardia, atrial extrasystoles, AF or AFl have also been noted.

Treatment Further doses of digoxin must be stopped at the earliest sign of toxicity; nothing more needs to be done in many patients, especially if the manifestations are only extracardiac.

Tachyarrhythmias can be treated with KCl infusion. For ventricular arrhythmias lidocaine is preferred, while propranolol is generally given for atrial arrhythmias. Atropine may be tried in case of severe bradycardia/A-V block. The *Fab* fragment of digoxin antibody is used to bind the glycoside and accelerate its elimination.

Interactions

1. *Diuretics*: cause hypokalemia which can precipitate digoxin-induced arrhythmias.
2. *Calcium*: synergises with digoxin → precipitates toxicity.
3. *Quinidine*: reduces binding of digoxin to tissue proteins as well as its renal and biliary clearance → plasma digoxin level is raised → toxicity can occur.
4. *Adrenergic drugs*: can induce arrhythmias in digitalized patients. *Plain lidocaine without Adr should be injected for dental anaesthesia.*
5. *Propranolol, verapamil, diltiazem and disopyramide:* may additively depress A-V conduction and oppose its positive inotropic action.

Uses

The two main indications of digoxin are CHF and control of ventricular rate in atrial fibrillation/flutter.

1. Congestive heart failure

CHF occurs when cardiac output is insufficient to meet the demands of tissue perfusion.

In heart failure there may be primary *systolic dysfunction*, i.e. ventricles are unable to develop sufficient wall tension (due to ischaemic heart disease, etc.) to eject adequate quantity of blood, or *diastolic dysfunction* in which ventricular wall is thickened (due to hypertension, etc.) and unable to relax properly during diastole to allow adequate ventricular filling (and later ejection), or both.

Cardiac glycosides primarily mitigate systolic dysfunction. Because of lower inotropic state, the failing heart is able to pump much less blood at the normal filling pressure (Fig. 12.3), more blood remains in the ventricles at the end of systole. The normal venous return is added to it and Frank-Starling compensation is utilized to increase filling pressure: the heart may be able to achieve the required stroke volume, but at a filling pressure which produces congestive symptoms (venous engorgement, edema, enlargement of liver, pulmonary congestion → dyspnoea, renal congestion → oliguria).

Digoxin-induced enhancement of contractility increases ventricular ejection and shifts the curve relating stroke output to filling pressure towards normal, so that adequate output may be obtained at a filling pressure that does not produce congestive symptoms. Improved tissue perfusion results in withdrawal of sympathetic overactivity → heart rate and central venous pressure (CVP)

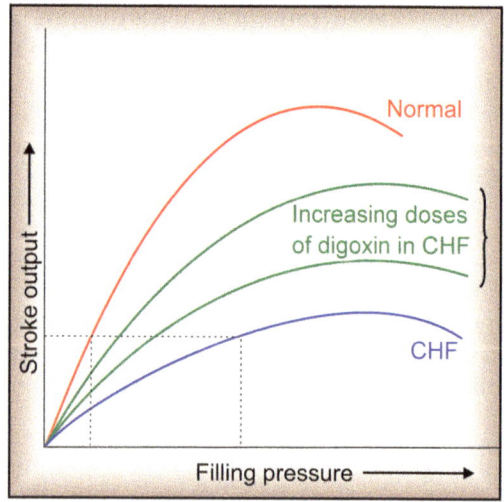

Fig. 12.3: Relationship between filling pressure and cardiac output in normal and failing heart. Digitalis tends to shift the curve towards normal

are lowered towards normal. Compensatory mechanisms retaining Na^+ and water are inactivated → diuresis occurs → edema is cleared. Liver regresses, pulmonary congestion is reduced → dyspnoea abates, cyanosis disappears. Low output symptoms like decreased capacity for muscular work are mitigated.

However, the two major limitations in the use of digoxin are low margin of safety and inability to reverse/retard the processes which cause the heart to fail. Digoxin does not afford any prognostic benefit or improve life expectancy.

2. Cardiac arrhythmias

Atrial fibrillation (AF), atrial flutter (AFl) Digoxin can be used for controlling ventricular rate in AF and AFl, but does not revert to sinus rhythm. A β blocker or verapamil or diltiazem are more commonly used for this purpose.

Digoxin reduces ventricular rate in AF and AFl by decreasing the number of impulses that are able to pass down the A-V node and bundle of His.

Paroxysmal supraventricular tachycardia (PSVT) The atrial rate in PSVT is 150–200/min with 1 : 1 A-V conduction. It is mostly due to reentry of impulses involving the SA or A-V node. Digoxin injected i.v. may terminate the arrhythmia by increasing vagal tone, but verapamil or adenosine or esmolol are more effective, less toxic and act faster. Digoxin is now reserved for preventing recurrences in selected cases.

TREATMENT OF CONGESTIVE HEART FAILURE

There are two distinct goals of drug therapy of congestive heart failure (CHF):
(a) Relief of congestive/low output symptoms and restoration of cardiac performance. This can be achieved by:
  Inotropic drugs—Digoxin, dobutamine/dopamine, inamrinone/milrinone
  Diuretics—Furosemide, metolazone, thiazides
  RAS inhibitors—ACE inhibitors, ARBs
  Vasodilators—Hydralazine, nitrate
  β blocker—Metoprolol, bisoprolol, carvedilol, nebivolol.
(b) Arrest/reversal of disease progression and prolongation of survival. This is possible with;
  ACE inhibitors/ARBs
  β blockers
  Aldosterone antagonist—Spironolactone, eplerenone.

Important nonpharmacological measures are rest and salt restriction. The pathophysiological mechanisms which perpetuate heart failure and contribute to disease progression, along with the sites of action of different categories of drugs are depicted in Fig. 12.4.

Diuretics

Almost all cases of symptomatic CHF are treated with a diuretic. High ceiling diuretics (furosemide, bumetanide) are the diuretics of choice for mobilizing edema fluid. Diuretics:
(a) Decrease preload and improve ventricular efficiency by reducing circulating volume.
(b) Remove peripheral edema and pulmonary congestion.

However, diuretics do not influence the disease process in CHF, though they may dramatically improve symptoms. Despite decades of experience, no prognostic benefit has been demonstrated for diuretics.

Renin-angiotensin system (RAS) inhibitors

Since RAS activation is pivotal to development of symptoms as well as disease progression in CHF, the ACE inhibitors and ARBs are the sheet anchor of drug therapy in CHF. They relieve symptoms by causing vasodilatation and afford disease modifying benefit in CHF by retarding/preventing ventricular

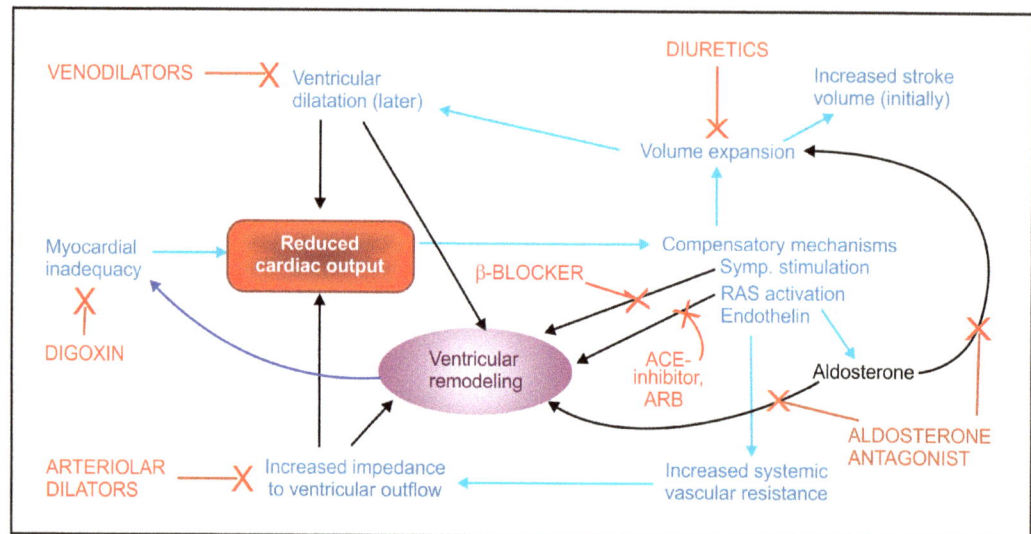

Fig. 12.4: The vicious cycle in heart failure: compensatory mechanisms evoked in response to reduced cardiac output themselves perpetuate failure and contribute to remodeling responsible for disease progression. The parameter which is improved by different therapeutic measures is indicated
ACE—Angiotensin converting enzyme; ARB—Angiotensin receptor blocker; RAS—Renin-angiotensin system

hypertrophy, myocardial cell apoptosis, fibrosis and remodeling. They are beneficial in all grades of CHF, *i.e.* asymptomatic systolic dysfunction through mild to severe symptomatic CHF.

Vasodilators

(i) *Nitrates* GTN and other nitrates are primarily venodilators, cause pooling of blood in systemic capacitance vessels and reduce preload on the failing heart. Controlled i.v. infusion of GTN rapidly relieves dyspnoea and other symptoms of acute left ventricular failure (LVF), particularly that attending MI. However, nitrates have no utility in the routine treatment of CHF.
(ii) *Hydralazine* It mainly dilates arterioles (resistance vessels) and reduces aortic impedance or afterload on heart, so that even weaker ventricular contractions are able to pump more blood. Though, it can afford short term symptom relief in low output failure, its utility in long term treatment of CHF is limited by its side effects causing tachycardia, fluid retention and worsening of myocardial ischaemia.
(iii) *Sodium nitroprusside* Administered by titrated i.v. infusion, sod. nitroprusside dilates both arterioles (resistance vessels) and veins (capacitance vessels). The action is very fast and short lasting. Employed in combination with a high ceiling diuretic and an i.v. inotropic drug it can help tide over crisis in very severe cases of CHF.

$β_1$-Adrenergic blockers

Though the early haemodynamic action of β blockers is to depress cardiac contractility and reduce ejection fraction, these parameters gradually improve over weeks when certain $β_1$ blockers, *Viz.* metoprolol, bisoprolol, nebivolol or β + $α_1$ blocker carvedilol are given to selected CHF patients. After a couple of months, ejection fraction is generally higher than baseline, and slow upward titration of dose further improves cardiac performance. The haemodynamic benefit is maintained over long term and hospitalization/mortality due to worsening cardiac failure, as well as all cause mortality is reduced. The benefits appear to be due to antagonism of ventricular wall stress enhancing, apoptosis promoting and pathological remodeling effects of excess sympathetic activity that occurs reflexly in CHF, as well as due to prevention of sinister arrhythmias. Incidence of sudden cardiac death, as well as that due to worsening heart failure is decreased.

Now, β blockers are part of standard therapy of most mild-to-moderate cases of CHF after compensation has been restored. However, β blocker therapy in CHF requires caution, proper patient selection and observance of several guidelines.

Aldosterone antagonist

Plasma aldosterone level has been found to be raised in CHF patients. Aldosterone, in addition to its well-known Na^+ and water retaining action, is an important contributor to progression of CHF by direct and indirect effects:
(a) Expansion of e.c.f. volume → increased cardiac preload.
(b) Fibrotic change in myocardium → worsening systolic dysfunction and pathological remodeling.
(c) Hypokalemia and hypomagnesemia → increased risk of ventricular arrhythmias and sudden cardiac death.

The aldosterone antagonists spironolactone and eplerenone are weak diuretics but can benefit CHF by antagonising the above effects of aldosterone. Because, eplerenone, is free of hormonal side effects, it is indicated as add-on therapy to ACE inhibitors ± other drugs in moderate-to-severe CHF. It can retard disease progression, reduce episodes of decompensation and death due to heart failure as well as sudden cardiac deaths over and above the protection afforded by ACE inhibitors/ARBs ± β blockers.

Sympathomimetic inotropic drugs

Drugs with β adrenergic and dopaminergic D_1 agonistic actions have positive inotropic and vasodilator properties which may be utilized to combat emergency pump failure. Dobutamine, a relatively selective $β_1$ agonist with prominent inotropic action, is the preferred drug for i.v. infusion in acute heart failure accompanying myocardial infarction (MI), cardiac surgery as well as to tide over crisis in advanced CHF. Dopamine has been used in cardiogenic shock due to MI and other causes. These drugs afford additional haemodynamic support over and above vasodilators, digoxin and diuretics, but benefits are short lasting. They have no role in the long-term management of CHF.

Phosphodiesterase III inhibitors

Amrinone (Inamrinone), Milrinone These are bipyridine derivatives, and selective phosphodiesterase III (PDE III) inhibitors. This isoenzyme is specific for intracellular degradation of cAMP in heart, blood vessels and bronchial smooth muscles. They increase myocardial cAMP and transmembrane influx of Ca^{2+}.

The two most important actions of inamrinone and milrinone are *positive inotropy* and direct *vasodilatation*. As such, they have been called 'inodilators'.

They are indicated only for short-term i.v. use in severe and refractory CHF, as additional drug to conventional therapy.

Levosimendan It is a new Ca^{2+} sensitizing inodilator which also inhibits PDE III. Infused i.v., it can be used for short-term treatment of acutely decompensated severe chronic heart failure.

ANTIARRHYTHMIC DRUGS

These are drugs used to prevent or treat irregularities of cardiac rhythm.

Cardiac arrhythmias arise due to abnormal impulse generation or abnormal impulse conduction or both. Ischaemia, electrolyte and pH imbalance, stretching, injury, neurogenic and drug influences, including antiarrhythmic drugs themselves, can cause arrhythmia by altering electrophysiological properties of cardiac fibres. The types of electrophysiological changes resulting in arrhythmias are:
1. Enhanced or ectopic pacemaker activity.
2. 'Early after-depolarizations' (associated with long Q-T interval due to slow repolarization) and 'delayed after-depolarizations' (due to Ca^{2+} overload) (Fig. 12.5).
3. Re-entry due to unidirectional conduction block of the impulse and its recirculation around an obstacle (infarcted or refractory myocardium) causing repetitive activation of the adjacent fibres (Fig. 12.6).
4. Fractionation of the impulse due to inhomogeneous refractory periods (RP) of different fibres; various fibres get activated asynchronously.
5. Slowing of impulse conduction through the A-V node producing partial to complete heart block.

The main categories of cardiac arrhythmias and their characteristics are:
1. *Extrasystoles (ES)* are premature beats due to abnormal automaticity or after-depolarization arising from an ectopic focus in the atrium (atrial ES), A-V node (nodal ES) or ventricle (ventricular ES).
2. *Paroxysmal supraventricular tachycardia (PSVT)* is sudden onset episodes of atrial tachycardia (rate 150–200/min) with 1:1 atrio-ventricular conduction:

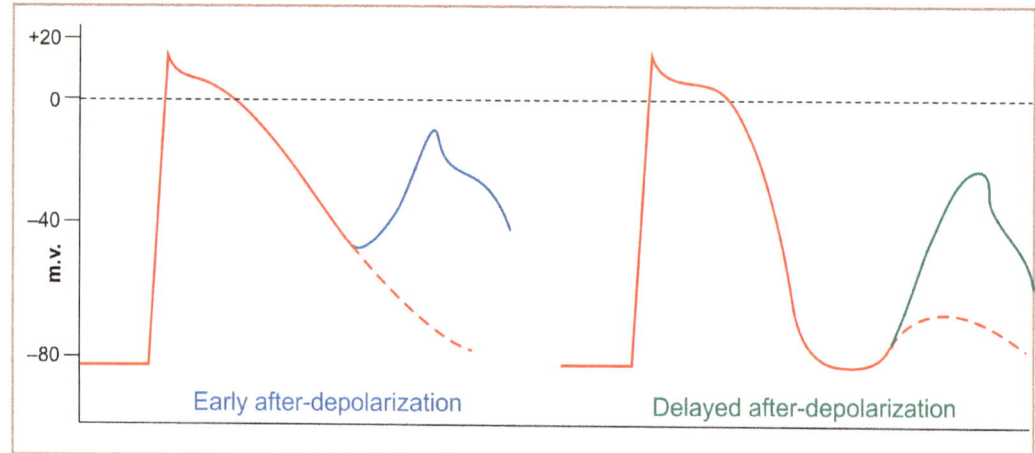

Fig. 12.5: Action potential in a nonautomatic ventricular fibre (in red) followed by early or delayed after-depolarizations

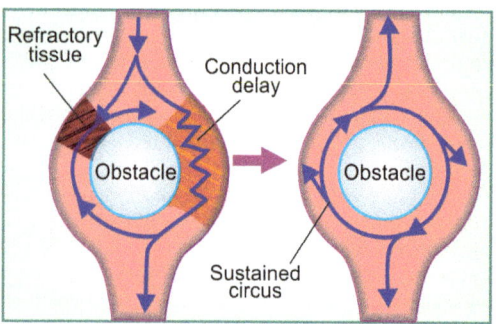

Fig. 12.6: Diagrammatic representation of circus movement re-entry in atrium

mostly due to circus movement type of re-entry involving the A-V node or SA node.

3. *Atrial flutter (AFl)* Atria beat at a rate of 220–350/min and there is a physiological 2:1 to 4:1 or higher, A-V block (because A-V node cannot transmit impulses faster than 200/min).
4. *Atrial fibrillation (AF)* Atrial fibres are activated asynchronously at a rate of 350–550/min (due to electrophysiological inhomogeneity of atrial fibres), associated with grossly irregular and often fast (100–160/min) ventricular response. Atria remain dilated and quiver like a bag of worms.
5. *Ventricular tachycardia* is a run of 4 or more consecutive ventricular extrasystoles.
6. *Ventricular fibrillation (VF)* is grossly irregular, rapid and fractionated activation of ventricles resulting in incoordinated contraction of its fibres with loss of pumping function. Ventricular fibrillation is fatal unless reverted within 2–5 min. It is the most common cause of sudden cardiac death.
7. *Atrio-ventricular (A-V) block* is due to depression of impulse conduction through the A-V node and bundle of His.
   First degree A-V block: Slowed conduction resulting in prolonged P-R interval.
   Second degree A-V block: Some supraventricular impulses are not conducted : drop beats.
   Third degree A-V block: No supraventricular complexes are conducted; ventricle generates its own impulse; also called complete heart block.

CLASSIFICATION

Antiarrhythmic drugs act by blocking myocardial Na^+, K^+ or Ca^{2+} channels. Some have additional or even primary autonomic effects. Classification of antiarrhythmic drugs has been difficult. Vaughan Williams and Singh (1969) proposed a 4 class system which takes into account the primary action of a drug.

CLASS I

The primary action of drugs in this class is to limit the conductance of Na^+ (and K^+) across cell membrane—a local anaesthetic action. These drugs also reduce rate of phase-4 depolarization responsible for impulse generation in automatic cells.

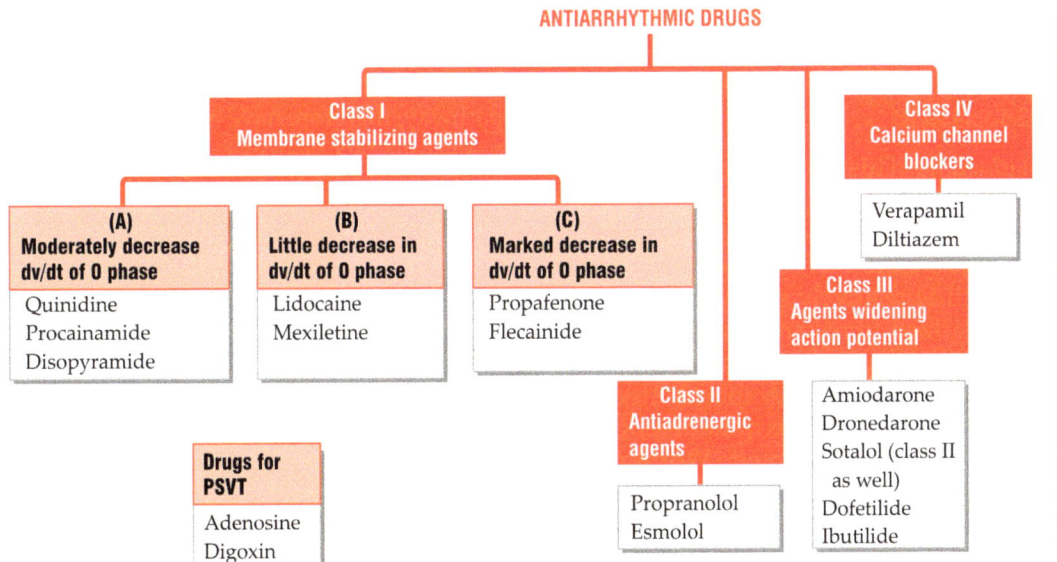

PSVT—Paroxysmal supraventricular tachycardia

Subclass IA

The subclass IA containing the oldest antiarrhythmic drugs *quinidine* and *procainamide* are open state Na⁺ channel blockers with little effect on resting channels. They also moderately delay channel recovery (1–10 s), suppress A–V conduction and prolong refractoriness. These actions serve to extinguish ectopic pacemakers that are often responsible for triggered arrhythmias and abolish re-entry by converting unidirectional block into bidirectional block.

Quinidine It is the oldest antiarrhythmic drug; has antivagal action which augments prolongation of atrial RP and minimises RP disparity of atrial fibres. Quinidine also decreases myocardial contractility: may precipitate failure in damaged hearts. It can cause fall in BP, decrease contractility of skeletal muscles, augment uterine contractions, induce vomiting and diarrhoea and produce neurological effects like ringing in ears, vertigo, deafness, visual disturbances and mental changes. Like its levoisomer quinine, it has antimalarial action.

Though quinidine is effective in many atrial and ventricular arrhythmias, it is not used to terminate them because of risk of adverse effects, including that of sudden cardiac arrest or VF. It is occasionally used to maintain sinus rhythm after termination of AF or AFl.

Procainamide This orally active amide derivative of the local anaesthetic procaine has cardiac electrophysiological actions similar to quinidine, but has minimal antivagal action, causes less depression of contractility, A-V conduction and BP. Prolonged use of procainamide can cause systemic lupus erythematosus. Cardiac toxicity is similar to quinidine; clinical use therefore is highly restricted.

Disopyramide It is a quinidine-like class IA drug which has prominent cardiac depressant and anticholinergic actions, but no α adrenergic blocking property. However, disopyramide produces less g.i. side effects and is better tolerated. It is a second line drug for preventing recurrences of ventricular arrhythmia and may be a better tolerated maintenance drug after cardioversion of AF or AFl.

Subclass IB

Lidocaine This most widely used local anaesthetic is the prototype member of subclass IB. It is a blocker of inactivated Na$^+$ channels more than that of open state. As such, it is relatively selective for partially depolarized fibres and those with longer action potential duration (APD), whose Na$^+$ channels remain inactivated for a longer period. Unlike quinidine, channel recovery is not delayed. While normal ventricular and conducting tissues are minimally affected, depolarized/damaged fibres are particularly depressed. The most prominent action of lidocaine is suppression of automaticity in ventricular ectopic foci and after-depolarizations. It is ineffective in atrial arrhythmias. Lidocaine does not depress A-V conduction and ventricular contractility or prolong refractoriness.

Lidocaine is inactive orally due to high first pass metabolism. Action of an i.v. bolus dose lasts only for 10–20 minutes because of rapid distribution, while elimination t½ is 1.5–2 hours due to metabolism. Lidocaine is used only in ventricular tachyarrhythmias by repeated i.v. injections or continuous i.v. infusion. Because of rapidly developing and titratable action, it is a good drug in the emergency setting, e.g. arrhythmias following MI or during cardiac surgery.

Mexiletine is an orally active congener of lidocaine with similar cardiac electrophysiological actions. Parenterally, it has been used as an alternative to lidocaine for postinfarction ventricular arrhythmias.

Subclass IC

The subclass IC drugs like *propafenone* and *flecainide* are the most potent Na$^+$ channel blockers with more prominent action on the open state and the longest channel recovery time (>10 s). They markedly delay conduction in A-V node as well as accessory pathway; therefore have been used in WPW re-entrant tachycardias. Propafenone has additional β adrenergic blocking property—can precipitate CHF and bronchospasm. Though class IC drugs are effective in many refractory arrhythmias, they also have high proarrhythmic potential. Chronic therapy in postinfarct patients has paradoxically increased the incidence of sudden cardiac death. Propaphenone is used mainly for maintaining sinus rhythm in patients of AF, and for prophylaxis of PSVT.

CLASS II

The primary action of class II drugs is to suppress adrenergically mediated ectopic activity and delayed after-depolarizations. Though some β blockers, e.g. *propranolol* (the most commonly used β blocker in arrhythmias) have quinidine like direct membrane stabilizing action at high doses, antiarrhythmic action is exerted clinically primarily by cardiac adrenergic blockade. The other important action is to prolong RP of A-V node. This impedes A-V conduction. As such, re-entrant arrhythmias that involve SA or A-V node (many PSVT) may be abolished.

The β blockers are very useful in treating inappropriate *sinus tachycardia, atrial and nodal extrasystoles provoked by emotion, exercise or stress (e.g. of dental procedure)*. Propranolol rarely abolishes AF or AFl, but can be used to control ventricular rate. β blockers are highly effective in sympathetically mediated arrhythmias occurring in pheochromocytoma or during anaesthesia with halothane. Digoxin-induced and thyrotoxic tachyarrhythmias usually respond. However, efficacy in chronic ventricular arrhythmias is low. Prophylactic treatment with β blockers reduces mortality in post-MI patients.

Esmolol is a quick and short-acting β₁ blocker that is used i.v. for emergency control of ventricular rate in AF/AFl. It can also terminate supraventricular tachycardia and arrhythmias associated with anaesthesia.

CLASS III

The characteristic action of class III antiarrhythmics is prolongation of repolarization: AP is widened which increases RP. Myocardial fibres remain refractory even after repolarization: re-entrant arrhythmias are terminated. Prolongation of APD is attributable to blockade of delayed rectifier K⁺ channels, which open during repolarization.

The most important member of this class *amiodarone* is an unusual iodine containing compound which in addition blocks inactivated Na⁺ channels and has noncompetitive β adrenergic blocking property. Amiodarone is highly lipophilic, extensively bound in tissues and exceptionally long acting (t½ 3–8 weeks). Given orally, its full action takes weeks to develop, but i.v. loading doses can rapidly terminate life-threatening arrhythmias. Amiodarone is effective in a wide range of ventricular and supraventricular arrhythmias, particularly resistant VT and recurrent VF. Despite prolongation of APD, the proarrhythmic potential of amiodarone is low. This, together with its broad spectrum efficacy and long duration of action makes it a commonly used antiarrhythmic. However, close supervision is needed because long term use carries the risk of hypothyroidism, photosensitization, peripheral neuropathy and pulmonary fibrosis.

Dronedarone is an orally active, less toxic as well as less effective congener of amiodarone which is primarily used to maintain sinus rhythm in selected patients of AF and for control of ventricular rate during AF.

Sotalol is a β blocker with prominent class III property of prolonging repolarization by blocking cardiac inward rectifier K⁺channels. It delays A-V conduction and prolongs nodal RP. Sotalol is effective in some cases of VT as well as for maintaining sinus rhythm in AF and AFl.

Dofetilide is a pure class III antiarrhythmic which has no other action than blocking delayed rectifier K⁺ channels. Its primary indication is to maintain sinus rhythm after conversion of AF and AFl.

Ibutilide Another similar drug, mainly used i.v. to terminate AF or AFl.

CLASS IV

The Ca²⁺ channel blockers *verapamil* and *diltiazem* (but not DHPs) exert antiarrhythmic action by depressing Ca²⁺ mediated depolarization. These drugs slow SA node pacemaker, depress A-V conduction and suppress re-entry through A-V node as well as in partially depolarized (ischaemic) tissue. Injected i.v., verapamil and diltiazem are second line drugs to adenosine for termination of PSVT. Given orally, they are suitable for prevention of its recurrences. The other use of verapamil is to control ventricular rate in AF and AFl. Efficacy of calcium channel blockers in ventricular arrhythmias is poor.

Adenosine Adenosine is an ultrashort acting endogenous purine signal molecule. Administered by rapid i.v. injection (over 1–3 sec) either as the free base or as ATP, it terminates within 30 seconds more than 90% episodes of PSVT involving the A-V node. Adenosine activates ACh sensitive K⁺ channels and causes membrane hyperpolarization through interaction with A1 type of adenosine receptors on SA node (resulting in pacemaker depression → bradycardia), A-V node (causing prolongation of RP → slowing of conduction) and atrium (leading to shortening of AP, reduced excitability). It indirectly reduces Ca²⁺ current in A-V node. Depression of the re-entrant circuit through A-V node is responsible for termination of PSVT.

Adenosine has a very short t½ in blood (~10 sec) due to uptake into RBCs and endothelial cells where it is converted to 5-AMP and inosine. Almost complete elimination occurs in a single passage through coronary circulation.

Adverse effects of adenosine are transient dyspnoea, chest pain, fall in BP and flushing in 30–60% patients; ventricular standstill for a few seconds or VF occurs in some patients. Bronchospasm may be precipitated in asthmatics. Adenosine has brief action, and has to be rapidly injected in a large vein. Therefore, it is not suitable for recurrent cases.

Other drugs that can be used i.v. to terminate PSVT are verapamil, diltiazem, esmolol and digoxin.

Drugs for A-V block

Atropine: When A-V block is due to vagal overactivity, e.g. digoxin toxicity and some cases of MI; it can be improved by atropine 0.6–1.2 mg i.m. Atropine abbreviates A-V node RP and increases conduction velocity in bundle of His.

Sympathomimetics (Adr, isoprenaline): These drugs may overcome partial heart block by facilitating A-V conduction and shortening RP of conducting tissues.

They may also be used in complete heart block to maintain a sufficient idioventricular rate (by increasing automaticity of ventricular pacemakers) till external pacemaker can be implanted.

Relevance to dentistry

Patients with history of recurrent cardiac arrhythmias, ischaemic heart disease or those on chronic digoxin therapy are at greater risk of precipitation of arrhythmias during dental procedure due to stress of the procedure and/or use of Adr containing local anaesthetic. A cardiologist should be consulted beforehand and the dentist should be prepared to provide first-line treatment of emergency arrhythmias such as PSVT, VT, VF, complete heart block, cardiac arrest, etc.

13 CHAPTER

Diuretics

RELEVANT PHYSIOLOGY OF URINE FORMATION

Urine formation starts from glomerular filtration (g.f.) in a prodigal way. Normally, about 180 L of fluid is filtered every day: all soluble constituents of blood minus the plasma proteins (along with substances bound to them) and lipids, are filtered at the glomerulus. More than 99% of the glomerular filtrate is reabsorbed in the tubules; about 1.5 L urine is produced in 24 hours. The diuretics act primarily by inhibiting tubular reabsorption: just 1% decrease in tubular reabsorption would more than double urine output.

The mechanisms that carryout ion movement across tubular cells are complex and involve a variety of energy dependent transmembrane pumps as well as channels in between the loose fitting cells of the proximal tubule (PT). All the Na^+ that enters tubular cells through the luminal membrane is pumped out of it into the renal interstitium at the basolateral membrane by $Na^+K^+ATPase$ energised Na^+-K^+ antiporter (*see* Figs 13.3 and 13.4). Because there is a large intracellular to extracellular gradient for K^+, it diffuses out through K^+ channels to be recirculated by the Na^+-K^+ antiporter. For simplification, tubular reabsorption can be divided into four sites (Fig. 13.1).

Site I: Proximal tubule Four mechanisms of Na^+ transport have been defined in this segment.

(a) Direct entry of Na^+ along a favourable electrochemical gradient. This is electrogenic.

(b) Transport of Na^+ and K^+ coupled to active reabsorption of glucose, amino acids, other organic anions and PO_4^{3-} through specific symporters.

(c) Exchange with H^+: The PT cells secrete H^+ with the help of cytosolic carbonic anhydrase (CAse-II) and a Na^+–H^+ antiporter (Fig. 13.2) located in the luminal membrane. This H^+ ion combines with luminal HCO_3^-. There is net reabsorption of HCO_3^- due to the activity of brush border CAse IV and a Na^+- HCO_3^- symporter at the basolateral membrane.

(d) The disproportionately large HCO_3^-, acetate, PO_4^{3-}, amino acid and other anion reabsorption create passive driving forces for Cl^- through the paracellular pathway. This also takes Na^+ and water along. Reabsorption in PT is isotonic because of high water permeability of this segment.

Major part of filtered K^+ is reabsorbed in the PT.

Site II: Thick ascending limb of loop of Henle
(TAL) The TAL is relatively impermeable to water but absorbs salt actively and thus dilutes the tubular fluid.

In the *medullary portion* a distinct luminal membrane carrier transports ions in the stoichiometric ratio of Na^+-K^+-$2Cl^-$ (Fig. 13.3). The Na^+ that enters the cell is pumped to e.c.f. by Na^+ $K^+ATPase$ at the basolateral membrane, while the excess intracellular K^+ back diffuses through K^+ channels. This

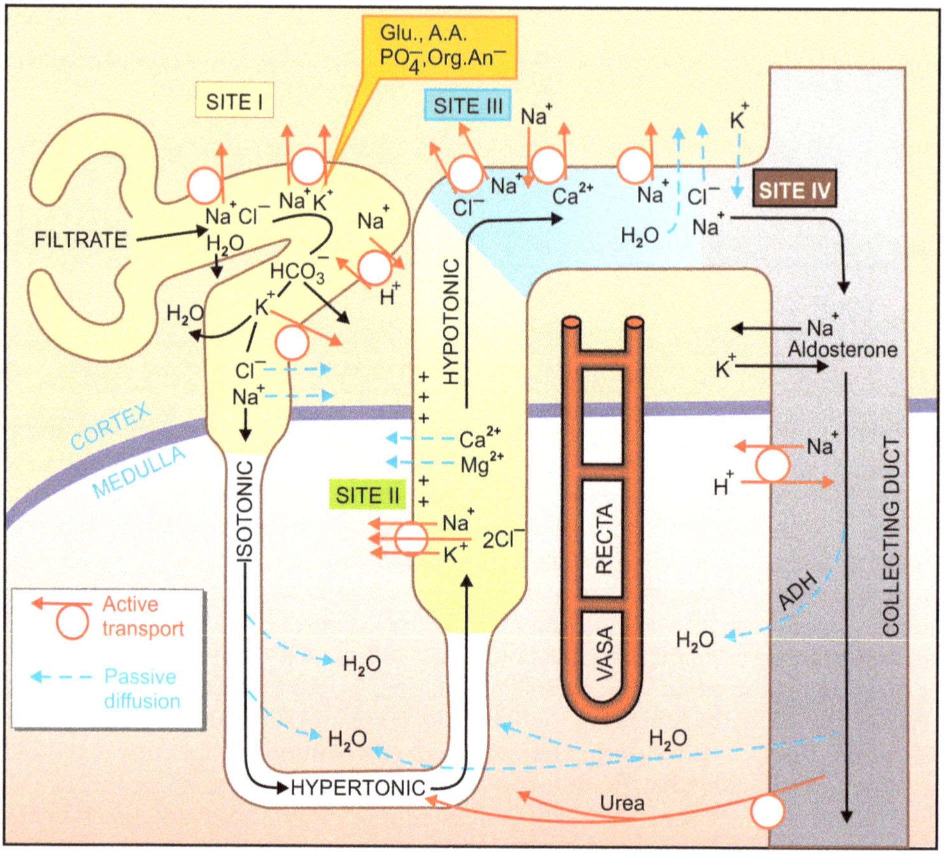

Fig. 13.1: Diagrammatic representation of nephron showing the four sites of solute reabsorption The thick ascending limb of loop of Henle (TAL) is impermeable to water; Glu.—Glucose; A.A.—Amino acid; Org. An.—Organic anions.

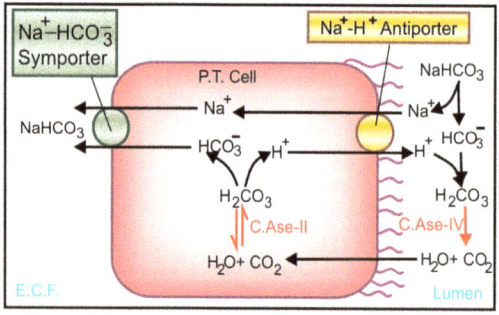

Fig. 13.2: The carbonic anhydrase (C.Ase) mediated bicarbonate absorption in proximal tubule (PT)

creates a lumen positive transepithelial potential which drives reabsorption of Ca^{2+} and Mg^{2+} (Fig. 13.3). A Na^+-Cl^- symporter moves Cl^- down its electrochemical gradient into e.c.f. and carries Na^+ along. As the tubular fluid traverses TAL, it progressively becomes hypotonic. Accumulation of NaCl in the medullary interstitium without accompanying water makes it hypertonic: a corticomedullary osmotic gradient is set up which is essential for production of both concentrated as well as dilute urine.

Site III: Cortical diluting segment of loop of Henle This segment, also impermeable to water, continues to absorb salt, but here it is through a Na^+-Cl^- symporter (Fig. 13.4). Tubular fluid gets further diluted.

Site IV: Distal tubule (DT) and collecting duct (CD) The principal cells in the late DT and CD do not express any Na^+ or K^+

transporter in their apical membranes. Rather, Na⁺ enters these cells through a specific amiloride sensitive *renal epithelial Na⁺ channel* without accompanying Cl⁻ or any other anion, thus creating a 10–15 mV lumen negative electrical potential. This drives paracellular Cl⁻ diffusion into the interstitium and K⁺ efflux. At this site, Na⁺ reabsorption is controlled by aldosterone (Fig. 13.5). This provides fine tuning to electrolyte excretion according to body needs.

Any diuretic acting proximal to the aldosterone sensitive ion exchange site causes an increased delivery of Na⁺ to the distal nephron—more exchange with K⁺ takes place. Thus, K⁺ is reabsorbed in PT and TAL, but secreted into the lumen of DT and CD. The net K⁺ loss is regulated by variations in the secretory process and depends on:

- The Na⁺ load delivered to distal segment
- Presence or absence of aldosterone
- Availability of H⁺
- Intracellular K⁺ stores.

The characteristic feature of cells lining CD is their responsiveness to antidiuretic hormone (ADH). If ADH is absent, the hypotonic fluid entering CD is passed as such → dilute urine is produced during water loading. If ADH levels are high, CD cells become fully permeable to water → equilibrate with hyperosmotic medulla → concentrated urine is passed, as occurs during water deprivation or hypertonic saline infusion.

ADH also promotes reabsorption of urea by inserting more urea transporter (UT_1 or VRUT) into the luminal membrane of CD cells. During water deprivation more urea is transported to the medullary interstitium, reinforcing the hypertonicity.

Relation to diuretic action

The relative magnitudes of Na⁺ reabsorption at different tubular sites are:

PT 65–70%;   TAL 20–25%;
DT 8–9%;   CD 2–3%.

The maximal natriuretic response to a diuretic can give a clue to its site of action. It may appear that diuretics acting on PT should be the most efficacious. However, these agents are either too weak or cause distortion of acid-base balance (as in the case of CAse inhibitors). Moreover, their effect is largely obscured by compensatory increase in reabsorption further down the nephron, because the reserve reabsorptive capacity of diluting segments is considerable and can overshadow more proximal actions.

A diuretic having primary action on TAL (furosemide) can produce substantial natriuresis because of limited capacity for salt absorption in DT and CD. This also explains why agents acting on DT and CD (K⁺ sparing diuretics) evoke only mild saluretic effect. Diuretics acting on cortical diluting segment (thiazides) are intermediate between these two.

DIURETICS

These are drugs which cause a net loss of Na⁺ and water in urine.

HIGH CEILING (LOOP) DIURETICS
(inhibitors of Na⁺-K⁺-2Cl⁻ Cotransport)

Furosemide (Frusemide) Prototype drug

The introduction of this orally and rapidly acting highly efficacious diuretic was a breakthrough. Its maximal natriuretic effect is much greater than diuretics of other classes. The diuretic response goes on increasing with increasing dose: up to 10 L of urine may be produced in a day. It is active even in patients with relatively severe renal failure. The onset of action is prompt (i.v. 2–5 min, i.m. 10–20 min, oral 20–40 min) and duration short (3–6 hours).

Chapter 13: Diuretics

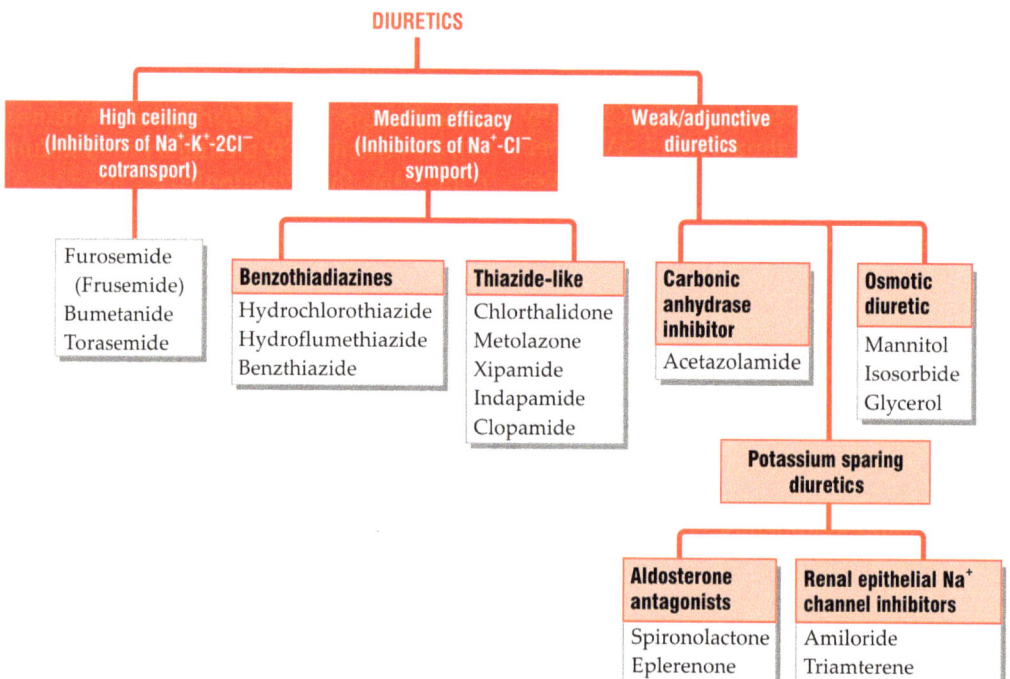

The major site of action is the TAL (site II) where furosemide inhibits Na^+-K^+-$2Cl^-$ cotransport (Fig. 13.3). It abolishes the corticomedullary osmotic gradient and blocks positive as well as negative free water clearance. K^+ excretion is increased, due to high Na^+ load reaching the DT.

Furosemide has weak CAse inhibitory action, therefore it increases HCO_3^- excretion as well. Its action is independent of acid-base balance of the body and it causes little distortion of the same.

In addition to its prominent tubular action, furosemide causes acute changes in renal and systemic haemodynamics. After 5 min of i.v. injection, renal blood flow is transiently increased, the result of which is decreased PT reabsorption. The intrarenal haemodynamic changes are brought about by enhanced local PG synthesis.

Intravenous furosemide causes prompt increase in systemic venous capacitance and decreases left ventricular filling pressure, even before the saluretic response is apparent. This is responsible for the quick relief it affords in LVF and pulmonary edema. This action may also be PG mediated.

Furosemide increases Ca^{2+} excretion (contrast thiazides which reduce it) as well as Mg^{2+} excretion. It tends to raise blood uric acid level by decreasing its renal excretion. A small rise in blood sugar level may be noted after regular use of furosemide, but this is less marked compared to that with thiazides.

Molecular mechanism of action: A glycoprotein with 12 membrane spanning domains has been found to function as the Na^+-K^+-$2Cl^-$ cotransporter in many epithelia including TAL. Furosemide attaches to the Cl^- binding site of this protein to inhibit its transport function.

Pharmacokinetics Furosemide is rapidly absorbed orally but bioavailability is about 60%. It is highly bound to plasma proteins,

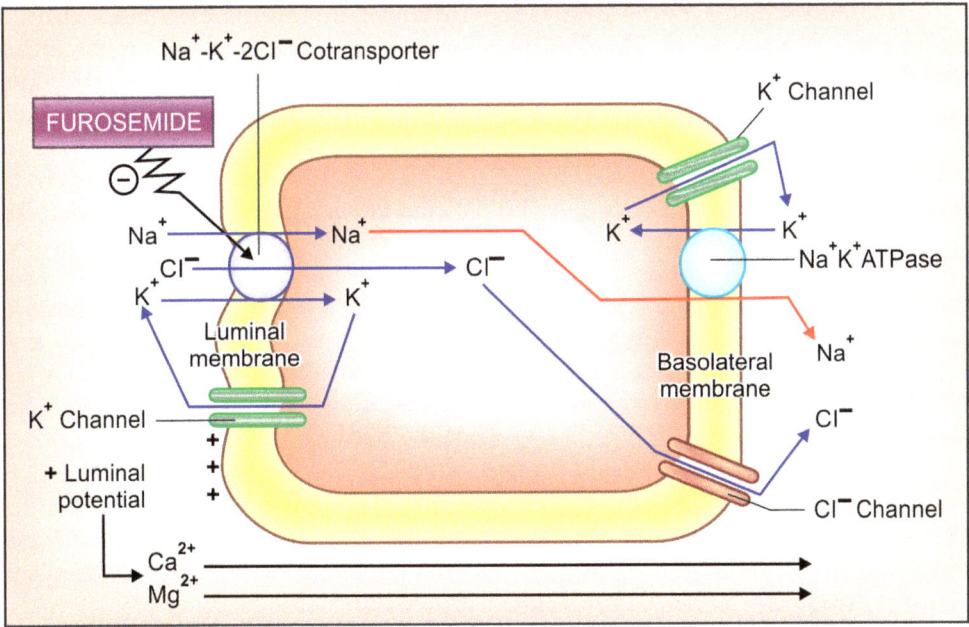

Fig. 13.3: Mechanism of salt reabsorption in the thick ascending limb of loop of Henle (TAL), and site of action of furosemide on the Na+-K+-2Cl− cotransporter

partly conjugated with glucuronic acid and excreted unchanged by glomerular filtration as well as tubular secretion. Plasma t½ is 1–2 hours.

Bumetanide It is similar to furosemide in all respects, but is 40 times more potent. Bumetanide induces very rapid diuresis and is highly effective in pulmonary edema. Hyperuricaemia, K+ loss, glucose intolerance and ototoxicity are claimed to be less marked than with furosemide, but, it may rarely cause myopathy.

Torasemide This high ceiling diuretic is dose to dose 3 times more potent than furosemide and longer acting.

Use of high ceiling diuretics

1. *Edema* Diuretics are used irrespective of etiology of edema—cardiac, hepatic or renal. The high ceiling diuretics are preferred initially in CHF for rapid mobilization of edema fluid. They are the diuretic of choice for nephrotic and other forms of resistant edema.

2. *Acute pulmonary edema (acute LVF, following MI)* Intravenous administration of furosemide produces prompt relief. This is due to selective vasodilator action that precedes the saluretic action.

3. *Cerebral edema* Though osmotic diuretics are preferred, furosemide may be employed by i.m. route.

4. *Hypertension* High ceiling diuretics are indicated only in presence of renal insufficiency, heart failure and in resistant cases or hypertensive emergencies; otherwise thiazides are preferred.

THIAZIDE AND RELATED DIURETICS
(Inhibitors of Na+-Cl− Symport)

These are medium efficacy diuretics with primary site of action in the cortical diluting segment or the early DT (Site III). Here they inhibit Na+–Cl− symport at the luminal membrane. Thiazides do not affect the corticomedullary osmotic gradient, indicating lack of action at the TAL. Positive free water clearance is reduced because tubular fluid is not maximally diluted (very dilute urine cannot be passed in the absence of ADH), but negative free water clearance (concentrated urine in the presence of ADH) is not affected.

Like the Na^+-K^+-$2Cl^-$ cotransporter, the Na^+-Cl^- symporter is also a glycoprotein with 12 membrane spanning domains which binds thiazides but not furosemide or any other class of diuretics. The site of action of thiazide diuretics is shown in Fig. 13.4.

Some of the thiazides and related drugs have additional CAse inhibitory property which may confer a secondary proximal tubular action to these drugs.

Under thiazide action, increased amount of Na^+ is presented to the distal nephron, more of it exchanges with K^+. As a result, urinary K^+ excretion is increased in parallel to the natriuretic response. The different thiazide and related diuretics have nearly the same maximal efficacy as hydrochlorothiazide, though potency (reflected in daily dose) differs markedly. Nevertheless, they are only moderately efficacious diuretics, because nearly, 90% of the glomerular filtrate has already been reabsorbed before it reaches their site of action. Thiazides have a flat dose response curve; little additional diuresis occurs when the dose is increased beyond 100 mg of hydrochlorothiazide or equivalent. No significant alteration in acid-base balance of the body is produced.

Renal Ca^{2+} excretion is diminished while Mg^{2+} excretion is enhanced by direct tubular action of thiazides. They decrease urate excretion by the same mechanism as furosemide.

The *extrarenal actions* of thiazides consist of a slowly developing fall in BP in hypertensives and elevation of blood sugar in some patients due to decreased insulin release.

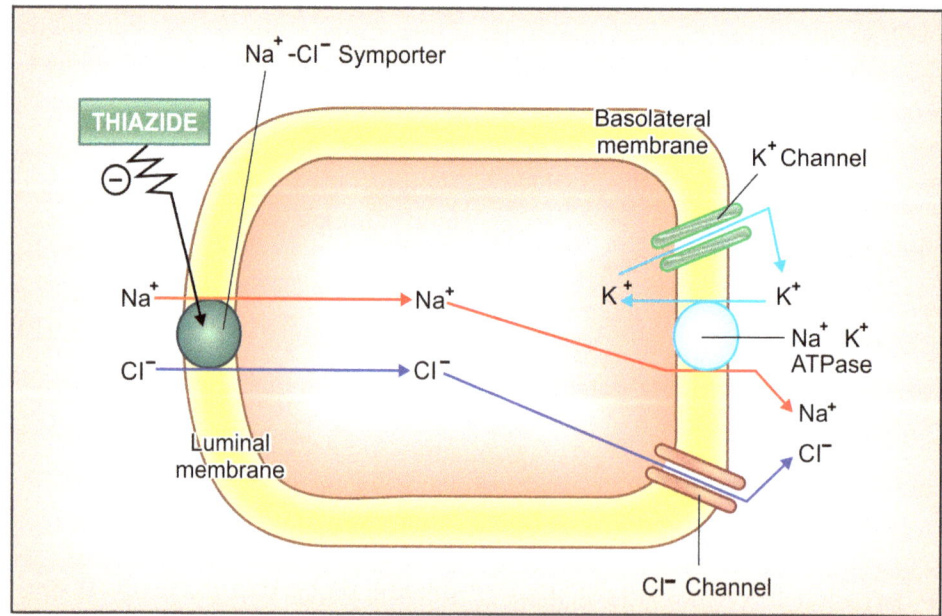

Fig. 13.4: Mechanism of salt reabsorption in early distal tubular cell and site of action of thiazide diuretics on Na^+Cl^- symporter

All thiazides and related drugs are well absorbed orally, and are administered only by this route. Their action starts within 1 hour, but the duration of action varies from 8–48 hours. Most of the agents undergo little hepatic metabolism and are largely excreted unchanged. They are filtered at the glomerulus as well as secreted in the PT by organic anion transport. Tubular reabsorption depends on lipid solubility: the more lipid soluble ones are highly reabsorbed—prolonging duration of action.

Uses

1. *Edema* Thiazides may be used for mild-to-moderate cases of edema. For mobilization of edema fluid more efficacious diuretics are employed initially, but thiazides are considered better for maintenance therapy. They are powerless in the presence of renal failure. Cirrhotics often develop refractoriness to thiazides due to development of secondary hyperaldosteronism.

2. *Hypertension* Thiazides are one of the first line drugs (*see* p. 191).

3. *Diabetes insipidus* Thiazides tend to reduce urine volume in this condition, but hypertonic urine cannot be passed.

Complications of high ceiling and thiazide-type diuretic therapy

Most of the adverse effects of these drugs are related to fluid and electrolyte changes caused by them. Usual side effects are weakness and tiredness. They are remarkably safe in low doses used over short periods.

1. *Hypokalaemia* This is the most significant problem. It is rare at low doses, but may be of grave consequence when brisk diuresis is induced or on prolonged therapy. The usual manifestations are weakness, fatigue, muscle cramps. Cardiac arrhythmias are the serious complications. It can be prevented and treated by:
(a) High dietary K^+ intake or
(b) Supplements of KCl (24–72 mEq/day) or
(c) Concurrent use of K^+ sparing diuretics.

2. *Acute saline depletion* Over enthusiastic use of diuretics, particularly high ceiling ones, may cause dehydration and fall in BP

3. *Dilutional hyponatremia* Can occur in CHF patients when vigorous diuresis is induced with high ceiling agents, rarely with thiazides.

4. *GIT and CNS disturbances* Nausea, vomiting, diarrhoea, headache, giddiness, weakness, paresthesias, impotence are the occasional complaints.

5. *Hearing loss* Occurs rarely, only with high ceiling diuretics.

6. *Allergic manifestations* Rashes, photosensitivity can occur, particularly in patients hypersensitive to sulfonamides.

7. Brisk diuresis induced in cirrhotics may precipitate mental disturbances and hepatic coma.

8. *Hyperuricaemia* Long-term use of thiazides in hypertension has caused rise in blood urate level, but is rare now due to use of lower doses.

9. *Hyperglycaemia and hyperlipidemia* Have occurred in the use of diuretics as antihypertensive. Use of lower doses now has minimized this complication.

10. *Magnesium depletion* It may develop after prolonged use of thiazides as well as loop diuretics.

Interactions

1. Thiazides and high ceiling diuretics potentiate all other antihypertensives.
2. Hypokalaemia induced by these diuretics:
   (a) Enhances digoxin toxicity.
   (b) Increases the risk of polymorphic ventricular tachycardia due to quinidine and other antiarrhythmics.

(c) Potentiates competitive neuromuscular blockers and reduces sulfonylurea action.
3. High ceiling diuretics and aminoglycoside antibiotics are both ototoxic; may produce additive toxicity.
4. Indomethacin and most NSAIDs diminish the action of high ceiling diuretics by inhibiting PG synthesis in the kidney. Antihypertensive action of thiazides and furosemide is also diminished by NSAIDs.
5. Probenecid competitively inhibits tubular secretion of furosemide and thiazides: decreases their action.
6. Serum lithium level rises when diuretic therapy is instituted. This is due to enhanced reabsorption of Li$^+$ in PT.

CARBONIC ANHYDRASE INHIBITORS
Acetazolamide

It is a sulfonamide derivative which noncompetitively but reversibly inhibits CAse (type II) in PT cells resulting in slowing of hydration of CO_2. This decreases availability of H$^+$ to exchange with luminal Na$^+$. Inhibition of brush border CAse (type IV) retards dehydration of H_2CO_3 in the tubular fluid so that less CO_2 diffuses back into the cells. The net effect is inhibition of HCO_3^- (and accompanying Na$^+$) reabsorption in PT producing mild alkaline diuresis.

Secretion of H$^+$ in DT and CD is also interfered. The distal Na$^+$ exchange takes place only with K$^+$ which is lost in excess. The urine produced under acetazolamide action is alkaline and rich in HCO_3^- which is matched by both Na$^+$ and K$^+$. Continued action of acetazolamide depletes body HCO_3^- and causes acidosis; less HCO_3^- (on which its diuretic action depends) is filtered at the glomerulus → self-limiting diuretic action. The extrarenal actions of acetazolamide are:
(i) Lowering of intraocular tension due to decreased formation of aqueous humour which is rich in HCO_3^-.
(ii) Raised level of CO_2 in brain and lowering of pH → elevation of seizure threshold.

Uses Because of self-limiting action, production of acidosis and hypokalaemia, acetazolamide is not used as diuretic. Its current clinical uses are:
1. Glaucoma: as adjuvant to other ocular hypotensives.
2. To alkalinise urine.
3. Epilepsy: as adjuvant drug in absence seizures.
4. Acute mountain sickness: for symptomatic relief as well as prophylaxis. Acetazolamide benefits probably by altering CO_2 transport in lungs, brain and other tissues, as well as by decreasing formation of CSF and lowering its pH.

Adverse effects are frequent. Acidosis, hypokalaemia, drowsiness, paresthesias, fatigue, abdominal discomfort. Hypersensitivity reactions—fever, rashes. Bone marrow depression is rare but serious.

POTASSIUM SPARING DIURETICS

Aldosterone antagonists and renal epithelial Na$^+$ channel inhibitors indirectly conserve K$^+$ while inducing mild natriuresis, and are called *potassium sparing diuretics*.

Aldosterone antagonists

Spironolactone

It is a steroid, chemically related to the mineralocorticoid aldosterone. Aldosterone acts on the late DT and CD cells (Fig. 13.5) by combining with an intracellular mineralocorticoid receptor (MR) → induces the formation of 'aldosterone-induced proteins' (AIPs). The AIPs promote Na$^+$ reabsorption by a number of mechanisms (*see* legend to Fig. 13.5) and K$^+$ secretion. Spironolactone combines with the MR and inhibits the formation of AIPs in a competitive manner. It has no effect on Na$^+$ and K$^+$

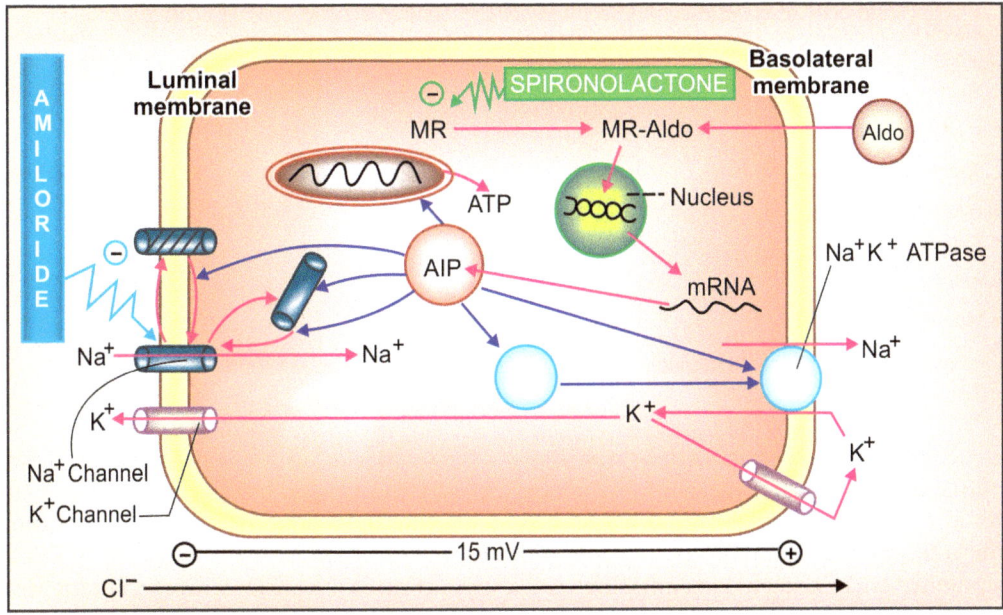

Fig. 13.5: Site and mechanism of action of potassium sparing diuretics on the late distal tubule/collecting duct cell
Aldosterone (Aldo) penetrates the cell from the interstitial side and combines with the mineralocorticoid receptor (MR). The complex translocates to the nucleus—promotes gene mediated mRNA synthesis. The mRNA then directs synthesis of aldosterone induced proteins (AIPs). The AIPs include Na⁺K⁺ ATPase and renal epithelial (amiloride sensitive) Na⁺ channels. More of these proteins are synthesized. The AIPs also activate these Na⁺ channels and, translocate them from cytosolic site to luminal membrane. They also translocate Na⁺K⁺ATPase to the basolateral membrane. AIPs increase ATP production by mitochondria. All these changes promote Na+ reabsorption. More K⁺ and H⁺ is secreted indirectly. Spironolactone binds to MR, prevents Aldo action and produces opposite effects.

Amiloride approaches the Na+ channel from the luminal side and blocks it—reducing the lumen negative transepithelial potential difference which governs K⁺ and H⁺ secretion

transport in the absence of aldosterone; while under normal circumstances, it increases Na⁺ and decreases K⁺ excretion.

Spironolactone is a mild saluretic because majority of Na⁺ has already been reabsorbed proximal to its site of action. However, it antagonises K⁺ loss induced by other diuretics and slightly adds to their natriuretic effect.

Pharmacokinetics The oral bioavailability of spironolactone from microfine powder tablet is 75%. It is highly bound to plasma proteins and completely metabolized in liver. Spironolactone is converted to active metabolites, the most important of which is *Canrenone*.

Use Spironolactone is a weak diuretic in its own right, and is used mostly in combination with other more efficacious diuretics.

1. To counteract K⁺ loss due to thiazide and loop diuretics.
2. Edema: Spironolactone is frequently added to a thiazide/loop diuretic in the treatment of ascites due to cirrhosis of liver. Resistance to thiazide and high ceiling diuretic due to secondary hyperaldosteronism is reversed.
3. Hypertension: As adjuvant to thiazides.
4. Heart failure: As additional drug to conventional therapy in moderate-to-severe CHF. It can retard disease progression and reduce mortality.

Interactions Given together with K⁺ supplements—dangerous hyperkalaemia can occur. Aspirin blocks spironolactone action by inhibiting tubular secretion of its active metabolite canrenone.

Chapter 13: Diuretics

Table 13.1: Urinary electrolyte pattern and natriuretic efficacy of some diuretics

Diuretic	Urinary electrolyte excretion				Max. % of filtered Na⁺ excreted	Efficacy
	Na^+	K^+	Cl^-	HCO_3^-		
1. Furosemide	↑↑↑	↑	↑↑	↑,−	25%	High
2. Thiazide	↑↑	↑	↑	↑	8%	Intermediate
3. Acetazolamide	↑	↑↑	↑,−	↑↑	5%	Mild
4. Spironolactone	↑	↓	↑	−,↑	3%	Low
5. Amiloride	↑	↓	↑	−,↑	3%	Low
6. Mannitol	↑↑	↑	↑	↑	20%	High

(↑ Increase; ↓ Decrease; — No change)

Adverse effects Side effects are drowsiness, confusion, abdominal upset. Spironolactone has antiandrogenic and other hormonal effects producing hirsutism, gynaecomastia, impotence and menstrual irregularities.

Most serious complication is hyperkalaemia.

Eplerenone A new more selective aldosterone antagonist which has lower affinity for androgen and progesterone receptors. It is less likely to cause gynaecomastia, impotence or menstrual irregularities. Eplerenone is the preferred aldosterone antagonist for use in CHF, post-infarction left ventricular dysfunction and hypertension.

Renal epithelial Na⁺ channel inhibitors

Amiloride, triamterine These are two nonsteroidal organic bases with similar actions. Their most important effect is to decrease K^+ excretion, particularly when it is high due to large K^+ intake or use of a diuretic that enhances K^+ loss. They also cause a small increase in Na^+ excretion. The effect on urinary electrolyte pattern is superficially similar to spironolactone, but their action is independent of aldosterone.

Mechanism of action: The luminal membrane of late DT and CD cells expresses a distinct 'renal epithelial' or 'amiloride sensitive' Na^+ channel through which Na^+ enters the cell down its electro-chemical gradient which is generated by Na^+K^+ ATPase operating at the basolateral membrane (Fig. 13.5). This Na^+ entry partially depolarizes the luminal membrane because it is not accompanied by Cl^- or HCO_3^- and creates a −15 mV transepithelial potential difference which promotes secretion of K^+ into the lumen through K^+ channels. Amiloride and triamterene block the luminal Na^+ channels— indirectly inhibit K^+ excretion, while the net excess loss of Na^+ is minor (most of it has already been absorbed).

Both triamterene and amiloride are used in conjunction with a thiazide type or a high ceiling diuretic to prevent hypokalaemia and slightly augment the natriuretic and antihypertensive response. These drugs should not be given along with K^+ supplements, because dangerous hyperkalaemia may develop. Hyperkalaemia is also more likely in patients receiving ACE inhibitors or ARBs, and in those with renal impairment.

Amiloride blocks entry of Li^+ through Na^+ channels in the CD cells and mitigates diabetes insipidus induced by lithium.

Dose to dose amiloride is 10 times more potent than triamterine.

OSMOTIC DIURETICS

Mannitol

Mannitol is a nonelectrolyte of low molecular weight (182) that is pharmacologically inert. Therefore, it can be given in large quantities sufficient to raise osmolarity of plasma and tubular fluid. It is not metabolized in the body, but freely filtered at the glomerulus and undergoes limited reabsorption; therefore, excellently suited to be used as osmotic diuretic. Mannitol appears to limit tubular water and electrolyte reabsorption by:

1. Retaining water iso-osmotically in PT and in descending limb of loop of Henle which are freely permeable to water. The diluted luminal fluid opposes NaCl reabsorption.
2. Inhibiting transport processes in the TAL by an unknown mechanism.
3. Expanding extracellular fluid volume—this increases g.f.r. and inhibits renin release.

Administration Mannitol is not absorbed orally; has to be given i.v. as 10–20% solution. It is excreted with a t½ of 0.5–1.5 hours.

Uses Mannitol is never used for the treatment of chronic edema or as a natriuretic. Its indications are:

1. Increased intracranial or intraocular tension (acute congestive glaucoma, head injury, stroke, etc.): by osmotic action it encourages movement of water from brain parenchyma, CSF and aqueous humour. Mannitol is also used before and after eye/brain surgery to prevent acute rise in intraocular/intracranial pressure.
2. To maintain g.f.r. and urine flow in impending acute renal failure.

Isosorbide and glycerol These are orally active osmotic diuretics which may be used to reduce intraocular or intracranial tension.

14

CHAPTER

Hormones and Related Drugs-1
Anterior Pituitary Hormones, Antidiabetic Drugs, Corticosteroids

INTRODUCTION

Hormone (Greek *hormaein*—to stir up) is a substance of intense biological activity that is produced by *specific cells* in the body and is transported *through circulation* to act on its target cells.

Hormones regulate body functions to bring about a programmed pattern of life events and maintain homeostasis in the face of markedly variable external and internal environment.

Body function	Major regulator hormone(s)
1. Availability of fuel	: Insulin, Glucagon, Growth hormone
2. Metabolic rate	: Triiodothyronine, Thyroxine
3. Somatic growth	: Growth hormone, Insulin-like growth factors
4. Sex and reproduction	: Gonadotropins Androgens, Estrogens, Progestins
5. Circulating volume	: Aldosterone, Antidiuretic hormone
6. Adaptation to stress	: Glucocorticoids, Adrenaline
7. Calcium balance	: Parathormone, Calcitonin, Vitamin D

Hormones are secreted by the *endocrine* or *ductless* glands. These are:

1. *Pituitary*

   (a) *Anterior*—Growth hormone (GH), Prolactin (Prl), Adrenocorticotropic hormone (ACTH), Thyroid stimulating hormone (TSH), Gonadotropins—Follicle stimulating hormone (FSH) and Luteinizing hormone (LH).

   (b) *Posterior*—Oxytocin, Antidiuretic hormone (ADH, Vasopressin).

2. *Thyroid* Thyroxine (T4), Triiodothyronine (T3), Calcitonin.

3. *Parathyroid* Parathormone (PTH).

4. *Pancreas* (Islets of Langerhans) Insulin, Glucagon.

5. *Adrenals*

   (a) *Cortex* Glucocorticoids (hydrocortisone) Mineralocorticoids (aldosterone) Sex steroids (dehydroepiandrosterone)

   (b) *Medulla* Adrenaline, Noradrenaline

6. *Gonads* Androgens (testosterone) Estrogens (estradiol) Progestins (progesterone)

In addition, hypothalamus, which is a part of the CNS and not a gland, produces many releasing and inhibitory hormones which control the secretion of anterior pituitary hormones.

Placenta also secretes many hormones:
- Chorionic gonadotropin
- Estrogens
- Placental lactogen
- Prolactin
- Progesterone

The natural hormones and in many cases their synthetic analogues which may be more suitable therapeutically, are used as drugs for substitution therapy as well as for pharmacotherapy. In addition, hormone antagonists and synthesis/release inhibitors are of therapeutic importance.

ANTERIOR PITUITARY HORMONES

Anterior pituitary (adenohypophysis), the master endocrine gland, which elaborates a number of important regulatory hormones. All of these are peptide in nature and act at extracellular receptors located on their target cells. Secretion of pituitary hormones is controlled by the hypothalamus through *releasing* and *release-inhibitory* hormones that are transported *via* hypothalamohypophyseal portal system, and is subjected to feedback inhibition by hormones of their target glands. Each anterior pituitary hormone is produced by a separate group of cells, which according to their staining characteristic are either acidophilic or basophilic.

The *acidophilic cells* secrete:
- Growth hormone (GH)
- Prolactin (Prl)

The *basophilic cells* secrete:
- Thyroid stimulating hormone (TSH)
- Adrenocorticotropic hormone (ACTH)
- Gonadotropins (Gns)
  - Follicle stimulating hormone (FSH)
  - Luteinizing hormone (LH)

Out of the above hormones, only GH and Gns are used therapeutically. Of greater clinical importance are the drugs which either inhibit or stimulate secretion of a particular anterior pituitary hormone. These are presented in the chart below.

Growth hormone (GH)

It is a 191 amino acid, single chain peptide of MW 22,000.

During childhood and adolescence, GH is required for normal development and attainment of adult stature. It promotes growth of all organs by inducing hyperplasia. In general, there is a proportionate increase in the size and mass of all parts; but in the absence of gonadotropins, sexual maturation does not take place. The growth of brain and eye is independent of GH. It promotes retention of nitrogen and other tissue constituents: more protoplasm is formed. The positive nitrogen balance results from increased uptake of amino acids by tissues and their synthesis into proteins.

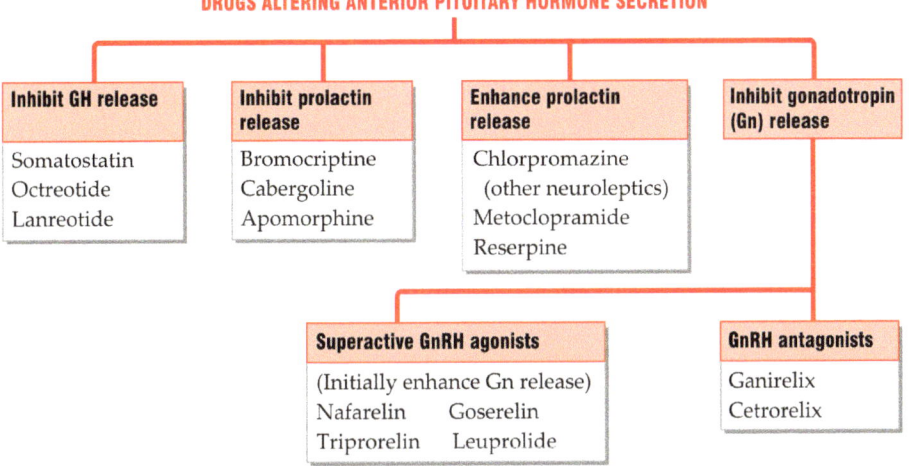

GH promotes utilization of fat and spares carbohydrates. The uptake of glucose by muscles is reduced while its output from liver is enhanced causing hyperglycaemia. Fat is broken down.

The growth promoting, nitrogen retaining and certain metabolic actions of GH are exerted *indirectly* through the elaboration of peptides called *Somatomedins* or *Insulin-like growth factors (IGF-1, also IGF-2)* which are extracellular mediators of GH response (*see* Fig. 14.1). GH acts directly as well.

Pathological involvements Excess production of GH is responsible for *gigantism* in childhood and *acromegaly* in adults. Hyposecretion of GH in children results in *pituitary dwarfism*.

Use The primary indication for GH is pituitary dwarfism. Human GH produced by recombinant DNA technique (*somatropin*) is used.

Other indications are catabolic states like severe burns, bedridden patients, chronic renal failure, Turner syndrome in girls, and GH deficiency in adults. It is now approved for AIDS-related wasting.

Somatostatin It is a 14 amino acid peptide produced by hypothalamus, pancreatic islets, etc. which inhibits the secretion of GH, prolactin, TSH, insulin, glucagon, gastrin and most gastrointestinal juices—can be beneficial in pancreatic, biliary and intestinal fistulae. It also constricts splanchnic, hepatic and renal blood vessels. Therefore, it can be used to control bleeding from esophageal varices and from peptic ulcer, but octreotide is preferred now.

Octreotide This synthetic octapeptide congener of somatostatin is longer acting and 40 times more potent except in inhibiting insulin secretion. It is preferred over somatostatin for acromegaly, esophageal variceal bleeding, and for certain secretory diarrhoeas.

Prolactin (Prl)

It is a 199 amino acid, single chain peptide of MW 23,000; quite similar chemically to GH.

Prolactin is the primary stimulus which, in conjunction with estrogens, progesterone and several other hormones, causes growth and development of breast during pregnancy. It promotes proliferation of ductal as well as acinar cells in the breast and induces synthesis of milk proteins and lactose. After parturition, Prl induces milk secretion because the inhibitory influence of high estrogen and progesterone levels is withdrawn.

Prolactin has an inhibitory effect on hypothalamo-pituitary-gonadal axis. Continued high level of Prl during breastfeeding is responsible for lactational amenorrhoea, inhibition of ovulation and infertility for several months postpartum.

Prolactin is under predominant inhibitory control of hypothalamus through dopamine that functions as the prolactin release inhibitory hormone (PRIH) and

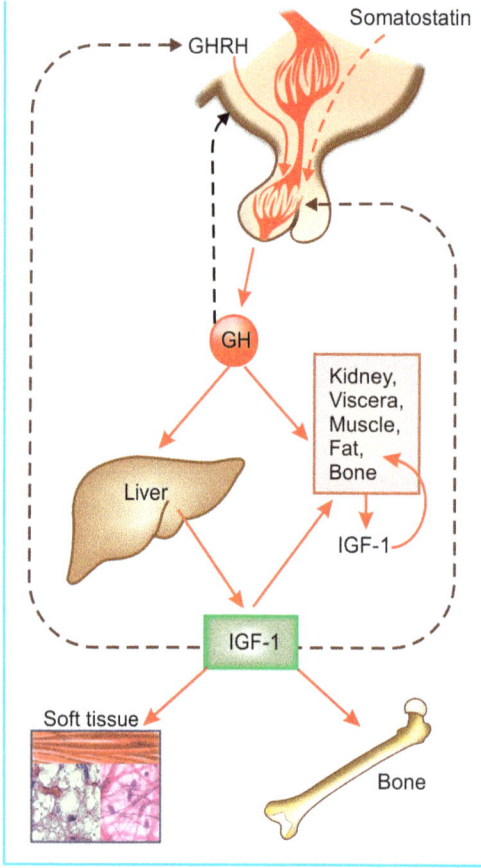

Fig. 14.1: Action of growth hormone (GH) and regulation of its secretion
GHRH—Growth hormone releasing hormone; IGF-1: Insulin like growth factor-1; Stimulation (⟶); Inhibition (- - -→)

acts on pituitary lactotrope D2 receptors. Dopaminergic agonists (DA, bromocriptine, cabergoline, apomorphine) lower plasma prolactin levels, while dopaminergic antagonists (chlorpromazine, haloperidol, metoclopramide) cause hyperprolactinaemia.

Hyperprolactinaemia is responsible for the galactorrhoea-amenorrhoea-infertility syndrome in women. In males it causes loss of libido and depressed fertility.

Bromocriptine

This synthetic ergot derivative is a potent dopamine agonist. It has greater action on D2 receptors, while at certain dopamine sites in the brain, it acts as a partial agonist or antagonist of D1 receptor. It is also a weak α adrenergic blocker but not an oxytocic.

Bromocriptine suppresses prolactin release and is indicated in hyperprolactinaemia causing galactorrhoea, amenorrhoea and infertility in women; gynaecomastia, impotence and sterility in men. Because bromocriptine decreases GH release from pituitary adenomas, it is an alternative drug for acromegaly. Due to its levodopa like action in the CNS, bromocriptine is an adjuvant drug for parkinsonism.

Bromocriptine produces nausea and vomiting by stimulating D2 receptors in CTZ. It has been largely replaced by the newer more potent and longer acting D2 receptor agonist cabergoline.

Cabergoline This newer bromocriptine congener is a longer acting (t½ > 60 hours), more potent and more selective D2 receptor agonist. It has superseded bromocriptine in the treatment of hyperprolactinaemia and acromegaly.

Gonadotropins (Gns)

The anterior pituitary secretes two Gns *viz.* FSH and LH. Both are two chain glycoproteins. FSH has a total of 203 AAs with MW 32000, while LH has 213 AAs and MW 30,000.

FSH and LH act in concert to promote gametogenesis and secretion of gonadal hormones.

FSH In the female it induces follicular growth, development of ovum and secretion of estrogens. In the male it supports spermatogenesis and has a trophic influence on seminiferous tubules. Ovarian and testicular atrophy occurs in the absence of FSH.

LH It induces preovulatory swelling of the ripe graafian follicle and triggers ovulation in females. It then brings about luteinization of the ruptured follicle and maintains corpus luteum till the next menstrual cycle. It is also probably responsible for atresia of the remaining follicles. Progesterone secretion occurs under the influence of LH. In the male LH stimulates testosterone secretion by the interstitial cells and is designated interstitial cell stimulating hormone (ICSH).

Disturbances of Gn secretion from pituitary may be responsible for delayed puberty or precocious puberty both in girls and boys.

Inadequate Gn secretion results in amenorrhoea and sterility in women; oligozoospermia, impotence and infertility in men. Excess production of Gn in adult women causes polycystic ovaries.

Gonadotropins are obtained either from urine of postmenopausal women (Menotropins FSH+LH or pure FSH) or urine of pregnant women (Human chorionic gonadotropin—HCG, which is equivalent to LH). Recombinant human FSH (Follitropin), recombinant human LH (Lutropin) and recombinant HCG (Choriogonadotropin) have also been produced. They can be used for:

1. Amenorrhoea and infertility in women due to deficient production of Gns by pituitary.
2. Hypogonadotrophic hypogonadism in males manifesting as delayed puberty or male sterility.
3. To aid *in vitro* fertilization.

Superactive/long acting GnRH agonists

Many analogues of GnRH, e.g. Goserelin, Leuprolide, Triptorelin, Nafarelin have been developed which are 15–150 times more potent than natural GnRH and longer acting because of high affinity for GnRH receptor and resistance to enzymatic hydrolysis. They initially increase Gn secretion, but after 1–2 weeks cause desensitization and down-regulation of GnRH receptors → inhibition of FSH and LH secretion → suppression of gonadal function. Spermatogenesis or ovulation cease and testosterone or estradiol levels fall to castration levels. Recovery occurs within 2 months of stopping treatment.

The superactive GnRH agonists are used as nasal spray or injected s.c./i.m. The resulting reversible pharmacological oophorectomy/orchiectomy is being used in precocious puberty, prostatic carcinoma, endometriosis, premenopausal breast cancer, uterine leiomyoma, polycystic ovarian disease and to assist induced ovulation.

GnRH antagonists
Some more extensively substituted GnRH analogues, e.g. *Ganirelix, Cetrorelix*, etc. act as GnRH receptor antagonists. They inhibit Gn secretion without causing initial stimulation, and produce quick Gn suppression. They are being used to aid *in vitro* fertilization, and for androgen withdrawal therapy of carcinoma prostate.

Thyroid stimulating hormone (TSH, thyrotropin)

It is a 210 amino acid, two chain glycoprotein, MW 30,000.

TSH stimulates thyroid to synthesize and secrete thyroxine (T_4) and triiodothyronine (T_3).
- It induces hyperplasia and hypertrophy of thyroid follicles and increases blood supply to the gland.
- It promotes trapping of iodide by the thyroid gland.
- It promotes organification of trapped iodine and its incorporation into T_3 and T_4 by enhancing peroxidase activity.
- It enhances endocytotic uptake of thyroid colloid by the follicular cells and proteolysis of thyroglobulin to release more of T_3 and T_4. This action starts within minutes of TSH administration.

Pathological involvement Only few cases of hypo- or hyperthyroidism are due to inappropriate TSH secretion. In majority of cases of myxoedema TSH levels are markedly elevated because of deficient feedback inhibition. Graves' disease is due to an immunoglobulin of the IgG class which attaches to the thyroid cells and stimulates them in the same way as TSH. Consequently, TSH levels are low.

Thyrotropin has no therapeutic use.

Adrenocorticotropic hormone (ACTH, corticotropin)

It is a 39 amino acid single chain peptide, MW 4,500, derived from a larger peptide *pro-opio melanocortin* (MW 30,000) which also gives rise to endorphins, two lipotropins and two melanocyte stimulating hormones.

ACTH promotes steroidogenesis in adrenal cortex by stimulating cAMP formation in cortical cells (through specific cell surface G protein coupled receptors). This rapidly increases the availability of cholesterol for conversion to pregnenolone which is the rate limiting step in the production of gluco, mineralo and weakly androgenic steroids. The stores of adrenal steroids are very limited and rate of synthesis primarily governs the rate of release. ACTH also exerts trophic influence on adrenal cortex (again through cAMP): high doses cause hypertrophy and hyperplasia. Absence of ACTH results in adrenal atrophy. However, zona glomerulosa is little affected because angiotensin II also exerts trophic influence on this layer and sustains aldosterone secretion.

Pathological involvement Excess production of ACTH from basophil pituitary tumours is responsible for some cases of Cushing's syndrome. Hypocorticism occurs in pituitary insufficiency due to low ACTH production. Iatrogenic suppression of ACTH secretion and the pituitary adrenal axis is the most common form of abnormality encountered currently due to the use of supraphysiological doses of glucocorticoids in nonendocrine diseases.

ACTH is not used therapeutically.

ANTIDIABETIC DRUGS

Diabetes mellitus (DM) It is a metabolic disorder characterized by hyperglycaemia, glycosuria, hyperlipidaemia, negative nitrogen balance and sometimes ketonaemia. A widespread pathological change is thickening of capillary basement membrane, increase in vessel wall matrix and cellular proliferation resulting in vascular complications like lumen narrowing, early atherosclerosis, sclerosis of glomerular capillaries, retinopathy, neuropathy and peripheral vascular insufficiency.

The two major types of diabetes mellitus are:

Type 1 Insulin-dependent diabetes mellitus (IDDM)/juvenile onset diabetes mellitus:

There is β cell destruction in pancreatic islets; majority of cases are autoimmune, but some are idiopathic. In all type 1 cases circulating insulin levels are low or very low, and patients are more prone to ketosis. This type is less common and has a low degree of genetic predisposition.

Type 2 Noninsulin-dependent diabetes mellitus (NIDDM)/maturity onset diabetes mellitus:

There is no loss or moderate reduction in β cell mass; insulin in circulation is either low or normal or even high, no anti-β-cell antibody is demonstrable. It has a high degree of genetic predisposition; generally has a late onset (past middle age). Over 90% cases of diabetes mellitus are type 2 DM. Causes may be:

- Abnormality in glucoreceptor of β cells so that they respond at higher glucose concentration; insulin secretion is impaired.
- Reduced sensitivity of peripheral tissues to insulin; down regulation of insulin receptors.
- Excess of hyperglycaemic hormones (glucagon, etc.)/obesity.

Most cases have relative insulin resistance as well as β cell insufficiency.

Approaches to drug therapy in type 2 DM	
Improve insulin availability	*Overcome insulin resistance*
Exogenous insulin Sulfonylureas Meglitinide/phenylalanine analogues Dipeptidyl peptidase-4 inhibitors (DPP-4Is) GLP-1 receptor agonists	Biguanides (Metformin) Thiazolidinediones (Pioglitazone) α glucosidase inhibitors (Acarbose)
Major limitations (except for DPP-4Is and GLP-1 agonists) Multiple daily injections (Insulins) Hypoglycaemic episodes Weight gain Concern about premature atherosclerosis due to hyperinsulinaemia	*Major limitations* Inability to achieve normoglycaemia by themselves in many patients, especially moderate-to-severe cases

INSULIN

The hypoglycaemic hormone insulin is synthesized in the β cells of pancreatic islets. It is a two chain polypeptide having 51 amino acids and MW about 6,000. The A-chain has 21 while B-chain has 30 amino acids. There are minor differences between human, pork and beef insulins:

Species	A-chain		B-chain
	8th AA	10th AA	30th AA
Human	THR	ILEU	THR
Pork	THR	ILEU	ALA
Beef	ALA	VAL	ALA

Under basal condition ~1 U insulin is secreted per hour by human pancreas. Much larger quantity is secreted after every meal. Secretion of insulin from β cells is regulated by chemical (primarily glucose, but also amino acids, fatty acids, ketone bodies), hormonal (growth hormone, corticosteroids, thyroxine, glucagon, somatostatin) and neural (adrenergic, cholinergic) mechanisms.

Actions of insulin

The overall effects of insulin are to dispose meal-derived glucose, amino acids and fatty acids, thus favour storage of fuel. The most prominent action of insulin is hypoglycaemia. It facilitates glucose transport across cell membrane (by enhancing insertion of glucose transporter GLUT4 into the cell membrane) and alters the activity of enzymes involved in carbohydrate, fat and protein metabolism in liver, muscle and adipose tissue to lower blood glucose level. Concurrently, the actions prevent rise in free fatty acid level, ketone body production and protein breakdown of the diabetic state (*see* box).

Most of the metabolic actions of insulin are exerted within seconds or minutes and are called the *rapid actions*. Others involving DNA mediated synthesis of glucose transporter and some enzymes of amino acid metabolism have a latency of few hours—the *intermediate* actions. In addition, insulin exerts major *long-term* effects on multiplication and differentiation of many types of cells.

Mechanism of action Insulin acts on specific receptors located on the cell membrane of practically all cells, liver and fat cells are very rich. The insulin receptor is a heterotetrameric glycoprotein consisting of 2 extracellular α and 2 transmembrane β subunits linked together by disulfide bonds. Its orientation across the membrane is depicted in Fig. 14.2. The α subunits carry insulin binding sites, while the β subunits have tyrosine protein kinase activity.

Binding of insulin to α subunits induces aggregation and internalization of the receptor along with the bound insulin molecules. This activates tyrosine kinase activity of the β subunits. Pairs of β subunits phosphorylate tyrosine residues of each other and then of Insulin Receptor Substrate proteins (IRS1, IRS2). In turn, a cascade of phosphorylation and dephosphorylation reactions is set into motion resulting in amplification of the signal and stimulation or inhibition of enzymes involved in the rapid metabolic actions of insulin.

Second messengers like phosphatidyl inositol tris-phosphate (PIP_3) also mediate the action of insulin on metabolic enzymes.

In addition, insulin enhances glucose transport across cell membrane by promoting ATP-dependent translocation of glucose transporter GLUT 4 to the cell membrane. In the long term, the genes for GLUT4 and many enzymes as well as carriers are upregulated while some are down regulated.

The internalized receptor-insulin complex is partly recycled to the surface and partly degraded intracellularly.

Fate of insulin

Insulin is distributed only extracellularly. It is a peptide, therefore degraded in the g.i.t. if given orally. Injected insulin or that released from pancreas is metabolized primarily in liver and to a smaller extent in kidney and muscles. The plasma t½ of insulin is 5–9 min.

Preparations of insulin

The older commercial insulin preparations were obtained from pork and beef pancreas. They contained proinsulin and other peptides which are potentially antigenic. These have now been replaced by highly

Actions of insulin producing hypoglycaemia		
Liver	Muscle	Adipose tissue
• Increases glucose uptake and glycogen synthesis • Inhibits glycogenolysis and glucose output • Inhibits gluconeogenesis from protein, pyruvate, FFA and glycerol	• Increases glucose uptake and utilization • Inhibits proteolysis and release of amino acids, pyruvate, lactate into blood which form the substrate for gluconeogenesis in liver	• Increases glucose uptake and storage as fat and glycogen • Inhibits lipolysis and release of FFA + glycerol which act as substrate for gluconeogenesis in liver

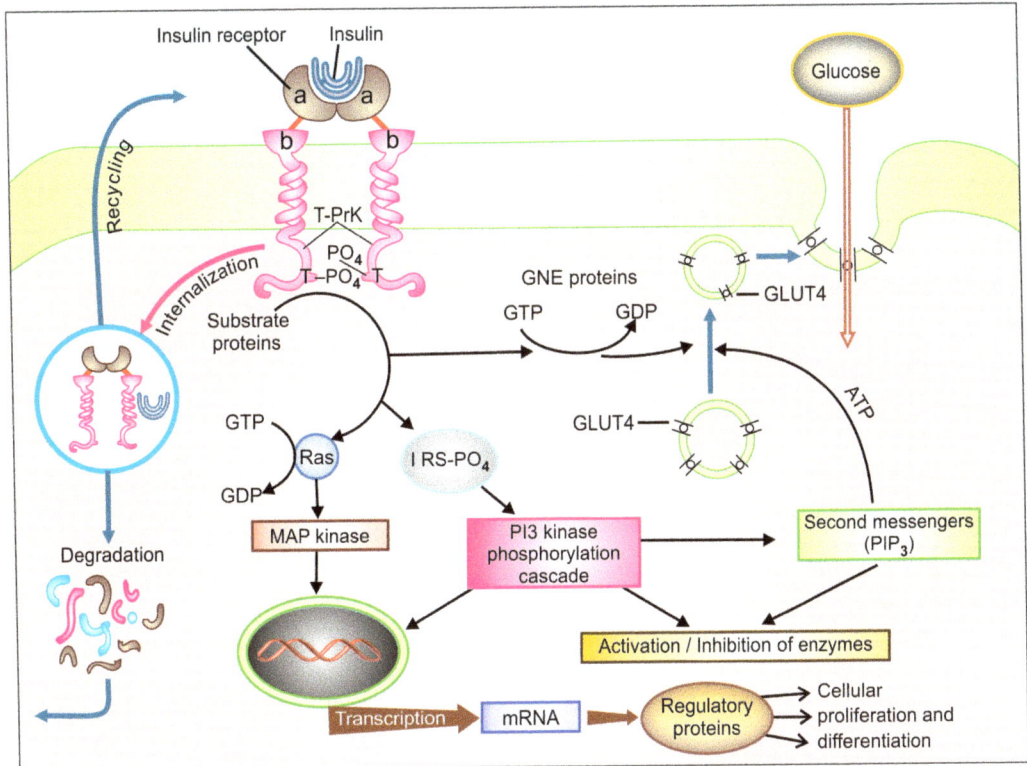

Fig. 14.2: A model of insulin receptor and mediation of its metabolic and cellular actions. T—Tyrosine residue; GLUT4—Insulin dependent glucose transporter; IRS—Insulin receptor substrate proteins; PIP_3—Phosphatidyl inositol trisphosphate; PI3 kinase—Phosphatidyl inositol 3 kinase; GNE proteins—Guanine nucleotide exchange proteins; MAP kinase—Mitogen-activated protein kinase; T-PrK—Tyrosine protein kinase; Ras—Regulator of cell division and differentiation (protooncogene product).

purified (monocomponent) pork insulins/human insulins/insulin analogues.

Highly purified pork insulins There are several types of insulin preparations. The regular (soluble) insulin is a buffered solution of unmodified insulin which needs to be injected s.c. 3-4 times daily and produces widely fluctuating blood levels. It has been modified by adding more zinc with or without protamine (a nonantigenic protein) to yield slowly absorbed and longer acting 'modified' or 'retard' preparations such as *lente insulin* and *isophane (NPH) insulin* (Table 14.1).

Human insulin produced by recombinant DNA technology or by enzymatic modification of pork insulin, has the same amino acid composition as that produced by human pancreas. It is now more extensively used than highly purified pork insulins. The human and purified pork insulin produce less allergic reaction, insulin resistance and injection site lipodystrophy. Human insulin has also been modified to produce 'lente' and 'isophane' perparations.

Insulin analogues Several analogues of human insulin produced by replacing 1-3 amino acids have the same pharmacodynamic actions but have modified pharmacokinetics after s.c. injection. They exhibit greater stability and consistency in time-course of action. *Insulin lispro, insulin aspart* and *insulin*

Chapter 14: Hormones and Related Drugs-1

Table 14.1: Types of insulin preparations and insulin analogues

Type	Appearance	Onset (hr)	Peak (hr)	Duration (hr)	Can be mixed with
Rapid acting					
Insulin lispro	Clear	0.2–0.3	1–1.5	3–5	Regular, NPH
Insulin aspart	Clear	0.2–0.3	1–1.5	3–5	Regular, NPH
Insulin glulisine	Clear	0.2–0.4	1–2	3–5	Regular, NPH
Short acting					
Regular (soluble) insulin	Clear	0.5–1	2–3	6–8	All preparations (except insulin glargine/detemir)
Intermediate acting					
Insulin zinc suspension or Lente*	Cloudy	1–2	8–10	12–20	Regular
Neutral protamine hagedorn (NPH) or isophane insulin	Cloudy	1–2	8–10	12–20	Regular
Long acting					
Insulin glarging	Clear	2–4	–	24	None
Insulin detemir	Clear	1–4	–	20–24	None

*Lente insulin is a 7:3 mixture of ultralente (crystalline) and semilente (amorphous) insulin zinc suspension. Ultralente (long-acting) and semilente (short-acting) are not separately marketed. The older protamine zinc insulin is also discontinued.

glulisine have a more rapid and predictable onset, peak and shorter duration of action than regular insulin. On the other hand, *insulin glargine* and *insulin detemir* are very slowly absorbed after s.c. injection. They are long acting; produce lower but smooth and 'peakless' blood insulin level. Once daily s.c. injection yields relatively constant background insulin action. The meal time glycaemia may be controlled by injecting a rapidly acting insulin preparation before each meal.

Reactions to insulin

1. *Hypoglycaemia* This is the most frequent and potentially the most serious reaction to insulin. Hypoglycaemia can occur in any diabetic following inadvertent injection of large doses or by *missing a meal (e.g. after a dental procedure)* or by performing vigorous exercise. The symptoms can be divided into those due to counter-regulatory sympathetic stimulation—sweating, anxiety, palpitation, tremor; and those due to deprivation of brain of its essential nutrient—glucose (neuroglucopenic symptoms)—dizziness, headache, behavioural changes, visual disturbances, hunger, fatigue, weakness, muscular incoordination and sometimes fall in BP. Generally, the reflex sympathetic symptoms occur before the neuroglucopenic symptoms.

Finally, when blood glucose falls further (to < 40 mg/dl) mental confusion, seizures and coma occur.

Treatment Glucose must be given orally or i.v. (for severe cases)—reverses the symptoms rapidly.

2. *Local reactions* Swelling, erythema and stinging sometimes occur at the injection site. *Localized*

lipodystrophy can occurs in the subcutaneous fat after long usage.

3. *Allergy* This is infrequent, and is due to contaminating proteins. Allergic reactions are very rare with human/highly purified insulins. Urticaria, angioedema and anaphylaxis are the manifestations.

Drug interactions

1. β adrenergic blockers prolong hypoglycaemia by inhibiting compensatory mechanisms operating through $β_2$ receptors ($β_1$ selective agents are less liable). Warning signs of hypoglycaemia like palpitation, tremor and anxiety are masked.

2. Thiazides, furosemide, corticosteroids, oral contraceptives and salbutamol tend to raise blood sugar and reduce effectiveness of insulin.

3. Heavy alcohol consumption can precipitate hypoglycaemia by depleting hepatic glycogen.

4. Lithium, theophylline and high dose aspirin may also accentuate hypoglycaemia by enhancing insulin secretion and peripheral glucose utilization.

Use of insulin in diabetes mellitus

The purpose of therapy in diabetes mellitus is to restore metabolism to normal, avoid symptoms due to hyperglycaemia and glucosuria, prevent short-term complications (infection, ketoacidosis, etc.) and long-term sequelae (cardiovascular, retinal, neurological, renal complications).

Insulin is effective in all forms of diabetes mellitus and is a must for type 1 cases. Many type 2 cases can be controlled by diet, reduction in body weight and appropriate exercise supplemented, if required, by oral hypoglycaemic drugs. Insulin is needed by such cases when:

- Not controlled by diet and exercise.
- Primary or secondary failure of oral antidiabetics.
- Underweight patients.
- Temporarily to tide over infections, trauma, surgery, pregnancy. In the perioperative period and during labour, monitored i.v. insulin infusion is preferable.
- Any complication of diabetes, e.g. ketoacidosis, diabetic or non-ketotic hyperosmolar coma, gangrene of extremities.

When instituted, insulin therapy is given by 2–4 daily s.c. injections of one or two types of insulin preparations. Regimens and doses are selected according to the requirement and response of the patient, determined by repeated blood-sugar and HbA_{1C} monitoring.

Insulin resistance

Insulin resistance refers to suboptimal response of the body tissues to physiological amounts of insulin. It is integral to the metabolic syndrome, of which hyperinsulinemia (with latent or overt type 2 diabetes), dyslipidaemia, hyperuricaemia and hypertension are important components. Advanced age, obesity and sedentary life style promote insulin resistance. *Infection, trauma, surgery and stress of dental procedure may produce low grade acute insulin resistance.* Insulin resistance can be overcome by increasing insulin dose.

Glucagon-like peptide-1 (GLP-1) receptor agonists

Taken orally glucose and other nutrients generate chemical signals called *incretins* from the gut which act on pancreatic β cells to trigger anticipatory release of insulin. Glucagon-like peptide-1 (GLP-1) is the most important incretin which induces insulin release, inhibits glucagon release, retards gastric emptying and suppresses appetite by acting on specific GLP-1 receptors. GLP-1 lowers blood glucose, but is not suitable for clinical use because it is degraded rapidly by the enzyme *dipeptidyl* peptidase-4 (DPP-4). Some stable analogues of GLP-1 like *exenatide* and *liraglutide* which are not susceptible to DPP-4 have been found clinically effective in type 2 DM. Exenatide injected s.c. twice daily is being used as add-on drug in patients not adequately controlled by oral antidiabetic drugs alone.

ORAL ANTIDIABETIC DRUGS

These drugs lower blood glucose level in diabetics and are effective orally.

Sulfonylureas
(K_{ATP} channel blockers)

The generic formula of sulfonylureas (SUs) is:

$$R_1-\text{C}_6\text{H}_4-SO_2-NH-CO-NH-R_2$$

SULFONYLUREA

All SUs have similar pharmacological profile. Their sole significant action is lowering of blood glucose level in normal subjects and in type 2 diabetics, but not in type 1 diabetics.

Sulfonylureas provoke release of insulin from pancreas, the mechanism of which is illustrated in Fig. 14.3. They act on a specific 'sulfonylurea receptor' (SUR1) on the pancreatic β cell membrane—cause depolarization by reducing conductance of ATP sensitive K⁺ channels. This enhances Ca^{2+} influx triggaring degranulation and insulin release. That they do not cause hypoglycaemia in pancreatectomised animals and in type 1 diabetics (presence of at least 30% functional β cells is essential for them to act), confirms their indirect action through pancreas.

After few months of use, the insulinaemic action of SUs declines, probably due to downregulation of SURs, but improvement in glucose tolerance is maintained. In this phase, they sensitize the target tissues (especially liver) to the action of insulin. It is hypothesized that long-term improvement in carbohydrate tolerance leads to lowering of circulating insulin concentration which reverses the down regulation of insulin receptors.

Pharmacokinetics All sulfonylureas are well absorbed orally. Their pharmacokinetic and distinctive features are given in Table 14.2.

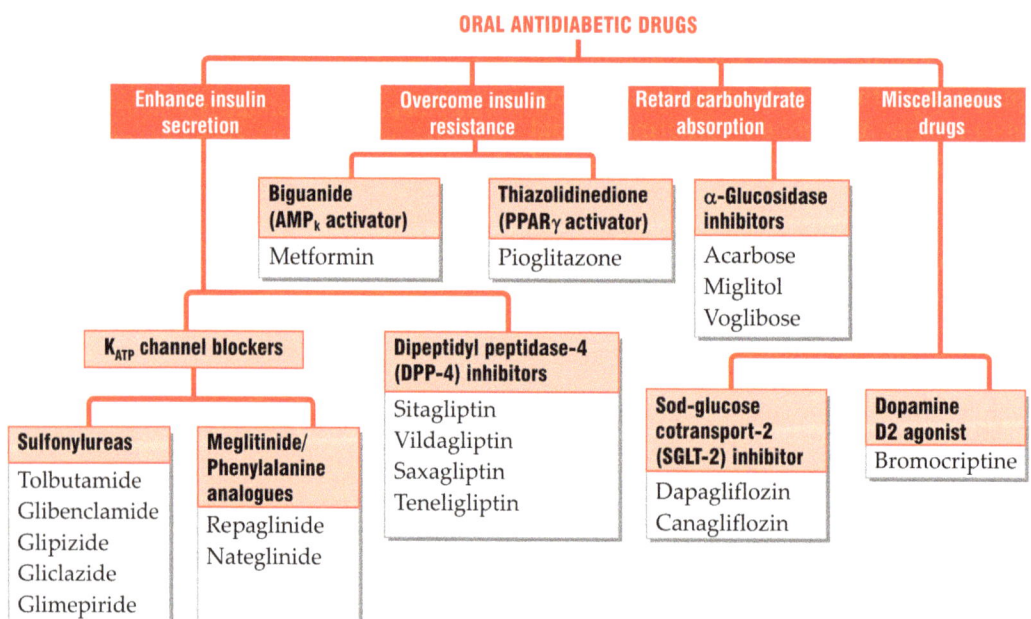

Antidiabetic Drugs

Table 14.2: Important features or oral antidiabetic drugs

Drug	Plasma t½ (hr)	Duration of action (hr)	Clearance route*	Daily dose	Remarks
SULFONYLUREAS					
1. Tolbutamide	6	6–8	L	0.5–3 g	Weaker, shorter acting, flexible dosage, safer in elderly and in those prone to hypoglycaemia
2. Glibenclamide (Glyburide)	2–4	24	L	2.5–15 mg	Potent but slow acting, higher incidence of hypoglycaemia, longer acting despite short t½ due to active metabolite and sequestration in β cells.
3. Glipizide	3–5	12	L	5–20 mg	Fast and shorter acting, hypoglycaemia and weight gain less likely, preferable in elderly
4. Gliclazide	8–20	12–24	L	40–240 mg	Has antiplatelet action, generates only inactive metabolite
5. Glimepiride	5–7	24	L	1–6 mg	Long acting, no active metabolite. Stronger extrapancreatic action.
MEGLITINIDE / PHENYLALANINE ANALOGUES					
1. Repaglinide	≤ 1	3–5	L	1–8 mg	Given 1/2 hr before each meal for limiting postprandial hyperglycaemia
2. Nateglinide	1.5	2–3	L	180–480 mg	Stimulates 1st phase insulin secretion, less likely to cause delayed hypoglycaemia
DPP-4 INHIBITORS					
1. Sitagliptin	~ 12	24	K	100 mg	Non-covalent binding to DPP-4; Low risk of hypoglycaemia. Body weight neutral
2. Vildagliptin	2–4	12–24	L, K	50–100 mg	Covalent binding to DPP-4; Metabolized in liver. Hepatotoxicity reported
BIGUANIDE					
1. Metformin	1.5–3	6–8	K	0.5–2.5 g	No hypoglycaemia. Not metabolized. Lactic acidosis rare, occurs only in kidney disease
THIAZOLIDINEDIONE					
1. Pioglitazone	3–5	24	L	15–45 mg	May improve lipid profile. Reverses insulin resistance. No hypoglycaemia, C/I in liver and heart disease

L—Metabolized in liver; K—Excreted unchanged by kidney.

Interactions

Drugs that enhance sulfonylurea action (may precipitate hypoglycaemia) are:

a. *By inhibiting SU metabolism/excretion:* Cimetidine, sulfonamides, ketoconazole, warfarin, chloramphenicol, acute alcohol intake.

b. *Synergise with or prolong pharmacodynamic action:* Propranolol, sympatholytic antihypertensives, lithium, theophylline, high dose aspirin.

Drugs that decrease sulfonylurea action (vitiate diabetes control) are:

a. *By inducing SU metabolism:* Phenobarbitone, phenytoin, rifampicin, chronic alcoholism.

b. *Produce opposite action/suppress insulin release:* Corticosteroids, thiazides, furosemide, oral contraceptives.

Adverse effects

1. *Hypoglycaemia* It is the commonest problem, may occasionally be severe and rarely fatal.

Treatment is to give glucose, may be for a few days because hypoglycaemia may recur.

2. *Nonspecific side effects* Weight gain, nausea, vomiting, flatulence, diarrhoea or constipation; paresthesias are infrequent.

3. *Hypersensitivity* Rashes, photosensitivity, purpura, transient leukopenia, rarely agranulocytosis.

Because safety of SUs during pregnancy is not established, changeover to insulin is advised.

Meglitinide/phenylalanine analogues

These are K_{ATP} channel blockers with quick and short lasting insulinemic action.

Repaglinide Though not a sulfonylurea, but a meglitinide analogue, it acts in an analogous manner by binding to sulfonylurea receptor → closure of ATP dependent K⁺ channels → depolarisation → insulin release.

Repaglinide induces rapid onset short-lasting insulin release. It is administered before each major meal to control postprandial hyperglycaemia; the dose may be omitted if a meal is missed. Because of short-lasting action, it carries a lower risk of serious hypoglycaemia. Side effects are mild headache, dyspepsia, arthralgia and weight gain.

Repaglinide is indicated only in selected type 2 DM patients who suffer pronounced post prandial hyperglycaemia, and is used along with metformin/long-acting insulin.

Nateglinide This phenylalanine derivative stimulates the 1st phase insulin secretion and has more rapid onset as well as shorter duration of hypoglycaemic action than repaglinide. There is little effect on fasting blood glucose level. Episodes of hypoglycaemia are less frequent than with sulfonylureas. Nateglinide is used only to control postprandial hyperglycaemia in type 2 diabetics.

Dipeptidyl-peptidase-4 (DPP-4) inhibitors

The enzyme DPP-4 expressed on capillary endothelial cells rapidly degrades the incretins *glucagon-like peptide-1* (GLP-1) and *glucose-dependent insulinotropic polypeptide* (GIP) which are peptides released from the gut in response to ingested glucose. They function to limit the postprandial glycaemia by releasing insulin from β cells and inhibiting glucagon secretion from α cells. They also suppress appetite and retard gastric emptying. *Sitagliptin, vildagliptin, saxagliptin, teneligliptin* and few others are orally active DPP-4 inhibitors which potentiate GLP-1 and GIP by preventing their degradation (Fig. 14.3). They have been found to limit postprandial hyperglycaemia as well as to lower fasting (basal) blood glucose level in type 2 diabetics, without producing hypoglycaemia in overdose or when a meal is missed. The DPP-4 inhibitors are now widely used to supplement metformin ± other hypoglycaemics in diabetics not adequately controlled by the other drugs. However, their blood sugar lowering efficacy is somewhat less than that of SUs. Monotherapy with DPP-4 inhibitors is advised only when metformin cannot be used. All DPP-4 inhibitors are well tolerated and neither increase, nor decrease body weight. Side effects are mild nausea, loose stools, headache, etc. Risk of hypoglycaemia is low, because GLP-1 evokes little insulin release at normal blood glucose levels. Nasopharyngitis has been reported with sitagliptin, and hepatotoxicity with vildagliptin.

Biguanide (AMPK activator)

Biguanides are one of the oldest oral hypoglycaemic drugs, of which only *metformin* is currently used.

Metformin It differs markedly from SUs, because it does not act by stimulating pancreatic β cells to secrete insulin and does

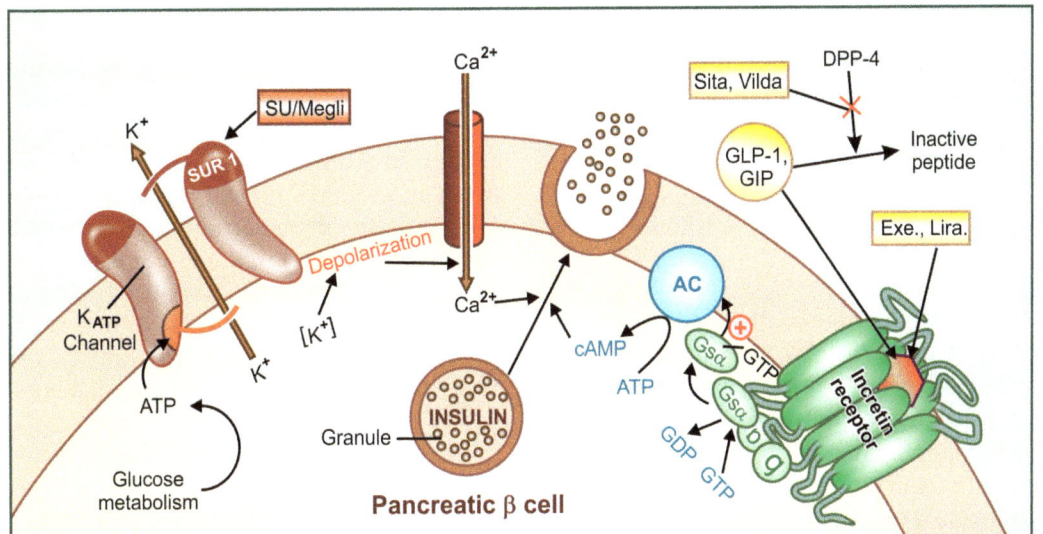

Fig. 14.3: Mechanism of action of insulin secretagogues
The sulfonylureas (SU) and meglitinide analogues (Megli) block the sulfonylurea receptor (SUR1) which constitutes a subunit of the inwardly rectifying ATP-sensitive K⁺ channel (K_{ATP}) in the membrane of pancreatic β cells. The outward flow of K⁺ ions is thereby restricted, intracellular K⁺ concentration rises and the membrane is partially depolarized augmenting Ca²⁺ channel opening as well as release of Ca²⁺ from intracellular stores. The Ca²⁺ ions promote fusion of insulin containing intracellular granules with the plasma membrane and exocytotic release of insulin.

Incretins such as glucagon-like peptide 1 (GLP1) and glucose-dependent insulinotropic polypeptide (GIP) act upon their own G-protein coupled receptors on the β cell membrane to activate adenylyl cyclase and generate cAMP, which also promotes exocytosis of insulin. Exenatide (Exe) and liraglutide (Lira) are GLP1 receptor agonists—produce the same response as GLP1. The incretins GLP1 and GIP are rapidly inactivated by the capillary endothelial enzyme dipeptidyl peptidase-4 (DPP-4). Their action is enhanced by DPP-4 inhibitors sitagliptin (sita) and vildagliptin (vilda). The DPP-4 inhibitors thus markedly accentuate the insulin response to ingested glucose/meal and attenuate post-prandial glycaemia.

not cause hypoglycaemia (lower blood sugar below normal) in nondiabetics as well as in diabetics, but lowers raised blood sugar in type 2 diabetics. It is thus, a 'normoglycaemic' rather than 'hypoglycaemic'. The mechanism of action of metformin is not clearly known, but appears to be through activation of AMP-dependent protein kinase (AMPK). Metformin:
- Suppresses hepatic gluconeogenesis and glucose output: This is the primary action which lowers blood sugar.
- Enhances insulin mediated glucose uptake in skeletal muscle and fat.
- Promotes peripheral glucose utilization through anaerobic glycolysis by interfering with mitochondrial respiratory chain.

Metformin is now established as a first choice drug for type 2 diabetics, except when not tolerated. Its advantages are:
- Has the potential to prevent microvascular as well as macrovascular complications of diabetes
- Low risk of hypoglycaemia
- Promotes weight reduction.
- Can prevent new onset type 2 diabetis in obese, middle aged subjects with impaired glucose tolerance.

The limiting feature of metformin is gastrointestinal side effects like abdominal pain, distention, nausea, loose stools, metallic taste and anorexia. Lactic acidosis is rare, except in alcoholics and in liver disease.

Thiazolidinediones (PPAR γ agonists)

This class of oral antidiabetic drugs are selective agonists for the nuclear *peroxisome proliferator-activated receptor γ* (PPARγ) expressed mainly in fat cells which enhances the transcription of several insulin responsive genes.

Pioglitazone is the only member of this class now available. It tends to reverse insulin resistance by stimulating GLUT4 expression and translocation to the cell membrane, so that entry of glucose into muscle and fat cells is improved. Insulin sensitivity of peripheral tissues is enhanced. Hepatic gluconeogenesis is suppressed while lipogenesis in adipocytes is promoted. Used alone it is a weaker hypoglycaemic than sulfonylureas and metformin, but when added to one of these—improved glycaemic control results in lowering of circulating HbA_{1c} and insulin levels in type 2 DM patients.

Pioglitazone, in addition, tends to lower serum triglycerides and raise HDL level, because it is a PPARα agonist as well; therefore it induces expression of reverse cholesterol transporter.

Pioglitazone is generally well tolerated; adverse effects are plasma volume expansion, edema, weight gain, headache, myalgia and mild anaemia; CHF may be precipitated or worsened. Monotherapy with pioglitazone is not associated with hypoglycaemic episodes.

Failure of oral contraception may occur during pioglitazone therapy. Ketoconazole inhibits and rifampin induces metabolism of pioglitazone.

Pioglitazone is indicated in type 2 DM, but not in type 1 DM. It is primarily used to supplement sulfonylureas/metformin, and in case of insulin resistance, but about 25% patients do not respond.

α Glucosidase inhibitors

Acarbose It is a complex oligosaccharide which reversibly inhibits α-glucosidases, the final enzymes for the digestion of carbohydrates in the brush border of small intestinal mucosa. It slows down and decreases digestion and absorption of polysaccharides (starch, etc.) and sucrose: postprandial glycaemia is reduced without increasing insulin levels. Long-term treatment with acarbose can reduce the occurrence of type 2 DM among prediabetics, and cardiovascular events in diabetics.

Acarbose is a mild antihyperglycaemic and not a hypoglycaemic. It may be used as an adjuvant to diet (with or without metformim/SUs) in obese diabetics. Flatulence, abdominal discomfort and loose stools are frequent side effects.

Miglitol and *Voglibose* are other α glucosidase inhibitors with similar properties, use and side effects as acarbose.

Sodium-glucose cotransport-2 (SGLT-2) inhibitors
All the glucose filtered at the glomerulus is reabsorbed in the proximal tubules, primarily by the transporter SGLT-2. *Dapagliflozin* and *Canagliflozin* are SGLT-2 inhibitors which produce glucosuria, reduce blood sugar level, cause weight loss and are approved for treating type-2 DM patients. Though these drugs can be used alone, they are mainly employed to supplement metformin ± SUs or other antidiabetic drugs. By causing glucosuria, they have the potential to predispose urogenital infections, produce electrolyte imbalance and ketoacidosis. Long-term safety of these drugs is not yet clear.

Oral antidiabetics in diabetes mellitus
Oral antidiabetics are indicated only in type 2 diabetes, when not controlled by diet and exercise alone. They are most useful in patients with—
1. Age above 40 years at onset of disease.
2. Obesity at the time of presentation.
3. Duration of disease < 5 years when starting treatment.
4. Fasting blood sugar < 200 mg/dl.
5. Insulin requirement < 40 U/day.

6. No ketoacidosis or a history of it, or any other complication.

The current recommendation is to institute metformin therapy as soon as diagnosis of type 2 DM is confirmed, because it has the potential to delay progression of diabetes and its complications. Many type-2 DM patients do not attain target level of glycaemia control by metformin alone, and a second drug is needed. The SUs are most commonly selected as the second drug. Pioglitazone is usually the 3rd choice drug; may be added to metformin ± a SU. Acarbose-like drugs are mostly given as supplementary drugs. The DPP-4 inhibitors are the latest hypoglycaemics which have gained popularity as second line/add-on antidiabetic drugs. A simplified treatment approach for diabetes mellitus is presented in Fig. 14.4.

Implications in dentistry Diabetes mellitus is associated with increased incidence of many dental problems like caries tooth, periodontal disease, oral candidiasis and other infections. Dental extractions and other simple procedures under local anaesthesia do not usually pose any special problems in diabetics, provided blood sugar levels are well controlled. If the diabetic who is being treated with insulin/oral hypoglycaemics is to miss the meals after a dental procedure, care should be taken that he/she does not develop hypoglycaemia. For more extensive dental procedures or those to be performed under general anaesthesia, it is advisable to monitor urine and blood sugar levels and

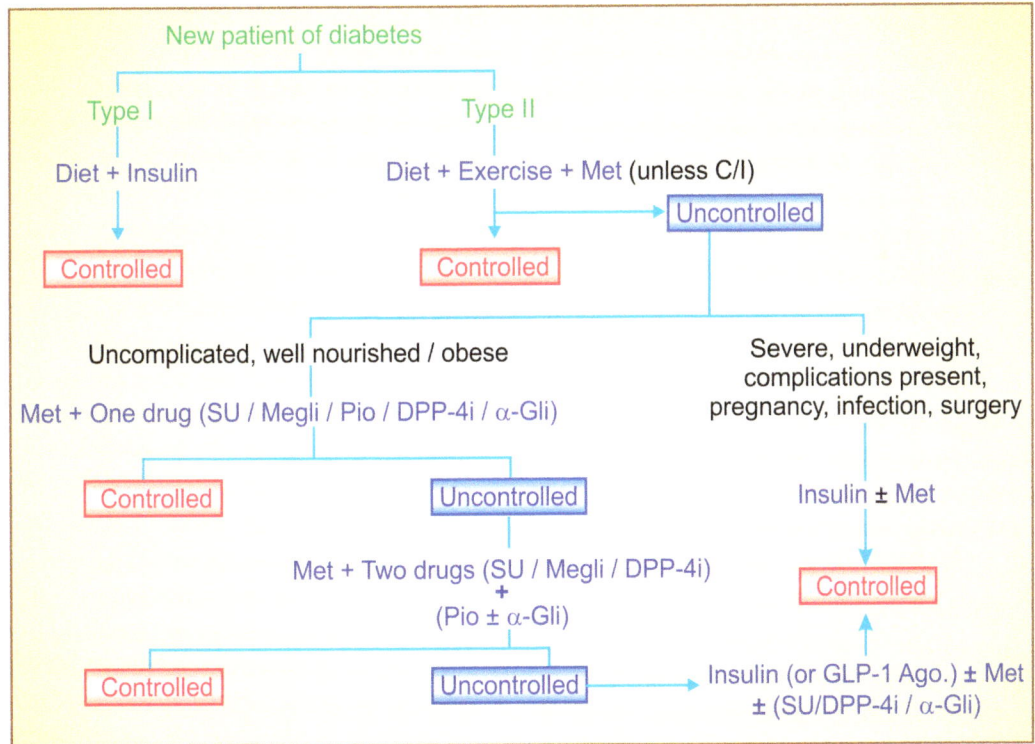

Fig. 14.4: Simplified flow chart of management approaches in diabetes mellitus.
Met—Metformin; SU—Sulfonylurea; Megli—Meglitinide/d-phenylalanine analogue; DPP-4i—Dipeptidyl peptidase-4 inhibitor; α Gli—α-Glucosidase inhibitor; Pio—Pioglitazone; GLP-1 Ago—GLP-1 receptor agonist.
Note: A meglitinide drug is indicated only in patients with predominant postprandial hyperglycaemia.
An α glucosidase inhibitor can be additional add on drug.

cover the perioperative period with regular insulin injected s.c. Severe/uncontrolled diabetics may be given an i.v. infusion of regular insulin along with 5% glucose solution during the procedure.

Prophylactic antibiotics should be given to cover dental procedures in diabetics, particularly if blood sugar level is poorly controlled.

CORTICOSTEROIDS

The adrenal cortex secretes steroidal hormones which have glucocorticoid, mineralocorticoid and weakly androgenic activities. Conventionally, the term 'corticosteroid' or 'corticoid' includes natural gluco- and mineralocorticoids and their synthetic analogues.

The corticoids (both gluco and mineralo) are 21 carbon compounds having a cyclopentanoperhydro-phenanthrene (steroid) nucleus. They are synthesized in the adrenal cortical cells from cholesterol. Adrenal steroidogenesis takes place under the influence of ACTH (see p. 232) which is under negative feed back regulation by circulating cortisol level (Fig. 14.5).

The normal rate of secretion of the two principal corticoids in man is—

Hydrocortisone (cortisol)	— 10-20 mg daily (nearly half of this in the few morning hours).
Aldosterone	— 0.125 mg daily.

Actions

The corticoids have widespread actions. They maintain fluid-electrolyte, cardiovascular and energy substrate homeostasis as well as functional status of skeletal muscles and nervous system. They prepare the body to withstand effects of all kinds of noxious stimuli and stress. The involvement of hypothalamo-pituitary-adrenal axis in corticosteroid production and in stress response is depicted in Fig. 14.5.

Actions of corticoids are divided into:

Glucocorticoid Effects on carbohydrate, protein and fat metabolism, and other actions that are inseparably linked to these.

Mineralocorticoid Effects on Na^+, K^+ and fluid balance.

Marked dissociation between these two types of actions is seen among natural as well as synthetic corticoids. Accordingly, compounds are labelled as 'glucocorticoid' or 'mineralocorticoid'.

Mineralocorticoid actions

Aldosterone is the natural mineralocorticoid. Enhancement of Na^+ reabsorption in the distal convoluted tubule of kidney associated with increased K^+ and H^+ excretion is the principal mineralocorticoid action. Excess of this action leads to Na^+ and water retention, edema, progressive rise in BP, hypokalaemia and alkalosis. Mineralocorticoid deficiency results in progressive Na^+ loss → dilutional hyponatraemia → cellular hydration → decreased blood volume. Hyperkalaemia and acidosis accompany. These distortions of fluid and electrolyte balance progress and contribute to the circulatory collapse that occurs in adrenal insufficiency if excess salt is not ingested. It is this action which makes adrenal cortex essential for survival.

The action of aldosterone is expressed by gene mediated increased transcription of m-RNA in renal tubular cells which directs synthesis of proteins (aldosterone-induced proteins—AIP). The Na^+K^+ ATPase of tubular basolateral membrane responsible for generating gradients for movement of cations in these cells is the major AIP (see Ch. 13). Aldosterone also promotes myocardial fibrosis in CHF, contributing to disease progression.

Glucocorticoid actions

1. **Carbohydrate and protein metabolism** Glucocorticoids promote glycogen

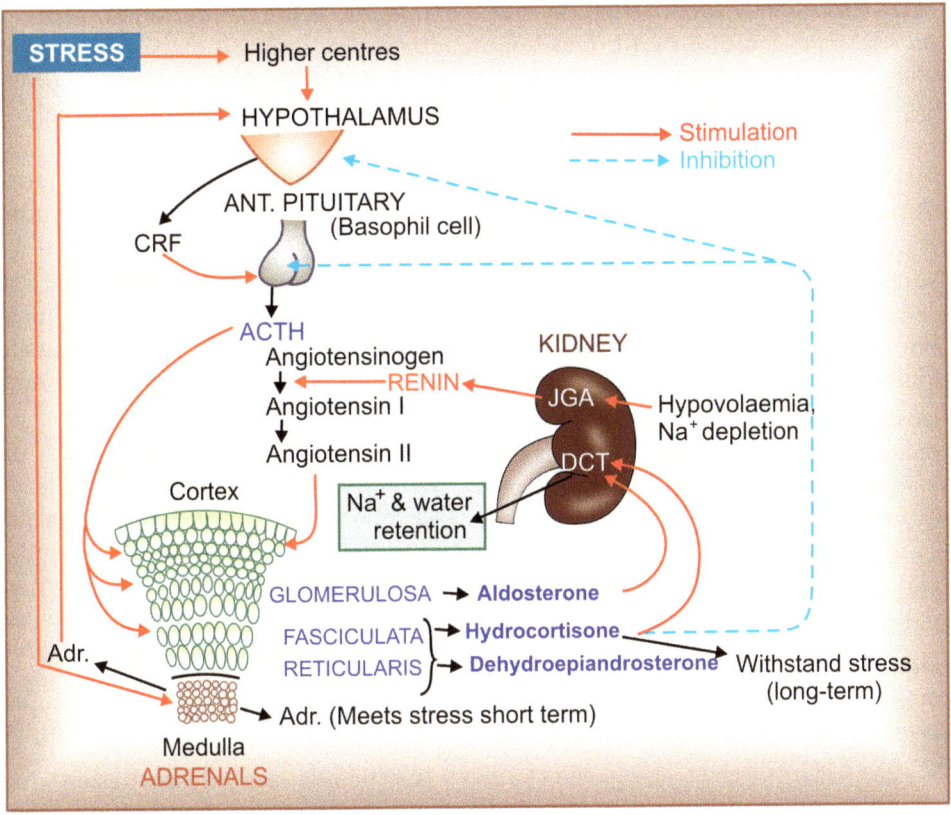

Fig. 14.5: Hypothalamo-pituitary-adrenal (HPA) axis; regulation of corticosteroid production and response to stress which overrides the negative feedback regulation of ACTH release

deposition in liver by inducing hepatic glycogen synthetase and promoting gluconeogenesis. They inhibit glucose utilization by peripheral tissues. This along with increased glucose release from liver results in hyperglycaemia, resistance to insulin and a diabetes-like state. Glucocorticoids also promote protein breakdown and amino acid mobilization from peripheral tissues which is responsible for side effects like muscle wasting, lympholysis, loss of osteoid from bone and thinning of skin. The amino acids so mobilized funnel into liver and are used up in gluconeogenesis, excess urea is produced resulting in negative nitrogen balance. Glucocorticoids are thus catabolic. Their function appears to be oriented to maintaining blood glucose levels during starvation—so that brain continues to get its nutrient.

Corticosteroids increase uric acid excretion.

2. Fat metabolism Corticoids promote lipolysis. Fat depots in different areas respond differently, so that redistribution of body fat occurs. Subcutaneous tissue over extremities loses fat which is deposited over face, neck and shoulder giving rise to the characteristic 'moon face', 'fish mouth', 'buffalo hump'.

3. Calcium metabolism Cortisol inhibits intestinal absorption and enhances renal excretion of Ca^{2+}. Loss of osteoid indirectly contributes to loss of Ca^{2+} from bone producing osteoporosis. Spongy bones (vertebrae, pelvis, ribs, etc.) are more sensitive.

4. **Water excretion** Glucocorticoids, but not aldosterone, maintain g.f.r. and help excreting excess water load.

5. **CVS** Glucocorticoids restrict capillary permeability, maintain tone of arterioles and myocardial contractility. They play a permissive role in the development of hypertension.

Adrenal insufficiency is attended by low cardiac output, arteriolar dilatation, poor response to Adr and increased permeability of capillaries.

6. **Skeletal muscles** Optimum level of cortisol is needed for normal muscular activity. Weakness occurs in both hypo- and hypercorticism, but the causes are different.

Hypocorticism: diminished work capacity and weakness are primarily due to hypodynamic circulation.

Hypercorticism: excess mineralocorticoid action → hypokalaemia → weakness; Excess glucocorticoid action → muscle wasting and myopathy → weakness.

7. **CNS** Mild euphoria is quite common with supraphysiological doses of glucocorticoids. This sometimes progresses to cause insomnia, anxiety or depression as side effect of corticosteroid therapy.

8. **Stomach** Secretion of gastric acid and pepsin is increased—may aggravate peptic ulcer.

9. **Lymphoid tissue** Glucocorticoids enhance the rate of destruction of lymphoid cells (T cells are more sensitive than B cells). A marked lytic response is shown by malignant lymphatic cells; therefore corticosteroids are palliative in lymphomas.

10. **Inflammatory responses** Irrespective of the type of injury or insult, the attending inflammatory response is suppressed by glucocorticoids. This is the basis of most of their clinical uses. The action is nonspecific and includes reduction of—increased capillary permeability, local exudation, cellular infiltration, phagocytic activity as well as late responses like capillary proliferation, collagen deposition, fibroblastic activity and ultimately scar formation. The action is direct and can be restricted to a site by local application. The cardinal signs of inflammation—redness, heat, swelling and pain are suppressed.

Glucocorticoids interfere at several steps in the inflammatory response, but the most important overall mechanism appears to be limitation of recruitment of inflammatory cells at the local site.

Production of PGs and several other mediators of inflammation like LTs, PAF, TNF_α and cytokines is interfered by negative regulation of COX and other relevant enzymes. Glucocorticoids induce formation of anti-inflammatory protein called *annexins* which inhibits phospholipase A that is responsible for release of arachidonic acid from membrane phospholipids for PG and LT synthesis.

Corticoids are only palliative, do not remove the cause of inflammation; the underlying disease continues to progress while manifestations are dampened. They favour spread of infections because capacity of defensive cells to kill microorganisms is impaired. They also interfere with healing and scar formation: peptic ulcer may perforate asymptomatically.

11. **Immunological and allergic responses** Glucocorticoids impair immunological competence. They suppress all types of hypersensitization and allergic phenomena. The clinical effect appears to be due to suppression of recruitment of leukocytes at the site of contact with the antigen, and of inflammatory response to immunological injury.

They cause greater suppression of cell mediated immunity (CMI) in which T cells are primarily involved, e.g. delayed hypersensitivity and graft rejection. This is the basis of use in autoimmune diseases and organ transplantation. Factors involved may be inhibition of IL-1 release from macrophages; inhibition of IL-2 formation and action, so that T cell proliferation is not stimulated; suppression of natural killer cells, etc. Overall, corticosteroids interrupt cooperative cell-to-cell communication between immunological cells.

Mechanism of action at cellular level

Corticosteroids penetrate cells and bind to a high affinity cytoplasmic receptor protein → a structural change occurs in the steroid-receptor complex that allows its migration into the nucleus and binding to the glucocorticoid response elements (GRE) on the chromatin → transcription of specific m-RNA → regulation of protein synthesis (*see* Fig. 3.9). This process takes at least 30-60 min. Therefore, effects of corticosteroid are not immediate, and once the appropriate proteins are synthesized—effects persist much longer than the steroid itself. In many tissues, the overall effect is catabolic, i.e. inhibition of protein synthesis. This may be a consequence of steroid directed synthesis of an inhibitory protein. The glucocorticoid receptor (GR) is very widely distributed (in practically all cells of the body). Therefore, effects of corticosteroids are widespread.

Pharmacokinetics

All natural and synthetic corticoids are absorbed by the oral route.

Hydrocortisone undergoes high first pass metabolism. Therefore, it has low oral: parenteral activity ratio. Oral bioavailability of synthetic corticoids is high.

Hydrocortisone is 90% bound to plasma protein, mostly to a specific cortisol-binding globulin (CBG or transcortin) as well as to albumin.

The steroids are metabolized primarily by hepatic microsomal enzymes. The metabolites are excreted in urine.

The plasma t½ of hydrocortisone is 1.5 hours. However, biological effect t½ is longer because of action through intracellular receptors and regulation of protein synthesis—effects that persist long after the steroid is removed from plasma.

The synthetic corticosteroids are more resistant to metabolism and are longer acting.

Phenobarbitone and phenytoin induce metabolism of hydrocortisone, prednisolone and dexamethasone, etc. to decrease their therapeutic effect.

Distinctive features

The relative potency and activity of different natural and synthetic corticosteroids employed systemically is compared in Table 14.3.

1. Hydrocortisone (cortisol) In addition to primary glucocorticoid, it has significant mineralocorticoid activity with rapid and short lasting action.

2. Prednisolone It is 4 times more potent than hydrocortisone; also more selective glucocorticoid, but fluid retention does occur with high doses. Has intermediate duration of action: causes less pituitary-adrenal suppression when a single morning dose or alternate day treatment is given. It is used for allergic, inflammatory, autoimmune diseases and in malignancies.

3. Methylprednisolone Slightly more potent and more selective than prednisolone.

Pulse therapy with high dose methylprednisolone (1 g infused i.v. every 6–8 weeks) has been tried in nonresponsive active rheumatoid arthritis, renal transplant, pemphigus, etc.

4. Triamcinolone Slightly more potent than prednisolone but highly selective glucocorticoid.

Chapter 14: Hormones and Related Drugs-1

Table 14.3: Relative activity of systemic corticosteroids

	Compound	Gluco	Mineralo	Equiv. dose (antiinflammatory)
GLUCOCORTICOIDS Short acting, (Biological t½ < 12 hr)	1. Hydrocortisone (cortisol)	1	1	20 mg
Intermediate acting, (Biological t½ 12–36 hr)	2. Prednisolone 3. Methyl-prednisolone 4. Triamcinolone 5. Deflazacort	4 5 5 3–4	0.8 0.5 0 0	5 mg 4 mg 4 mg 6 mg
Long acting, (Biological t½ > 36 hr)	6. Dexamethasone 7. Betamethasone	25 25	0 0	0.75 mg 0.75 mg
MINERALO-CORTICOIDS				Equiv. salt retaining dose
	8. Desoxycortico-sterone acetate (DOCA) 9. Fludrocortisone 10. Aldosterone	0 10 0.3	100 150 3,000	2.5 mg (sublingual) 0.2 mg not used clinically

5. Dexamethasone Very potent and highly selective glucocorticoid. Long acting, causes marked pituitary-adrenal suppression, but fluid retention and hypertension are not a problem.

It is used for inflammatory and allergic conditions, shock, cerebral edema, etc.

6. Betamethasone Similar to dexamethasone. Dexamethasone or betamethasone are preferred in cerebral edema and other states in which fluid retention must be avoided.

7. Deflazacort It is a highly selective glucocorticoid, dose-to-dose slightly less potent than prednisolone, but lacks mineralocorticoid activity. It is claimed to produce fewer adverse effects and less growth retardation in children.

Adverse effects

Adverse effects are extension of the pharmacological action of corticosteroids that become prominent with prolonged therapy, and are a great limitation to their use in chronic diseases.

A. Mineralocorticoid Sodium and water retention, edema, hypokalaemic alkalosis and a progressive rise in BP is a consequence of mineralocorticoid action. This is infrequent now, because more selective glucocorticoids are generally used.

Gradual rise in BP occurs due to excess glucocorticoid action as well.

B. Glucocorticoid
1. Cushing's habitus: characteristic appearance with rounded face, narrow mouth, supraclavicular hump, obesity of trunk with relatively thin limbs.
2. Fragile skin, purple striae—easy bruising, telengiectasis, hirsutism. Cutaneous atrophy occurs with topical application of the steroid as well.
3. Hyperglycaemia, precipitation of diabetes.
4. Muscular weakness, especially of proximal limb muscles; myopathy occurs occasionally.
5. Susceptibility to infection; opportunistic infections with low-grade pathogens (*Candida*, etc.).

6. Delayed healing of wounds.
7. Peptic ulceration.
8. Osteoporosis: Specially involving vertebrae and other flat spongy bones.
9. Growth retardation: in children occurs even with small doses if given for long periods.
10. Foetal abnormalities: Cleft palate and other defects are produced in animals, but have not been encountered in pregnant women.
11. Psychiatric disturbances.
12. Suppression of hypothalamo-pituitary-adrenal (HPA) axis: occurs depending both on dose and duration of therapy. In time, adrenal cortex atrophies and stoppage of exogenous steroid precipitates a withdrawal syndrome producing malaise, anorexia, nausea, postural hypotension, weakness, etc. and reactivation of the disease. Subjected to stress, these patients may go into acute adrenal insufficiency.

Any patient who has received > 20– 25 mg/day hydrocortisone or equivalent such as ≥ 5 mg prednisolone/day for longer than 2–3 weeks should be put on a scheme of gradual withdrawal. Such patients may need protection with steroids if a stressful situation develops up to one year after withdrawal.

If a patient on corticosteroid therapy develops an infection—the *steroid should not be discontinued* despite its propensity to weaken host defence. Rather, the dose may have to be increased to meet the stress of the infection.

Measures that minimise HPA axis suppression are:
a. Use shorter acting steroids (hydrocortisone, prednisolone) at the lowest possible dose.
b. Use steroids for the shortest period of time possible.
c. Give the entire daily dose at one time in the morning.
d. Switch to alternate-day therapy if the condition does not deteriorate on the 'off' day.
e. If appropriate, use local (dermal, inhaled, ocular, nasal, buccal, rectal, intrasynovial) preparations.

Uses

Systemic as well as topical corticosteroids have one of the widest spectrum of medical uses for their anti-inflammatory and immunosuppressive properties. They are powerful drugs: have the potential to cause dramatic improvement in many severe diseases, but can produce equally serious adverse effects. Important conditions in which they are used are:

1. Collagen and autoimmune diseases, e.g. systemic lupus erythematosus, polyarteritis nodosa, nephrotic syndrome, glomerulonephritis, rheumatoid arthritis, rheumatic fever, acute gouty arthritis, haemolytic anaemia, thrombocytopenia, myasthenia gravis, etc.
2. Severe allergic reactions: Anaphylaxis, angioneurotic edema, urticaria, serum sickness.
3. Bronchial asthma: Majority of cases are treated with inhaled steroids. Other lung conditions benefited by corticosteroids are pulmonary edema, aspiration pneumonia, allergic rhinitis. Dexamethasone/betamethasone given to pregnant women before premature delivery, prevent respiratory distress syndrome in the neonate.
4. Eye diseases: Allergic conjunctivitis, iridocyclitis, keratitis, uveitis, retinitis, optic neuritis, etc.
5. Skin diseases: Mostly topical use in dermatitis; systemic steroids are needed in pemphigus vulgaris, exfoliative dermatitis, Stevens-Johnson syndrome and other serious disorders.

6. Inflammatory bowel disease: Ulcerative colitis, Crohn's disease.
7. Infective diseases: Only in serious/life-threatening infective diseases under effective antimicrobial cover, e.g. in bacterial/tubercular meningitis, miliary tuberculosis, severe lepra reaction, etc.
8. Neurological conditions: Like cerebral edema due to tubercular meningitis/ cerebral tumours, Bells' palsy, neurocysticercosis.
9. Malignancies: acute lymphatic leukaemia, Hodgkin's disease, lymphomas, etc.
10. Nausea and vomiting: Dexamethasone injected i.v. is used to augment the antiemetic effect of ondansetron against cancer chemotherapy induced vomiting.
11. Renal and other organ transplantation, skin allograft.
12. Substitution therapy in acute and chronic adrenal insufficiency and congenital adrenal hyperplasia.

Contraindications

The following diseases are aggravated by corticosteroids. Since steroids may have to be used as a life-saving measure, all of these are relative contraindications. In patients with these conditions, corticosteroids may be used only under compelling circumstances and with due precautions.

1. Peptic ulcer
2. Diabetes mellitus
3. Hypertension
4. Viral and fungal infections
5. Tuberculosis and other infections
6. Osteoporosis
7. Herpes simplex keratitis
8. Psychosis
9. Epilepsy
10. CHF
11. Renal failure.

Implications in dentistry

Application of corticosteroids in dental conditions is rather limited. Recurrent oral ulceration may be treated with topical steroids, but maintaining long enough contact between the steroid and the oral lesion is often difficult. Severe oral lesions like pemphigus, erosive lichen planus, etc. need to be treated with systemic corticosteroids. Pain from exposed dental pulp is occasionally treated with locally applied steroids. Intra-articular hydrocortisone may be injected in the temporomandibular joint to relieve refractory pain and stiffness. Only rarely a corticosteroid is needed to suppress pain and swelling due to dental surgery, (e.g. impacted third molar extraction), for which NSAIDs are the first line drugs.

In the case of patients who are/have been in recent past on long-term corticosteroid therapy, consideration has to be given to the need for supplementary prophylactic corticoid to cover a dental procedure. In general, simple extractions and other mildly traumatic surgeries do not warrant additional steroid dose. For traumatic procedures and those to be performed under general anaesthesia, supplementary steroids may be needed, particularly if the dose and duration of steroid therapy are such as to have caused significant adrenal suppression, or the patient is excessively anxious. Monitoring of BP of such patients during surgery is required. In case BP falls, hydrocortisone should be injected i.v. immediately.

Chapter 15

Hormones and Related Drugs-2
Androgens, Anabolic Steroids, Estrogens, Progestins and Contraceptives

The gonads produce steroidal hormones which have androgenic, estrogenic and progestational activities. Their synthetic analogues have similar or antagonistic actions and form an important class of drugs.

ANDROGENS (Male sex hormones)

These are substances which cause development of secondary sex characters in the castrated male. *Testosterone* produced by the testes is the principal androgen, a part of which is converted in extra-glandular tissues by the enzyme steroid 5α reductase to the more active compound *dihydrotestosterone*. Whereas in most target tissues dihydrotestosterone is the active androgen, testosterone itself is active at the spermatogenic (in testes) and erythropoietic (in bone marrow) cells, and for feedback inhibition of LH at the hypothalamic/pituitary site.

Actions

1. *Sex organs and secondary sex characters (Androgenic)* Testosterone is responsible for all the changes that occur in a boy at puberty: Growth of genitals—penis, scrotum, seminal vesicles, prostate.
Growth of hair—pubic, axillary, beard, moustache, body hair and male pattern of its distribution.
Thickening of skin, proliferation and increased activity of sebaceous glands—especially on the face, acne vulgaris. Larynx grows and voice deepens.
Behavioral effects are—increased physical vigour, aggressiveness, penile erections.

Testosterone is also important for the intrauterine development of the male phenotype.

2. *Testes* Testosterone is needed for normal spermatogenesis and maturation of spermatozoa. However, larger doses administered exogenously cause testicular atrophy by inhibiting Gn secretion from pituitary.

3. *Skeleton and skeletal muscles (Anabolic)* Testosterone is responsible for the pubertal spurt of growth in boys and to a smaller extent in girls. There is rapid bone growth. After puberty, the epiphyses fuse and linear growth comes to a halt. Testosterone also promotes muscle building, especially if aided by exercise. Appetite is improved and a sense of well-being prevails. There is accretion of nitrogen, minerals (Na, K, Ca, P, S) and water—body weight increases rapidly, more protoplasm is built.

4. *Erythropoiesis* Testosterone accelerates erythropoiesis by increasing erythropoietin production and probably direct action on haeme synthesis.

Mechanism of action Testosterone can largely be regarded as the circulating prohormone.

In most target cells its 4–5 double bond is reduced producing *dihydrotestosterone*, which binds more avidly with the cytoplasmic androgen receptor (AR). This complex migrates to the nucleus, combines with the 'androgen response elements', DNA transcription is enhanced or repressed, and the effects are expressed through modification of protein synthesis.

Pharmacokinetics

Testosterone is inactive orally due to high first pass metabolism in liver. Slowly absorbed esters of testosterone are used by the i.m. route. A transdermal gel formulation is also available.

The major metabolic products of testosterone are androsterone and etiocholanolone which are excreted in urine. Small quantities of estradiol are also produced from testosterone by aromatization of A ring in extraglandular tissues. Plasma t½ of testosterone is 10–20 min.

Side effects

1. Virilization and menstrual irregularities in women.
2. Acne: in males and females.
3. Frequent, sustained and often painful erections.
4. Oligozoospermia with moderate doses given for a few weeks.
5. Precocious puberty and shortening of stature.
6. Cholestatic jaundice: occurs with 17-alkyl substituted derivatives but not with parenterally used esters of testosterone.

Androgens accelerate growth of carcinoma prostate and that of male breast.

Uses

Testosterone is used for replacement therapy in case of primary or secondary testicular failure resulting in delayed puberty, loss of libido and impotence. However, impotence due to psychological and other factors, and not testosterone deficiency, does not respond.

The anabolic effect of testosterone can be used to improve weakness and muscle wasting in AIDS patients.

Attacks of hereditary angioneurotic edema can be prevented by 17α-alkylated androgens (methyltestosterone, stanozolol, danazol) but not by testosterone. They act by increasing synthesis of complement (C1) esterase inhibitor.

Anabolic steroids

These are synthetic androgens with supposedly higher anabolic and lower androgenic activity. However, the anabolic selectivity of these steroids is modest. Drugs are *Nandrolone, Oxymetholone, Stanozolol, Methandienone* and others.

The anabolic steroids have been used for osteoporosis in elderly males, in catabolic states like severe trauma, major surgery, during convalescence and in hypoplastic or malignancy associated anaemia. Use of anabolic steroids for promoting suboptimal growth in children is controversial. Misuse by athletes to enhance physical ability is illegal.

Antiandrogens

Cyproterone acetate This is a steroidal antiandrogen with progestational activity. It antagonises actions of testosterone, and in addition inhibits LH secretion by its progestational action. Cyproterone acetate can be used for precocious puberty in boys, inappropriate sexual behaviour in men, and for severe cases of acne vulgaris in women.

Flutamide It is a nonsteroidal androgen antagonist with no other hormonal activity. Flutamide competitively blocks androgen action on accessory sex organs as well as on pituitary—increases LH secretion by blocking feedback inhibition. Combined with castration or a GnRH agonist (to suppress LH secretion), it has been used for palliative therapy of advanced carcinoma prostate. Liver damage is reported.

Bicalutamide It is a longer acting and more potent congener of flutamide that is less hepatotoxic and better tolerated. As such, it is preferred over flutamide for palliative treatment of metastatic carcinoma prostate.

5 α-reductase inhibitor

Finasteride A competitive inhibitor of the enzyme 5 α-reductase which converts testosterone into more active dihydrotestosterone responsible for androgen action in many tissues including the prostate gland and hair follicles. During finasteride treatment testosterone levels remain unchanged: libido and potency are largely preserved.

Treatment with finasteride has resulted in decreased prostate size and increased peak urinary flow rate after few months in patients with symptomatic benign hypertrophy of prostate (BHP).

Concurrent treatment with α_1 adrenergic blocker + finasteride produces greater symptomatic relief.

Finasteride has also been found effective in male pattern baldness.

Dutasteride An exceptionally long acting (plasma t½ ~ 9 weeks) congener of finasteride which is, similarly useful in BHP and male pattern baldness.

ESTROGENS

The estrogens, its receptor agonists and antagonists, and synthesis blockers are classified in the following chart:

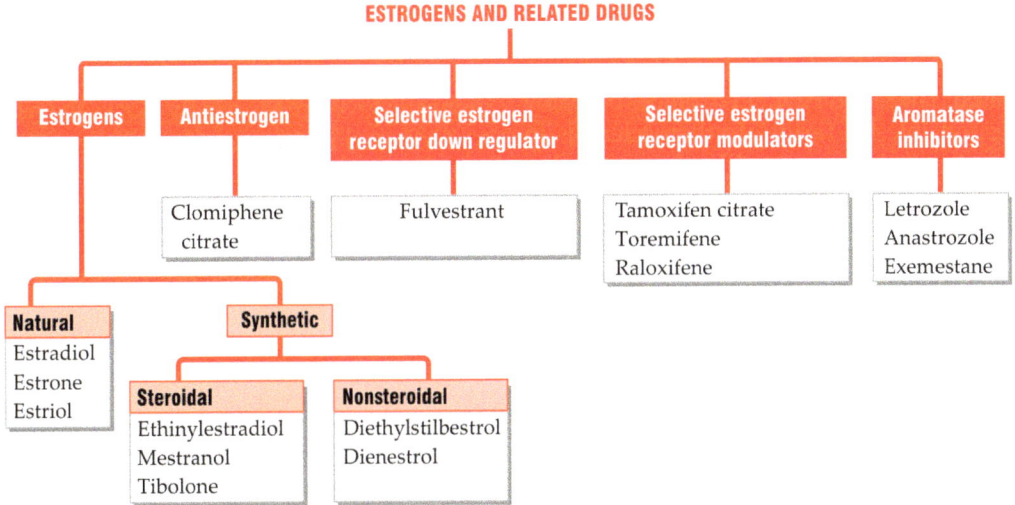

Estrogens are substances which can induce estrus in spayed (ovariectomised) animals.

Estradiol is the major estrogen secreted by the ovary. It is synthesized in the graafian follicle, corpus luteum and placenta from cholesterol.

Estradiol is rapidly oxidized in liver to *estrone* which is hydroxylated to form *estriol*. All three are found in the blood, but estrone and estriol have much lower affinity for the estrogen receptor (ER) than estradiol.

Natural estrogens are inactive orally and have a short duration of action due to rapid metabolism in the liver.

Actions

1. *Sex organs* The estrogens bring about pubertal changes in the female; promote growth of uterus, fallopian tubes and vagina. Vaginal epithelium gets thickened, stratified and cornified. Estrogens are responsible for the proliferation of endometrium in the preovulatory phase, and it is only in concert with estrogens that progesterone brings about secretory changes.

Estrogens increase rhythmic contractions of the fallopian tubes and uterus, and induce a watery alkaline secretion from the cervix which is favourable to sperm penetration. They also sensitize the uterus to oxytocin.

Deficiency of estrogens is responsible for the atrophic changes in the female reproductive tract that occur after menopause.

2. *Secondary sex characters* Estrogens produced at puberty cause growth of breasts. The pubic and axillary hair appear, feminine body contours and behaviour are influenced.

3. *Metabolic effects* Estrogens are anabolic, similar to but weaker than testosterone. Continued action of estrogen promotes fusion of epiphyses. They are important in maintaining bone mass primarily by retarding bone resorption and promoting positive calcium balance.

Estrogens decrease plasma LDL cholesterol while HDL and triglyceride levels are raised. The raised HDL : LDL ratio is probably responsible for rarity of atherosclerosis in premenopausal women. Blood coagulability is increased by estrogens due to induction of synthesis of clotting factors. They increase lithogenicity of bile.

Mechanism of action Estrogens act by binding to specific *estrogen receptors* (ERs) located normally in the nucleus of the target cells, thereby regulating protein synthesis through interaction with certain *coactivator* and *corepressor* proteins. Two distinct ERs designated ERα and ERβ have been identified which probably have different pattern of interaction with coactivators and corepressors.

Pharmacokinetics Estrogens are well absorbed orally and transdermally, but natural estrogens are inactive orally due to rapid metabolism in liver. Transdermal estradiol (Estradiol-TTS) bypasses first pass metabolism in the liver; the patch applied over skin is active for 3-4 days. Estradiol esters injected i.m. are slowly absorbed and exert prolonged action.

Natural estrogens (estradiol, estrone, estriol) are conjugated with glucuronic acid and sulfate—excreted in urine and bile. Considerable enterohepatic circulation occurs due to deconjugation in intestines and reabsorption.

Ethinylestradiol is metabolized very slowly. It is orally active and more potent.

Adverse effects Most of the adverse effects of estrogens are described with oral contraceptives (*see* p. 260).

In addition, adverse effects noted when use is made for other indications are:
1. Suppression of libido, gynaecomastia and feminization when given to males.
2. Fusion of epiphyses and reduction of adult stature when given to children.
3. In postmenopausal women, estrogens can increase the risk of endometrial carcinoma. A progestin given concurrently blocks the risk.
4. Increased incidence of breast cancer is a risk with higher doses.
5. Long-term estrogen therapy doubles the incidence of gallstones.
6. Estrogens increase the incidence of thromboembolic diseases.
7. Migraine and endometriosis may be worsened by estrogens.

Uses Currently, the two major uses of estrogens are as contraceptives and for hormone replacement therapy (HRT) in postmenopausal women. The dose of estrogen used for HRT is substantially lower than that for contraception.

Estrogen HRT is highly efficacious in suppressing the menopausal syndrome. Hot flushes, palpitation, mood changes and other symptoms are mitigated. HRT improves general physical, mental and sexual well being. Atrophic genital changes are arrested. The vulval and urinary symptoms are effectively relieved.

HRT restores calcium balance and further bone loss is prevented.

However, the benefits of long term HRT must be weighed against the risks (predisposition to endometrial/breast cancer, gallstones, venous thromboembolism, worsening of migraine, etc.) in individual women. Now HRT is generally restricted to a limited duration of 6–24 months in women below 60 years of age or within 10 years of menopause, and aimed only for relief of menopausal symptoms.

Other indications of estrogens are senile vaginitis, dysfunctional uterine bleeding (as adjuvant to progestin), and as substitution therapy for delayed puberty in girls.

Antiestrogen

Clomiphene citrate It acts as a pure estrogen antagonist in all human tissues and induces Gn secretion in women by blocking estrogenic feed-back inhibition of pituitary. In response, the ovaries enlarge and ovulation occurs if the ovaries are responsive to Gn. Antagonism of peripheral actions of estrogen results in hot flushes. Endometrium and cervical mucus may be modified.

The chief use of clomiphene is in infertility due to failure of ovulation. Many women who previously were amenorrhoeic or had anovular cycles conceive after clomiphene treatment.

Polycystic ovaries, multiple pregnancy, hot flushes are the adverse effects.

Selective estrogen receptor down-regulator

Fulvestrant It is a new drug designated as 'pure estrogen antagonist' or 'selective estrogen receptor downregulator' (SERD), which is used for palliative treatment of metastatic ER positive breast cancer in postmenopausal women, particularly those who have stopped responding to tamoxifen.

Selective estrogen receptor modulators (SERMs)

Tamoxifen citrate It acts as potent estrogen antagonist in breast carcinoma cells, blood vessels and at some peripheral sites, but as partial agonist in uterus, bone, liver and pituitary. Inhibition of human breast cancer cells and hot flushes reflect antiestrogenic action, while the weak estrogen agonistic action manifests as stimulation of endometrial proliferation, lowering of Gn and prolactin levels in postmenopausal women as well as improvement in their bone density. Similar to estrogen HRT, it increases the risk of deep vein thrombosis by 2–3 times.

Tamoxifen is used for hormonal treatment of breast cancer in both pre- and post-menopausal women. It is also approved for primary prophylaxis of breast cancer in high-risk women. However, endometrial thickening occurs and risk of endometrial carcinoma is increased 2 to 3-fold.

Side effects are hot flushes, vomiting, vaginal bleeding and menstrual irregularities.

Raloxifene This SERM is an estrogen partial agonist in bone, on lipid metabolism and cardiovascular system, but an antagonist in endometrium and breast.

Raloxifene prevents bone loss in postmenopausal women; bone mineral density (BMD) may even increase. It also reduces the risk of breast cancer.

Raloxifene does not stimulate endometrial proliferation and there is no increase in risk of endometrial carcinoma.

Hot flushes, leg cramps are mild side effects. The only serious concern is 3-fold increase in risk of deep vein thrombosis and pulmonary embolism.

Raloxifene is an alternative to HRT for prevention and treatment of osteoporosis in postmenopausal women. However, bisphosphonates are now the preferred drugs.

Aromatase inhibitors

Aromatization (introduction of double bonds) of 'A' ring in testosterone produces estradiol. Inhibition of the aromatase enzyme leads to arrest of estrogen production in the body, which can have palliative effect in breast cancer. *Letrozole, Anastrozole and Exemestane* are orally active aromatase inhibitors which have demonstrated clinical superiority over tamoxifen in the treatment of breast cancer. They also do not increase the risk of thromboembolism and endometrial cancer. While letrozole and anastrozole are nonsteroidal and reversible aromatase inhibitors, exemestane is a steroidal and irreversible inhibitor. They cause nearly total estrogen deprivation of breast carcinoma cells arresting their proliferation. Letrozole and anastrozole are now first line drugs for adjuvant therapy after mastectomy in early ER +ve breast cancer, as well as for palliative therapy in advanced cases. Hot flushes, vaginal dryness, nausea, dyspepsia, acceleration of bone loss and joint pain are the important side effects.

PROGESTINS

These are substances which convert the estrogen primed proliferative endometrium into secretory endometrium and maintain pregnancy in animals spayed after conception (*Progestin* = favouring pregnancy).

Progesterone, a 21 carbon steroid, is the natural progestin. It is secreted by the corpus luteum in the later half of menstrual cycle under the influence of LH. Its production declines a few days before the next menstrual flow. If the ovum gets fertilized and implants—the blastocyst immediately starts producing chorionic gonadotropin which is absorbed into maternal circulation and sustains the corpus luteum in early pregnancy. Placenta starts secreting lots of estrogens and progesterone from 2nd trimester till term.

A number of synthetic progestins which are active by the oral route have been produced. These are either progesterone derivatives (21 C) or 19-nortestosterone derivatives (18 C, also called 'estranes'). Estranes with 13-ethyl substitution are called 'gonanes', and are more potent. The progesterone derivatives are almost pure progestins, have weaker antiovulatory action and are used primarily as adjuvants to estrogens in HRT, as well as for threatened abortion, endometriosis, etc. Some of the 19-nortestosterone derivatives have additional weak estrogenic, androgenic, anabolic and potent antiovulatory action. They are used primarily in combined contraceptive pills.

Progesterone derivatives	
Medroxyprogesterone acetate	
Megestrol acetate	
Dydrogesterone	
Hydroxyprogesterone caproate	
Newer compound	
Nomegestrol acetate	

19-Nortestosterone derivatives	
Estranes	Gonanes
Norethindrone (Norethisterone)	Levonorgestrel
	Desogestrel
Lynestrenol (Ethinylestrenol)	Norgestimate
	Gestodene
Allylestrenol	

Actions

The main function of progesterone is preparation of uterus for nidation and maintenance of pregnancy. The latter is due to prevention of endometrial shedding, decreased uterine motility and inhibition of immunological rejection of the foetus, because progesterone depresses T-cell function and cell-mediated immunity (CMI).

1. Progesterone brings about secretory changes in the estrogen primed endometrium while epithelial proliferation is halted. It is withdrawal of progestational support which causes mucosal shedding during menstruation.

2. It converts the watery cervical secretion induced by estrogens to viscid, scanty and cellular secretion which is hostile to sperm penetration.

3. Progesterone induces pregnancy like changes in the vaginal mucosa. *The pregnancy associated increased incidence of gingival inflammation has been ascribed to high levels of progesterone.*
4. Progesterone causes proliferation of acini in the mammary glands. Acting in concert with estrogens, it prepares the breast for lactation. Withdrawal of these hormones after delivery causes release of prolactin from pituitary and milk secretion starts.
5. It causes a slight (0.5°C) rise in body temperature by resetting the hypothalamic thermostat and increasing heat production. This is responsible for the higher body temperature seen during the luteal phase.
6. Prolonged use of oral contraceptives impairs glucose tolerance in some women. This has been ascribed to the progestational component. Progestins tend to raise LDL and lower HDL cholesterol levels.
7. Progesterone is a weak inhibitor of Gn secretion from pituitary. Administration of progestin during follicular phase suppresses the preovulatory LH surge. Thus, it synergises with estrogen to prevent ovulation.

Progesterone acts by binding to the progesterone receptor (PR) located in the nucleus of the target cells, thereby regulating gene transcription. The distribution of PR in the body is restricted to the female genital tract, breast, CNS and pituitary.

Pharmacokinetics

Progesterone, unless specially formulated, is inactive orally because of high first pass metabolism in liver. It is mostly injected i.m. in oily solution. Even after an i.m. dose, it is rapidly cleared from plasma, has a short t½ (5–7 min). Progesterone is nearly completely degraded in the liver.

A micronized formulation of progesterone (referred to as '*natural progesterone*') has been developed for oral administration.

Most of the synthetic progestins are orally active and are metabolized slowly. They have plasma t½ ranging from 8–24 hours.

Adverse effects

- Breast engorgement, headache, rise in body temperature, esophageal reflux, and mood swings may occur with higher doses.
- Irregular bleeding or amenorrhoea can occur if a progestin is given continuously.
- Blood sugar may rise and diabetes may be precipitated.
- Long-term use of progestin in HRT may increase the risk of breast cancer.

Uses

1. *As contraceptive*: Most common use.
2. *Hormone replacement therapy (HRT)*: To counteract the risk of inducing endometrial carcinoma by the estrogen given alone.
3. *Dysfunctional uterine bleeding:* A progestin in relatively large doses promptly stops bleeding and keeps it in abeyance as long as given.
4. *Endometriosis:* This condition is due to the presence of ectopic endometrium; manifestations are dysmenorrhoea, painful pelvic swellings and infertility. Continued administration of progestins affords symptomatic relief.
5. *Threatened / habitual abortion:* Progestins are almost routinely prescribed, but benefit only when there is progestin deficiency.
6. *Endometrial carcinoma:* Progestins are palliative.
7. Progesterone treatment *may improve oral aphthous ulcers that are related to menstruation in women.*

Antiprogestin

Mifepristone It is a 19-norsteroid which acts as a potent progesterone antagonist with weak agonistic action in the absence of progesterone. In addition, mifepristone has significant antiglucocorticoid and antiandrogenic activity.

Given during the follicular phase, its antiprogestin action results in attenuation of the midcycle Gn surge from pituitary. This causes slowing of follicular development and delay/failure of ovulation. Given during the luteal phase, it prevents secretory changes normally brought about by progesterone. Later in the cycle, it blocks progesterone support to the endometrium, and stimulates uterine contractions by unrestraining PG release. Mifepristone also sensitizes myometrium to PGs and induces menstruation. If implantation has occurred, it blocks decidualization, so that the conceptus is dislodged and abortion occurs.

The antiglucocorticoid action is usually not manifest because antagonism of the negative feed-back at hypothalamic-pituitary level elicits ACTH release → plasma cortisol rises and overcomes the direct antiglucocorticoid action. Larger doses do ameliorate Cushing's syndrome.

Uses of mifepristone are:
1. Termination of pregnancy of up to 7 weeks.
2. To induce cervical ripening before attempting abortion/induction of labour.
3. As postcoital contraceptive within 72 hours of intercourse. It has also been tried as once-a-month contraceptive.
4. Cushing's syndrome: for its antiglucocorticoid property.

Ulipristal It is a newer *selective progesterone receptor modulator* developed for use as postcoital/emergency contraceptive. Given in the preovulatory phase, it suppresses LH surge and follicular rupture, while it interferes with implantation if given after ovulation has occurred. Some trials have found that ulipristal continues to act as postcoital contraceptive even when the drug is taken 5 days after intercourse. Thus, it may be an effective alternative to mifepristone or levonorgestrel, if the woman misses to take the drug within 72 hours of intercourse.

HORMONAL CONTRACEPTIVES

These are hormonal preparations used for reversible suppression of fertility.

Over 100 million women worldwide are currently using hormonal contraceptives. With these drugs, fertility can be suppressed at will, for as long as desired, with almost 100% confidence and complete return of fertility on discontinuation. The efficacy, convenience, low cost and overall safety of oral contraceptives (OCs) has allowed women to decide whether and when they want to become pregnant and to plan their activities. A variety of oral and parenteral preparations are now available offering individual choices.

The oral contraceptive preparations are listed in Table 15.1.

Types of methods

1. Combined pill It contains an estrogen and a progestin. With accumulated experience, it has been possible to reduce the amount of estrogen and progestin in the 'second generation' OC pills without compromising efficacy, but reducing side effects and complications. Ethinylestradiol 30 µg daily is considered threshold but can be reduced to 20 µg/day if a progestin with potent antiovulatory action (such as desogestrel) is included. While both estrogens and progestins synergise to inhibit ovulation, the progestin ensures prompt bleeding at the end of a cycle and blocks the risk of developing endometrial carcinoma due to the estrogen given alone. One tablet is taken daily for 21

Hormonal Contraceptives

Table 15.1: Oral contraceptive preparations

PROGESTIN		ESTROGEN		TRADE NAME
COMBINED PILLS				
1. Norgestrel	0.3 mg	Ethinylestradiol	30 µg	MALA–D (21 tabs + 7 ferrous sulfate 60 mg tabs)
2. Norgestrel	0.5 mg	Ethinylestradiol	50 µg	OVRAL-G 20 tabs
3. Levonorgestrel	0.25 mg	Ethinylestradiol	50 µg	OVRAL, DUOLUTON-L 21 tabs
4. Levonorgestrel	0.15 mg	Ethinylestradiol	30 µg	OVRAL-L, OVIPAUZ 21 tabs
5. Levonorgestrel	0.1 mg	Ethinylestradiol	20 µg	LOETTE, OVILOW, COMBEE 21 tabs
6. Desogestrel	0.15 mg	Ethinylestradiol	30 µg	NOVELON 21 tabs
7. Desogestrel	0.15 mg	Ethinylestradiol	20 µg	FEMILON 21 tabs
PHASED PILL				
1. Levonorgestrel	50–75 –125 µg	Ethinylestradiol	30–40 –30 µg	TRIQUILAR (6 + 5 + 10 tabs)
2. Norethindrone	0.5–0.75 –1.0 mg	Ethinylestradiol	35–35 –35 µg	ORTHONOVUM 7/7/7 (7 + 7 + 7 tabs)
POSTCOITAL PILL				
1. Levonorgestrel	0.25 mg	Ethinylestradiol	50 µg	OVRAL, DUOLUTON-L (2 + 2 tabs)
2. Levonorgestrel	0.75 mg 1.5 mg	-Nil -Nil-	—	NORLEVO, ECEE2 (1 + 1 tab)— iPILL, NOFEAR-72, OH GOD (1 tab)
MINI PILLS				
1. Norethindrone	0.35 mg	-Nil-	—	MICRONOR*, NOR-QD*
2. Norgestrel	75 µg	-Nil-	—	OVRETTE*

*Not marketed in India.

days, starting on the 5th day of menstruation. The next course is started after a gap of 7 days in which bleeding occurs. Thus, a cycle of 28 days is maintained. Calendar packs of pills are available. This is the most popular and most efficacious method.

2. Phased pill Triphasic pills have been introduced to permit reduction in total steroid dose. The estrogen dose is kept constant (or varied slightly between 30–40 µg), while the amount of progestin is low in the first phase and progressively higher in the second and third phases.

3. Progesterone only pill (Minipill) A low-dose progestin only pill is taken daily continuously without any gap. The menstrual cycle tends to become irregular and ovulation occurs in 20–30% women, but other mechanisms contribute to the contraceptive action. The efficacy of this pill is lower (96–98%) compared to 98–99.9% with the combined pill.

4. Postcoital (emergency) pill
This is for use in a woman not taking any contraceptive, who has a sexual intercourse risking unwanted pregnancy.
Currently 3 regimens are in use:
(a) Levonorgestrel 0.75 mg 2 doses taken at 12 hour interval (or 1.5 mg single dose) within 72 hours of unprotected intercourse. This is the most popular method; recommended by WHO as well.
(b) Mifepristone 600 mg single dose taken within 72 hours of intercourse.
(c) Ulipristal 30 mg single dose as soon as possible, but within 120 hours of intercourse.

Emergency postcoital contraception should be reserved for unexpected or accidental exposure (rape, condom rupture) only and not practiced routinely.

Injectable These have been developed to obviate the need for daily ingestion of pills. The contraceptives are injected i.m. as oily solution, and are highly effective.

Two *long acting progestin* only injections are in use. These are:

(a) Depot medroxyprogesterone acetate (DMPA) 150 mg at 3-month intervals.

(b) Norethindrone (Norethisterone) enanthate (NEE) 200 mg at 2-month intervals. The most important drawback is complete disruption of menstrual bleeding pattern and total amenorrhoea in many cases.

Mechanism of action

Hormonal contraceptives interfere with fertility in many ways. The relative importance of each mechanism depends on the type of method.

1. Inhibition of Gn release from pituitary. When the combined pill is taken, release of both FSH and LH is reduced and the midcycle LH surge is abolished. As a result, follicles fail to develop and fail to rupture— *ovulation does not occur*. This is the primary mechanism of action of the combined pill.

2. Thick *cervical mucus* secretion *hostile to sperm penetration* is evoked by progestin action. This mechanism operates with all types of pills except in case of postcoital pill.

3. Even if ovulation and fertilization occur, the blastocyst may fail to implant because *endometrium* is *out of phase* with fertilization, and is not suitable for nidation. This action is most important in case of progestin only pill and postcoital pill.

4. *Uterine and tubal contractions* may be modified to disfavour fertilization.

5. The postcoital pill may *dislodge* a just implanted blastocyst.

Adverse effects

Since contraceptives are used in otherwise healthy and young women, adverse effects, especially long-term consequences, assume great significance. The present-day low-dose preparations carry relatively minor risk.

A. Nonserious side effects
These are frequent, especially in the first 1–3 cycles and then disappear gradually.

1. Nausea and vomiting.
2. Headache; migraine may be precipitated or worsened.
3. Breakthrough bleeding or spotting. Amenorrhoea may occur in few.
4. Breast discomfort.

B. Side effects that appear later
1. Weight gain, acne and increased body hair.
2. Chloasma: pigmentation of cheeks.
3. Pruritus vulvae.
4. Carbohydrate intolerance and precipitation of diabetes.
5. Mood swings, abdominal distention.

C. Serious complications
1. *Leg vein thrombosis and pulmonary embolism*: Significant risk in women >35 years of age, diabetics, hypertensives and in those who smoke.
2. *Coronary and cerebral thrombosis* resulting in *myocardial infarction or stroke*: A 2 to 6-fold increase in risk was estimated earlier, when relatively higher dose pills were used. However, recent studies have found no increased incidence with the low dose pills in the absence of other risk factors.
3. *Rise in BP*: This again is less frequent and smaller in magnitude with the low-dose pills of today.
4. *Genital carcinoma*: Risk of developing genital carcinoma is increased in predisposed individuals but not in the general population.

Growth of already existing hormone-dependent tumour may be hastened.

Epidemiological data has recorded minor increase in breast cancer incidence among current OC users.

5. *Gallstones:* Incidence of gallstones is slightly higher in women on OCs.

Contraindications

The combined oral contraceptive pill is absolutely contraindicated in:
1. Thromboembolic, coronary and cerebrovascular disease or a history of it.
2. Moderate-to-severe hypertension; hyperlipidaemia.
3. Active liver disease, hepatoma or h/o jaundice during past pregnancy.
4. Suspected/overt malignancy of genitals/breast.
5. Impending major surgery—to avoid postoperative thromboembolism.

Interactions Contraceptive failure may occur if the following drugs are used concurrently:

(a) *Enzyme inducers:* phenytoin, phenobarbitone, primidone, carbamazepine, rifampin.

(b) *Suppression of intestinal microflora:* tetracyclines, ampicillin, etc. When these antibiotics are given orally, deconjugation of estrogens excreted in bile does not occur. As a result, their enterohepatic circulation is interrupted → blood level of the drugs fall and ovulation may occur.

Ormeloxifene (Centchroman) It is a nonsteroidal SERM developed at CDRI, India as an oral contraceptive. By antiestrogenic action, it suppresses endometrial proliferation. The contraceptive effect appears to be due to utero-embryonic asynchrony and failure of implantation, while pituitary-ovarian functions are largely unaffected. However, failure rate is higher than with combined estrogen-progestin pill. Ormeloxifene is also approved for reducing dysfunctional uterine bleeding.

16

Hormones and Related Drugs-3
Thyroid Hormone and Thyroid Inhibitors, Hormones Regulating Calcium Balance

THYROID HORMONE

The thyroid gland secretes 3 hormones—thyroxine (T_4), triiodothyronine (T_3) and calcitonin. The former 2 are produced by thyroid follicles, have similar biological activity and the term 'thyroid hormone' is restricted to these only. *Calcitonin* produced by interfollicular 'C' cells is chemically and biologically entirely different. It regulates calcium metabolism.

Chemistry, synthesis and metabolism

Both T_4 and T_3 are iodine containing derivatives of *thyronine* which is a condensation product of two molecules of the amino acid *tyrosine*.

The thyroid hormones are synthesized and stored in the thyroid follicles as part of *thyroglobulin* molecule—which is a glycoprotein. The synthesis, storage and release of T_4 and T_3 is summarized in Fig. 16.1 and involves the following processes:

1. Iodide uptake into the thyroid by active transport through Na^+: Iodide symporter (NIS) which is activated by thyroid stimulating hormone (TSH).
2. Oxidation of the trapped iodide by thyroid peroxidase enzyme to forms of iodine *viz*. iodinium ions (I^+), hypoiodous acid (HOI) or enzyme-linked hypoiodate (E-OI) which combine avidly with tyrosil residues of thyroglobulin to form monoiodotyrosine (MIT) and diiodotyrosine (DIT).
3. Coupling of MIT and DIT with the aid of the same peroxidase enzyme to form T_3 and T_4.
4. Storage of T_3, T_4, MIT and DIT residues containing thyroglobulin as thyroid colloid in the interior of the follicles till it is taken back into the cells by endocytosis and broken down by lysosomal proteases. The T_4 and T_3 so released are secreted into the circulation.
5. Peripheral conversion of a portion of T_4 into T_3 by deiodination in several tissues, especially liver and kidney.

Thyroid hormones are avidly bound to plasma proteins—only 0.03–0.08% of T_4 and 0.2–0.5% of T_3 are in the free form.

Only the free hormone is available for action as well as for metabolism and excretion. Metabolic inactivation of T_4 and T_3 occurs by deiodination and glucuronide/sulfate conjugation of the hormones as well as of their deiodinated products. Liver is the primary site. The conjugates are excreted in bile. A significant fraction of this is deconjugated in intestines and reabsorbed (enterohepatic circulation) to be finally excreted in urine.

Plasma t½ of T_4 is 6–7 days, while that of T_3 is 1–2 days.

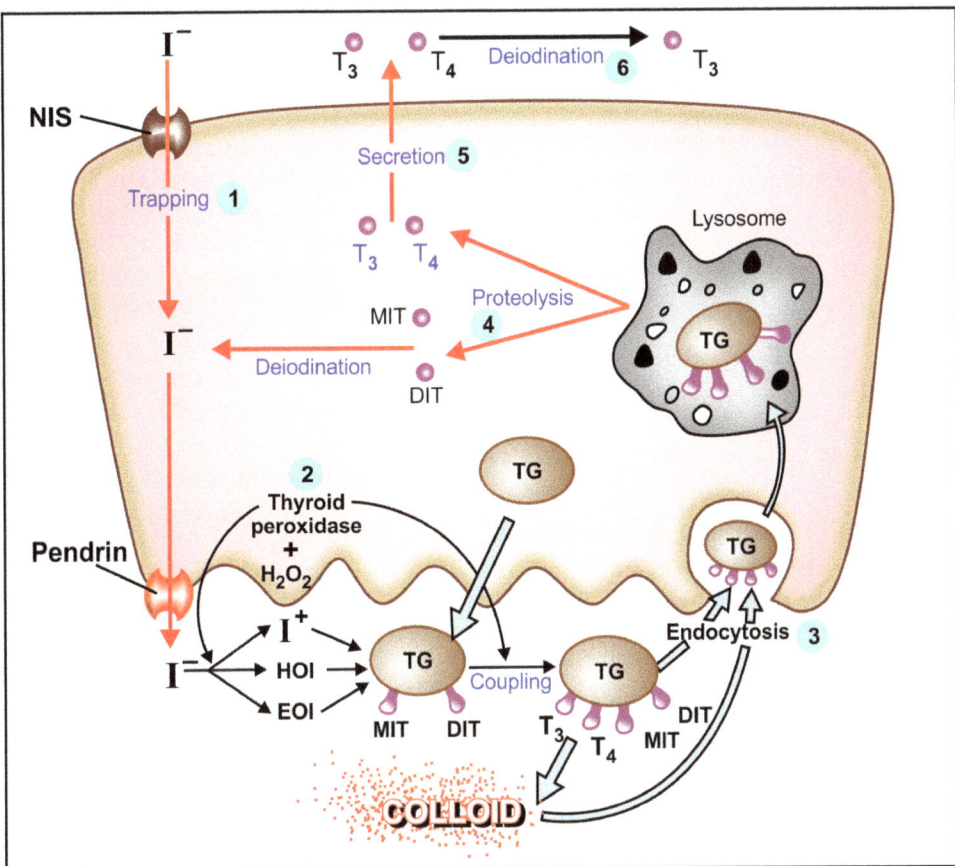

Fig. 16.1: Synthesis, storage and secretion of thyroid hormone
TG—Thyroglobulin; MIT—Monoiodotyrosine; DIT—Diiodotyrosine; T_3—Triiodothyronine; T_4—Thyroxine (Tetraiodothyronine); HOI—Hypoiodous acid; EOI—Enzyme-linked hypoiodate; NIS–Na^+ iodide symporter
Thyroid-stimulating hormone (TSH) activates steps 1, 2, 3, 4, and 5; Ionic inhibitors block step 1; Excess iodide interferes with steps 1, 2, 3 and 5 with primary action on step 3 and 5; Propylthiouracil inhibits steps 2 and 6; Carbimazole inhibits step 2 only.

Actions

The actions of T_4 and T_3 are qualitatively similar and are nicely depicted in the features of hypo- and hyperthyroidism. These hormones affect the function of practically everybody cell.

1. *Growth and development* T_4 and T_3 are essential for normal growth and development. The action is exerted through a critical control of protein synthesis in the translation of the genetic code. Congenital deficiency of T_4 and T_3 resulting in cretinism emphasizes their importance. The milestones of development are delayed and practically every organ and tissue of the body suffers. The greatest sufferer, however, is the nervous system. Retardation and nervous deficit is a consequence of paucity of axonal and dendritic ramification, synapse formation and impaired myelination. In adult hypothyroidism also, intelligence is impaired and movements are slow.

2. *Intermediary metabolism* Thyroid hormones have marked effect on lipid, carbohydrate and protein metabolism. Lipolysis and cholesterol metabolism are accelerated, more cholesterol is converted to bile acids.

Though utilization of sugar by tissues is increased, glycogenolysis and gluconeogenesis in liver more than compensate it causing hyperglycaemia and diabetes like state.

Synthesis of certain proteins is increased, but the overall effect of T_3 is catabolic—increased amounts of protein being used as energy source. Prolonged action results in negative nitrogen balance and tissue wasting.

3. *Calorigenesis* T_3/T_4 increase BMR by stimulation of cellular metabolism and resetting of the energystat. This is important for maintaining body temperature.

4. *Organ systems* Heart rate, cardiac contractility and output are increased resulting in a fast, bounding pulse. T_3/T_4 stimulate heart by direct action on contractile elements as well as by upregulation of β adrenergic receptors. Atrial fibrillation and other irregularities are common in hyperthyroidism. Angina and CHF may be precipitated due to the hyperdynamic state of circulation.

The T_3/T_4 have profound functional effect on CNS. Mental retardation is the hallmark of cretinism; sluggishness and other behavioral features are seen in myxoedema. Hyperthyroid individuals are anxious, nervous, excitable, exhibit tremors and hyperreflexia.

Muscles are flabby and weak in myxoedema, while thyrotoxicosis produces increased muscle tone. Propulsive activity of gut is increased by T_3/T_4. Hypothyroid patients are often constipated, while diarrhoea is common in hyperthyroidism. Thyroid hormones are facilitatory to erythropoiesis and reproduction.

Mechanism of action T_3 (and T_4) penetrate cells by active transport and combine with

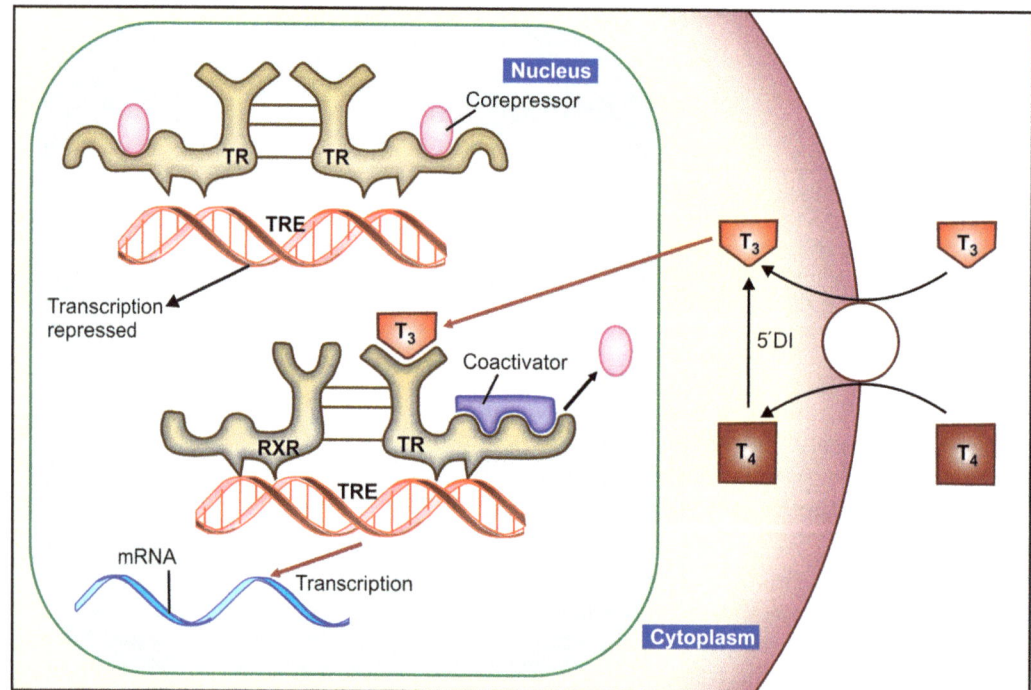

Fig. 16.2: Mechanism of action of thyroid hormone on nuclear thyroid hormone receptor (TR) T_3—Triiodothyronine; T_4—Thyroxine; TRE—Thyroid hormone response element; RXR—Retinoid X receptor; mRNA—Messenger ribonucleic acid; 5'DI—5'Deiodinase (See text for explanation).

a nuclear thyroid hormone receptor (TR). A specific DNA sequence called *'thyroid hormone response element'* has been identified in the regulatory region of specific genes to which the T_3-receptor complex binds causing derepression of gene transcription or in some cases direct activation of gene transcription (Fig. 16.2). This results in expression of predetermined genetically coded pattern of protein synthesis producing various metabolic and anatomic effects.

Many of the manifestations, e.g. tachycardia, arrhythmias, raised BP, tremor, hyperglycaemia are mediated, at least partly, by sensitization of adrenergic receptors to catecholamines. In the thyrotoxic patient, *Adr mixed local anaesthetic should be avoided for dental anaesthesia.*

Because T_3 binds more avidly to the intracellular receptor and is 5 times more potent as well as faster acting than T_4, in most tissues, it is the major active hormone, while T_4 is mainly the transport form or prohormone.

Uses The most important uses of thyroid hormone are as *replacement therapy* in cretinism (congenital hypothyroidism) and myxoedema (adult hypothyroidism). Levothyroxine (T_4) given orally is the preparation of choice and the benefits are most gratifying. Nontoxic goiter is due to relative thyroid hormone deficiency which triggers excess TSH secretion—causing thyroid enlargement, more efficient iodide trapping and T_3 synthesis, so that enough hormone to meet peripheral demand is produced, and the patient is clinically not hypothyroid. Treatment with T_4 normalises TSH level and tends to regress the goiter if the enlargement was recent and diffuse. Endemic goiter and endemic cretinism can be prevented by iodizing table salt.

Thyroxine has palliative effect in certain benign functioning thyroid nodules and in papillary carcinoma of thyroid by lowering TSH levels. Myxoedema coma is an emergency that is treated with l-thyroxine (T_4) injected i.v. followed by oral dosing. Due to higher risk of arrhythmias and angina, i.v. liothyronine (T_3) is not employed now, though it acts faster.

THYROID INHIBITORS

These are drugs used to lower the functional capacity of the hyperactive thyroid gland.

Thyrotoxicosis is due to excessive secretion of thyroid hormones. The two main causes are Graves' disease and toxic nodular goiter. Graves' disease is an autoimmune disorder in which IgG class of antibodies are produced which bind to the TSH receptor and stimulate thyroid cells, as well as produce other TSH like effects. Due to feedback inhibition, TSH levels are low.

Toxic nodular goiter, which produces thyroid hormone independent of TSH, mostly supervenes on old nontoxic goiters.

Thioamides (Antithyroid drugs)

By convention, the synthesis inhibitors are also called 'antithyroid drugs', though this term should apply to all thyroid inhibitors.

The thioamides bind to the thyroid peroxidase and prevent oxidation of iodide and iodotyrosyl residues, thereby;

(i) Inhibit iodination of tyrosine residues of thyroglobulin molecule.
(ii) Inhibit coupling of iodotyrosine residues to form T_3 and T_4.

Thyroid colloid is gradually depleted and blood level of T_4/T_3 is lowered. Effects of antithyroid drugs are not apparent till the thyroid is depleted of its hormone content.

Propylthiouracil inhibits peripheral conversion of T_4 to T_3 as well. This may partly contribute to its effects. Methimazole and carbimazole do not have this action.

Pharmacokinetics All antithyroid drugs are quickly absorbed orally, widely distributed in the body, enter milk and cross placenta, are

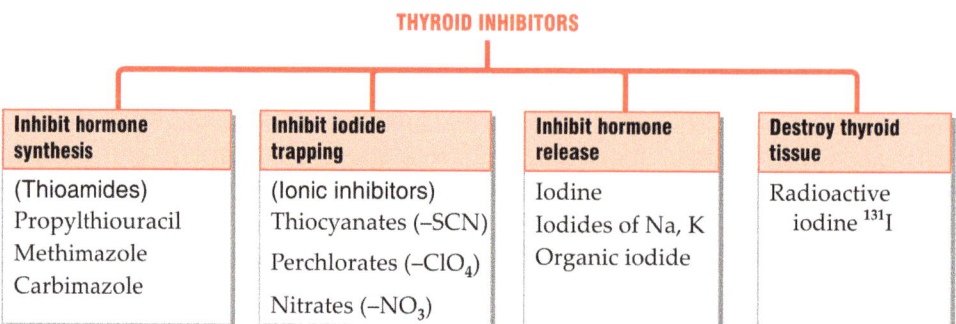

metabolized in liver and excreted in urine, primarily as metabolites.

Adverse effects Hypothyroidism and goiter can occur due to overtreatment, but this is reversible on stopping the drug.

Important side effects are: g.i. intolerance, skin rashes and joint pain. Liver damage is infrequent.

A rare but serious adverse effect is agranulocytosis.

Use Thioamide antithyroid drugs control thyrotoxicosis in both Graves' disease as well as in toxic nodular goiter. Clinical improvement starts after 1–2 weeks or more and may take 1–3 months for full control. These drugs may be used for short periods before partial thyroidectomy (surgery in thyrotoxic patient is risky) or while awaiting response to radioactive iodine. Thioamides can also be used as definitive therapy at lower (maintenance) doses for long periods.

Ionic inhibitors These monovalent ions inhibit iodide trapping by thyroid cells so that T_3/T_4 cannot be synthesized. However, they are toxic and not used clinically.

Iodine and iodides

Though iodine is a constituent of thyroid hormone, it is the fastest acting thyroid inhibitor. Iodine is reduced in the intestines to iodide and the response to iodine or iodides is identical. In Graves' disease the gland, if enlarged, shrinks, becomes firm and less vascular. The thyroid status starts returning to normal at a rate commensurate with complete stoppage of hormone release from the gland. Peak effects are seen in 10–15 days, after which 'thyroid escape' occurs, T_3/T_4 synthesis resumes and thyrotoxicosis may return with greater vengeance.

All facets of thyroid function seem to be affected, but the most important action is inhibition of hormone release. Endocytosis of colloid and proteolysis of thyroglobulin comes to a halt.

In thyrotoxicosis, iodine is primarily used for about 10 days just preceding thyroid surgery to make the gland firm, less vascular and easier to operate on, as well as to somewhat reduce thyrotoxicosis symptoms. It is not employed for long term treatment of hyperthyroidism. Iodine may also be given to stop thyroid storm.

Incidence of endemic goiter in iodine deficient areas has been reduced by iodizing table salt.

Potassium iodide is an expectorant. Tincture iodine is used externally as an antiseptic.

Adverse effects Long-term ingestion of high doses of iodine/iodides can cause hypothyroidism and goiter. Chronic overdose also results in inflammation of mucous membranes. An acute reaction consisting of swelling of lips, eyes, angioedema, fever, thrombocytopenia, etc. can develop in sensitive individuals.

Radioactive iodine

The stable isotope of iodine is ^{127}I. Its radioactive isotope ^{131}I has a physical half-life of 8 days, and this isotope is most commonly used in medicine.

^{131}I emits γ-rays as well as β particles. The former are useful in tracer studies, while the latter are utilized for their destructive effect on thyroid cells. ^{131}I is concentrated by thyroid and incorporated in the colloid. Thus, it emits radiation from within the follicles. The β particles penetrate only 0.5–2 mm of tissue. The thyroid follicular cells are affected from within, undergo pyknosis and necrosis followed by fibrosis when a sufficiently large dose has been administered, without damage to neighbouring tissues. With carefully selected doses, it is possible to achieve partial ablation of thyroid.

Radioactive iodine is used as sodium salt of ^{131}I dissolved in water and taken orally.

Diagnostic 25–100 µ curie is given; counting or scanning is done at intervals. No damage to thyroid cells occurs at this dose.

Therapeutic The most common indication of ^{131}I is hyperthyroidism. The average therapeutic dose is 3–6 m curie. This is calculated on the basis of previous tracer studies and thyroid size. The response is slow—starts after 2 weeks and gradually increases, reaching peak at 3 months or so.

Treatment with ^{131}I is simple, conveniently given on outpatient basis and inexpensive. Once hyperthyroidism is controlled, cure is permanent.

The biggest disadvantage of ^{131}I therapy is development of life-long hypothyroidism in many recipients, especially of Graves' disease. Long latent period of response is another drawback. Radioactive iodine may be palliative in metastatic carcinoma of thyroid.

β-Adrenergic blockers

Propranolol (and other nonselective β blockers) have emerged as an important form of therapy to rapidly alleviate manifestations of thyrotoxicosis that are due to sympathetic overactivity *viz.* palpitation, tremor, nervousness, severe myopathy, sweating. They are valuable in thyroid storm as well. However, they have little effect on thyroid function and the hypermetabolic state. Thus, they are used for symptomatic relief only while awaiting response to carbimazole or ^{131}I, and along with iodine before subtotal thyroidectomy.

HORMONES REGULATING CALCIUM

CALCIUM

After C, O, H and N, calcium is the 5th most abundant body constituent, making up about 2% of body weight: 1–1.5 kg in an adult. About 98% of this is stored in bones (and teeth), the rest being distributed in the plasma, all tissues and cells, and serves important physiological roles.

1. Calcium controls excitability of nerves and muscles and regulates permeability of cell membranes and cell adhesion.

2. Ca^{2+} ions are essential for excitation-contraction coupling in all types of muscles and excitation-secretion coupling in exocrine and endocrine glands, release of transmitters from nerve ending and other release reactions.

3. Ca^{2+} is an intracellular messenger for hormones, autacoids and transmitters.

4. Ca^{2+} controls impulse generation in heart—determines level of automaticity and A-V conduction.

5. Ca^{2+} is essential for coagulation of blood.
6. Calcium serves structural function in bone and teeth; abnormalities of calcium balance affect teeth indirectly.

Plasma calcium level is precisely regulated by 3 hormones almost exclusively devoted to this function viz. *parathormone* (PTH), *calcitonin* and *calcitriol* (active form of vit D). These regulators control its intestinal absorption, exchange with bone and renal excretion as summarized in Fig. 16.3. In addition, glucocorticoids, sex steroids, thyroid hormone and growth hormone affect calcium homeostasis as secondary regulators.

Normal plasma calcium is 9–11 mg/dl. Of this, about 40% is bound to plasma proteins—chiefly albumin; 10% is complexed with citrate, phosphate and carbonate in an undissociable form; the remaining (about 50%) is ionized and physiologically important.

Calcium turnover Major fraction of calcium in the bone is stored as crystalline hydroxyapatite deposited on the organic bone matrix *osteoid*, while a small labile pool is in dynamic equilibrium with plasma. Even the fully laid down parts of the bone undergo constant *remodeling* by way of two closely coupled but directionally opposite processes of resorption and new bone formation (Fig. 16.4). Millions of tiny remodeling units are working on the surface of bone trabeculae and Haversian canals to dig micropits by osteoclastic activity and then repair by osteoblastic activity. Initially collagen and other proteins (osteoid) are deposited in the micropits, followed by mineralization; the full cycle taking 4–6 months.

Absorption and excretion Calcium is absorbed by facilitated diffusion from the entire small intestine. In addition, a carrier-mediated active transport operates in the duodenum under the influence of vit D. Phytates, phosphates, oxalates, tetracyclines, glucocorticoids and phenytoin reduce calcium absorption.

Ionized calcium is totally filtered at the glomerulus and most of it is reabsorbed in the tubules. Vit D increases and calcitonin decreases proximal tubular reabsorption, while PTH increases distal tubular reabsorption of Ca^{2+}. About 300 mg of endogenous calcium is excreted daily: half in urine and half in faeces. To maintain calcium balance, the same amount has to be absorbed in the small intestine

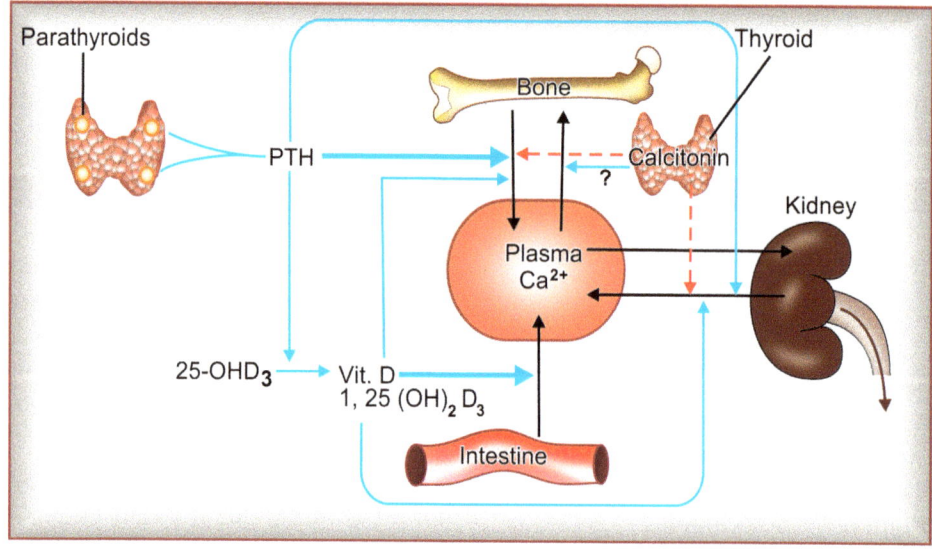

Fig. 16.3: Regulation of plasma level of calcium
⎯→ stimulation, ⎯ ⎯ ⎯→ Inhibition; Bold arrow—major action.
PTH—Parathormone; 25-OHD$_3$—Calcifediol; 1,25 (OH)$_2$D$_3$—Calcitriol

from the diet. Because normally only 1/3rd of ingested calcium is absorbed, the dietary allowance for calcium is 0.8–1.5 g per day. Calcium is administered as one of its salts.

1. *Calcium carbonate* (40% Ca) is the most commonly used salt. It is insoluble, tasteless and nonirritating, but gastric acid is required to convert it into the absorbable chloride salt; systemic availability may be low. It also acts as antacid.
2. *Calcium citrate* (as tetrahydrate, 21% Ca) dissolves well in the presence of HCl, is better absorbed and is nonirritating.
3. *Calcium gluconate* (9% Ca) It is used both as oral tablets and as 10% solution for slow i.v. injection, which is nonirritating to the vascular endothelium, but imparts a sense of warmth.
4. *Calcium dibasic phosphate* (23% Ca) It is also insoluble, nonirritating and requires gastric HCl for absorption.

Side effects Calcium supplements are usually well tolerated; only g.i. side effects like constipation, bloating and excess gas have been reported.

Use

1. *As dietary supplement* especially in growing children, pregnant, lactating and menopausal women. *Abnormalities of dentition can be reduced by avoiding calcium deficiency.*
2. *Osteoporosis* Calcium + vit D_3 have adjuvant role to HRT/raloxifene/bisphosphonates in prevention and treatment of osteoporosis.
3. To prevent and treat tetany which occurs due to hypocalcaemia.
4. As antacid (Calcium carbonate).

PARATHYROID HORMONE (Parathormone)

Parathyroid hormone (PTH) is the hypercalcaemic hormone. It is a single chain 84 amino acid polypeptide, MW 9,500. Secretion of PTH is regulated by plasma Ca^{2+} concentration; there is no trophic hormone for it. Fall in plasma Ca^{2+} induces PTH release and rise inhibits secretion. Changes in plasma phosphate concentration affect PTH secretion indirectly by altering Ca^{2+} concentration.

PTH raises plasma calcium levels by:

1. Increasing resorption of calcium from bone (Fig. 16.4). This is the most prominent action of PTH.
   PTH enhances proliferation and differentiation of preosteoblasts and deposition of osteoid as well. Bone resorption predominates when high concentrations of PTH are present continuously, but intermittent exposure to low concentrations has the opposite effect.
2. Increasing calcium reabsorption in the distal tubule. PTH also promotes phosphate excretion which tends to supplement the hypercalcaemic effect.
3. Enhancing the formation of calcitriol (active form of vit D) in the kidney, which then increases intestinal absorption of calcium.

Hypoparathyroidism Manifestations are:
Low plasma calcium levels, tetany, convulsions, laryngospasm, paresthesias, cataract and psychiatric changes. Pseudohypoparathyroidism occurs due to reduced sensitivity of target cells to PTH. Hypoparathyroidism is treated with Vit D, because PTH has to be given parenterally and is expensive.

Hyperparathyroidism It is mostly due to parathyroid tumour. It produces:
Hypercalcaemia, decalcification of bone—deformities and fractures (osteitis fibrosa generalisata), metastatic calcification, renal stones, muscle weakness, constipation and anorexia.

Treatment It is surgical removal of the parathyroid tumour.

Cinacalcet It is an orally active calcimimetic compound which activates Ca^{2+} sensing receptor in the parathyroids and decreases PTH secretion. Cinacalcet is indicated in secondary hyperparathyroidism due to renal disease, and for inoperable cases of parathyroid cancer.

Teriparatide It is a recombinant preparation of 1-34 amino acids of human PTH which duplicates the actions of PTH, and has been approved for the treatment of severe osteoporosis.
Teriparatide is short acting (plasma t½ after s.c. injection is 1 hour). Injected once daily, it acts intermittently, and the bone forming action predominantes over bone resorbing action. As such, it increases bone mineral density in osteoporotic women and men. Teriparatide

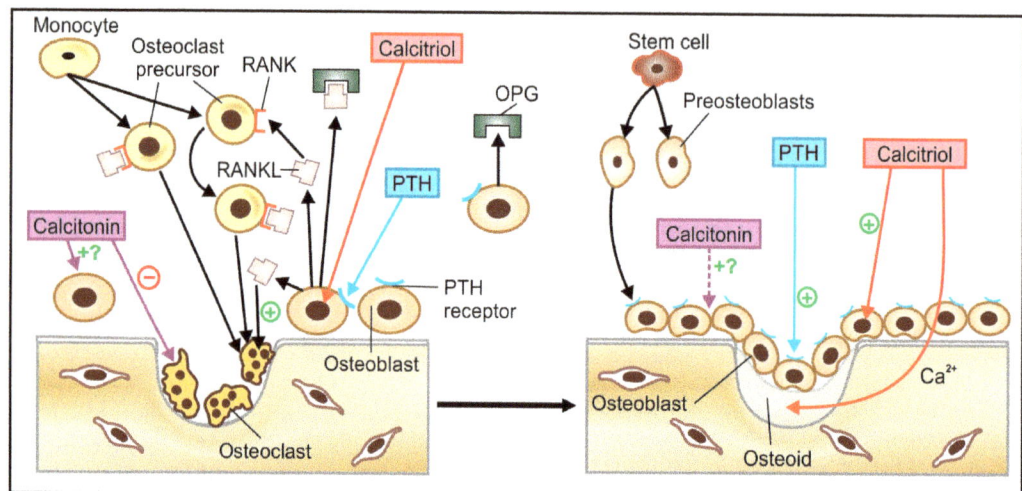

Fig. 16.4: Hormonal regulation of bone remodeling unit
The monocyte osteoclast precursor cells in the marrow near the bony surface are activated to proliferate and fuse to form multinucleated osteoclasts. The osteoclast-precursors express a 'receptor for activation of nuclear factor-κ B' (RANK) on their surface. The osteoblasts on activation release a protein RANK-ligand (RANKL). When RANKL is bound to RANK on the surface of osteoclast-precursors they are transformed into mature osteoclasts and develop bone lysing ruffled surface. A bone resorption pit is dug out by secretion of acid and proteolytic acid hydrolases.

Osteoblasts produce another protein osteoprotegerin (OPG) as well, which can bind RANKL and prevent it from combining with RANK to activate osteoclasts. Thus, osteoblasts by producing RANKL and OPG regulate bone resorption.

After formation of the remodeling pit, preosteoblasts from bone marrow stem cells proliferate, migrate to the base of the pit, transform into mature osteoblasts and laydown new osteoid, which is later mineralized.

Parathormone (PTH) acts on PTH-receptor located on the osteoblast membrane and induces RANKL production—indirectly activating osteoclast differentiation and function. Subsequently PTH promotes new bone formation as well.

Calcitriol also induces RANKL in osteoblasts to indirectly activate osteoclasts. Similarly, it promotes laying of osteoid as well as bone mineralization.

Calcitonin directly inhibits osteoclast function and probably enhances osteoblastic new bone formation.

is the only agent which stimulates bone formation, and acts faster than bisphosphonates, that only check bone resorption. Teriparatide reduces risk of minimal trauma fractures in osteoporotic men as well as women.

CALCITONIN

Calcitonin is the hypocalcaemic hormone. It is a 32 amino acid single chain polypeptide (MW 3,600) produced by parafollicular 'C' cells of thyroid gland.

Synthesis and secretion of calcitonin is regulated by plasma Ca^{2+} concentration itself: rise in plasma Ca^{2+} increases, while fall in plasma Ca^{2+} decreases calcitonin release. However, the physiological role of calcitonin in regulating plasma Ca^{2+} appears to be minor. The plasma t½ of calcitonin is 10 min, but its action lasts for ~ 8 hours.

The actions of calcitonin are generally opposite to that of PTH.

Calcitonin inhibits bone resorption by direct action on osteoclasts—decreasing their ruffled surface which forms contact with the resorptive pit.

Calcitonin inhibits proximal tubular calcium and phosphate reabsorption by direct action on the kidney.

Calcitonin is rarely used clinically; indications are Paget's disease of bone and hypercalcaemic states like hypervitaminosis D, osteolytic bony metastasis, etc. It has to be injected i.m. or s.c.

A nasal spray formulation of calcitonin has been used for postmenopausal osteoporosis, but is not recommended now.

VITAMIN D

Vitamin D is the collective name given to antirachitic substances synthesized in the body and found in foods activated by UV radiation.

Vit D_3: cholecalciferol — synthesized in the skin under the influence of UV rays.

Vit D_2: calciferol—present in irradiated food—yeasts, fungi, bread, milk.

In man, vit D_2 and D_3 are equally active and *calcitriol* (active form of D_3) is more important physiologically. Calcifediol (25-OH-D_3) is released in blood from liver. Its final hydroxylation in kidney is the rate limiting step and is controlled by many factors. This step is activated or induced by calcium deficiency and/or vit D deficiency, as well as by PTH, estrogens and prolactin, while calcitriol inhibits it in a feedback manner.

Thus, vit D should be considered a hormone because:
(a) It is synthesized in skin: (under ideal conditions, it is not required in diet).
(b) It is transported by blood, activated in the body and then acts on specific receptors in target tissues.
(c) Feedback regulation of vit D activation occurs by plasma Ca^{2+} level and by the active form itself.

Actions

1. Calcitriol enhances absorption of calcium and phosphate from *intestine*. This is brought about by increasing synthesis of calcium channels and a carrier protein for Ca^{2+} called 'calcium binding protein' (Ca BP) or Calbindin. Calcitriol acts in the same manner as the steroid hormones; *i.e.* it binds to a cytoplasmic receptor → translocates to the nucleus → increases synthesis of specific mRNA → regulation of protein synthesis. At least part of vit D action is quick (within minutes) and, therefore, appears to be exerted by mechanisms not involving gene regulation.

2. Calcitriol enhances resorption of calcium and phosphate from *bone* to raise its plasma concentration. It appears to help bone mineralization indirectly by maintaining normal plasma calcium and phosphate level. Calcitriol also activates osteoblastic cells to lay down osteoid. Its action is independent of but facilitated by PTH.

3. It enhances tubular reabsorption of both calcium and phosphate in *kidney*.

Vit D deficiency Plasma calcium and phosphate tend to fall due to inadequate intestinal absorption. As a consequence, PTH is secreted which mobilizes calcium from bone in order to restore plasma Ca^{2+} level. The bone fails to mineralize normally in the newly laid area, becomes soft producing rickets in children

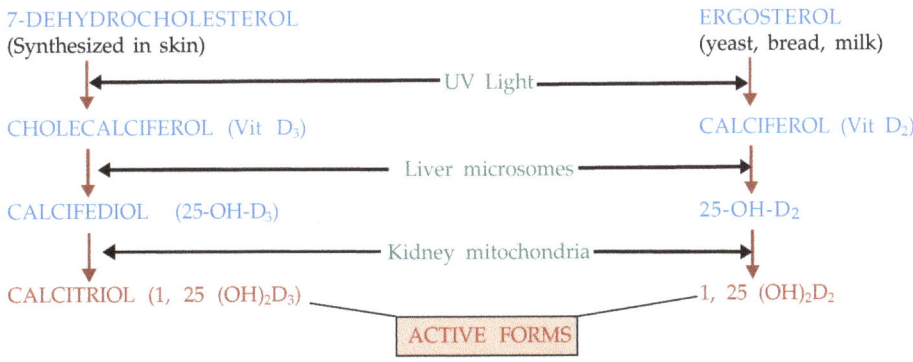

and osteomalacia in adults. However, in contrast to osteoporosis, the organic matrix (osteoid) is normal in osteomalacia.

Retarded development of mandible, delayed/faulty eruption of teeth and defective tooth enamel are the dental complications of vit D deficiency.

Hypervitaminosis D It may occur due to chronic ingestion of large doses (~50,000 IU/day) or due to increased sensitivity of tissues to vit D. Manifestations are due to elevated plasma calcium and its ectopic deposition.

Hypercalcaemia, weakness, fatigue, vomiting, diarrhoea, sluggishness, polyuria, albuminuria, ectopic Ca^{2+} deposition (in soft tissues, blood vessels, parenchymal organs), renal stones, hypertension and growth retardation in children.

Treatment: consists of withholding the vitamin, low calcium diet, plenty of fluids and corticosteroids.

Pharmacokinetics Vit D is well absorbed from intestines in the presence of bile salts. Malabsorption and steatorrhoea interfere with its absorption.

In the circulation, it is bound to a specific α globulin and is stored in the body, mostly in adipose tissues, for many months. It is hydroxylated in liver to both active and inactive metabolites. The t½ of different forms of vit D varies from 1–18 days: 25-OHD$_3$ (calcifediol), having the longest t½, constitutes the primary circulating form. Metabolites of vit D are excreted mainly in bile.

1 µg of cholecalciferol = 40 IU of vit D.

The daily requirement of vit D varies, depending on exposure to sunlight. It is estimated that if no vit D$_3$ is synthesized in the body, a dietary allowance of 400 IU/day will prevent deficiency symptoms.

Use

1. *Prophylaxis* (400 IU/day) and *treatment* (3,000–4,000 IU/day) of *nutritional vit D deficiency:* Vit D is used to prevent as well as to treat rickets in children and osteomalacia in adults.

2. *Metabolic rickets* These are a group of conditions in which tissues do not respond to normal doses of vit D. The active forms of vit D *Calcitriol* or *Alfacalcidol*, which do not need hydroxylation by kidney, are effective in these conditions.

3. *Senile or postmenopausal osteoporosis* Age-related decrease in calcium absorption from gut has been noted. Vit D$_3$ + calcium have been shown to improve calcium balance in osteoporotic females as well as in elderly males. However, benefit in terms of improved bone mass or reduced fracture risk is marginal, unless combined with bisphosphonate therapy.

4. *Hypoparathyroidism* Calcitriol/alfacalcidol are more effective than vit D$_2$ or D$_3$ because they act quickly and directly without the need for hydroxylation in kidney which needs PTH.

Interactions Long-term treatment with phenytoin and phenobarbitone can cause rickets/osteomalacia, probably by reducing tissue response to calcitriol.

BISPHOSPHONATES

Bisphosphonates (BPNs) are analogues of pyrophosphate in which carbon atom replaces oxygen in the P-O-P skeleton. They inhibit bone resorption and have attracted considerable attention because of their ability to prevent and check osteoporosis in addition to their usefulness in metabolic bone diseases and hypercalcaemia. They are the most effective antiresorptive drugs. Chronologically and according to potency, the BPNs can be grouped into 3 generations (*see* box). Only the second and third generation BPNs, which have higher efficacy and additional mode of action, are used now.

The BPNs have strong affinity for calcium phosphate, therefore exert selective action in calcified tissue by getting internalized into osteoclasts alongwith Ca^{2+} ions in the bone remodeling pit. They affect isoprenoid lipid synthesis as well. The net result is:

- Accelerated apoptosis of osteoclasts reducing their number.
- Disruption of cytoskeleton and ruffled border of osteoclasts.

In addition, BPNs appear to affect osteoclast precursors and inhibit their differentiation by suppressing IL-6. Interference with mevalonate pathway may also impart antitumor action on bony metastasis.

The BPNs are useful in conditions characterized by enhanced bone turnover.

1. *Osteoporosis* The second and third generation BPNs (alendronate, ibandronate, risedronate) are the most effective oral drugs for preventing and treating postmenopausal osteoporosis in women as well as idiopathic and steroid-induced osteoporosis in both men and women. Risk of vertebral and hip fracture is reduced by about 50%.

BPNs (along with Calcium + Vit D) may have adjuvant value in the treatment of *teeth attrition* or *tooth decay* due to osteoporosis, particularly in postmenopausal women.

Bisphosphonate	Relative potency
First generation BPN	
Etidronate	1
Second generation BPNs	
Pamidronate	100
Alendronate	100–500
Ibandronate	500–1000
Third generation BPNs	
Risedronate	1000
Zoledronate	5000

Bisphosphonate

2. *Paget's disease* This disease due to abnormal osteoclast function producing disordered bone architecture is benefited by BPNs. These drugs arrest osteolytic lesions, reduce bone pain and improve secondary symptoms.

3. *Osteolytic bone metastasis* Parenteral pamidronate/zoledronate arrest osteolytic lesions and reduce bone pain (most commonly secondary to prostate cancer). Potent BPNs, especially zoledronate, have shown independent antitumour property.

4. *Hypercalcaemia of malignancy* Pamidronate or zoledronate injected i.v. after repletion of plasma volume normalise plasma Ca^{2+} level in this medical emergency.

Alendronate, ibandronate and risedronate are oral BPNs used mainly in osteoporosis. They are to be taken on empty stomach in the morning with plenty of water once a week. The patient is instructed not to lie down or take food for at least 30 min, to prevent contact of the BPN with esophageal mucosa to avoid esophagitis. Calcium or iron preparations or NSAIDs should not be administered with these drugs. The oral bioavailability of alendronate and risedronate is only 1%, but they get sequestrated in bone with terminal elimination t½ of ~10 years. In osteoporosis they conserve bone mineral density and cutdown risk of fracture by ~50%.

Pamidronate and Zoledronate are administered only by i.v. infusion. They are indicated in bony metastasis, hypercalcaemia of malignancy and in Pagets' disease. Zoledronate is more potent in suppressing osteoclastic activity and can be infused i.v. over a shorter time than pamidronate. In case of bony metastasis from prostate/breast cancer and in multiple myeloma, zoledronate exerts additional antitumour effect by interfering with mevalonate pathway. Bone pain and a flu-like reaction are the common adverse effects.

CHAPTER 17

Drugs Affecting Blood

HAEMATINICS

Haematinics are substances required in the formation of blood, and are used for treatment of anaemias.

Anaemia occurs when the balance between production and destruction of RBCs is disturbed by:
(a) Blood loss (acute or chronic).
(b) Impaired red cell formation due to:
- Deficiency of essential factors, i.e. iron, vitamin B_{12}, folic acid.
- Bone marrow depression (hypoplastic anaemia), erythropoietin deficiency.
(c) Increased destruction of RBCs (haemolytic anaemia).

IRON

Iron is an essential body constituent. Total body iron in an adult is 2.5–5 g (average 3.5 g). It is more in men (50 mg/kg) than in women (38 mg/kg) and is distributed into:

Haemoglobin (Hb)	62%
Iron stores as ferritin and haemosiderin	25%
Myoglobin (in muscles)	7%
Parenchymal iron (enzymes, etc.)	6%

To raise the Hb level of blood by 1 g/dl—about 200 mg of elemental iron is needed. Though the primary reflection of iron deficiency occurs in blood, severe deficiency affects practically every cell. Oral ulceration, stomatitis, glossitis may even be early manifestations of iron deficiency. The daily iron requirement is:

Adult male	:	0.5–1 mg (13 µg/kg)
Adult female	:	1–2 mg (21 µg/kg)
Infants	:	60 µg/kg
Children	:	25 µg/kg
Pregnancy	:	3–5 mg (80 µg/kg).

Iron absorption, transport and excretion

Iron absorption occurs all over the intestine, but major portion in the upper part. Dietary iron is present either as heme or as inorganic iron. Heme iron is absorbed better (up to 35%) and without the aid of a carrier (Fig. 17.1), than inorganic (~5% absorbed), but the former is a smaller fraction of the dietary iron. Inorganic iron is mostly in the ferric form; needs to be reduced to ferrous form before it can be absorbed. Two separate iron transporters in the intestinal mucosal cells function to effect iron absorption. At the luminal membrane the *divalent metal transporter* 1 (DMT1) carries ferrous iron into the mucosal cell. This along with the iron released from heme is transported across the basolateral membrane by another iron transporter *ferroportin* (FP). These iron transporters are regulated according to the body needs. Absorption of heme iron is largely independent of other foods simultaneously ingested, but that of inorganic iron is affected by several factors. Gastric acid, reducing substances (ascorbic acid) and amino acids facilitate iron absorption, while antacids,

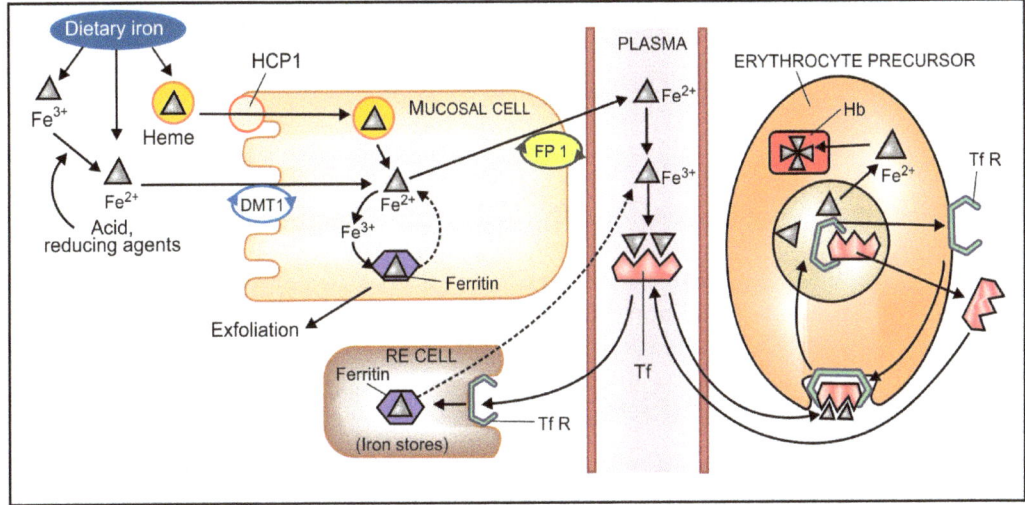

Fig. 17.1: Schematic depiction of intestinal absorption, transport, utilization and storage of iron
Fe^{2+}—Ferrous iron; Fe^{3+}—Ferric iron; DMT1—Divalent metal transporter 1; HCP1—Heme carrier protein 1; Hb—Haemoglobin; RE cell—Reticuloendothelial cell; FP1—Ferroportin; Tf—Transferrin; TfR—Transferrin receptor

tetracyclines, phosphates and phytates impede iron absorption.

Mucosal block The gut has a mechanism to prevent entry of excess iron in the body. Iron reaching inside mucosal cell is either transported to plasma or oxidised to ferric form and complexed with apoferritin to form ferritin (Fig. 17.1). This ferritin generally remains stored in the mucosal cells and is lost when they are shed (lifespan 2–4 days). This is called the 'Ferritin Curtain'.

The iron status of the body and erythropoietic activity govern the balance between these two processes, a larger percentage is absorbed during iron deficiency.

Because free iron is highly toxic, it is carried in blood in combination with a glycoprotein *transferrin (Tf)*. Iron is transported inside the cells through attachment of transferrin to specific membrane bound transferrin receptors (TfRs). In iron deficiency the erythron becomes selectively more efficient in trapping iron. Iron is stored in RE cells in liver, spleen, bone marrow, also in hepatocytes and myocytes as ferritin and haemosiderin. Plasma iron derived from destruction of old RBCs (lifespan–120 days), from iron stores and from intestinal absorption forms a common pool that is available for erythropoiesis and to all other cells as well as for restorage.

Oral iron preparations

The preferred route of iron administration is oral in the form of dissociable ferrous salts.
1. Ferrous sulfate: (hydrated salt 20% iron, dried salt 32% iron) is the cheapest. It often leaves a metallic taste in the mouth.
2. Ferrous gluconate (12% iron).
3. Ferrous fumarate (33% iron): is less water soluble than ferrous sulfate but tasteless.
4. Colloidal ferric hydroxide (50% iron).

Other forms of iron present in oral formulations are:

Ferrous succinate (35% iron)
Iron calcium complex (5% iron)
Ferric ammonium citrate (20% iron)
Ferric hydroxy polymaltose
Ferrous aminoate (10% iron)

Carbonyl iron (metallic iron in very fine powder form)

These compounds of iron are claimed to be better absorbed and/or produce less bowel upset, but this is primarily due to lower iron content.

The elemental iron content and not the quantity of iron compound per dose unit should be taken into consideration.

A total of 200 mg elemental iron (infants and children 3–5 mg/kg) given daily in 3 divided doses produces the maximal haemopoietic response. Prophylactic dose is 30 mg iron daily.

Adverse effects of oral iron These are common and related to the elemental iron content of the formulation, but individuals differ in susceptibility.

Epigastric pain, heart burn, nausea, vomiting, bloating, staining of teeth, metallic taste are the common side effects.

Constipation is more common (believed to be due to astringent action of iron) than diarrhoea (thought to reflect irritant action). However, these side effects may be caused by alteration of intestinal flora as well.

Parenteral iron preparations

Iron therapy by injection is indicated only when:
1. Oral iron is not tolerated: bowel upset is too much.
2. Failure to absorb oral iron.
3. Non-compliance to oral iron.
4. In presence of severe deficiency with chronic bleeding.
5. Along with erythropoietin: to meet the accelerated demand.

The rate of response with parenteral iron is not faster than that with optimal doses given orally provided such oral doses are tolerated by the patient. However, stores can be replenished in a shorter time by parenteral therapy.

Four organically complexed iron preparations are now available for i.m. or i.v. injection.

1. *Iron-dextran* It is a high molecular weight colloidal solution containing 50 mg elemental iron/ml. It is generally given i.m. using Z track technique to avoid staining of overlying skin. Absorption occurs through lymphatics. Iron-dextran can also be injected i.v., either 2 ml daily injections or by i.v. infusion of total dose over 6–8 hours. Local pain, abscess formation at i.m. injection site, fever, flushing, palpitation, chest pain and anaphylactoid reaction are the adverse effects.

2. *Ferrous-sucrose* This newer formulation is a high molecular weight complex of iron hydroxide for slow i.v. injection (not i.m.) once daily to once weekly. It is better tolerated and safer than the older formulation. Side effects are mild and incidence of hypersensitivity reaction is low.

3. *Ferric carboxymaltose* Another new formulation containing ferric hydroxide in a macromolecular carbohydrate shell. On i.v. injection it is taken up into RE cells and then delivered to the erythropoietic cells. Side effects are milder and anaphylactoid reaction is infrequent.

4. *Iron isomaltoside-100* This is the latest injectable iron formulation. After i.v. injection, it is rapidly taken up into the RE cells, and then slowly released for utilization by erythropoeitic cells. The remarkable feature of this formulation is that a large single i.v. dose (1–2 g) can be injected over 15–30 min, permitting correction of full iron deficit by a single short duration infusion. Alternatively, 100–200 mg may be injected over 5 min daily. Iron isomaltoside-1000 is well tolerated, and has low immunogenicity. Adverse effects are nausia, epigastric pain and abdominal cramps. Anaphylactoid reaction is very rare.

Use

Prophylaxis and treatment of iron deficiency anaemia is the most important indication for medicinal iron. A rise in Hb level by 0.5–1 g/dl per week is an optimum response to iron therapy. Treatment should be continued till normal Hb level is attained (generally takes 1–3 months depending on the severity) and 2–4 months thereafter to replenish the stores, because after correction of anaemia, iron absorption is slow.

Prophylactic administration of supplemental iron is routinely advised during later part of pregnancy and to infants. It may also be needed in menorrhagic women and during chronic illnesses.

Iron is given in megaloblastic anaemia along with vit B_{12}/folic acid so that existing iron deficiency may not be unmasked when brisk haemopoiesis is induced by the maturation factors.

Ferric chloride is used in throat paint as an astringent.

Maturation factors

VITAMIN B_{12}

Cyanocobalamin and hydroxocobalamin are complex cobalt containing compounds present in the diet and referred to as vit B_{12}.

Vit B_{12} occurs as water soluble, thermostable red crystals. It is synthesized in nature only by microorganisms; plants and animals acquire it from them. Vit B_{12} is synthesized by the colonic microflora, but this is not available for absorption in man.

Daily requirement: is 1–3 µg; during pregnancy and lactation it is 3–5 µg.

Metabolic functions Vit B_{12} is intricately linked with folate metabolism in many ways; megaloblastic anaemia occurring due to deficiency of either is indistinguishable. In addition, vit B_{12} has some independent metabolic functions as well. The active coenzyme forms of B_{12} generated in the body are deoxyadenosyl-cobalamin (DAB_{12}) and methyl-cobalamin (methyl B_{12}).

(i) Vit B_{12} is essential for the conversion of homocysteine to methionine

$$\text{methyl-THFA} \rightarrow \text{B}_{12} \rightarrow \text{methionine}$$
$$\text{THFA} \leftarrow \text{methyl-B}_{12} \leftarrow \text{homocysteine}$$

Methionine is needed as a methyl group donor in many metabolic reactions and for protein synthesis. This reaction is also critical in making tetrahydrofolic acid (THFA) available for reutilization. In B_{12} deficiency THFA gets trapped in the methyl form and a number of *one carbon* transfer reactions suffer.

(ii) Purine and pyrimidine synthesis is affected primarily due to defective 'one carbon' transfer because of 'folate trap'. The most important of these is nonavailability of thymidylate for DNA production.

(iii) Malonic acid $\xrightarrow{DAB_{12}}$ Succinic acid: is an important step in propionic acid metabolism. This reaction does not require folate.

(iv) Deoxyadenosyl B_{12} is needed for the reaction:

Methionine $\xrightarrow{DAB_{12}}$ S-adenosyl methionine

Interference with this reaction may be responsible for the neurological damage of B_{12} deficiency, because it is needed in the synthesis of phospholipids and myelin.

(v) Vit B_{12} is essential for cell growth and multiplication.

Utilization of vit B_{12} Intrinsic factor (a glycoprotein) secreted by stomach is essential for the absorption of B_{12} ingested in physiological amounts. The B_{12}-intrinsic factor complex attaches to specific mucosal receptors and is internalized by an active carrier. In the blood, B_{12} is transported in combination with a specific β globulin *transcobalamin II* (TCII).

Vit B_{12} is not degraded in the body. It is excreted mainly in bile (3–7 µg/day), all but 0.5–1 µg of this is reabsorbed. Thus, in the absence of intrinsic factor or when there is malabsorption, B_{12} deficiency develops much more rapidly than when it is due to nutritional deficiency.

Vit B_{12} is completely absorbed after i.m. or deep s.c. injection. Normally, only traces of B_{12} are excreted in urine, but when pharmacological doses (> 100 µg) are given orally or parenterally—a large part is excreted in urine.

Deficiency B_{12} deficiency occurs due to absence of intrinsic factor secretion by stomach (pernicious anaemia in which there is autoimmune gastric mucosal damage). Chronic gastritis, gastric carcinoma, malabsorption, increased demand or nutritional deficiency are the other causes.

Manifestations of deficiency are:
(a) Megaloblastic anaemia, neutrophils with hypersegmented nuclei, giant platelets.
(b) Glossitis, g.i. disturbances: damage to epithelial structures.
(c) Neurological: subacute combined degeneration of spinal cord; peripheral neuritis, paresthesias, depressed stretch reflexes; mental changes—poor memory, mood changes, hallucinations, etc.

Uses
1. Prevention and treatment of B_{12} deficiency: Confirmed B_{12} deficiency should be treated by i.m./s.c injection of cyanocobalamin/ hydroxocobalamin because its absorption from oral route is not reliable. When B_{12} deficiency is due to lack of intrinsic factor (pernicious anaemia, gastric carcinoma, etc.), it must be given parenterally to bypass the defective absorptive mechanism. It is wise to add 1–5 mg of oral folic acid and an iron preparation, because reinstitution of brisk haemopoiesis may unmask deficiency of these factors. Prophylactic oral cyanocobalamin needs to be given only to subjects at risk of developing B_{12} deficiency.
2. Mega doses of B_{12} have been used in neuropathies, psychiatric disorders, cutaneous sarcoid and as a general tonic to allay fatigue, improve growth. Value of such use is questionable.

Methylcobalamine, an active coenzyme form of vit B_{12} has been especially advocated for neurological defects in diabetic and other forms of neuropathy.

FOLIC ACID

Chemically, it is *Pteroyl glutamic acid (PGA)* consisting of pteridine + paraaminobenzoic acid (PABA) + glutamic acid. Folic acid occurs as yellow crystals.

Daily requirement of an adult is < 0.1 mg, but dietary allowance of 0.2 mg/day is recommended. During pregnancy, lactation or any condition of high metabolic activity, 0.8 mg/day is considered appropriate.

Utilization Small, physiological amounts of folic acid are absorbed by specific carrier-mediated active transport in the intestinal mucosa. Large pharmacological doses may gain entry by passive diffusion, but only a fraction is absorbed.

Folic acid is rapidly extracted by tissues and stored in cells as polyglutamates. Liver takes up a large part and secretes methyl-THFA in bile which is mostly reabsorbed. Normally, only traces are excreted, but when pharmacological doses are given, 50–90% of a dose may be excreted in urine.

Metabolic functions Folic acid is inactive as such and is reduced to the coenzyme form in two steps: FA → DHFA → THFA by folate reductase (FRase) and dihydrofolate reductase (DHFRase) enzymes. THFA mediates a number of one carbon transfer reactions by carrying a methyl group as an adduct.

1. Conversion of homocysteine to methionine.
2. Generation of thymidylate, an essential constituent of DNA:

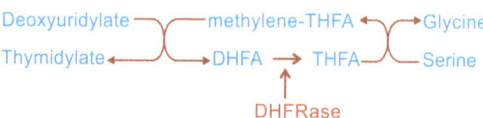

3. Conversion of serine to glycine: needs THFA and results in the formation of methylene-THFA which is utilized in thymidylate synthesis.
4. Purine synthesis: *de novo* building of purine ring requires formyl-THFA and methenyl-THFA.
5. Generation and utilization of 'formate pool'.
6. Histidine metabolism.

Deficiency Folate deficiency occurs due to:
(a) Inadequate dietary intake
(b) Malabsorption: coeliac disease, tropical sprue, regional ileitis, etc.
(c) Chronic alcoholism.

(d) Increased demand: pregnancy, lactation, rapid growth periods, haemolytic anaemia.
(e) Drug induced: prolonged therapy with anticonvulsants (phenytoin, phenobarbitone, primidone) and oral contraceptives which interfere with absorption and storage of folate.

Manifestations of deficiency are:
(i) Megaloblastic anaemia, indistinguishable from that due to B_{12} deficiency.
(ii) Epithelial damage: glossitis, enteritis, diarrhoea, steatorrhoea.
(iii) General debility, weight loss, sterility.

Uses
1. *Megaloblastic anaemia* due to nutritional folate deficiency and that occurring due to increased folate demand, or malabsorption or antiepileptic therapy can be treated by oral folic acid, but in acutely ill patients, it may be injected initially.

Folic acid should never be given alone to patients with B_{12} deficiency, because haematological response may occur, but neurological defect may progress due to diversion of meagre amount of B_{12} present in body to haemopoiesis.

2. *Prophylaxis* of folate deficiency: when definite predisposing factors are present. Routine folate supplementation is advised during pregnancy to reduce the risk of neural tube defects in the newborn.

3. *Methotrexate toxicity*: Folinic acid (Leucovorin, citrovorum factor, 5-formyl-THFA) which is an active coenzyme form, is used in this condition. Methotrexate is a DHFRase inhibitor; its toxicity is not counteracted by folic acid, but antagonized by folinic acid.

4. *Citrovorum factor rescue*: In certain malignancies, high dose of methotrexate is injected i.v. and is followed within ½–2 hours with 1–3 mg i.v. of folinic acid to rescue the normal cells.

COAGULANTS

These are substances which promote coagulation, and are indicated in haemorrhagic states.

Haemostasis (arrest of blood loss) and blood coagulation involve complex interactions between the injured vessel wall, platelets and coagulation factors. A cascading series of proteolytic reactions (Fig. 17.2) is started by:
(i) Contact activation of Hageman factor: *intrinsic system*, in which all factors needed for coagulation are present in the plasma. Blood kept in a glass tube clots through this pathway. It is slow and takes several minutes to activate factor X.
(ii) Tissue thromboplastin: *extrinsic system*, needs a tissue factor, but activates factor X in seconds. Coagulation after injury to vessel wall occurs normally by this pathway.

The subsequent events are common in the two systems and result in the formation of fibrin meshwork in which blood cells are trapped and clot is formed.

Most clotting factors are proteins present in plasma in the inactive (zymogen) form. By partial proteolysis, they themselves become active proteases and activate the next factor. On the other hand, factors like *antithrombin, protein C, antithromboplastin* and the *fibrinolysin system* tend to oppose coagulation and lyse formed clot. Thus, a check and balance system operates to maintain blood in a fluid state while in circulation and allows rapid haemostasis following injury.

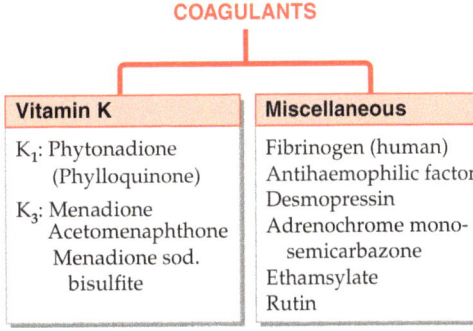

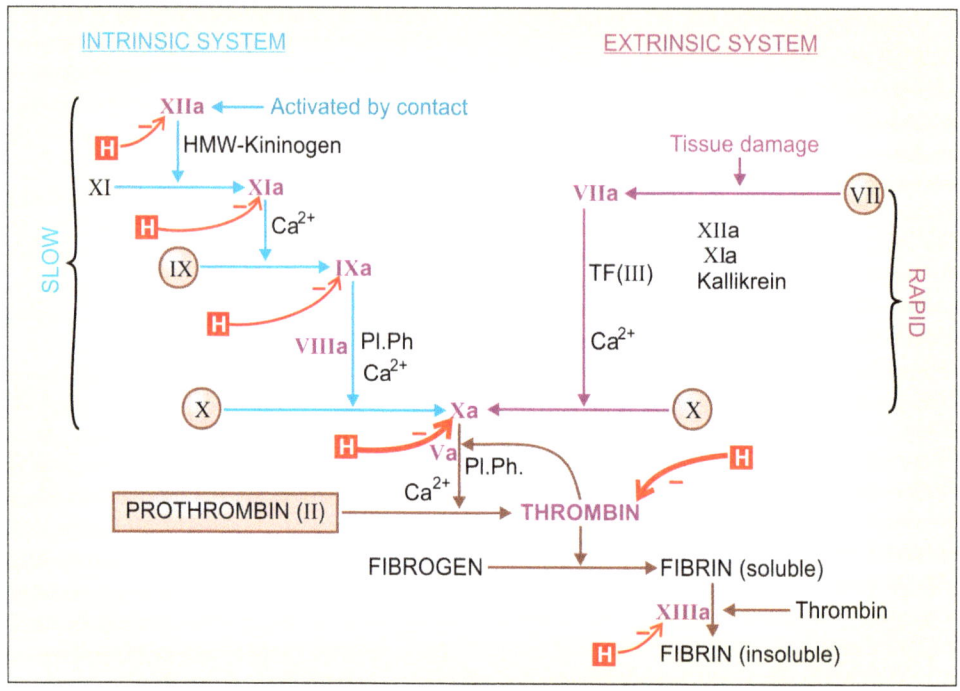

Fig. 17.2: The coagulation cascade. The vit. K dependent factors (II, VII, IX, and X) have been encircled; Factors inactivated by heparin (H) are in red; the more important inhibited steps are highlighted by thick arrow. a—activated form; Pl.Ph.—Platelet phospholipid; HMW—High molecular weight; TF—Tissue factor (factor III)

Fresh whole blood or plasma provide all the factors needed for coagulation and are the best therapy for deficiency of any clotting factor. Moreover, they act immediately.

Vitamin K

It is a fat-soluble dietary principle required for the synthesis of clotting factors. Vit K has a basic naphthoquinone structure, with or without a side chain.

Daily requirement of vit K is uncertain, because a variable amount becomes available from colonic bacteria. Even 3–10 μg/day external source may be sufficient. However, the total requirement of an adult has been estimated to be 50–100 μg/day.

Vit K acts as a cofactor at a late stage in the synthesis of coagulation proteins, *viz.* prothrombin, factors VII, IX and X occurring in the liver. The vit K dependent change (γ carboxylation of glutamate residues of these zymogen proteins; see Fig. 17.3) confers on them the capacity to bind Ca^{2+} and to get bound to phospholipid surfaces—properties essential for participation in the coagulation cascade.

Fat-soluble forms of vit K are absorbed from intestine *via* lymph and require bile salts for absorption, while water-soluble forms are absorbed directly into portal blood. Vit K is only briefly concentrated in liver, but there are no significant stores of vit K in the body. It is metabolized in liver by side chain cleavage and glucuronide conjugation; metabolites are excreted in bile and urine.

Deficiency Deficiency of vit K occurs due to liver disease, obstructive jaundice, malabsorption, long-term antimicrobial therapy which alters intestinal flora. However, deficient diet is rarely responsible. The most important manifestation is bleeding tendency due to lowering of the levels of prothrombin and other clotting factors in blood. Haematuria is usually first to occur; other common sites of bleeding are g.i.t., gums, nose and under the skin—ecchymoses.

Use The only use of vit K is in prophylaxis and treatment of bleeding due to deficiency of clotting factors in the above situations.

All newborns have low levels of prothrombin and other clotting factors. Vit K 1 mg i.m. soon after birth has been recommended routinely. Menadione (K_3) should not be used for this purpose (*see* below).

The most important indication of vit K is to reverse the effect of overdose of oral coumarin anticoagulants: Phytonadione (K_1) is the preparation of choice, because it acts most rapidly. The dose of vit K depends on the severity of hypoprothrombinaemia (measured INR) and bleeding. Unnecessary high dose is to be avoided because it will render the patient unresponsive to oral anticoagulants for several days.

Menadione and its water-soluble derivatives can cause haemolysis in a dose-dependent manner. Patients with G-6-PD deficiency and neonates are specially susceptible. In the newborn menadione or its salts can precipitate kernicterus:
(a) by inducing haemolysis and increasing bilirubin load.
(b) by competitively inhibiting glucuronidation of bilirubin.

Fibrinogen The fibrinogen fraction of human plasma is employed to control bleeding in haemophilia, antihaemophilic globulin (AHG) deficiency and in acute afibrinogenemic states; 0.5 g is infused i.v.

Antihaemophilic factor It is concentrated human AHG prepared from pooled human plasma. It is indicated (along with human fibrinogen) in haemophilia and AHG deficiency. It is highly effective in controlling bleeding episodes, but action is short lasting (1 to 2 days).

Desmopressin This V_2 receptor agonist analogue of vasopressin checks bleeding in haemophilia and von Willebrand's disease by releasing factor VIII and von Willebrand's factor (vWF) from the vascular endothelium.

Ethamsylate It is a synthetic compound which reduces capillary bleeding when platelets are adequate; probably by correcting abnormalities of platelet adhesion, but does not stabilize fibrin (not an antifibrinolytic). Ethamsylate has been used in the prevention and treatment of capillary bleeding in menorrhagia, after abortion, epistaxis, malena, hematuria and after *tooth extraction*. Side effects are nausea, rash, headache, and fall in BP (only after i.v. injection).

Dose: 250-500 mg TDS oral/i.v.; ETHAMSYL, HEMSYL, K. STAT 250, 500 mg tabs, 250 mg/2 ml inj.

Haemostasis in dentistry

Many dental procedures cause at least some bleeding: the dentist has to routinely deal with haemostasis (arrest of blood loss). After tooth extraction or similar procedures, bleeding occurs due to disruption of arterioles and smaller blood vessels that cannot be sutured. Normal haemostasis occurs successively by

- contraction of injured vessel wall (lasting few minutes)
- adhesion and aggregation of platelets to form a plug
- formation of a blood clot, and finally in due course
- dissolution of the clot by fibrinolysis.

Postextraction bleeding from the tooth socket is usually arrested by a cotton-gauze pressure pack held for 20 to 30 min. Suturing may be required if bleeding is due to tear around the socket. However, control of bleeding may need to be aided by the use of local haemostatics.

Local Haemostatics (styptics) are substances used to stop bleeding from a local and approachable site. They are particularly effective on oozing surfaces, e.g. tooth socket, abrasions, etc. Absorbable materials like *fibrin* (prepared from human plasma and dried as sheet or foam), *gelatin foam, oxidized cellulose* (as strips which can be cut and placed in the socket) provide a meshwork which activates the clotting mechanism and checks bleeding. Left in situ these materials are absorbed in 1–4 weeks and generally cause no foreign body reaction. *Thrombin* obtained from bovine plasma may be applied as dry powder or freshly prepared solution to the bleeding surface in haemophiliacs. *Vasoconstrictors* like 1% Adr solution may be soaked in sterile cotton-gauze and packed in the bleeding socket (or nose in case of epistaxis) to check bleeding when vasoconstriction is inadequate. Astringents such as tannic acid or metallic salts (e.g. alum, ferric chloride) are occasionally applied for bleeding gums, bleeding piles, etc.

Many diseases and drugs can affect the vascular response to injury, platelet function or coagulation to create haemostatic problems. When dental surgery is contemplated in patients with such defects, careful planning and consultation with their physician are needed.

1. Vitamin C deficiency impairs collagen synthesis and causes bleeding gums, excessive postextraction blood loss. Scurvy should be corrected before elective dental surgery. In case of emergency surgery, careful packing and pressure can stop the bleed. Long-term corticosteroid therapy can also compromise haemostasis by impairing vessel retraction as well as by reducing platelet count.
2. Platelet function may be deficient due to thrombocytopenia (count<100,000/mL) or use of drugs which inhibit platelet aggregation. Transfusion of platelet-rich plasma is indicated before dental surgery in patients with low platelet count. Corticosteroid therapy helps to restore platelet count in idiopathic thrombocytopenic purpura. Aspirin and other NSAIDs are the most important drugs that inhibit platelet aggregation. A large number of older individuals now receive long-term low-dose aspirin prophylaxis for ischaemic heart disease or stroke. Many others receive long term clopidogrel for a variety of thromboembolic disorders. Several patients of arthritis regularly take NSAIDs. Discontinuation of aspirin for 5 days (other antiplatelet drugs for periods appropriate to their duration of action) before dental surgery should be considered. In case this is not possible, proper packing and use of local haemostatics is needed to prevent excess bleeding.
3. Even minor dental procedures (like scaling) put the haemophiliac patient at great risk of bleeding. The patient should be covered before and after the procedure with i.v. infusion of antihaemophilic factor (AHG or factor VIII) along with fibrinogen. The antifibrinolytic drug *tranexaemic acid* has adjuvant value by reducing the requirement of AHG. *Desmopressin* injected i.v. also helps in checking dental bleeding in haemophiliacs as well as in von Willebrand's disease by releasing factor VIII and von Willebrand's factor from the vascular endothelium.
4. Any oral surgery in patients on anticoagulant medication requires due care to avoid excessive bleeding. Since the action of i.v. heparin lasts for only 4–6 hours, tooth extraction can be scheduled at a time when anticoagulation is minimal. Low dose s.c. heparin and LMW heparin therapy ordinarily does not increase dental surgery associated bleeding. The heparin antagonist *protamine* may be given i.v. in case of emergency bleed.

In patients treated with oral anticoagulants, due consultation with their physician and monitoring of their INR prior to dental surgery is essential. An INR of <3 generally does not increase bleeding due to simple extractions, but in case of more invasive procedures, it may be advisable to stop the anticoagulant for 2–3 days or temporarily switch over the patient to heparin. In case of emergency dental bleed, the effect of oral anticoagulant is reversed by i.v. infusion of fresh frozen plasma (containing all coagulation factors). Vit. K may be injected in addition. Adequate packing and local measures must be applied.

ANTICOAGULANTS

These are drugs used to reduce the coagulability of blood. They are classified in the chart:

Heparin

Heparin is a non-uniform mixture of straight chain mucopolysaccharides with MW 10,000 to 20,000. It contains polymers of two sulfated disaccharide units:

D-glucosamine-L-iduronic acid
D-glucosamine-D-glucuronic acid
} chain length and proportion of the two disaccharide units varies. Some glucosamine residues are N-acetylated.

Heparin carries strong electronegative charges and is the strongest organic acid present in the body. It occurs in mast cells and is loosely bound to the granular protein. Commercially, heparin is produced from ox lung and pig intestinal mucosa.

Actions

1. *Anticoagulant* Heparin is a powerful and instantaneously acting anticoagulant, effective both *in vivo* and *in vitro*. It acts indirectly by activating plasma antithrombin III (AT III, a serine proteinase inhibitor). The heparin-AT III complex then binds to clotting factors of the intrinsic and common pathways (Xa, IIa, IXa, XIa, XIIa and XIIIa) and inactivates them but not factor VIIa operative in the extrinsic pathway. At low concentrations of heparin, factor Xa mediated conversion of prothrombin to thrombin is selectively affected. The anticoagulant action is exerted mainly by inhibition of factor Xa as

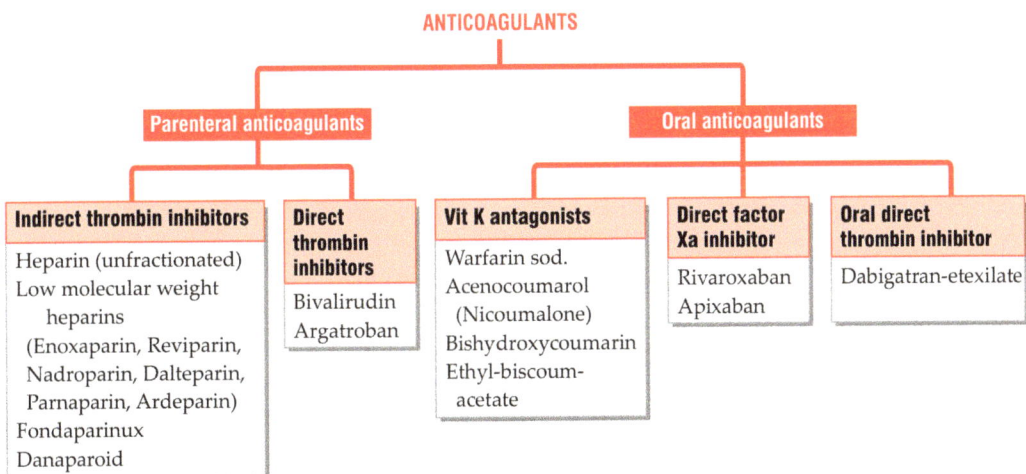

well as thrombin (IIa) mediated conversion of fibrinogen to fibrin.

Low concentrations of heparin prolong activated partial thromboplastin time (aPTT) without significantly prolonging prothrombin time (PT). High concentrations prolong both. Thus, low concentrations interfere selectively with the intrinsic pathway, affecting amplification and continuation of clotting, while high concentrations affect the common pathway as well.

2. *Antiplatelet* Heparin in higher doses inhibits platelet aggregation and prolongs bleeding time.

3. *Lipaemia clearing* Injection of heparin clears turbid post-prandial lipaemic plasma by releasing a lipoprotein lipase from the vessel wall and tissues, which hydrolyses triglycerides of chylomicra and very low density lipoproteins to free fatty acids (FFAs); these then pass into tissues and the plasma looks clear.

Pharmacokinetics Heparin is a large, highly ionized molecule; therefore not absorbed orally. Injected i.v. it acts instantaneously, but after s.c. injection anticoagulant effect develops after ~60 min. Heparin does not cross blood-brain barrier or placenta. It is metabolized in liver by heparinase and fragments are excreted in urine. Heparin is not a physiologically circulating anticoagulant.

After i.v. injection, dose-dependent inactivation is seen and t½ varies from 1–4 hours.

Heparin is conventionally given i.v. in a bolus dose of 5,000–10,000 U followed by continuous infusion. The rate of infusion is regulated by aPTT measurement which is kept at 50–80 sec. or 1.5–2.5 times the patient's pretreatment value.

Low dose (s.c.) regimen 5,000 U is injected s.c. every 8–12 hours; started before surgery and continued for 7–10 days or till the patient starts moving about. This regimen has been found to prevent postoperative deep vein thrombosis without increasing surgical bleeding. It also does not prolong aPTT or clotting time.

Adverse effects

1. Bleeding due to overdose is the most serious complication of heparin therapy. Aspirin, other NSAIDs and antiplatelet drugs enhance heparin-induced bleeding.
2. Heparin induced thrombocytopenia (HIT) is another common problem.

Low molecular weight (LMW) heparins

Heparin has been fractionated into LMW forms (MW 3,000–7,000) by different techniques. LMW heparins have a different anticoagulant profile. They selectively inhibit factor Xa with little effect on IIa. As a result, LMW heparins have smaller effect on aPTT and whole blood clotting time than unfractionated heparin (UFH) relative to antifactor Xa activity. Also, LMW heparins appear to have lesser antiplatelet action—less interference with haemostasis. The more important advantages of LMW heparins are pharmacokinetic:
- Better subcutaneous bioavailability; less variable response
- Longer and more consistent t½: once daily s.c. administration.
- Since aPTT/clotting times are not prolonged, laboratory monitoring is not needed.

Indications of LMW heparins are:
1. Prophylaxis of deep vein thrombosis (DVT) and pulmonary embolism (PE) in high-risk patients undergoing surgery, stroke or other immobilized patients.
2. Treatment of established DVT.
3. Unstable angina.
4. To maintain patency of cannulae and shunts in dialysis patients, and in extracorporeal circulation.

A number of LMW heparins (Enoxaparin, Raviparin, Dalteparin, Nadroparin, etc.) have been marketed.

Fondaparinux It is synthetically produced pentasaccharide segment present in heparin molecules which binds to AT III with high affinity to selectively inactivate factor Xa without binding to thrombin (factor IIa). Fondaparinux is 100% bioavailable on s.c. injection, longer acting, less likely to cause thrombocytopenia and bleeding. It is indicated for prophylaxis and treatment of DVT, PE and in selected cases of acute coronary syndromes (ACS). It does not require laboratory monitoring.

Danaparoid This is a heparin-like substance obtained from pig gut mucosa which can be used in patients who develop thrombocytopenia with heparin.

Heparin antagonist
Protamine sulfate is a strongly basic, low molecular weight protein obtained from the sperm of certain fish. Given i.v. it neutralises heparin weight for weight, i.e. 1 mg is needed for every 100 U of heparin. It is used when heparin action needs to be terminated rapidly, e.g. after cardiac or vascular surgery and for heparin-induced bleeding.

Direct thrombin inhibitors
Unlike heparin which inactivates thrombin indirectly by activating AT III, these newer anticoagulants bind directly to thrombin and inactivate it.

Bivalirudin It is a synthetic peptide congener of *hirudin* which is a polypeptide anticoaglulant secreted by the salivary gland of leech. Bivalirudin binds firmly to thrombin and inactivates it directly. It has a quick onset and short duration (t½ 25 min) anticoagulant action, which is not antagonized by protamine. Bivalirudin is used for percutaneous coronary intervention (PCI), unstable angina (UA) and MI. It is particularly valuable for patients prone to develop HIT, because it does not cause thrombocytopenia.

Argatroban This is a synthetic nonpeptide direct inhibitor of thrombin which acts by reversibly binding to its catalytic site. Injected i.v. as a bolus followed by slow infusion, argatroban produces rapid onset short duration antithrombin action which is used for propylaxis and treatment of thrombosis and to cover PCI in patients with HIT.

ORAL ANTICOAGULANTS

Vitamin K antagonists
Warfarin and its congeners act as anticoagulants only *in vivo*, not *in vitro*. This is so because they act indirectly by interfering with the synthesis of vit K dependent clotting factors in liver. They reduce the plasma levels of functional clotting factors in a dose-dependent manner. In fact, they inhibit the enzyme *vit K epoxide reductase (VKOR)* and interfere with regeneration of the active hydroquinone form of vit K (Fig. 17.3) which acts as a cofactor for the enzyme γ-glutamyl carboxylase that carries out the final step of γ carboxylating glutamate residues of prothrombin and factors VII, IX and X. This carboxylation is essential for the ability of the clotting factors to bind Ca^{2+} and to get bound to phospholipid surfaces, necessary for the coagulation sequence to proceed.

Factor VII has the shortest plasma t½ (6 hr), its level falls first when warfarin is given, followed by factor IX (t½ 24 hr), factor X (t½ 40 hr) and prothrombin (t½ 60 hr). The anticoagulant effect develops gradually over 1–3 days as the levels of the clotting factors

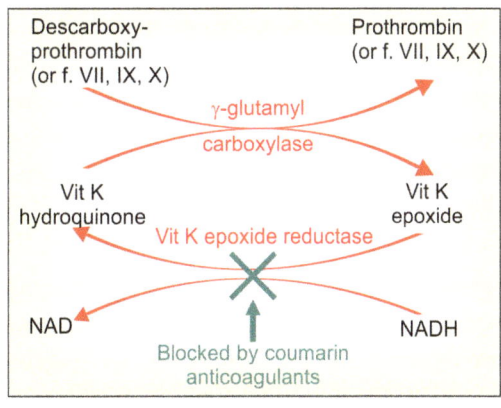

Fig. 17.3: Mechanism of action of coumarin oral anticoagulants
NAD—Nicotinamide adenine dinucleotide; NADH—its reduced form

already present in plasma decline according to their t½s. Thus, there is always a delay between administration of these drugs and the anticoagulant effect.

The differences between different coumarin anticoagulants are primarily pharmacokinetic and in the adverse side effects produced by them.

Warfarin sod It is the most commonly used oral anticoagulant. Its action develops over 2-3 days and lasts for 3-6 days. Alopecia and dermatitis are infrequent side effects.

Acenocoumarol (nicoumalone) It is relatively faster and shorter acting, used occasionally. Oral ulceration, bowel upset and dermatitis are the side effects.

Bishydroxycoumarin and Ethyl biscoumacetate are not preferred now.

Bleeding as a result of extension of the pharmacological action is the most important adverse effect, causing ecchymosis, epistaxis, hematuria, bleeding in the g.i.t., intracranial or other internal haemorrhages, which may be fatal.

Treatment: of bleeding due to coumarin anticoagulants consists of:
- Withhold the anticoagulant.
- Give fresh blood transfusion. Alternatively, fresh frozen plasma may be used as a source of clotting factors.
- Give vit K_1—specific antidote, but it takes 6–24 hours for the clotting factors to be resynthesized and released in blood after vit K administration.

Dose regulation The dose of coumarin anticoagulant must be individualized by repeated measurement of *prothrombin time*; the aim is to achieve a therapeutic effect without unduly increasing the chances of bleeding. A standardized system called the International Normalized Ratio (INR) has been developed by WHO to quantify the effect of oral anticoagulants. An INR of 2–4.5 is considered therapeutic for different indications.

Drug interactions A large number of drugs interact with coumarin anticoagulants and either enhance or decrease their effect. These interactions are clinically important (may be fatal if bleeding occurs).

A. *Enhanced anticoagulant action*
1. Broad-spectrum antibiotics: inhibit gut flora and reduce vit K production.
2. Certain cephalosporins (ceftriaxone, cefoperazone) cause hypoprothrombinaemia by the same mechanism as warfarin —additive action.
3. Aspirin: inhibits platelet aggregation and causes g.i. bleeding—this may be hazardous in anticoagulated patients.
4. Sulfonamides, indomethacin, phenytoin displace warfarin from plasma protein binding.
5. Metronidazole, chloramphenicol, erythromycin, cimetidine, allopurinol and amiodarone inhibit warfarin metabolism.

B. *Reduced anticoagulant action*
1. Barbiturates, carbamazepine, rifampin and griseofulvin induce the metabolism of warfarin.
2. Oral contraceptives: increase blood levels of clotting factors.

Direct factor Xa inhibitors

Rivaroxaban In contrast to the older coumarin anticoagulants which inhibit the synthesis of clotting factors, this new compound directly binds to and inactivates factor Xa. Therefore, it acts rapidly (within 3-4 hours) without a lag period, and has a shorter duration of action (~24 hours). Moreover, no laboratory monitoring is needed. Rivaroxaban is now routinely used for prophylaxis of DVT and PE following knee/hip replacement surgery. It is also indicated for preventing stroke in patients with atrial fibrillation as well as to treat DVT and PE.

Apixaban This is another orally active factor Xa inhibitor which is approved for:
- Prevention of venous thromboembolism (VTE) following knee/hip replacement.

- Prophylaxis of stroke in AF patients.
- Treatment of DVT and PE.

Oral direct thrombin inhibitor

Dabigatran etexilate This oral anticoagulant binds directly to the catalytic site of thrombin inhibiting it reversibly. The action of dabigatran etexilate is rapid and consistent, so that no laboratory monitoring is needed. It is being used for prevention of post knee replacement venous thromboembolism, as well as stroke due to atrial fibrillation.

Uses of anticoagulants

The aim of using anticoagulants is to prevent thrombus extension and embolic complications by reducing the rate of fibrin formation. They do not dissolve already formed clot, but prevent recurrences. Conditions in which they are indicated are:

1. Prophylaxis of DVT and PE following knee/hip replacement surgery, and in high-risk bed ridden, elderly, postpartum, post stroke and leg fracture patients.
2. Treatment of existing DVT and PE.
3. Prophylaxis of stroke and systemic embolism in patients of nonvalvular atrial fibrillation.
4. To cover percutaneous coronary intervention (PCI) in patients of MI and high-risk UA.
5. As adjuvants to antiplatelet drugs aspirin ± clopidogrel to prevent reocclusion of coronary arteries following fibrinolytic therapy of MI.
6. Anticoagulants are combined with antiplatelet drugs in patients with prosthetic heart valves, and in those undergoing vascular surgery or haemodialysis.
7. To maintain patency of intravascular cannulae/catheters.
8. To preserve clotting factors in defibrination syndrome.

The important features of heparin and warfarin are compared in Table 17.1.

Table 17.1: Some comparative aspects of heparin and warfarin.

	Heparin	Warfarin
1. Chemistry	Mucopolysaccharide	Coumarin derivative
2. Source	Hog lung, pig intestine	Synthetic
3. Route of admin.	Parenteral (i.v., s.c.)	Oral
4. Onset of action	Immediate	Delayed (1–3 days)
5. Duration of action	4–6 hrs	3–6 days
6. Activity	In vitro and in vivo	In vivo only
7. Mechanism	Blocks action of factor X and thrombin	Inhibits synthesis of clotting factors
8. Antagonist	Protamine sulphate	Vit K
9. Variability in response	Little	Marked
10. Lab. control	aPTT/clotting time (desirable)	Prothrombin time/INR (essential)
11. Drug interactions	Few and not significant	Many and significant
12. Use	To initiate therapy	For maintenance

FIBRINOLYTIC DRUGS (Thrombolytics)

These are drugs which dissolve thrombi/clot to recanalize occluded blood vessels (mainly coronary artery). They work by activating the natural fibrinolytic system.

Haemostatic plug of platelets formed at the site of injury to blood vessels is reinforced by fibrin deposition to form a thrombus. Once repair is over, the fibrinolytic system is activated to remove the fibrin. The enzyme responsible for digesting fibrin is a serine protease *Plasmin* generated from *plasminogen* by tissue plasminogen activator (t-PA). Plasminogen circulates in plasma as well as remains bound to fibrin. The t-PA selectively activates fibrin bound plasminogen within the thrombus.

Fibrinolytics like *Streptokinase, Urokinase, Alteplase* (recombinant t-PA or rt-PA), *Reteplace* and *Tenecteplase* have been produced. Tenecteplase, a genetically engineered mutant of t-PA, is the latest and most favoured fibrinolytic now because of several desirable features. All fibrinolytics are administered by i.v. injection. Haemorrhage is their major complication.

Uses of fibrinolytics

1. *Acute myocardial infarction* is the prime indication of fibrinolytics. They are an alternative to emergency percutaneous coronary intervention (PCI) with stent placement. Fibrinolytics benefit by recanalizing the occluded vessel. Best results are obtained if thrombolysis is achieved within 1-2 hours of symptom onset.
2. *Deep vein thrombosis* in leg, pelvis, shoulder, etc.; up to 60% patients can be successfully treated.
3. *Pulmonary embolism* Fibrinolytic therapy is indicated in large, life-threatening pulmonary embolism.
4. *Stroke* Thrombolysis with alteplace is recommended only for carefully selected patients of ischaemic stroke. These drugs are absolutely contraindicated in haemorrhagic stroke.

ANTIFIBRINOLYTIC DRUGS

These are drugs which inhibit plasminogen activation and dissolution of clot. They are used to check bleeding due to fibrinolysis.

Epsilon amino-caproic acid (EACA) It is an analogue of the amino acid lysine, which combines with the lysine binding sites of plasminogen and plasmin so that the latter is not able to bind to fibrin and lyse it. EACA is a specific antidote for fibrinolytic agents, and has been used in many hyperplasminaemic states associated with excessive intravascular fibrinolysis resulting in bleeding.

Tranexaemic acid Like EACA, it binds to the lysine binding site on plasminogen and prevents its combination with fibrin, and is 7 times more potent. Therefore, it is preferred for prevention/control of excessive bleeding due to:
- Fibrinolytic drugs.
- Tooth extraction, tonsillectomy, prostate surgery in haemophiliacs.
- Cardio-pulmonary bypass surgery.
- Menorrhagia, IUCD.
- Recurrent epistaxis, ocular trauma.

Main side effects are nausea and diarrhoea. Headache, giddiness and thrombophlebitis of injected vein are other adverse effects.

ANTIPLATELET DRUGS (Antithrombotic drugs)

These are drugs which interfere with platelet function and are useful in the prophylaxis of thromboembolic disorders. However, all of them *are likely to accentuate dental surgery related bleeding*.

Platelets stick to the damaged vessel wall, then they stick to each other (aggregate) and release ADP, thromboxane A_2 (TXA_2) which promote further aggregation. Thus, a 'platelet plug' is formed.

Prostacyclin (PGI_2), synthesized in the intima of blood vessels, is a strong inhibitor of platelet aggregation. A balance between TXA_2 released from platelets and PGI_2 released from vessel wall appears to control intravascular thrombus formation.

Drugs interfering with platelet function are classified in the chart.

Aspirin It acetylates the enzyme cyclooxygenase (COX) and TX-synthetase—inactivating them irreversibly. Because TXA_2 is the major arachidonic acid product generated by platelets, and that platelets are exposed to aspirin in the portal circulation before it is deacetylated during first pass in liver, as well as because platelets cannot synthesize fresh enzyme (have no nuclei), TXA_2 formation is suppressed at very low doses and till fresh

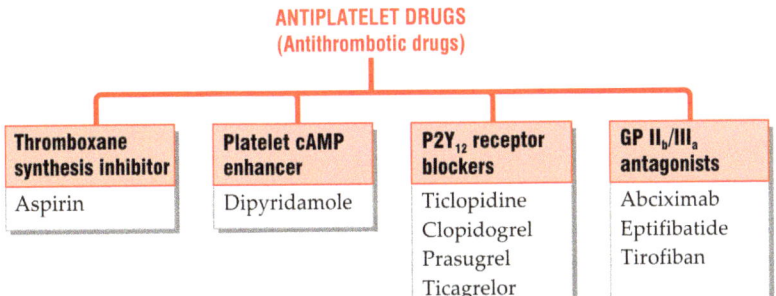

platelets are formed. Thus, aspirin induced prolongation of bleeding time lasts for 5–7 days. Effect of daily doses cumulates and it has now been shown that doses as low as 40 mg/day have an effect on platelet aggregation. Maximal inhibition of platelet function occurs at ~160 mg aspirin per day.

Aspirin also inhibits PGI_2 synthesis in vessel wall. However, since intimal cells can synthesize fresh enzyme, activity returns rapidly. At low doses (75–150 mg/day), TXA_2 formation by platelets is selectively suppressed, whereas higher doses (> 900 mg/day) may decrease both TXA_2 and PGI_2 production.

Aspirin inhibits the release of ADP from platelets and their sticking to each other. However, it has no effect on platelet survival time and their adhesion to damaged vessel wall.

Other NSAIDs are reversible inhibitors of COX, produce short-lasting inhibition of platelet function—are not clinically useful but can prolong bleeding time for variable periods.

Dipyridamole It is a vasodilator which inhibits the enzyme phosphodiesterase and blocks the uptake of adenosine to increase platelet cAMP. This potentiates PGI_2 and interferes with aggregation.

Dipyridamole given along with warfarin decreases the incidence of thromboembolism in patients with prosthetic heart valves.

Risk of stroke in patients with transient ischaemic attacks (TIAs) may be additively reduced when dipyridamole is combined with aspirin, because it enhances the antiplatelet action of aspirin.

Ticlopidine It is the first thienopyridine which alters surface receptors on platelets and inhibits ADP as well as fibrinogen-induced platelet aggregation. It acts by blocking the $P2Y_{12}$ subtype of purinergic receptors through which ADP inhibits adenylyl cyclase in platelets. As a result, platelet activation is interfered.

Ticlopidine was found to have prophylactic effect in TIAs, stroke, MI and to synergize with aspirin in reducing incidence of restenosis after PCI. However, it produced more side effects and some serious reactions like neutropenia, haemolysis and jaundice. Ticlopidine has been superseded by safer congeners like clopidogrel.

Clopidogrel This more potent congener of ticlopidine has similar mechanism of action, *viz.* irreversibly blocks the $P2Y_{12}$ subtype of purinergic receptors on the surface of platelets, thereby inhibiting platelet aggregation. Therapeutic efficacy of clopidogrel is similar to ticlopidine, but it is safer and better tolerated. However, clopidogrel is a prodrug; only a fraction of the administered dose is slowly activated in the liver. Therefore, the antiplatelet action takes at least 4 hours to start and develops over several days. Some patients fail to activate it, and are unresponsive. Nevertheless, clopidogrel is now extensively used for TIAs, unstable angina, prevention of stroke and recurrence of MI. Combined with aspirin, it has markedly lowered the incidence of restenosis after coronary angioplasty and stent thrombosis. Side effects are diarrhoea, epigastric pain and rashes.

Clopidogrel has replaced ticlopidine.

Prasugrel This is a newer, still more potent and faster acting $P2Y_{12}$ purinergic receptor blocker that is being used in MI, unstable angina, and to cover coronary angioplasty.

Though prasugrel is also a prodrug, it is more rapidly absorbed and more completely activated resulting in more consistent and reliable antiplatelet action. Bleeding complications are also more.

Ticagrelor This is the latest $P2Y_{12}$ receptor blocker which acts directly without need for activation in the body. Unlike clopidogrel and prasugrel, the action of ticagrelor is reversible. Therefore, it has a faster onset and quicker offset of action, needing twice daily dosing. In acute coronary syndromes (ACS), ticagrelor has been found to achieve greater reduction in mortality compared to clopidogrel. As such, prophylactic ticagrelor is now recommended in all high risk ACS patients. Side effects of ticagrelor are shortness of breath, tightness in chest, nausea and dizziness.

Glycoprotein (GP) II$_b$/III$_a$ receptor antagonists

GP II$_b$/III$_a$ antagonists are a class of potent platelet aggregation inhibitors which act by blocking the key receptor involved in platelet aggregation. The GP II$_b$/III$_a$ is an adhesive receptor on platelet surface for fibrinogen and vWF through which agonists like collagen, thrombin, TXA_2, ADP, etc. induce platelet aggregation. Thus, GP II$_b$/III$_a$ antagonists block aggregation induced by all platelet agonists. They are used only in patients of acute coronary syndromes (ACS) and to cover PCI or coronary artery bypass grafting (CABG).

Abciximab It is the Fab fragment of a chimeric monoclonal antibody against GP II$_b$/III$_a$, which is given along with aspirin + heparin during coronary angioplasty. It has markedly reduced the incidence of restenosis, subsequent MI and death. Unstable angina is another indication.

Eptifibatide It is a synthetic cyclic peptide GPIIb/IIIa antagonist which strongly inhibits platelet aggregation, and is used as a better suited alternative to abciximab for i.v. infusion before and after coronary angioplasty and in acute coronary syndromes.

Tirofiban This is a synthetic nonpeptide GPIIb/IIIa antagonist that has antiplatelet action similar to eptifibatide. Infused i.v. for 24–72 hours, it is used in acute coronary syndromes and coronary angioplasty.

Uses of antiplatelet drugs

Antiplatelet drugs are used to prevent intravascular thrombus formation and embolization with as low risk of haemorrhage as possible. The intensity of antiplatelet therapy is selected according to the condition being treated.

1. *Coronary artery disease* Long term low dose aspirin is now recommended in all subjects with evidence of coronary artery disease as well as in those with risk factors for the same. Aspirin/clopidogrel prophylaxis in post-MI patients reduces reinfarction and mortality.

2. *Acute coronary syndromes* Aspirin and LMW heparin are given at presentation to all patients of unstable angina and MI. Clopidogrel can be used in place of aspirin, and a combination of the two is more potective. Prasugrel or ticagrelor + aspirin is now being preferred to cover coronary angioplasty. The most powerful antiplatelet drugs GP II$_b$/III$_a$ inhibitors are indicated in high risk patients undergoing angioplasty or coronary bypass surgery.

3. *Cerebrovascular disease* Antiplatelet drugs do not alter the course of stroke due to cerebral thrombosis. However, aspirin has reduced the incidence of TIAs, of stroke in patients with TIAs or persistent atrial fibrillation and in those with history of stroke in the past. Clopidogrel also reduces TIAs and stroke.

4. *Prosthetic heart valves and arteriovenous shunts* Antiplatelet drugs, used with warfarin reduce formation of microthrombi on artificial heart valves and the incidence of embolism. Antiplatelet drugs also prolong the patency of chronic arteriovenous shunts.

5. *Peripheral vascular disease* Aspirin/clopidogrel may produce some improvement in intermittent claudication and reduce the incidence of thromboembolism.

HYPOLIPIDAEMIC DRUGS

These are drugs which lower the levels of lipids and lipoproteins in blood, and have potential to prevent cardiovascular disease by retarding the accelerated atherosclerosis in hyperlipidaemic individuals.

Whereas, raised low density lipoprotein-cholesterol (LDL-CH) is atherogenic, an increased level of high density lipoprotein-cholesterol (HDL-CH) is either itself protective or indicates a low atherogenic state. Elevated plasma triglyceride (TG) level also poses risk of coronary artery disease (CAD) and stroke, irrespective of cholesterol level.

The mechanism of action and profile of lipid lowering effect of important classes of hypolipidaemic drugs is summarized in Table 17.2.

HMG-CoA reductase inhibitors (Statins)

These are the most efficacious, most extensively used and best tolerated hypolipidaemic drugs. They competitively inhibit conversion of 3-Hydroxy-3-methyl glutaryl coenzyme A (HMG-CoA) to mevalonate, the rate limiting step in cholesterol (CH) synthesis, by the enzyme HMG-CoA reductase. Therapeutic doses reduce CH synthesis by 20–50%. This results in compensatory increase in LDL receptor expression on liver cells thereby enhancing receptor mediated uptake and catabolism of intermediate density lipoprotein (IDL) and LDL. Consequently, dose-dependent lowering of LDL-CH level occurs.

At their maximum recommended doses, atorvastatin and rosuvastatin can reduce LDL-CH by up to 45–55%, while the ceiling effect of lovastatin and pravastatin is 35–40% LDL-CH reduction.

A concurrent fall by 10–30% in plasma TG level, probably due to reduction of very low density lipoprotein (VLDL) occurs. A rise in HDL-CH by 5–15% is also noted. Statins are not useful when TG alone is markedly raised.

All statins are remarkably well tolerated; overall incidence of side effects not differing from placebo. Side effects are headache, nausea, bowel upset, rashes and sleep disturbances. Muscle tenderness is the commonest side effect. Rise in CPK level and hepatic injury are infrequent. Myopathy is the only serious reaction, but is rare.

Statins are the first choice drugs for lowering raised LDL and total CH levels, with or without raised TG levels. Efficacy of statins in reducing raised LDL-CH associated mortality and morbidity is now well established. Venous thromboembolism

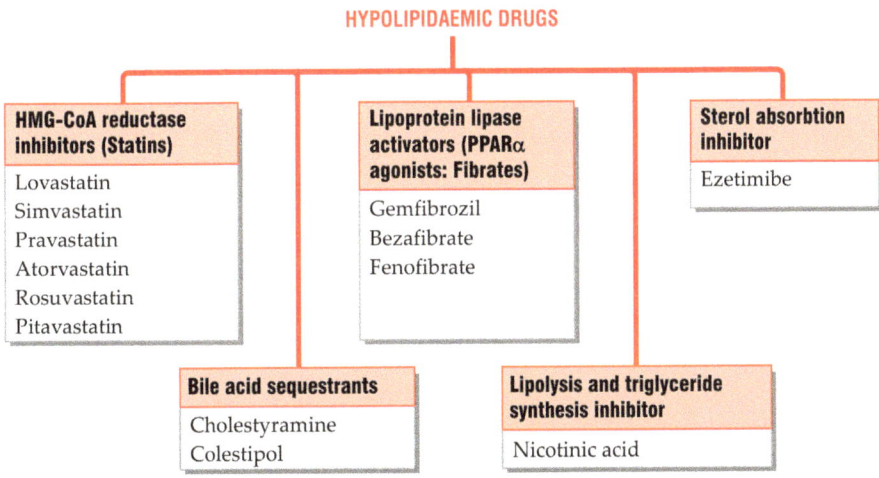

Table 17.2: Mechanism of action and pattern of lipid lowering effect of important classes of hypolipidaemic drugs

Drug	Mechanism of action	Effect on lipid levels (%)
HMG-CoA reductase inhibitors	↓ CH synthesis by inhibition of rate limiting HMG-CoA reductase	LDL ↓ 20–55 HDL ↑ 5–15 TG ↓ 10–35
Fibric acid derivatives	↑ Activity of lipoprotein lipase, ↓ release of fatty acids from adipose tissue	LDL ↓ 5–15 HDL ↑ 10–20 TG ↓ 20–50
Nicotinic acid	↓ Production of VLDL, ↓ lipolysis in adipocytes	LDL ↓ 15–25 HDL ↑ 20–35 TG ↓ 20–50
Ezetimibe	↓ Intestinal absorption of CH and phytosterols	LDL ↓ 15–20 HDL ↑ 5 TG ↓ —

CH–cholestrol; LDL–low density lipoprotein; HDL–high density lipoprotein; TG–triglycerides; VLDL–very low density lipoprotein

following knee replacement is reduced by rosuvastatin.

Improvement in endothelial function, reduction in LDL oxidation and an antiinflammatory effect are proposed as additional mechanisms by which statins may exert antiatherosclerotic action.

Bile acid sequestrants (Resins)

Cholestyramine and Colestipol are basic ion exchange resins supplied in the chloride form. They bind bile acids in the intestine interrupting their enterohepatic circulation. Faecal excretion of bile salts and CH is increased. This indirectly leads to enhanced hepatic metabolism of CH to bile acids and lowering of LDL-CH level. However, resins are unpalatable and produce g.i. symptoms, therefore rarely used.

Lipoprotein-lipase activators (Fibrates)

The fibrates (isobutyric acid derivatives) activate lipoprotein lipase which is a key enzyme in the degradation of VLDL resulting in lowering of circulating TGs. This effect is exerted through nuclear *paroxisome proliferator-activated receptor α (PPARα)* which is a gene transcription regulating receptor that enhances lipoprotein lipase synthesis and fatty acid oxidation. PPARα may also mediate enhanced LDL receptor expression in liver. Fibrates decrease hepatic TG synthesis as well. Drugs in this class primarily lower TG levels by 20–50%, generally accompanied by 10–15% decrease in LDL-CH and a 10–15% increase in HDL-CH.

Fibrates are the hypolipidaemic drugs of choice for patients with raised TG levels, whether or not CH levels are also raised. In hypercholesterolaemia, they may be used as adjuvants to statins. Reduction in coronary events and slowing of atherosclerotic process has been noted in post-MI subjects. Their main side effects are g.i. upset, rashes, bodyache, rarely myopathy (particularly when combined with statins).

Nicotinic acid

It is a B group vitamin which in much higher doses (2-4 g/day) reduces plasma lipids. This action is unrelated to its vitamin activity and not present in nicotinamide. When nicotinic acid is given, TGs and VLDL decrease rapidly, followed by a modest fall in LDL-CH and total CH. A 20–50% reduction in plasma TGs and 15–25% reduction in CH levels has been recorded. It is the most effective drug to raise HDL-CH; a 20–30% increase is generally obtained.

Nicotinic acid inhibits lipolysis in adipose tissue and reduces flow of free fatty acids

(FFAs) from adipocytes to liver, restricting availability of FFAs for production of TGs and VLDL by the liver. Direct depression of TG synthesis in hepatocytes is also possible.

Adverse effects The large doses needed for hypolipidaemic action are poorly tolerated. Only about half of the patients are able to take the full doses. Marked flushing, heat and itching (especially in the blush area) occur after every dose. Since this is associated with release of PG D_2 in the skin, aspirin taken before each dose subdues the reaction. *Laropiprant*, a prostanoid receptor inhibitor, also reduces flushing.

Dyspepsia is very common; vomiting and diarrhoea occur when full doses are given. Peptic ulcer may be activated. Long term use can cause liver dysfunction and precipitate diabetes.

Risk of myopathy due to statins is increased.

Use Nicotinic acid is primarily used to lower raised plasma TGs and VLDL. The most important indication is to control as well as prevent pancreatitis associated with severe hypertriglyceridaemia. Benefit of nicotinic acid therapy for prevention of atherosclerotic cardiovascular disease is uncertain, and not recommended now by some guidelines. Because of marked side effects, use of nicotinic acid is restricted to high-risk cases only.

Ezetimibe

This drug interferes with a specific CH transport protein NPC1C1 in the intestinal mucosa and thus reduces absorption of both dietary and biliary CH by a mechanism different from that of resins. The LDL-CH level is lowered by 15–20%. Used alone, ezetimibe is a weak hypocholesterolemic drug, but it synergises with statins. The combination of ezetimibe + low dose statin causes as much LDL-CH lowering as high dose of statin alone. However, additional cardiovascular event reduction achieved by adding ezetimibe to statin appears to be minimal or uncertain. Ezetimibe is generally well tolerated.

CHAPTER 18

Drugs for Gastrointestinal Disorders

DRUGS FOR PEPTIC ULCER AND REFLUX DISEASE

Peptic ulcer It occurs in that part of the gastrointestinal tract (g.i.t.) which is exposed to gastric acid and pepsin, i.e., the stomach and duodenum. The etiology of peptic ulcer is not clearly known. It results probably due to an imbalance between the *aggressive* (acid, pepsin and *H. pylori*) and the *defensive* (gastric mucus and bicarbonate secretion, prostaglandins, nitric oxide, innate resistance of the mucosal cells) factors. A variety of psychosomatic, humoral and vascular derangements have been implicated and the causative role of *Helicobacter pylori* infection in ulcer formation as well as in recurrence has been recognized.

In peptic ulcer patients gastric acid secretion may be high or normal or even low, but it does contribute to ulceration as an aggressive factor, reduction of which is the main approach to ulcer treatment.

Gastroesophageal reflux disease (GERD) It is a very common problem presenting as 'heartburn', acid eructation, sensation of stomach contents coming back in the foodpipe, especially after a large meal, aggravated by stooping or lying flat. Some cases have an anatomical defect (hiatus hernia) but majority are only functional in which lower esophageal sphincter (LES) relaxation occurs even while not swallowing. The disease severity varies: symptoms may be occasional to frequent or even persistent.

Repeated reflux of acid gastric contents into lower 1/3rd of esophagus causes esophagitis, erosions, ulcers, strictures, and increases the risk of esophageal carcinoma.

Though GERD is primarily a g.i. motility disorder, acidity of gastric contents is the most important aggressive factor in causing symptoms and esophageal lesions.

Regulation of gastric acid secretion The mechanisms operating at the gastric parietal cells are summarized in Fig. 18.1. The terminal enzyme $H^+K^+ATPase$ (proton pump) which secretes H^+ ions in the apical canaliculi of parietal cells can be activated by histamine, ACh and gastrin acting *via* their own receptors located on the basolateral membrane of these cells. Out of the three physiological secretagogues, histamine, acting through H_2 receptors, plays the dominant role, because the other two, gastrin and ACh act partly directly and partly indirectly by releasing histamine from paracrine enterochromaffin-like (ECL) cells located in the oxyntic glands.

H_2 ANTAGONISTS

These are the first class of highly effective drugs for acid-peptic disease, but have been largely superseded by the proton pump inhibitors (PPIs). Cimetidine was the first H_2 blocker to be introduced clinically and is described as the prototype.

Pharmacological actions
Cimetidine and all other H_2 antagonists block histamine-induced gastric secretion. They attenuate fall in BP due to histamine, especially the late phase response seen with high doses. This is due to blockade of relaxant

Drugs for Peptic Ulcer and Reflux Disease

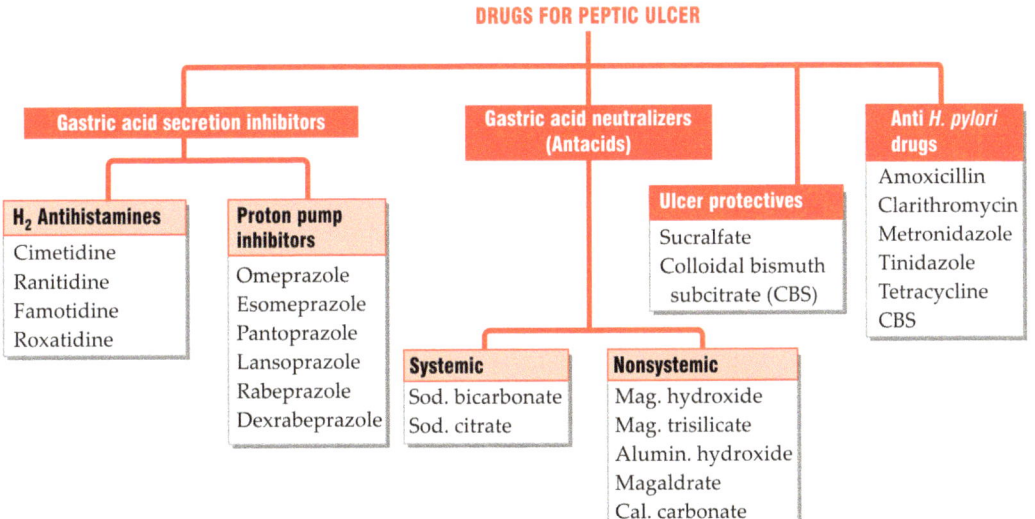

H_2 receptors located directly on vascular smooth muscle. Other H_2 receptor actions prominent in isolated organs (stimulation of guinea pig heart, relaxation of rat uterus) are also blocked. These antagonists are highly selective: have no effect on H_1 mediated responses or on action of other transmitters/autacoids.

The only significant *in vivo* action of H_2 blockers is marked inhibition of gastric secretion. All phases (basal, psychic, neurogenic, gastric) of secretion are suppressed dose-dependently. Secretory responses to not only histamine but also all other stimuli (ACh, gastrin, insulin, alcohol, food) are attenuated. This reflects the permissive role of histamine in amplifying responses to other secretagogues.

The usual ulcer healing doses produce 60–70% inhibition of 24-hour acid output. The H_2 blockers have antiulcerogenic effect. Gastric ulceration due to stress and drugs (NSAIDs) is prevented.

Pharmacokinetics Cimetidine is adequately absorbed orally. About 2/3rd of a dose is excreted unchanged in urine and bile, the rest as oxidized metabolites. The elimination t½ is 2–3 hr.

Adverse effects Cimetidine is well tolerated by most patients: adverse effects occur in ~5%. Side effects like headache, dizziness, bowel upset and dry mouth are generally mild. High dose or rapid i.v. injection can cause confusional state, hallucinations, cardiac arrhythmias or cardiac arrest.

Cimetidine (but not other H_2 blockers) has antiandrogenic action. High doses given for long periods have produced gynaecomastia, loss of libido, impotence and temporary decrease in sperm count.

Interactions Cimetidine inhibits cytochrome P-450 and reduces hepatic blood flow. It inhibits the metabolism of many drugs so that they can accumulate to toxic levels, e.g. metronidazole, theophylline, phenytoin, phenobarbitone, sulfonylureas, warfarin, imipramine, lidocaine.

Antacids reduce absorption of all H_2 blockers.

Ranitidine This H_2 blocker has several desirable features compared to cimetidine:
- About 5 times more potent than cimetidine.
- No antiandrogenic action, does not increase prolactin secretion or spare

Chapter 18: Drugs for Gastrointestinal Disorders

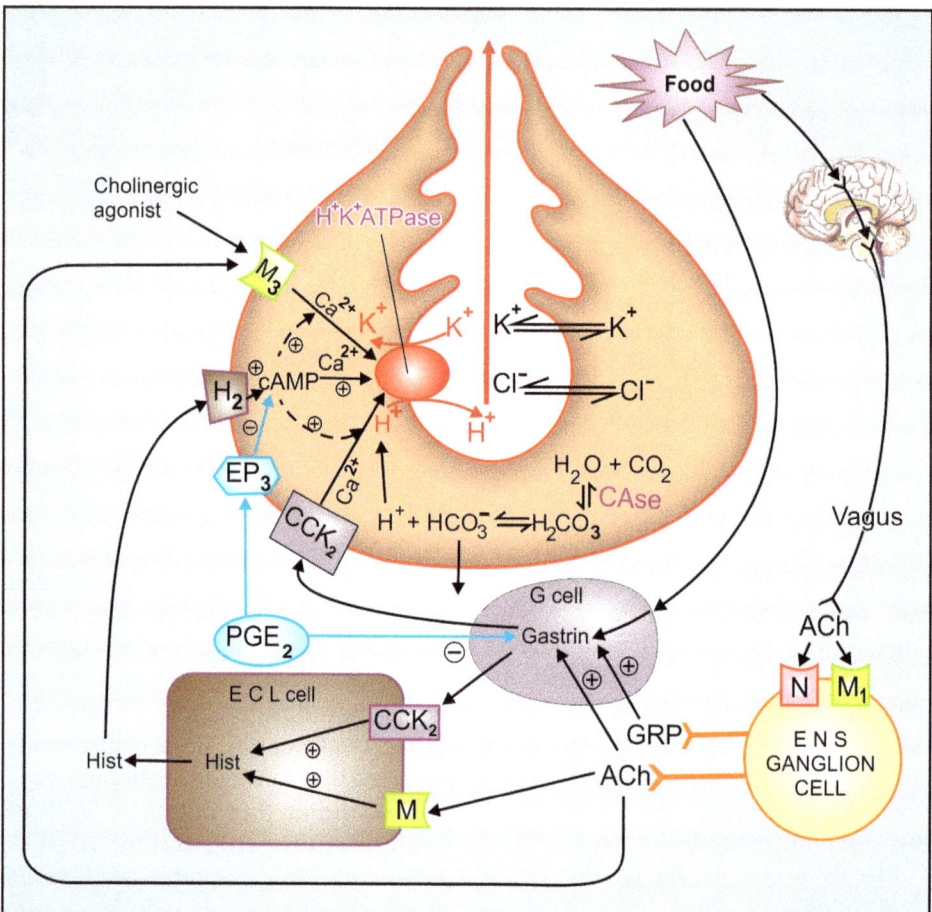

Fig. 18.1: Secretion of HCl by gastric parietal cell and its regulation
C.Ase.—Carbonic anhydrase; Hist.—Histamine; ACh.—Acetylcholine; CCK_2—Gastrin/cholecystokinin receptor; M.—Muscarinic receptor; N—Nicotinic receptor; H_2—Histamine H_2 receptor; EP_3—Prostaglandin receptor; ENS—Enteric nervous system; ECL cell—Enterochromaffin-like cell; GRP—Gastrin releasing peptide;
+ = Stimulation; − = Inhibition.

estradiol from hepatic metabolism—no effect on male sexual function or gynaecomastia.
- Lesser permeability into the brain: lower propensity to cause CNS effects.
- Does not significantly inhibit hepatic metabolism of other drugs; drug interactions mostly have no clinical relevance.
- Overall incidence of side effects is lower.

Famotidine It is 5–8 times more potent than ranitidine and has no antiandrogenic action. Because of low affinity for cytochrome P450 and the low dose, drug metabolism modifying propensity is minimal.

PROTON PUMP INHIBITORS (PPIs)

Developed a decade after H_2 blockers, this class of potent acid suppressant drugs are one of the most commonly used medications now.

Omeprazole It is the prototype member of substituted benzimidazoles which inhibit the final common step in gastric acid secretion. The PPIs have overtaken H_2 blockers for treating acid-peptic disorders.

The only significant pharmacological action of omeprazole is dose-dependent suppression of gastric acid secretion; without blocking any transmitter receptor. It is a powerful inhibitor of gastric acid which can totally abolish HCl secretion, both resting as well as that stimulated by any of the secretagogues, without much effect on the secretion of pepsin, intrinsic factor and juice volume or gastric motility.

Omeprazole is inactive at neutral pH, but at acidic pH < 5 it rearranges into two charged cationic forms that react covalently with SH groups of the H^+K^+ATPase enzyme and inactivate it irreversibly, especially when two molecules of omeprazole react with one molecule of the enzyme. After diffusing into the parietal cell from blood, it gets concentrated in the acidic pH of the canaliculi because the charged forms generated there at the acidic pH are unable to diffuse back. Moreover, it gets tightly bound to the enzyme. These features and the specific localization of H^+K^+ATPase to the apical membrane of parietal cells confer high degree of selectivity of action to omeprazole and other PPIs. Acid secretion resumes only when new H^+K^+ATPase molecules are synthesized.

All PPIs are administered orally in enteric coated form because they are unstable at acidic pH; bioavailability from omeprazole tablet is ~ 50%. As the gastric pH rises, a higher fraction (up to 3/4) may be absorbed. PPIs should be administered in empty stomach, followed 1 hour later by food to activate the H^+K^+ ATPase at a time when plasma concentration of the PPI is maximal.

Omeprazole is highly plasma protein bound, rapidly metabolised in liver by CYP2C19 and CYP3A4 (plasma t½ ~1 hr) and metabolites are excreted in urine. Since only actively secreting proton pumps are inhibited by the PPIs, and only few pumps may be active during the brief interval when the drug is present in plasma, repeated doses produce cumulative acid suppression. After a single dose, inhibition of HCl secretion occurs within 1 hr, reaches maximum at 2 hr, is still half maximal at 24 hr and lasts for 2–3 days. At steady-state after repeated dosing the PPIs produce 80–98% suppression of 24 hour acid output.

Adverse effects PPIs are very safe drugs. Side effects are minimal: nausea, loose stools, headache, abdominal pain, muscle and joint pain, dizziness.

Interactions Omeprazole inhibits oxidation of certain drugs. Levels of diazepam, phenytoin and warfarin may be increased.

Lansoprazole, pantoprazole and rabeprazole are other PPIs with only minor differences from omeprazole. *Esomeprazole, S-Pantoprazole* and *Dexrabeprazole* are single active enantiomers respectively of omeprazole, pantoprazole and rabeprazole.

Uses of proton pump inhibitors and H_2 blockers

The PPIs and H_2 blockers are used in conditions in which it is profitable to suppress gastric acid secretion.

1. *Peptic ulcer* Both PPIs and H_2 blockers produce excellent and rapid (within 2–3 days) pain relief and promote healing of ulcers. The PPIs are more effective and faster acting than H_2 blockers. With PPIs some duodenal ulcers heal even at 2 weeks and majority in 4 weeks, but healing rates are lower with H_2 blockers and may take 8 weeks or more. Gastric ulcers take longer to heal, but majority respond to PPI therapy in 8 weeks. The PPIs are the drugs of choice for NSAIDs induced gastric/duodenal ulcers, and are more effective than H_2 blockers or misoprostol. Maintenance therapy with either a PPI or a H_2 blocker

reduces ulcer recurrence. The PPIs are an integral component of anti-*H. pylori* therapy.

2. **Bleeding peptic ulcer** Intravenous PPI (pantoprazole or rabeprazole or esomeprazole) infusion helps to control bleeding from peptic ulcer.

3. *Stress ulcers and gastritis* Acutely stressful situations like severe burns and trauma, prolonged surgery, etc. are associated with gastric erosions and bleeding. Intravenous infusion of a H_2 blocker or PPI prevents the gastric lesions and haemorrhage.

4. *Gastroesophageal reflux disease (GERD)* The PPIs are the most effective drugs, both for symptomatic relief as well as for healing of esophageal lesions. More complete suppression of round the clock acid secretion is required for healing of esophagitis than for peptic ulcer. This level of acid suppression can be consistently achieved only by PPIs. Therefore, PPIs are the drugs of choice for patients with all stages of GERD, particularly severe cases. Prolonged therapy is required in chronic cases, because symptoms recur a few days after drug stoppage.

The H_2 blockers cause less complete acid suppression. Their use in GERD is restricted to milder cases as alternative to PPIs.

Use of *antacids* in GERD is limited to intercurrent relief of heartburn, and not for lasting relief or healing of esophagitis.

Prokinetic drugs are believed to relieve regurgitation and heartburn by increasing LES tone and facilitating gastric emptying. However, they afford only minor symptom relief and do not promote healing of esophageal lesions. Domperidone or metoclopramide are commonly added to PPI therapy, but whether this improves outcome is uncertain.

5. *Prophylaxis of aspiration pneumonia* H_2 blockers given preoperatively (evening before and then in the morning) reduce risk of aspiration of acidic gastric contents during anaesthesia and prolonged surgery. PPIs are the alternative drugs.

6. *Zollinger-Ellison syndrome* It is a gastric hyperseretory state due to a rare tumour which secretes gastrin. High dose PPI given 2–3 times daily is the most effective medical therapy for inoperable cases. H_2 blockers are less effective and used only when a PPI cannot be given.

PROSTAGLANDIN ANALOGUES

PGE_2 and PGI_2 are produced in the gastric mucosa and serve a protective role by inhibiting acid secretion as well as by promoting mucus and HCO_3 secretion. In addition, PGs increase mucosal blood flow and have an ill-defined "cytoprotective" action.

Misoprostol, a stable PG analogue, inhibits acid secretion and promotes ulcer healing. However, it is less effective in relieving ulcer pain.

Major problems in using misoprostol for ulcer healing is that it causes diarrhoea, abdominal cramps, uterine bleeding, and needs to be given by multiple daily doses. Patient acceptability is poor. Misoprostol is rarely used now for prevention and treatment of NSAID associated gastrointestinal injury and blood loss, because PPIs are more effective, more convenient, better tolerated and cheaper.

In ulcer patients, dentists should take care not to prescribe aspirin or other NSAIDs; instead choose paracetamol/codeine/selective COX-2 inhibitor for pain relief.

ANTACIDS

These are basic substances which neutralize gastric acid and raise pH of gastric contents. Peptic activity is indirectly reduced when the pH rises above 4, because optimum pH for pepsin action is between 2–4.

Antacids do not decrease acid production; rather, agents that raise the antral pH to > 4 evoke reflex gastrin release → more acid is secreted, especially in patients with hyperacidity and duodenal ulcer. As a result "acid rebound" occurs and gastric motility is increased.

The potency of an antacid is generally expressed in terms of its *acid neutralizing capacity* (ANC), which is defined as number of mEq of 1N HCl that are brought to pH 3.5 in 15 min (or 60 min in some tests) by a unit dose of the antacid preparation.

Systemic antacids

Sodium bicarbonate It is water soluble, acts instantaneously, but the duration of action is short. It is a potent neutralizer (1 g neutralizes 12 mEq HCl), pH may rise above 7. However, it has several demerits:
(a) Absorbed systemically: large doses will induce alkalosis.
(b) Produces CO_2 in stomach → distention, discomfort, belching, risk of ulcer perforation.
(c) Acid rebound occurs, but is usually short lasting.
(d) Increases Na^+ load: may worsen edema and CHF.
Use of sod. bicarbonate is restricted to casual treatment of heart burn. It provides quick symptomatic relief. Other uses are to alkalinize urine and to treat acidosis.

Sodium citrate Properties similar to sod. bicarbonate; 1 g neutralizes 10 mEq HCl; CO_2 is not evolved.

Nonsystemic antacids

These are insoluble and poorly absorbed basic compounds that react in stomach to form the corresponding chloride salt. The chloride salt again reacts with the intestinal bicarbonate so that HCO_3 is not spared for absorption—no acid-base disturbance occurs.

Mag. hydroxide has low water solubility but reacts with HCl promptly and is an efficacious antacid (1 g neutralizes 30 mEq HCl).

Magnesium trisilicate has low solubility and reactivity; clinically neutralizes only about 1 mEq acid per gram due to slow action. All Mg salts have a laxative action—by generating osmotically active $MgCl_2$ in the stomach and through Mg^{2+} ion induced cholecystokinin release.

Aluminium hydroxide gel It is a bland, weak and slowly reacting antacid. On keeping it slowly polymerizes to variable extents into still less reactive forms. Thus, the ANC of a preparation gradually declines on storage. ANC usually varies from 1–2.5 mEq/g. Thus, 5 ml of its suspension may neutralize just 1 mEq HCl.

The Al^{3+} ions relax smooth muscle. Thus, it delays gastric emptying. Alum. hydrox. frequently causes constipation due to its smooth muscle relaxant and mucosal astringent action. By binding phosphate in the intestine, it can cause hypophosphataemia after prolonged use.

Magaldrate It is a hydrated complex of hydroxy-magnesium aluminate that initially reacts rapidly with acid and releases alum. hydrox. which then reacts more slowly. Thus, magaldrate cannot be equated to a physical mixture of mag. and alum. hydroxides. It is a good antacid with prompt and sustained neutralizing action.

Calcium carbonate It is a potent and rapidly acting acid neutralizer, but ANC of the commercial preparations is variable and usually low due to differing crystal structure. It slowly liberates CO_2 in the stomach. The Ca^{2+} ions that diffuse into the gastric mucosa can increase acid production and cause acid rebound. Mild constipation is often complained. It is also used as a calcium supplement.

Antacid combinations A combination of two or more antacids is frequently used. Combinations may be superior to any single agent on the following accounts:
(a) Fast (Mag. hydrox.) and slow (Alum. hydrox.) acting components yield prompt as well as sustained effect.
(b) Mag. salts are laxative, while Alum. salts are constipating: combination may annul each other's action and bowel movement may be least affected.
(c) Dose of individual components is reduced; systemic toxicity (dependent on fractional absorption) is minimized.

Drug interactions By raising gastric pH and by forming complexes, the non-absorbable antacids decrease the absorption of many drugs, especially tetracyclines, iron salts, fluoroquinolones, ketoconazole, H_2 blockers, diazepam, phenothiazines, indomethacin, phenytoin, isoniazid, ethambutol and nitrofurantoin. If any of these drugs is to be given along with an antacid, their administration should be staggered by 2 hours. The efficacy of nitrofurantoin is reduced by alkalinization of urine.

Uses Antacids are no longer used for healing peptic ulcer because they are needed in large and frequent doses, are inconvenient, can cause acid rebound and bowel upset, afford little nocturnal protection and have poor patient acceptability. They are now employed only for intercurrent pain relief and acidity, mostly self- prescribed by the patients. They continue to be used for nonulcer dyspepsia and minor episodes of heartburn, acid eructation or reflux.

ULCER PROTECTIVES

Sucralfate It is a basic aluminium salt of sulfated sucrose; a drug of its own kind. Sucralfate polymerizes at pH < 4 by cross linking of molecules, assuming a sticky gel-like consistency. It preferentially and strongly adheres to the ulcer base, especially duodenal ulcer and acts as a physical barrier preventing acid, pepsin and bile from coming in contact with the ulcer base. Dietary proteins get deposited on this coat, forming another layer.

Sucralfate has no acid neutralizing action, but may augment gastric mucosal PG synthesis. It is minimally absorbed after oral administration. Though, it promotes healing of both duodenal and gastric ulcers, it is infrequently used now because of need for 4 large well-timed daily doses and the availability of simpler H_2 blockers/PPIs. As a suspension in glycerol, sucralfate is used as a protective in stomatitis.

Side effects are few; constipation is reported by 2% patients.

Interactions Sucralfate adsorbs many drugs and interferes with the absorption of tetracyclines, fluoroquinolones, cimetidine, phenytoin and digoxin. Antacids given concurrently reduce the efficacy of sucralfate.

Colloidal bismuth subcitrate (CBS; Tripotassium dicitratobismuthate)
It is a colloidal bismuth compound; water soluble but precipitates at pH < 5. It is not an antacid, but heals 60% ulcers at 4 weeks and 80–90% at 8 weeks. The mechanism of action of CBS is not clear; probabilities are:
- Stimulation of mucosal PGE_2 and bicarbonate production.
- Creating a diffusion barrier by coating the ulcer.
- Anti-*H. pylori* action.

Gastritis and nonulcer dyspepsia associated with *H. pylori* are also improved by CBS. Patient acceptance of CBS is compromised by blackening of tongue, dentures and stools; by variable and delayed symptom control and inconvenience of dosing schedule. Presently, it is used occasionally as a component of triple drug anti-*H. pylori* regimen.

ANTI-*HELICOBACTER PYLORI* DRUGS

H. pylori is a gram-negative bacillus uniquely adapted to survival in the hostile environment of stomach. It attaches to the surface epithelium beneath the mucus, has high urease activity—produces ammonia which maintains a neutral microenvironment around the bacteria, and promotes back diffusion of H^+ ions. *H. pylori* has been found as a commensal in 20–70% normal individuals, and is now accepted as an important contributor to the causation of chronic gastritis, dyspepsia, peptic ulcer, gastric lymphoma and gastric carcinoma. Up to 90% patients of duodenal and gastric ulcer have tested positive for *H. pylori*.

Eradication of *H. pylori* concurrently with H_2 blocker/PPI therapy of peptic ulcer has been associated with faster ulcer healing and lower relapse rate. Anti-*H. pylori* therapy is, therefore, now recommended in all ulcer patients who test positive for *H. pylori*. If *H. pylori* testing is not available, all cases with failed conventional ulcer therapy and relapse cases may be given the benefit of *H. pylori* eradication.

Antimicrobials that have been found clinically effective against *H. pylori* are: amoxicillin, clarithromycin, tetracycline and metronidazole/tinidazole. However, any single antibiotic is relatively ineffective. Resistance develops rapidly, especially to metronidazole/tinidazole and clarithromycin, but amoxicillin resistance is infrequent. In tropical countries, metronidazole resistance is more common than clarithromycin resistance. Since bismuth (CBS) is active against *H. pylori* and resistance does not develop to it, combination regimens including bismuth may be employed, but have poor patient acceptability, and are infrequently used now.

It is observed that PPI monotherapy reduces the population of *H. pylori* in the gastric antrum, probably by altering the acid environment as well as by a direct inhibitory effect. One of the PPIs is an integral component of all anti-*H. pylori* regimens along with 2 antimicrobials out of amoxicillin, clarithromycin and metronidazole/tinidazole (triple drug regimen). A number of 3-drug regimens of 1 or 2 weeks duration have been tested reporting 60–96% eradication rates. In India a one week regimen is generally employed, while the 2 week regimens are reserved for cases who fail to achieve complete eradication.

The US-FDA approved regimen is: lansoprazole 30 mg + amoxicillin 1000 mg + clarithromycin 500 mg all given twice daily for 2 weeks. It has achieved 86–92% eradication rate. Long-term benefits of *H. pylori* eradication therapy include lowering of ulcer disease prevalence and prevention of gastric carcinoma/lymphoma. However, benefits in nonulcer dyspepsia are equivocal.

ANTIEMETIC DRUGS

These are drugs used to prevent or suppress vomiting (emesis).

Emesis Vomiting occurs due to stimulation of the *emetic (vomiting) centre* situated in the medulla oblongata. Multiple pathways can elicit vomiting (Fig. 18.2). The *chemoreceptor trigger zone (CTZ)* located in the area postrema and the *nucleus tractus solitarius (NTS)* are the most important relay areas for afferent impulses arising in the g.i.t, throat and other viscera. The CTZ is accessible to blood-borne drugs, mediators, hormones, toxins, because it is unprotected by the blood-brain barrier. Cytotoxic drugs, radiation and other g.i. irritants release 5-HT from enterochromaffin cells in the gut which acts on 5-HT$_3$ receptors present on vagal afferents and sends impulses to NTS and CTZ. However, 5-HT is not the only mediator of such signals: many peptides and other messengers are also involved.

The CTZ and NTS express a variety of receptors, Viz. histamine H$_1$, dopamine D2, serotonin 5-HT$_3$, neurokinin NK$_1$ (activated by substance P), cannabinoid CB$_1$, cholinergic M and opioid µ receptor through which the emetic signals are relayed and which could be targets of antiemetic drug action.

The vestibular apparatus generates impulses when body is rotated or equilibrium is disturbed, or when ototoxic drugs act. These impulses reach the vomiting centre mainly relayed from the cerebellum and utilize muscarinic as well as H$_1$ receptors.

ANTICHOLINERGIC DRUGS (*See* Ch. 5)

Hyoscine is the most effective drug for motion sickness. However, it has a brief duration of action; produces sedation, dry mouth and other anticholinergic side effects and is suitable only for short brisk journies. Hyoscine acts probably by blocking conduction of nerve impulses across a cholinergic link in the pathway leading from the vestibular apparatus to the vomiting centre. It is not effective in vomiting of other etiologies.

Dicyclomine This oral antimuscarinic drug has been used for prophylaxis of motion sickness and for morning sickness.

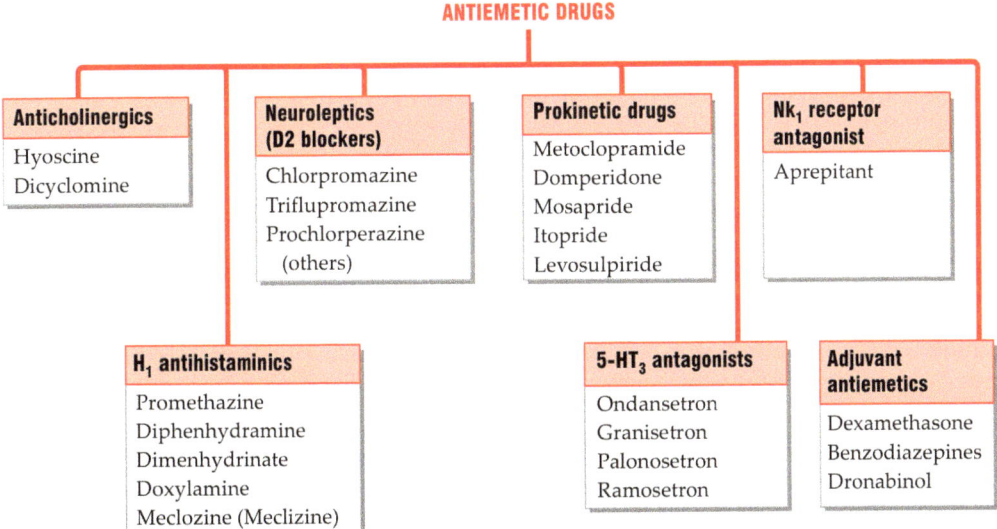

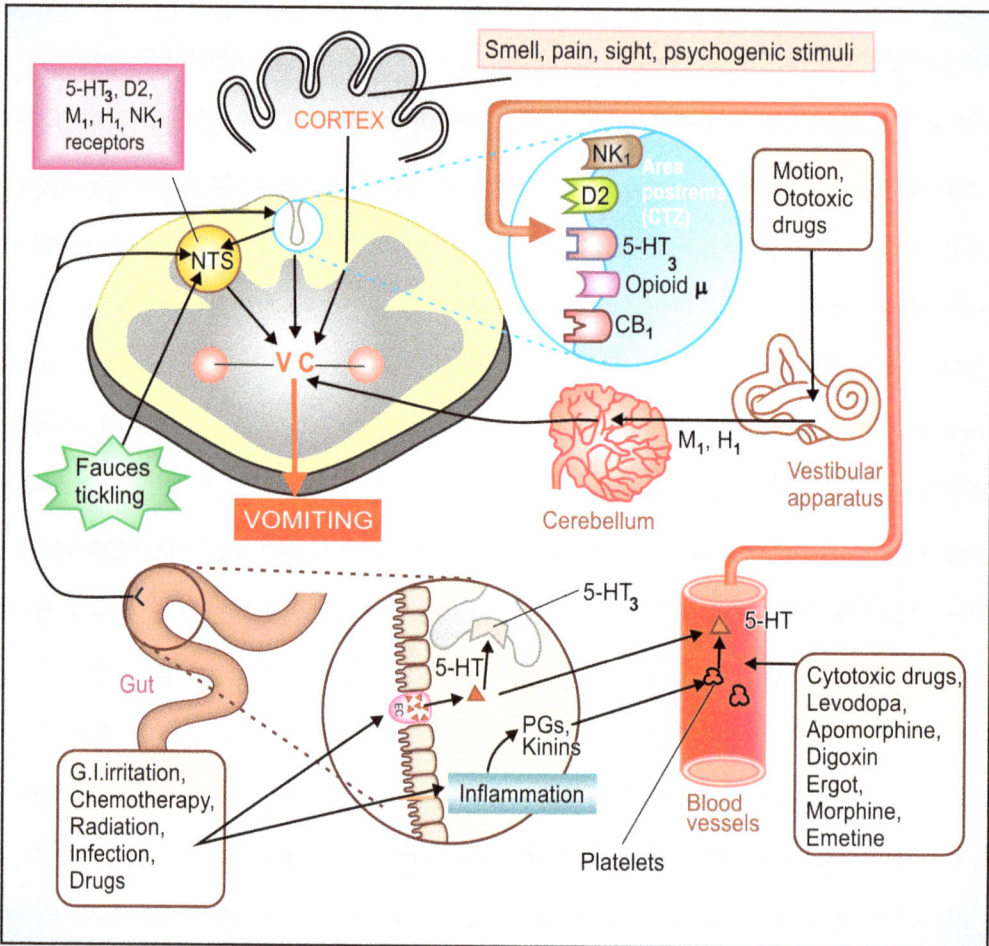

Fig. 18.2: Major central and visceral structures involved in emesis and the neurohumoral receptors mediating the emetic response.
NTS—Nucleus tractus solitarius; VC—vomiting centre; CTZ—chemoreceptor trigger zone; 5-HT—5HT$_3$ receptor; H$_1$—histamine H$_1$ receptor; D2—dopamine D2 receptor; M$_1$—muscarinic M$_1$ receptor; NK$_1$—Neurokinin 1 receptor; CB$_1$—cannabinoid 1 receptor

H$_1$ ANTIHISTAMINICS (*See* Ch. 7)

Some antihistaminics have antiemetic property. They are useful mainly in motion sickness and to a lesser extent in morning sickness, postoperative and some other forms of vomiting. Their antiemetic effect appears to be based on anticholinergic, antihistaminic and sedative properties.

Promethazine, diphenhydramine, dimenhydrinate afford protection from motion sickness for 4–6 hours, but produce sedation and dryness of mouth. Promethazine is a phenothiazine; therefore has weak central antidopaminergic action as well. Its theoclate salt is specifically promoted as antiemetic.

Meclozine (meclizine) is less sedative and less anticholinergic. Meclozine is long acting, protects against sea sickness for nearly 24 hours.

Doxylamine This H$_1$ antihistaminic has prominent sedative and anticholinergic properties. In combination with pyridoxine,

Antiemetic Drugs

it is specifically promoted for morning sickness.

Motion sickness Anticholinergic-antihistamics are the preferred antiemetics for motion sickness. These drugs are more effective when taken ½–1 hour before commencing journey. Once sickness has started, it is more difficult to control; higher doses/parenteral administration may be needed.

NEUROLEPTICS (*See* Ch. 10)

These are potent antiemetics; act by blocking D2 receptors in the CTZ. They have broad-spectrum antiemetic action in:
(a) Drug induced and postoperative nausea and vomiting (PONV).
(b) Disease induced vomiting: gastroenteritis, uraemia, liver disease, migraine, etc.
(c) Malignancy associated and mild intensity cancer chemotherapy induced nausea and vomiting (CINV).
(d) Radiation sickness vomiting (less effective).
(e) Morning sickness: Neuroleptics should not be used except in hyperemesis gravidarum.

Neuroleptics are *not* effective in motion sickness: the vestibular pathway probably does not involve dopaminergic link.

Most of these drugs produce significant degree of sedation. Acute muscle dystonia may occur after a single dose, especially in children and girls. The antiemetic dose is generally much lower than antipsychotic doses.

Prochlorperazine This D2 receptor blocking phenothiazine is a labyrinthine suppressant, has selective antivertigo and antiemetic actions. It is highly effective when given by injection in vertigo associated with vomiting, and to some extent in CINV.

PROKINETIC DRUGS

These are drugs which promote gastro-intestinal transit and hasten gastric emptying.

Metoclopramide

Introduced in early 1970s as a 'gastric hurrying' agent, metoclopramide is a commonly used antiemetic.

Metoclopramide increases gastric peristalsis while relaxing the pylorus and the first part of duodenum. Thus, it speeds gastric emptying, especially when the same was slow. The tone of LES is increased and gastroesophageal reflux is opposed. Metoclopramide increases intestinal peristalsis to some extent, but has no significant action on colonic motility and on gastric secretion.

Metoclopramide acts as an antiemetic; by blocking D2 receptors in CTZ. The gastrokinetic action may contribute to the antiemetic effect. Other manifestations of D2 receptor blockade are chlorpromazine like extrapyramidal side effects and hyperprolactinaemia, but no antipsychotic effect is exerted. The gastric hurrying and LES tonic effects are mainly due to activation of 5-HT$_4$ receptors on myenteric interneurones which enhance ACh release from primary motor neurones innervating the gastric and LES smooth muscles. Because dopamine acts as an inhibitory transmitter in the g.i.t., the D2 receptor blocking action also contributes to the gastrokinetic effects.

Pharmacokinetics Metoclopramide is rapidly absorbed orally, enters brain, crosses placenta and is secreted in milk. It is partly conjugated in liver and excreted in urine within 24 hours; t½ is 3–6 hours. Orally, it acts in ½–1 hr, but within 10 min after i.m. and 2 min after i.v. injection. Action lasts for 4–6 hours.

Interactions Metoclopramide hastens the absorption of many drugs, e.g. aspirin, diazepam, etc. by facilitating gastric emptying. It reduces the extent of absorption of digoxin by allowing less time for it.

By blocking dopamine receptors in basal ganglia, it abolishes the therapeutic effect of levodopa.

Adverse effects Metoclopramide is generally well tolerated.

Sedation, dizziness, loose motion, muscle dystonias (especially in children) are the main side effects. Long-term use can cause parkinsonism, galactorrhoea and gynaecomastia.

Uses

1. *Antiemetic:* Metoclopramide can be used for many types of vomiting—postoperative, drug induced, disease associated (especially migraine), radiation sickness, etc. but is less effective in motion sickness. Though ondansetron is preferred, metoclopramide continues to be used for mild to moderate CINV.
2. *Gastrokinetic:* To accelerate gastric emptying:
- When emergency general anaesthesia has to be given and the patient has taken food less than 4 hours before.
- To relieve postvagotomy or diabetes associated gastric stasis.
- To facilitate duodenal intubation.
3. *Dyspepsia* and other functional g.i. disorders.
4. *Gastroesophageal reflux disease (GERD):* Metoclopramide may afford symptomatic relief in milder cases of GERD, but is much less effective than PPIs/H_2 blockers. It does not aid healing of esophagitis.

Domperidone This D2 receptor antagonist is chemically related to haloperidol, but pharmacologically related to metoclopramide. The antiemetic and prokinetic actions have a lower ceiling. Unlike metoclopramide, its prokinetic action is not attenuated by atropine and is based only on D2 receptor blockade in upper g.i.t. Domperidone poorly crosses blood-brain barrier, accordingly, extrapyramidal side effects are rare, but hyperprolactinaemia can occur. However, it does act on CTZ which is not protected by blood-brain barrier, though antiemetic efficacy is lower than metoclopramide.

Domperidone is used for drug and disease induced vomiting, and as gastrokinetic for dyspepsia and GERD. Side effects of domperidone are fewer and milder than with metoclopramide: dry mouth, loose stools, headache, rashes, galactorrhoea.

Mosapride It is a prokinetic drug with weak antiemetic action, because the D2 receptor blocking property is absent. Its effects on gastric motility resemble those of metoclopramide and are due to $5\text{-}HT_4$ agonism which promotes ACh release from myenteric neurones. However, mosapride augments peristalsis throughout the g.i.t. and often produces loose stools. It is devoid of action on the CTZ, and does not produce extrapyramidal side effects or hyperprolactinaemia. Unlike its predecessor cisapride (which has been banned) it has not caused QTc prolongation or cardiac arrhythmias. Mosapride has no clinically useful antiemetic action, and is used only as prokinetic in g.i. motility disorders, dyspepsia and GERD.

Itopride It is a new prokinetic drug having dopaminergic D2 blocking and ACh potentiating action, but low affinity for $5\text{-}HT_4$ receptor. Thus, the basis of its prokinetic action is different from that of mosapride. No QTc prolonging and arrhythmogenic effect has been observed. Side effects are abdominal pain, loose motion and headache. Indications of itopride are similar to those of mosapride.

$5\text{-}HT_3$ ANTAGONISTS

Ondansetron It is the prototype of a class of antiemetic drugs developed to control cancer chemotherapy/radiotherapy induced vomiting and later found to be highly effective in PONV, disease and drug-induced vomiting as well. Ondansetron blocks the depolarizing action of 5-HT through $5\text{-}HT_3$ receptors on vagal afferents in the g.i.t. as well as in the NTS and CTZ. Cytotoxic drugs and radiation produce nausea and vomiting by causing cellular damage → release of mediators including 5-HT from intestinal mucosa → activation of vagal afferents in the gut triggaring transmission of emetogenic impulses to the NTS and CTZ. Ondansetron blocks emetogenic impulses both at their peripheral origin and at their central relay.

Pharmacokinetics: Oral bioavailability of ondansetron is 60–70% due to first pass metabolism. No clinically significant drug interactions have been noted. It is eliminated in urine and faeces, mostly as metabolites; t½ being 3–5 hrs, and duration of action is 8–12 hr.

Indications of ondansetron include prophylaxis and treatment of chemotherapy/radiotherapy induced vomiting, PONV, vomiting associated with drug overdosage, gastrointestinal disorders, uraemia, neurological injuries etc., but not motion sickness.

Side effects: Ondansetron is generally well tolerated: The only common side effect is headache. Mild constipation or diarrhoea and abdominal discomfort occur in a few patients. Rashes and allergic reactions are possible, especially after i.v. injection.

Granisetron It is 10 times more potent than ondansetron and probably more effective during the repeat cycle of chemotherapy. It is also longer acting.

Palonosetron This is the longest acting (elimination t½ 40 hrs) and highly potent 5-HT$_3$ blocker, equally effective against acute phase CINV as ondansetron, and more effective in suppressing delayed vomiting that occurs between 2nd to 5th day. Palonosetron is administered by a single i.v. dose before chemotherapy, and is not to be repeated before 7 days.

Ramosetron Another potent 5-HT$_3$ antagonist effective in preventing CINV as well as PONV. Ramosetron is also indicated for symptomatic relief in diarrhoea predominant irritable bowel syndrome.

NK$_1$ RECEPTOR ANTAGONIST

Aprepitant Since substance P released in the body due to emetogenic chemotherapy and other stimuli plays a role in the causation of vomiting by activating neurokinin (NK$_1$) receptors in the CTZ and NTS, selective antagonists of this receptor have been produced and found to possess antiemetic property. Aprepitant is the first and prototype member of this class. Oral aprepitant (3 doses over 3 days) given along with standard i.v. ondansetron + dexamethasone regimen significantly enhances the antiemetic efficacy against highly emetogenic cisplatin based chemotherapy. Greater protection is afforded against delayed vomiting, and in patients undergoing multiple cycles of chemotherapy. A single dose given before surgery suppresses PONV as well.

ADJUVANT ANTIEMETICS

Corticosteroids (e.g. dexamethasone 8–20 mg i.v. before chemotherapy) can partly alleviate nausea and vomiting due to moderately emetogenic chemotherapy, but are more often employed to augment the efficacy of the primary antiemetics like metoclopramide or ondansetron against highly emetogenic chemotherapy. Oral dexamethasone 8 mg/day from 2nd to 5th day helps to alleviate delayed vomiting.

Benzodiazepines The weak antiemetic property of benzodiazepines is primarily based on the sedative action. Used as adjuvant to metoclopramide/ondansetron, they help by alleviating the psychogenic component, anticipatory vomiting and produce amnesia for the unpleasant procedure.

Cannabinoids Δ^9 Tetrahydrocannabinol (Δ^9 THC) is the active principle of the hallucinogen *Cannabis indica*. It possesses antiemetic activity.

Dronabinol is pure Δ^9 THC produced synthetically or extracted from *Cannabis*. It has been used for chemotherapy induced vomiting in patients who cannot tolerate other antiemetics or are unresponsive to them. Its hallucinogenic and disorienting actions are a limitation.

LAXATIVES (Aperients, Purgatives, Cathartics)

These are drugs which promote evacuation of bowels. A distinction is sometimes made according to the intensity of action.
(a) *Laxative or aperient*: milder action, elimination of soft but formed stools.
(b) *Purgative or cathartic*: stronger action resulting in more fluid evacuation.

Many drugs in low doses act as laxative and in larger doses as purgative. Thus, the distinction is vague

Chapter 18: Drugs for Gastrointestinal Disorders

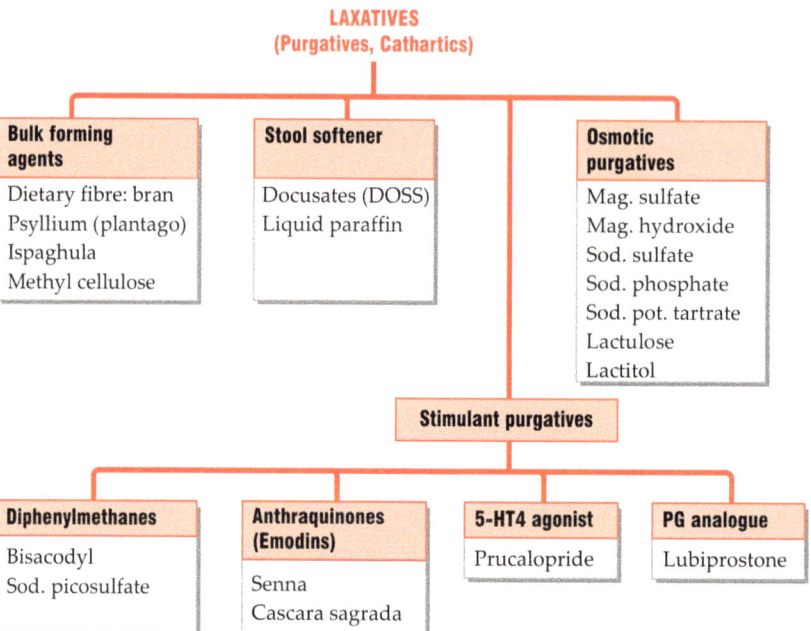

MECHANISM OF ACTION

All purgatives increase water content of the faeces by:
(a) A hydrophilic or osmotic action, retaining water and electrolytes in the intestinal lumen. This increases volume of colonic content and makes it easily propelled.
(b) Acting on intestinal mucosa to decrease net absorption of water and electrolyte; intestinal transit is enhanced indirectly by the fluid bulk.
(c) Enhancing propulsive activity as primary action—allowing less time for absorption of salt and water as a secondary effect.

Net fluid output from the mucosal cell can be enhanced by:
- Inhibiting $Na^+ K^+$ ATPase in villous cells.
- Stimulating adenylyl cyclase in crypt cells.
- Enhancing PG synthesis in mucosa, which promotes secretion.
- Increasing mucosal NO synthesis.

Bulk forming laxatives

Bran is the residual byproduct of flour industry which consists of ~ 40% dietary fibre containing unabsorbable cell wall and other constituents of cereals, *viz.* cellulose, pectins, glycoproteins and other polysaccharides. It absorbs water in the intestines, swells, increases water content of faeces and facilitates colonic transit.

Psyllium and ispaghula husk These substances contain natural colloidal mucilage which absorbs water, swells and forms a bulky gelatinous mass in the intestines. This increases water content of faeces—softens it and facilitates colonic transit.

Bulk forming laxatives are the most appropriate method for prevention and treatment of functional constipation. They are the first line approach for most patients of simple constipation. Full effect requires daily administration for at least 3–4 days. In patients of irritable bowel syndrome (IBS), regular intake of ispaghula and other soluble fibres reduces rectosigmoid intraluminal pressure which helps to relieve the symptoms.

Generous amounts of water must be taken with all bulk forming agents.

Stool softener

Docusates (Dioctyl sodium sulfosuccinate: DOSS) is an anionic detergent. It softens the stools by net water accumulation in the lumen due to an action on the intestinal mucosa. It emulsifies the colonic contents and increases penetration of water into the faeces. A mild laxative effect is produced, and it is especially indicated when straining at stools must be avoided. Side effects are cramps and abdominal pain.

Liquid paraffin is a viscous liquid; a mixture of petroleum hydrocarbons. It is pharmacologically inert. Taken for 2–3 days, it softens stools and is said to lubricate hard scybali by coating them. However, it is unpleasant to swallow and has many drawbacks such as interference with absorption of fat-soluble vitamins, likelihood of leakage past the anus, lipid pneumonia if it trickles into the airway, or foreign body granulomas in mesenteric lymph nodes if it is absorbed.

Stimulant purgatives

These are powerful purgatives: often produce griping. Though some of them do primarily increase gut motility by acting on myenteric plexuses, the more important mechanism of action is accumulation of water and electrolytes in the lumen by altering absorptive and secretory activity of the mucosal cell. They inhibit Na$^+$K$^+$ATPase at the basolateral membrane of villous cells—transport of Na$^+$ and accompanying water across the cell to the interstitium is reduced. Secretion is enhanced by activation of cAMP in crypt cells and by increased PG synthesis.

Larger doses of stimulant purgatives can cause excess purgation which may lead to fluid and electrolyte imbalance. Hypokalaemia can occur on regular use. Routine and long-term use must be discouraged; produces colonic atony.

Bisacodyl is a synthetic diphenylmethane which primarily acts in the colon. At optimum doses it produces one or two semiformed motions after 6–8 hours. However, the same dose may be ineffective in some individuals but cause fluid evacuations and cramps in others. Bisacodyl can also be used as suppository.

Sodium picosulfate is another diphenylmethane which is hydrolysed by the colonic bacteria to release the active form that activates the myenteric neurones. Bowel movement generally occurs after 6–12 hours.

Senna and Cascara sagrada These are plant products containing anthraquinone glycosides (also called emodins). Unabsorbed in the small intestine, they are passed to the colon where bacteria liberate the active *anthrol* form which acts locally or is absorbed into circulation to be excreted in bile and act on small intestine. Thus, these purgatives take 6–8 hours to produce action.

Taken at bedtime—a single, soft but formed evacuation generally occurs in the morning. Cramps and excessive purging occur in some cases. The active principle is believed to act on the myenteric plexus to increase peristalsis and decrease segmentation. They also inhibit salt and water absorption in the colon.

Skin rashes and fixed drug eruption are produced occasionally by both anthraquinones and diphenylmethanes.

Prucalopride It is a new selective 5-HT$_4$ receptor agonist which activates 5-HT$_4$ receptors on prejunctional enteric neurones promoting release of ACh from them. Propulsive contractions, especially in the colon, are enhanced. Colonic transit is hastened and stool frequency is improved in constipation predominant IBS. It is being used to treat chronic constipation in women, when other laxatives have failed.

Lubiprostone This PG analogue is a prostanoid EP$_4$ receptor agonist which stimulates Cl$^-$ channels in the gut mucosa to increase Cl$^-$ rich intestinal secretion and accelerate colonic transit. Lubiprostone is effective in the treatment of constipation-predominant IBS and idiopathic chronic constipation. It is recommended for patients who have not responded satisfactorily to other laxatives. Side effects are nausea, dyspepsia and diarrhoea.

Osmotic purgatives

Solutes that are not absorbed in the intestine retain water osmotically, distend the bowel and increase peristalsis indirectly. Magnesium ions release cholecystokinin which augments motility as well as secretion and thus contributes to the purgative action of Mag. salts. All inorganic salts used as osmotic purgatives have similar action but differ in dose, palatability and risk of systemic toxicity. The saline purgatives produce 1–2 fluid evacuations within 1–3 hours with mild cramping; cause nearly complete emptying of bowels. Smaller doses may have a milder laxative action. Repeated use of saline purgatives can cause fluid and electrolyte imbalance.

Saline purgatives are seldom used for the treatment of constipation, because they are unpleasant, produce watery stools and cause after-constipation. However, they may be preferred for preparation of bowel before surgery and colonoscopy; in food/drug poisoning and as after-purge in the treatment of tapeworm infestation.

Lactulose It is a semisynthetic disaccharide of fructose and lactose which is neither digested nor absorbed in the small intestine—retains water. Further, it is broken down in the colon by bacteria to osmotically more active products. In a dose of 10 g twice a day taken with plenty of water, lactulose produces soft formed stools in 8–12 hours. Flatulence is common, cramps occur in few. Some patients feel nauseated by its peculiar sweet taste. Lactulose is an alternative to bulk forming laxatives for treatment of constipation.

Lactulose is also used to decrease blood NH_3 level in hepatic encephalopathy, because its acidic breakdown products generated in the colon react with NH_3 to form ionized NH_4 salts that are not absorbed.

Lactitol It is a disaccharide alcohol which, like lactulose, is neither absorbed nor digested in the ileum, but gets fermented by colonic bacteria into osmotically active and weakly acidic products. The laxative efficacy of lactitol is comparable to that of lactulose, and many subjects find it more palatable than the latter. Lactitol also discourages NH_3 production by colonic bacteria and reduces its absorption. Thus, it is an alternative to lactulose for the treatment of constipation and hepatic encephalopathy.

USES OF PURGATIVES

Laxatives are as important for their harmfulness when used habitually as they are for their value in medicine.

The primary indication of laxatives is prevention and treatment of constipation.

1. *Functional constipation* Constipation is infrequent production of hard stools requiring straining to pass, or a sense of incomplete evacuation.

Constipation may be spastic or atonic.
(i) *Spastic constipation* (irritable bowel): The stools are hard, rounded, stone like and difficult to pass. The first choice laxative is ispaghula or any of the soluble fibres taken over weeks/months. Lactulose/lactitol is an alternative. Stimulant purgatives are contraindicated.
(ii) *Atonic constipation* (sluggish bowel): Non-drug measures like plenty of fluids, exercise, regular habits and reassurance should be tried. In resistant cases a bulk forming agent or lactulose should be prescribed. In case of poor compliance or if the patient is not satisfied—bisacodyl or senna may be given once or twice a week for as short a period as possible.

2. *Bedridden patients* (myocardial infarction, stroke, fractures, postoperative).

To prevent constipation: Give bulk forming agents on a regular schedule; docusates or lactulose is an alternative.

To treat constipation: Enema (soap-water/glycerine) is preferred; bisacodyl, senna or lactulose may be used otherwise.

3. *To avoid straining at stools* (hernia, cardiovascular disease, eye surgery) and in perianal afflictions (piles, fissure, anal

surgery) use adequate dose of a bulk forming agent, lactulose/lactitol or docusates.

4. *Preparation of bowel for surgery, colonoscopy, abdominal X-ray* The bowel needs to be emptied of the contents including gas. Saline purgative, bisacodyl or senna may be used.

5. *After certain anthelmintics* (especially for tape-worm) Saline purgative or senna may be used to flush out the worm and the anthelmintic drug.

The choice of a purgative depends on the latency of action and type of stools desired. This is given in Table 18.1.

Table 18.1: Type of stools and latency of action of purgatives employed in usually recommended doses

Soft, formed faeces (take 1–3 days)	Semifluid stools (take 6–8 hr)	Watery evacuation (within 1–3 hr)
Bulk forming Docusates Liquid paraffin Lactulose	Bisacodyl Sod. picosulfate Senna	Saline purgatives

TREATMENT OF DIARRHOEAS

Diarrhoea is too frequent, often too precipitate passage of poorly formed stools. The WHO has defined diarrhoea as 3 or more loose or watery stools in a 24 hours period. In pathological terms, it occurs due to passage of excess water in the faeces.

Diarrhoeal diseases constitute a major cause of morbidity and mortality worldwide; especially in developing countries and in children. It is estimated that in India 13 children die of diarrhoea every hour. Even mild diarrhoea, and that in adults, is a disabling symptom and an inconvenience.

Rational management of diarrhoea depends on establishing the underlying cause and instituting specific therapy only if necessary. Therapeutic measures for diarrhoea may be grouped into:
(a) Rehydration
(b) Antimicrobial drugs
(c) Probiotics
(d) Nonspecific antidiarrhoeal drugs
(e) Drugs for inflammatory bowel disease (IBD).

ORAL REHYDRATION

In majority of cases this is the only measure needed, especially if the fluid loss is mild (5–7% BW).

Oral rehydration is possible if glucose is added with salt. It capitalizes on the intactness of glucose coupled Na^+ absorption, even when other mechanisms have failed or when intestinal secretion is excessive. The secreted fluid lacks glucose and cannot be reabsorbed otherwise.

After extensive field studies in developing countries and trying the standard formula oral rehydration solution (ORS), the WHO in 2002 recommended a new formula ORS for universal use in children as well as in adult patients of diarrhoea. Its composition is given in the box.

New formula WHO-ORS			
Content		Concentrations	
NaCl	: 2.6 g	Na^+	— 75 mM
KCl	: 1.5 g	K^+	— 20 mM
Trisod. citrate	: 2.9 g	Cl^-	— 65 mM
Glucose	: 13.5 g	Citrate	— 10 mM
Water	: 1 L	Glucose	— 75 mM
Total osmolarity 245 mOsm/L			

The rate of administration of ORS depends on the degree of dehydration and the capacity of the patient to drink it. Patients are encouraged to drink small quantities every hour till fluid loss has been made up. Subsequently, it is left to the demand of the patient.

Oral rehydration therapy (ORT) is not designed to stop diarrhoea, but to restore and maintain hydration, electrolyte and pH balance until diarrhoea ceases, mostly spontaneously.

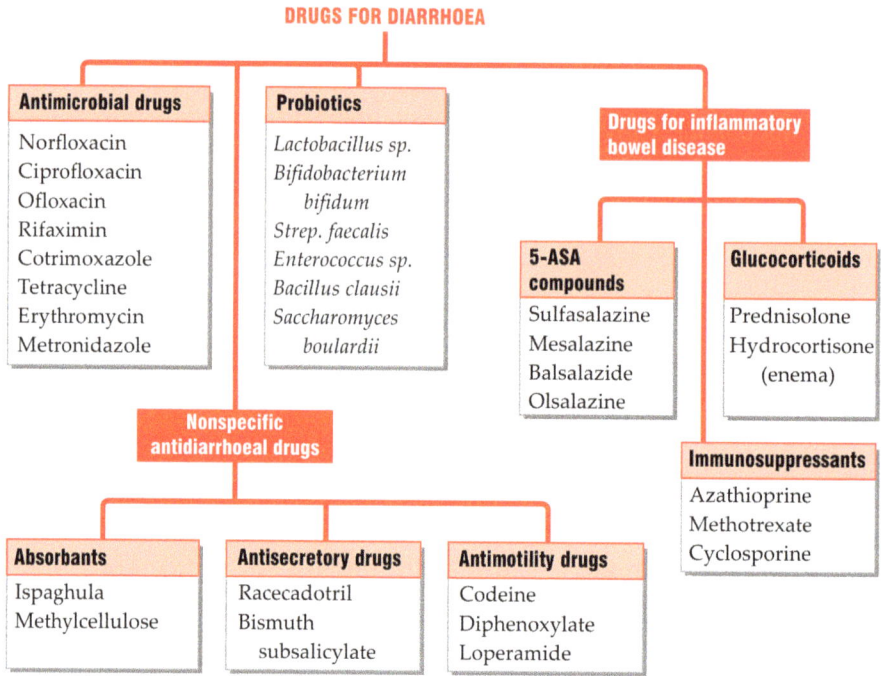

ANTIMICROBIAL DRUGS

One or more antimicrobial agent is almost routinely prescribed to every patient of diarrhoea. However, such drugs alter the course of the diarrhoeal illness only in selected cases, because:
- Bacterial pathogen is causative only in some patients.
- Even in bacterial diarrhoea, antimicrobials reduce the duration/intensity of only certain types of diarrhoeas.

A. Antimicrobials are of no value In diarrhoea due to *noninfective causes*, such as irritable bowel syndrome, coeliac disease, pancreatic enzyme deficiency, thyrotoxicosis as well as infective diarrhoea due to rotavirus or other diarrhoea causing viruses, antimicrobials have no beneficial effect. Mild *Salmonella* food poisoning is also a self-limiting disease.

B. Antimicrobials are useful in severe disease (but not in mild cases) in case of:
(i) Travellers' diarrhoea: mostly due to enterotoxigenic *E.coli* (ETEC), *Campylobacter* or viruses: Ciprofloxacin, norfloxacin, doxycycline reduce the duration of diarrhoea and total fluid needed only in severe cases.

Another antibiotic *Rifaximin* has recently become available for the emperic treatment of traveller's diarrhoea caused mostly by ETEC. It is a minimally absorbed congener of rifampin which acts locally in the gut lumen; no systemic effect/toxicity has been noted. Rifaximin is also being used for preparation of gut for surgery and to reduce recurrence of hepatic encephalopathy by suppressing ammonia producing gut bacteria.

(ii) Invasive diarrhoea: Severe cases with blood and mucus in stools, fever, cramps caused by enteropathogenic *E. coli* (EPEC), nontyphoid *Salmonella, Yersinia enterocolitica, Shigella*, etc. need to be treated empirically with ciprofloxacin, ofloxacin, cotrimoxazole or doxycycline.

C. Antimicrobials are useful in all cases:
- Cholera: Though only fluid replacement is life saving, tetracyclines reduce stool

volume to nearly ½. Cotrimoxazole, norfloxacin and erythromycin are the alternatives.
- *Campylobacter jejuni:* Norfloxacin and other fluoroquinolones control diarrhoea. Erythromycin is fairly effective.
- *Clostridium difficile:* produces antibiotic associated psuedo-membranous enterocolitis. The drug of choice for it is metronidazole.
- *Amoebiasis* ⎫ metronidazole,
- *Giardiasis* ⎭ diloxanide furoate are effective drugs.

PROBIOTICS

These are microbial cell preparations, either live cultures or lyophillised powders, that are intended to restore and maintain healthy gut flora or have other health benefits. Diarrhoeal illnesses and antibiotic use (for diarrhoea or for other purposes) are associated with alteration in the population, composition and balance of gut microflora. Recolonization of the gut by nonpathogenic, mostly lactic acid forming bacteria, and/or yeast is believed to help restore this balance. A variety of preparations containing single to multiple species of the microorganisms are being used for this purpose. The organisms included are *Lactobacillus sp., Bifidobacterium, Streptococcus faecalis, Enterococcus sp.* and the yeast *Saccharomyces boulardii,* etc.

Several studies have suggested that probiotics significantly reduce antibiotic-associated diarrhoea, acute infective diarrhoea and risk of traveller's diarrhoea.

While probiotics appear to be useful adjuncts to conventional therapy of acute infectious diarrhoea, convincing evidence of their efficacy is lacking. Stronger evidence of efficacy has emerged against antibiotic-associated diarrhoea, but there is no justification yet for routine inclusion of probiotics while prescribing antibiotics. Natural curd/yogurt is an abundant source of lactic acid producing organisms, which can serve as probiotic.

NONSPECIFIC ANTIDIARRHOEAL DRUGS

1. Antisecretory drugs

Racecadotril It is a recently introduced prodrug which after conversion to the active form *thiorphan* in the body inhibits the enzyme enkephalinase. Degradation of enkephalins, which are mainly δ opioid receptor agonists, is prevented—resulting in attenuation of intestinal hypersecretion. It can be given to young children as well, while the antimotility drug loperamide is contraindicated in them. Racecadotril is indicated for the short-term treatment of acute secretory diarrhoeas.

Bismuth subsalicylate Taken as a suspension 3–4 times a day, it decreases intestinal secretion to benefit traveller's diarrhoea, but is inconvenient, and seldom used in India.

2. Antimotility drugs

These are opioid drugs which increase tone and segmenting activity of the bowel, reduce propulsive movements and diminish intestinal secretions while enhancing absorption. The major action appears to be mediated through μ opioid receptors located on enteric neuronal network, but direct action on intestinal smooth muscle and secretory/absorptive epithelium has also been demonstrated.

Codeine This opium alkaloid has prominent constipating action. Though its dependence producing liability is low, but it is a restricted drug. Due to availability of loperamide it is not used now to control diarrhoea.

Diphenoxylate is a synthetic opioid used exclusively as constipating agent. Its action is similar to that of codeine. Because it is absorbed systemically and crosses blood-brain barrier—CNS effects do occur. Therefore, atropine is added to its tablet in subpharmacological dose to discourage abuse. It has been largely replaced by loperamide.

Loperamide is an opiate analogue with major peripheral μ opioid agonistic and additional weak anticholinergic property. As a constipating agent, it is much more potent than codeine. Because of poor water solubility—little is absorbed from the intestines. Entry into brain is negligible—CNS effects are rare. Loperamide has no analgesic action and abuse liability.

In addition to its opiate like action on motility, loperamide also inhibits intestinal secretion.

Abdominal cramps and rashes are the most common side effects. Paralytic ileus, toxic megacolon with abdominal distension is a serious complication in young children. Therefore, loperamide is contraindicated in children < 4 years.

The utility of antimotility drugs in diarrhoea is limited to symptomatic relief in noninvasive diarrhoea, mild travellers' diarrhoea and when diarrhoea is exhausting. Their use is a short-term measure.

Antimotility drugs are contraindicated in acute infective diarrhoeas because they delay clearance of the pathogen from the intestine. If invasive organisms (*Shigella*, EPEC, EH, etc.) are present, antimotility drugs can be disastrous.

Antimotility drugs can be used to induce deliberate short-term constipation, e.g. after anal surgery.

DRUGS FOR INFLAMMATORY BOWEL DISEASE

Inflammatory bowel disease (IBD) is a chronic relapsing inflammatory disorder of the ileum, colon or both, that may be associated with systemic manifestations. It is an idiopathic, probably autoimmune disorder which presents in two main types, viz. Ulcerative colitis (UC) and Crohn's disease (CrD). The former affects only the colon, and the lesions are mucosal, while the latter may affect several segments of the g.i.t (even oral ulcers can occur) and the lesions are transmural.

Drugs used for IBD are:

Sulfasalazine It is a compound of 5-aminosalicylic acid (5-ASA) with sulfapyridine, linked through an azo bond.

$$HOOC-\underset{5\text{-ASA}}{\underset{HO-}{\bigcirc}}-\underset{AZO\ bond}{N=N}-\underset{Sulfapyridine}{\bigcirc-SO_2NH-\bigcirc_N}$$

SULFASALAZINE

Taken orally, it traverses without being absorbed through the ileum to the colon where the azo bond is split by colonic bacteria to release 5-ASA and sulfapyridine. The former exerts a local anti-inflammatory effect in the colon, affording symptomatic relief in UC. Sulfasalazine is less effective than corticosteroids in controlling acute phase of UC, but induces remission when continued for few weeks. Maintenance therapy with sulfasalazine delays relapses of UC in majority of cases.

The released sulfapyridine is partially absorbed in the colon contributing to adverse effects like fever, rashes, joint pain, mild anaemia and blood dyscrasias. It also interferes with folate absorption; folic acid supplementation is given routinely with it.

Sulfasalazine is also used in rheumatoid arthritis as a disease modifying antirheumatic drug (DMARD).

Mesalazine (Mesalamine) Realizing that 5-ASA is the active moiety for UC, this moiety has been formulated as a late release preparation, or coated with acrylic polymer so as to deliver 5-ASA to the distal small bowel and colon.

In UC, mesalazine has the same efficacy as sulfasalazine, without producing adverse effects that are due to sulfapyridine. The primary role of mesalazine is to prevent relapses in UC, but it is also being used as an adjunct to corticosteroids for controlling an exacerbation.

Balsalazide This is 5-ASA linked to another carrier 4-aminobenzoyl-β-alanine in place of sulfapyridine. Balsalazide releases 5-ASA in the colon; the carrier is inert, and not absorbed. It is a better tolerated alternative to sulfasalazine.

Coticosteroids Prednisolone 40–60 mg/day (or equivalent) is highly effective in controlling acute symptoms of both UC and CrD, as well as in inducing remission. However, corticosteroids are neither effective in maintaining remission nor suitable for this purpose. Because of the adverse consequences of long-term steroid therapy, these drugs are gradually withdrawn after a remission is induced, while mesalazine started concurrently is continued for years.

Immunosuppressants

Azathioprine It is the most effective immunosuppressant in both UC and CrD. It has good remission maintaining and steroid sparing property. However, it (and other immunosuppressants) is not useful for controlling acute symptoms and inducing remission, because its action takes 1–3 months to develop. Azathioprine is indicated in patients of IBD who experience repeated flareups, and is continued for at least for 2–3 years.

Methotrexate (Mtx) This dihydrofolate reductase inhibitor has immunosuppressant and anti-inflammatory property. Mtx. is a 2nd line drug in IBD, particularly in CrD. It acts faster than azathioprine, and has remission inducing property as well.

Cyclosporine This potent immunosuppressant is a reserve drug in severe and unresponsive UC and CrD.

CHAPTER 19

Drugs for Respiratory Disorders

DRUGS FOR COUGH

Cough is a protective reflex, its purpose being expulsion of respiratory secretions and foreign particles from air passages. It occurs due to stimulation of mechano- or chemoreceptors in throat, respiratory passages or stretch receptors in the lungs. Cough may be useful or useless. Useless (nonproductive) cough should be suppressed. Useful (productive) cough serves to drain the airway, its suppression is not desirable, may even be harmful. Apart from specific remedies (antibiotics, etc.), cough may be treated as a symptom (nonspecific therapy) with:

Pharyngeal demulcents sooth the throat and reduce afferent impulses from the inflamed/irritated pharyngeal mucosa, thus provide symptomatic relief in dry cough arising from throat.

Expectorants (Mucokinetics) are drugs believed to increase bronchial secretion or reduce its viscosity, facilitating its removal by coughing.

Guaiphenesin, vasaka, tolu balsam are plant products which are supposed to enhance bronchial secretion and mucociliary function

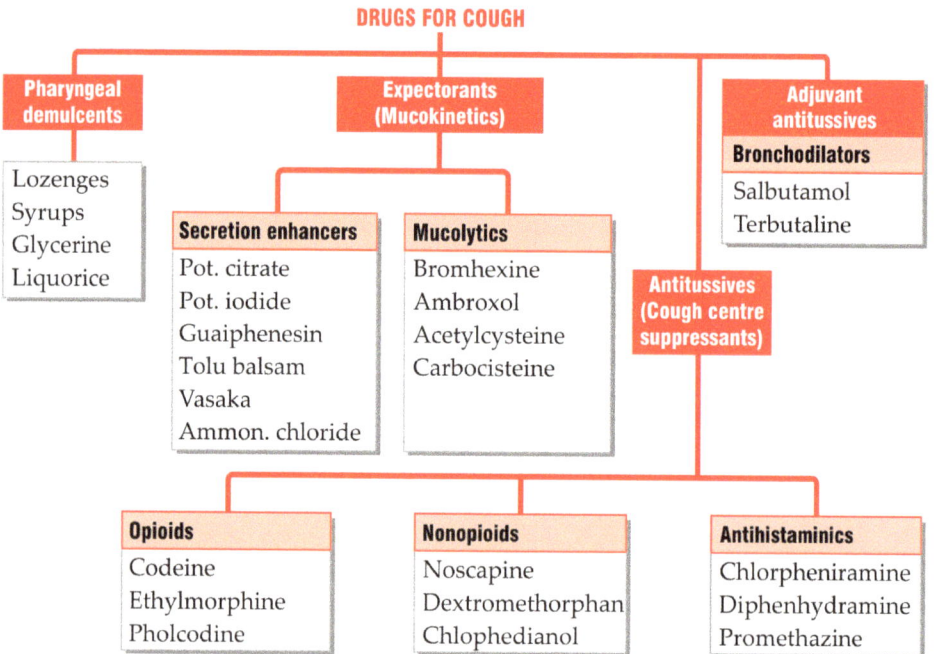

while being secreted by tracheobronchial glands. Ammonium salts are nauseating—reflexly increase respiratory secretions. A variety of expectorant formulations containing an assortment of the above ingredients, often in combination with antitussives/antihistaminics are marketed and briskly promoted, but objective evidence of efficacy of these is non-conclusive.

Bromhexine A derivative of the alkaloid vasicine, obtained from vasaka, bromhexine is a potent mucolytic and mucokinetic capable of inducing thin copious bronchial secretion. It depolymerises mucopolysaccharides, and is particularly useful if mucus plugs are present.

Ambroxol A metabolite of bromhexine having similar mucolytic action, uses and side effects.

Acetylcysteine, Carbocisteine These drugs liquefy viscid sputum by opening disulfide bonds in mucoproteins. Some patients of chronic bronchitis are benefited.

ANTITUSSIVES

These are drugs that act in the CNS to raise the threshold of cough centre. Because they aim to control rather than eliminate cough, antitussives should be used only for dry nonproductive cough or if it is unduly tiring, disturbs sleep or is hazardous (as in patients with hernia, piles, cardiac disease, ocular surgery).

Codeine (see Ch. 24) It is an opium alkaloid, qualitatively similar to but less potent than morphine. Codeine is more selective for the cough centre and is treated as the standard antitussive. It suppresses cough for about 6 hours. The antitussive. It action is blocked by naloxone indicating that it is exerted through opioid receptors in the brain. Abuse liability is low, but present; constipation is the chief drawback.

Ethylmorphine Like codeine, it has selective antitussive and respiratory depressant action, but is believed to be less constipating.

Pholcodine It has practically no analgesic or addicting property, but is similar in efficacy as antitussive to codeine and is longer acting—acts for 12 hours.

Noscapine (Narcotine) An opium alkaloid of the benzoisoquinoline series, noscapine depresses cough but has no narcotic, analgesic or dependence inducing properties. It is nearly equipotent antitussive to codeine, and is especially useful in spasmodic cough.

Dextromethorphan A synthetic NMDA receptor antagonist whose *d*-isomer has antitussive action (raises threshold of cough centre). Dextromethorphan does not depress mucociliary function of the airway mucosa and is practically devoid of constipating action.

Chlophedianol It is a centrally acting antitussive with slow onset and longer duration of antitussive action.

Antihistamines Some older H_1 antihistamines (e.g. chlorpheniramine) have been conventionally added to antitussive/expectorant formulations. They afford relief in cough due to their sedative and anticholinergic actions, but lack selectivity for the cough centre. These antihistaminics have no expectorant property, may even reduce secretions by anticholinergic action. They have been specially promoted for cough in respiratory allergic states.

Bronchodilators Bronchospasm can induce or aggravate cough. Stimulation of pulmonary receptors can trigger both cough and bronchoconstriction, especially in individuals with bronchial hyperreactivity. Bronchodilators relieve cough in such individuals and improve the effectiveness of cough in clearing secretions by increasing surface velocity of airflow during cough. They should be used only when an element of bronchoconstriction is present and not routinely.

DRUGS FOR BRONCHIAL ASTHMA

Bronchial asthma is characterised by hyper-responsiveness of tracheobronchial smooth muscle to a variety of stimuli, resulting in narrowing of air tubes, often accompanied by increased secretion, mucosal edema and mucus plugging.

Asthma is now recognized to be a primarily inflammatory condition: inflammation underlying the hyperreactivity. An allergic basis can be demonstrated in many adult, and higher percentage of pediatric patients. In others, a variety of trigger factors (infection, irritants, pollution, exercise, exposure to cold air, psychogenic) may be involved.

The inflammation in bronchial asthma is initiated by mast cells (present in lungs), and the infiltrate is dominated by eosinophils, lymphocytes and mast cells. The initial inflammatory reaction produces a multitude of mediators, *viz.* histamine, TNFα, PGs, LTs, PAF, interleukins, etc. which constrict bronchial smooth muscle, cause mucosal edema, hyperemia and produce viscid secretions, all resulting in reversible airway obstruction. In the long term, airway remodeling occurs which progressively worsens the disease.

Chronic obstructive pulmonary disease (COPD) It is also an inflammatory disease of the airways and lungs which is dominated by neutrophills, macrophages and cytotoxic lymphocytes. COPD is characterized by progressive emphysema (alveolar destruction) and bronchiolar fibrosis in variable proportions. The expiratory airflow limitation does not fluctuate markedly over long periods of time, but there are exacerbations precipitated by respiratory infections, pollutants, etc. It is clearly related to smoking and characteristically starts after the age of 40.

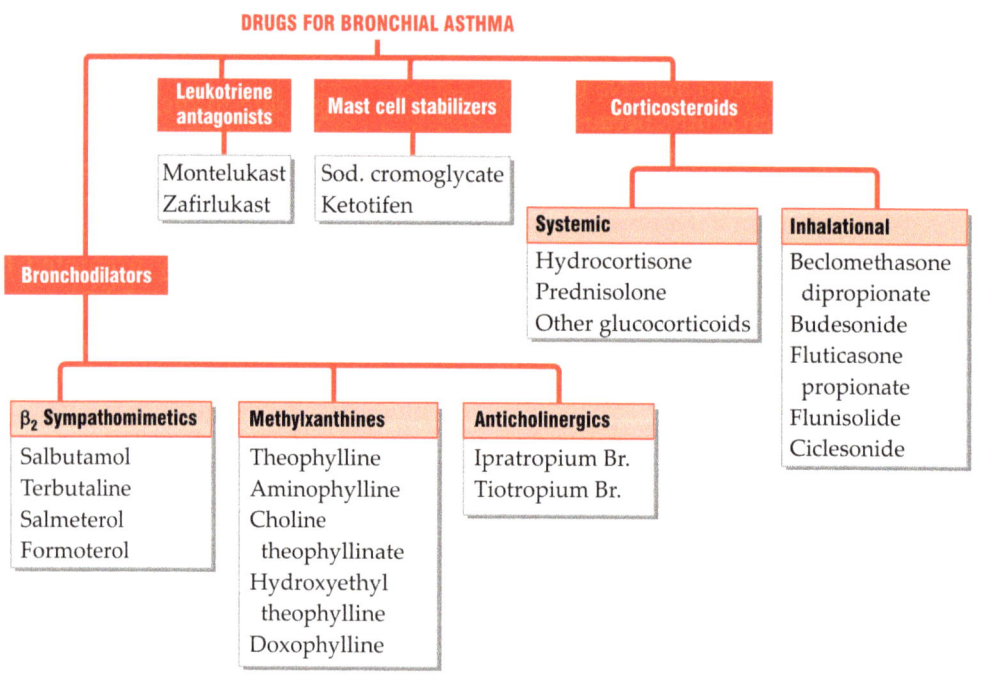

SYMPATHOMIMETIC DRUGS (*See* Ch. 6)

Adrenergic drugs cause bronchodilatation through β_2 receptor stimulation and increased cAMP formation in bronchial muscle cell resulting in relaxation. Adrenergic drugs are the mainstay of treatment of reversible airway obstruction. They are the fastest acting bronchodilators when inhaled.

The highly selective β_2 agonists like *salbutamol* and *terbutaline* are used in asthma to minimize side effects due to cardiac stimulation. Selectivity is further increased by inhaling the drug. Inhaled salbutamol produces bronchodilatation within 5 min and the action lasts for 2 to 4 hours. It is, therefore, used to abort and terminate attacks of asthma but is not suitable for round-the-clock prophylaxis. Muscle tremors are the dose-related side effect. Palpitation, restlessness, nervousness, throat irritation can also occur. Oral salbutamol acts for 4–6 hours.

Because of more frequent side effects, oral β_2 agonist therapy is reserved for patients who cannot correctly use inhalers, and during severe asthma exacerbations.

However, β_2 agonists do not reduce bronchial hyperreactivity: may even worsen it—this may be responsible for the diminished responsiveness seen after long-term use. Regular use also down-regulates bronchial β_2 receptors. It is advised that patients requiring regular β_2 agonists should be treated with inhaled steroids and use of β_2 agonist inhalers should be restricted to symptomatic relief of wheezing.

Salmeterol It is the first long-acting selective β_2 agonist with a slow onset of action. It is used by inhalation on a twice daily schedule for maintenance therapy and for nocturnal asthma, but not for acute symptoms. Concurrent use of inhaled glucocorticoid with salmeterol is advocated.

Long-acting β_2 agonists are superior to short-acting ones in COPD.

Formoterol is another long-acting selective β_2 agonist which has a faster onset of action within 10 min, generally used on a regular morning-evening schedule.

METHYLXANTHINES

Theophylline is one of the three naturally occurring methylated xanthine alkaloids *caffeine, theophylline* and *theobromine*. The chemical relation between the three is depicted below:

THEOPHYLLINE (1,3, Dimethylxanthine)

THEOBROMINE (3,7, Dimethylxanthine)

CAFFEINE (1,3,7, Trimethylxanthine)

They are consumed as beverages. The source and average alkaloid content of the beverages, as they are usually prepared is given in the box below. Theophylline has the most prominent bronchodilator action.

Source	Alkaloid content in beverage		
1. Thea sinensis (Tea leaves)	Caffeine Theophylline	50 mg 1 mg	in an average cup of tea
2. Coffea arabica (Coffee seeds)	Caffeine	75 mg	in an average cup of coffee
3. Theobroma cacao (Cocoa, chocolate)	Theobromine Caffeine	200 mg 4 mg	in an average cup of cocoa
4. Cola acuminata (Guru nuts)	Caffeine	30 mg	in 200 ml bottle of cola drink

Pharmacological actions

1. *CNS* Caffeine and theophylline are CNS stimulants, primarily affect the higher centres. Caffeine produces a sense of well-being, alertness, beats boredom, allays fatigue, thinking becomes clearer. It tends to improve performance and increase motor activity. Higher doses cause nervousness, restlessness, panic, insomnia and excitement. Still higher doses produce tremors, delirium and convulsions. Theophylline has greater propensity to produce these adverse effects at higher doses and is definitely more toxic than caffeine.

2. *CVS* Methylxanthines stimulate the heart and increase force of myocardial contractions without interacting with β adrenergic receptors. They tend to increase heart rate by direct action, but decrease it by causing vagal stimulation—net effect is variable. Tachycardia is more common with theophylline. At high doses, cardiac arrhythmias may be produced.

Methylxanthines, especially theophylline, dilate systemic blood vessels by direct action. However, cranial vessels are constricted, especially by caffeine. This is one of the basis for its use in migraine.

Effect on BP is variable and unpredictable.

3. *Smooth muscles* All smooth muscles are relaxed; most prominent effect is exerted on bronchi, especially in asthmatics. Theophylline is more potent bronchodilator than caffeine. Slow but sustained broncho-dilatation is produced.

4. *Skeletal muscles* Caffeine enhances contractile power of skeletal muscles. Enhanced diaphragmatic contractility probably contributes to the beneficial effects of theophylline in dyspnoea.

5. *Mast cells and inflammatory cells* Theophylline decreases the release of histamine and other mediators from mast cells and other activated inflammatory cells. This may contribute to its therapeutic effect in bronchial asthma and in COPD.

Other minor actions of methylxanthines are mild diuresis, gastric irritation, increased gastric secretion and increased BMR.

Mechanism of action Three distinct cellular actions of methylxanthines have been defined—

(a) Release of Ca^{2+} from sarcoplasmic reticulum, especially in skeletal and cardiac muscle.

(b) Inhibition of phosphodiesterase (PDE) which degrades cyclic nucleotides intracellularly.

ATP	*adenylylcyclase*	cAMP	*phosphodiesterase*	5-AMP
or	→	or	→	or
GTP	*guanylylcyclase*	cGMP	INHIBITED BY THEOPHYLLINE	5-GMP

Thus, the concentration of cyclic nucleotides is increased. Bronchodilatation, cardiac stimulation and vasodilatation occur when cAMP level rises in the concerned cells.

(c) Blockade of adenosine receptors: adenosine acts as a local mediator in CNS, CVS and other organs. It contracts smooth muscles, especially bronchial; dilates cerebral blood vessels, depresses cardiac pacemaker and inhibits gastric secretion. Methylxanthines produce opposite effects.

Action (c) and action (b) are exerted at concentrations in the therapeutic range and may be more important in mediating bronchodilatation.

Pharmacokinetics Theophylline is well absorbed orally. It is extensively metabolized in liver by demethylation and oxidation. Only 10% is excreted unchanged in urine. At therapeutic concentrations, the t½ in adults is 7–12 hours. Children eliminate it much faster and elderly more slowly.

Theophylline metabolizing enzymes are saturable, t½ is prolonged with higher doses as kinetics changes from first to zero order: plasma concentrations, therefore, increase disproportionately.

Adverse effects Theophylline has a narrow margin of safety. Adverse effects are primarily referable to g.i.t., CNS and CVS, *viz* dyspepsia, vomiting, nervousness, tremor, delirium, hypotension, arrhythmias and convulsions.

Interactions
1. Agents which induce theophylline metabolism and lower its plasma level are—smoking, phenytoin, rifampicin, phenobarbitone, charcoal broiled meat meal.
2. Drugs which inhibit theophylline metabolism and raise its plasma level are—erythromycin, ciprofloxacin, cimetidine, oral contraceptives, allopurinol; dose of theophylline should be reduced to 2/3rd.
3. Theophylline enhances the effects of—furosemide, sympathomimetics, digoxin, warfarin and hypoglycaemics.

Uses
1. *Bronchial asthma and COPD*: Theophylline benefits mainly by causing bronchodilatation. Other actions of theophylline which may add to the response are—stimulation of respiratory drive, augmentation of diaphragmatic contractility and attenuation of release of inflammatory mediators. However, because of narrow margin of safety, wide individual variability and limited efficacy, its use has declined. Sustained release theophylline can be used in mild-to-moderately severe asthma, as an adjuvant drug. Theophylline is more useful in COPD.
2. *Apnoea in premature infant*: Theophylline reduces the frequency and duration of episodes of apnoea that occur in some preterm infants.

ANTICHOLINERGIC DRUGS (*See* Ch. 5)

Atropinic drugs cause bronchodilatation by blocking M_3 receptor mediated cholinergic constrictor tone. They act primarily in the larger airways (Fig. 19.1).

In bronchial asthma inhaled ipratropium bromide is less efficacious than inhaled

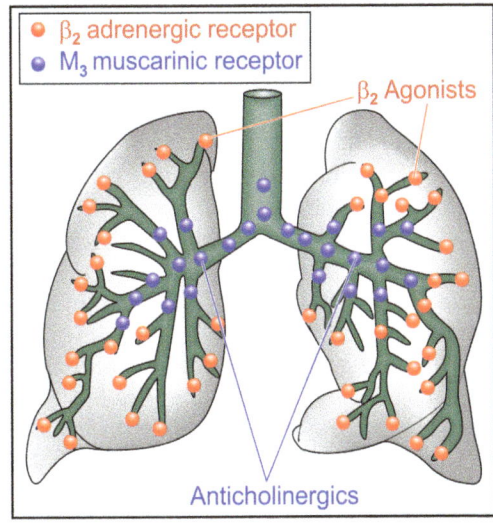

Fig. 19.1: Primary sites of bronchodilator action of inhaled adrenergic β_2 agonists and inhaled anticholinergics. Salbutamol mainly relaxes bronchiolar smooth muscle; Ipratropium blocks bronchoconstriction mainly in the larger airways

β_2 agonists but can add to their response. Patients of asthmatic bronchitis, COPD and psychogenic asthma respond better to anticholinergics. Inhaled ipratropium/tiotropium are the bronchodilators of choice in COPD. They produce slower response than inhaled β_2 agonists and are better suited for regular prophylactic use than for quick relief of breathlessness. Nebulized ipratropium mixed with salbutamol is employed in refractory asthma.

LEUKOTRIENE ANTAGONISTS

Since it was realized that cystenyl leukotrienes (LT-C_4/D_4) are important mediators of bronchial asthma, efforts were made to develop their antagonists and synthesis inhibitors. Two cysLT$_1$ receptor antagonists *montelukast* and *zafirlukast* are now established drugs for asthma.

Montelukast and Zafirlukast Both have similar actions and clinical utility. They competitively antagonise cysLT$_1$ receptor mediated bronchoconstriction, airway mucus secretion, increased vascular permeability and recruitment of eosinophils. Bronchodilatation, reduced sputum eosinophil count, suppression of bronchial inflammation and hyperreactivity are noted in asthma patients. Parameters of lung function show improvement, but to variable extent.

Montelukast and zafirlukast are indicated for prophylactic therapy of mild-to-moderate asthma as alternatives to inhaled glucocorticoids, but their efficacy is lower. In severe asthma, they may permit reduction in steroid dose. However, they are not to be used for terminating asthma episodes and for COPD.

Montelukast and zafirlukast are well absorbed orally. The plasma t½ of montelukast is 3 to 6 hours, while that of zafirlukast is 8 to 12 hours.

MAST CELL STABILIZERS
Sodium cromoglycate (Cromolyn sod.)
It is a synthetic chromone derivative which inhibits degranulation of mast cells by trigger stimuli. Release of mediators of asthma like histamine, LTs, PAF, interleukins, etc. from mast cells as well as other inflammatory cells is attenuated. Bronchospasm induced by allergens, irritants, cold air and exercise may be reduced. It is not a bronchodilator and does not antagonise the constrictor action of histamine, ACh, LTs, etc. Therefore, it is ineffective if given during an asthmatic attack.

Sod. cromoglycate is not absorbed orally. It is administered as an aerosol through metered dose inhaler. Because of lower and inconsistent efficacy, and availability of inhaled steroids, sod. cromoglycate is seldom used now.

Ketotifen It is an antihistaminic (H_1) with some cromoglycate like action, so that mediator release is attenuated. It is not a bronchodilator but produces sedation.

After regular use, symptomatic improvement may occur in asthma patients, but improvement in lung function is marginal. It may produce some symptomatic relief in atopic dermatitis, perennial rhinitis, conjunctivitis, urticaria and food allergy as well.

CORTICOSTEROIDS

Glucocorticoids are not bronchodilators. They benefit asthma by inhibiting inflammatory cytokine production, infiltration of lungs as well as by reducing bronchial hyper-reactivity, and mucosal edema. They suppress inflammatory response to AG:AB reaction or other trigger stimuli. Their mechanism of action is detailed in Ch. 14.

The realization that asthma is primarily an inflammatory disorder which, if not controlled, accentuates with time, and the availability of inhaled corticosteroids (ICS) which produce few adverse effects, has led to early introduction and more extensive use of glucocorticoids in asthma. Corticosteroids afford more complete and sustained symptomatic relief than bronchodilators, reverse refractoriness to β_2 agonists, suppress bronchial hyperreactivity, and retard disease progression.

Systemic steroid therapy It is resorted to in asthma under the following two situations:

(i) Severe chronic asthma: not controlled by bronchodilators and ICS, or when there are frequent recurrences of increasing severity. Few patients require long-term oral steroids—in them dose should be kept at minimum.

(ii) Status asthmaticus / acute asthma exacerbation: This refers to asthma attack not respnding to intensive bronchodilator therapy: start with high dose of a rapidly acting i.v. glucocorticoid which generally acts in 6–24 hours. When the exacerbation subsides, shift to oral steroid therapy for 5 to 7 days and then discontinue abruptly or taper rapidly.

COPD A short course of oral glucocorticoid may benefit COPD during an exacerbation.

Inhaled corticosteroids These glucocorticoids have high topical and low systemic activity (due to poor absorption and/or marked first pass metabolism). *Beclomethasone dipropionate, Budesonide* and *Fluticasone* have similar properties. *Ciclesonide* is a later addition. Because airway inflammation is present even in early mild disease as well, and bronchial remodeling starts developing from the beginning, it has been suggested that inhaled steroids should be the 'step one' for all asthma patients. However, currently inhaled steroids are not considered necessary for patients with mild and episodic asthma. They are indicated when inhaled β_2 agonists are required almost daily, or when the disease is not only episodic.

Inhaled steroids suppress bronchial inflammation, increase peak expiratory flow rate, reduce need for rescue β_2-agonist inhalations and prevent episodes of acute asthma. However, ICS have no role during an acute attack or in status asthmaticus.

COPD: High dose ICS are beneficial in advanced COPD with frequent exacerbations. They should not be used in early/mild cases.

Hoarseness of voice, dysphonia, sore throat, asymptomatic or symptomatic oropharyngeal candidiasis are the most common side effects. These side effects can be minimized by use of a spacer and gargling after every dose.

Choice of treatment

A stepwise guideline to the treatment of asthma as per needs of the patient has been recommended:

1. *Mild episodic asthma* (symptoms less than once daily, normal in between attacks): Inhaled short-acting β_2 agonist at onset of each episode. No regular prophylactic therapy (Step 1).

2. *Seasonal asthma* Start regular low dose ICS 3–4 weeks before anticipated seasonal attacks and continue till 3–4 weeks after the season is over. Alternatively, oral montelukast/zafirlukast may be tried. Treat individual episodes with inhaled short-acting β_2 agonist.

3. *Mild chronic asthma with occasional exacerbations* (symptoms once daily or so) Regular low-dose ICS. Alternatively, daily oral montelukast/zafirlukast may be tried, but appears to be less effective. Oral theophylline is another alternative. (Step 2). Episode treatment with inhaled short-acting β_2 agonist.

4. *Moderate asthma with frequent exacerbations* (attacks affect activity, occur > 1 per day or mild baseline symptoms) low-to-medium doses of ICS + inhaled long-acting β_2 agonist (Step 3). Leukotriene antagonists or sustained release theophylline may be tried as additional/alternative drug. Episode treatment with inhaled short-acting β_2 agonist.

5. *Severe asthma* (continuous symptoms; activity limitation; frequent exacerbations/hospitalization) Regular high dose ICS through a large volume spacer device + inhaled long-acting β_2 agonist twice daily. Additional treatment with one or more of the following (Step 4): Sustained release oral theophylline/inhaled ipratropium bromide/leukotriene antagonist/oral β_2 agonist.

In patients not adequately controlled or those needing frequent emergency care—institute oral steroid therapy (Step 5). Periodically attempt withdrawing oral steroids.

6. *Status asthmaticus/Refractory asthma*
- High flow humidified oxygen inhalation.
- Hydrocortisone hemisuccinate 100 mg i.v. *stat* followed by 100–200 mg/8 hr infusion.
- Nebulized salbutamol + ipratropium bromide intermittent inhalations.
- Salbutamol/terbutaline 0.4 mg i.m./s.c. may be added since inhaled drug may not reach smaller bronchi due to severe narrowing/plugging.
- Treat chest infection with intensive antibiotic therapy.
- Correct dehydration and acidosis with saline + sod. bicarbonate/lactate infusion.

Vitamins

Vitamins are nonenergy yielding organic compounds, essential for normal human metabolism, that must be supplied in small quantities in the diet. This definition excludes the inorganic essential trace minerals and essential amino acids and fatty acids which are required in much larger quantities.

The importance of vitamins as drugs is primarily in the prevention and treatment of deficiency diseases. *Deficiency of many vitamins produces oro-dental manifestations*, i.e.
- Stomatitis/glossitis/sore mouth/oral ulcers in riboflavin, niacin, pyridoxine or vit A deficiency.
- Spongy and bleeding gums/gingivitis/loose and deformed teeth in vit C deficiency.

As such, dentists have the responsibility to recognise and treat these deficiencies.

Some vitamins do have other empirical uses in pharmacological (larger) doses. Vitamins, as a class, are overpromoted, over- prescribed and overused. Myths like 'they energise the body', 'any physical illness is accompanied by vitamin deficiency', 'vitamin intake in normal diet is precariously marginal', 'they are harmless' are rampant.

Vitamins are traditionally divided into two groups:

(a) *Fat soluble* (A, D, E, K): These (except vit K) are stored in the body for prolonged periods and are liable to cause cumulative toxicity after regular ingestion of large amounts. Some (vit A and D) interact with specific cellular receptors analogous to hormones.

(b) *Water soluble* (B complex, C): These are meagerly stored in the body; excess is excreted with little chance of toxicity. They act as cofactors for specific enzymes of intermediary metabolism.

Vitamin D (Ch. 16), vit K, folic acid and B_{12} (Ch. 17) have already been considered. Some relevant information is tabulated in Table 20.1.

FAT-SOLUBLE VITAMINS

VITAMIN A

Vitamin A occurs in nature in several forms, viz. retinol, retinal, dehydroretinal in fish liver oils, egg, milk, butter. The plant pigment β carotene is a provitamin found in carrot, turnip, spinach, etc.

Retinol is absorbed from the intestines by a carrier-mediated transport. Absorption is aided by bile and is normally complete. Retinol ester circulates in chylomicrons and is stored in liver cells. Free retinol released by hepatocytes combines with *retinol binding protein* (*RBP* a plasma globulin) and is transported to the target cells. On entering them, it gets bound to the *cellular retinol binding protein* (*CRBP*). Small amount is conjugated with glucuronic acid, excreted in bile, undergoes enterohepatic circulation.

Table 20.1: Chemical forms, stability and daily allowance of vitamins

Vitamin	Chemical forms	Thermostability	Daily allowance (adult males)
Fat-soluble vitamins			
A	Retinol (A_1) Dehydroretinol (A_2) β-Carotene (provit.)	Stable in absence of air	1000 μg (4,000 IU)
D	Calciferol (D_2) Cholecalciferol (D_3) Calcitriol	Stable	5 μg (200 IU) 1 μg
E	α-Tocopherol	Stable; air & UV light decompose it	10 mg
K	Phytonadione (K_1) (Phylloquinone) Menaquinones (K_2) Menadione (K_3) Acetomenaphthone	Stable, decomposed by light	50–100 μg
Water-soluble vitamins			
B_1	Thiamine	Relatively labile	1.5 mg
B_2	Riboflavin	Relatively stable	1.7 mg
B_3	Nicotinic acid } Niacin Nicotinamide Tryptophan (provit.)	Stable	20 mg
B_6	Pyridoxine Pyridoxal Pyridoxamine	Stable in absence of air	2 mg
	Pantothenic acid	Labile	4–7 mg
	Biotin	Stable	0.1–0.2 mg
	Folic acid Folinic acid	Labile	0.2 mg
B_{12}	Cyanocobalamin Hydroxocobalamin Methylcobalamin	Stable	2 μg
C	Ascorbic acid	Labile in solution	60 mg

In contrast to retinol, only 30% of dietary β carotene is absorbed. It is split into two molecules of *retinal* in the intestinal wall; only half of this is reduced to retinol and utilized.

Physiological role and actions

(a) *Visual cycle* Retinal generated by reversible oxidation of retinol is a component of the light sensitive pigment *Rhodopsin* which is synthesized by rods during dark adaptation. This pigment gets bleached and split into its components by dim light and in the process generates a nerve impulse (Fig. 20.1). Retinal so released is reutilized. In vit. A deficiency rods are affected more than cones; irreversible structural changes with permanent night blindness occur if the deprivation is long term.

(b) *Epithelial tissue* Vit A promotes differentiation and maintains structural integrity of epithelia all over the body. It also promotes mucus secretion, inhibits keratinization and

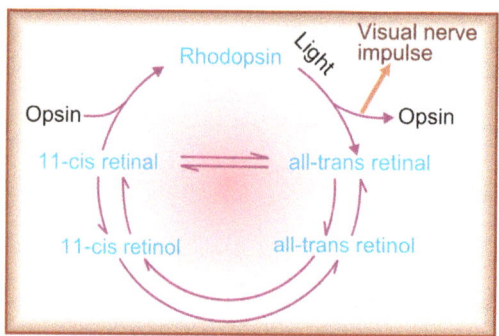

Fig. 20.1: The role of vit A in visual cycle

improves resistance to infection. Vit A appears to have the ability to retard development of malignancies of epithelial structures. Vit A is also required for bone growth.

(c) *Reproduction* Retinol is needed for maintenance of spermatogenesis and foetal development.

(d) *Immunity* Increased susceptibility to infection occurs in vit A deficiency. Physiological amount of vit A appears to be required for proper antibody response, normal lymphocyte proliferation and killer cell function.

Deficiency and use Vit A deficiency is quite prevalent, especially among infants and children in developing countries. Manifestations are:
- Xerosis (dryness) of eye, 'Bitot's spots', keratomalacia (softening of cornea), corneal opacities, night blindness (nyctalopia) progressing to total blindness.
- Dry and rough skin with papules (phrynoderma), hyperkeratinization, atrophy of sweat glands.
- Keratinization of bronchopulmonary epithelium, increased susceptibility to infection.
- Unhealthy gastrointestinal mucosa, diarrhoea.
- Increased tendency to urinary stone formation due to shedding of ureteric epithelial lining which acts as nidus.
- Sterility due to faulty spermatogenesis, abortions, foetal malformations.
- Growth retardation, impairment of special senses.

Vit A (3000–5000 IU/day) is used for prophylaxis of Vit A deficiency, particularly during infancy, early childhood, pregnancy, lactation and hepatobiliary diseases. Under the National Vit-A mass prophylaxis program in India, 200,000 IU Vit A is administered orally every 6 months to all children from age 9 months to 5 years (total 9 mega doses). For treatment of established Vit A deficiency 50,000–200,000 IU Vit A is given orally/i.m. daily for 5 days, followed by intermittent supplemental doses.

Retinoic acid and 2nd or 3rd generation retinoids are used for acne, psoriasis, etc.

Hypervitaminosis A Regular ingestion of gross excess of retinol (100,000 IU daily for months) has produced toxicity—nausea, vomiting, itching, erythema, dermatitis, exfoliation, hair loss, bone and joint pains, loss of appetite, irritability, bleeding, increased intracranial tension and chronic liver disease. Excess retinol is also teratogenic in animals and man. Daily intake should not exceed 20,000 IU.

Acute poisoning has been described after consumption of polar bear liver which contains 30,000 IU/g vit A.

Retinoic acid (vit A acid) Retinoic acid has vit A activity in epithelial tissues and promotes growth, but is inactive in eye and reproductive organs. All-trans retinoic acid (Tretinoin) is used topically, while 13–cis retinoic acid (Isotretinoin) is given orally for acne.

Retinoid receptors Retinol and retinoic acid act through *nuclear retinoid receptors* which function in a manner analogous to the steroid receptors. Their activation results in modulation of protein synthesis in the target cells (epithelial, gonadal, fibroblast). Two distinct families of retinoid receptors, viz. *Retinoic acid receptors (RARs)* and *Retinoid X receptors (RXRs)* have been identified with differing affinities for different retinoids.

VITAMIN E

A number of tocopherols, of which α tocopherol is the most abundant and potent, have vit E activity. Wheat germ oil is the richest source of vit E; other sources are cereals, nuts, spinach and egg yolk.

Vit E is absorbed from the intestine through lymph with the help of bile; it circulates in plasma in association with β-lipoprotein, is stored in tissues and excreted slowly in bile and urine as metabolites.

Physiological role and actions Vit E acts as *antioxidant*, protecting unsaturated lipids in cell membranes, coenzyme Q, etc. from free radical oxidation damage and curbing generation of toxic peroxidation products. However, vit E might be having some more specific action or a structural role in biological membranes.

Deficiency Experimental vit E deficiency in animals produces recurrent abortion, degenerative changes in spinal cord, skeletal muscles and heart, and haemolytic anaemia. No clear-cut vit E deficiency syndrome has been described in humans, but vit E deficiency has been implicated in certain neuromuscular diseases in children, neurological defects in hepatobiliary disease and in some cases of haemolytic anaemia.

Uses Supplemental doses of vit E have been given prophylactically to patients with hepatobiliary disease, haemolytic anaemia, to premature infants and subjects with G-6-PD deficiency or acanthocytosis.

Large doses (400–600 mg/day) have been reported to afford symptomatic improvement in intermittent claudication, fibrocystic breast disease and in nocturnal muscle cramps.

For its antioxidant property, vit E has been promoted for recurrent abortion, sterility, menopausal syndrome, toxaemia of pregnancy, atherosclerosis, ischaemic heart disease, cancer prevention, several skin diseases, prevention of neurodegenerative disorders, and many other conditions, but without convincing evidence of benefit.

Toxicity Even large doses of vit E for long periods have not produced any significant toxicity, but creatinuria and impaired wound healing have been reported. Abdominal cramps, loose motions and lethargy have been described as side effects of vit E.

Vit E can interfere with iron therapy.

WATER-SOLUBLE VITAMINS

THE VITAMIN B COMPLEX GROUP
Thiamine (Aneurine, Vit B$_1$)

Thiamine is a pyrimidine compound present in the outer layers of cereals (rice polishing), pulses, nuts, green vegetables, yeasts, egg and meat.

Physiological amounts are absorbed by active transport. When large doses are given orally, some passive diffusion also occurs. Limited amounts are stored in tissues; excess is rapidly excreted in urine.

Physiological role After conversion in the body to *Thiamine pyrophosphate,* it acts as a coenzyme in carbohydrate metabolism; participates in decarboxylation of ketoacids and in hexose monophosphate shunt. Its requirement is dependent upon carbohydrate intake. It also appears to play some role in neuromuscular transmission.

Deficiency symptoms The syndrome of thiamine deficiency called 'beriberi' is seen in *dry* and *wet* forms:

Dry Beriberi: Neurological symptoms are prominent—polyneuritis with numbness, tingling, hyperesthesia, muscular weakness and atrophy resulting in 'wrist drop', 'foot drop', mental changes, sluggishness, poor memory, loss of appetite and constipation.

Wet Beriberi: Cardiovascular system is primarily affected—palpitation, breathlessness, high output cardiac failure and ECG changes. Protein deficiency is commonly associated along with thiamine deficiency, and adds to the generalised edema due to CHF.

Therapeutic uses
1. Prophylactically (2–10 mg daily) in infants, pregnant women, chronic diarrhoeas, patients on parenteral alimentation.
2. Treatment of Beriberi—100 mg/day i.m. or i.v.
3. Chronic alcoholics: Most neurological symptoms in alcoholics are due to thiamine deficiency.
4. In neurological and cardiovascular disorders, hyperemesis gravidarum, chronic anorexia and obstinate constipation—symptoms improve dramatically if thiamine deficiency has been causative.

Thiamine is nontoxic.

Riboflavin (Vit B_2)

Riboflavin is a yellow flavone compound found in milk, egg, liver, green leafy vegetables and grains. It is well absorbed by active transport and phosphorylated in the intestine. Riboflavin phosphate (Flavin mononucleotide: FMN) is formed in other tissues as well. Body does not significantly store riboflavin; larger doses are excreted unchanged in urine.

Actions and physiological role Flavin adenine dinucleotide (FAD) and flavin mononucleotide (FMN) are coenzymes for flavoproteins involved in many oxidation-reduction reactions.

Deficiency symptoms Riboflavin deficiency generally occurs in association with other deficiencies. Characteristic lesions are angular stomatitis; sore and raw tongue, lips, throat, ulcers in mouth; vascularization of cornea. Dry scaly skin, loss of hair; anaemia and neuropathy develop later.

Riboflavin is used to prevent and treat ariboflavinosis.

Niacin (Vit B_3)

Niacin refers to *Nicotinic acid* as well as *Nicotinamide* which are pyridine compounds found in liver, fish, meat, cereal husk, nuts and pulses. The amino acid *tryptophan* (mainly from animal protein) can be regarded as a provitamin, because it is partially converted in the body to nicotinic acid.

Niacin is completely absorbed from the gastrointestinal tract. Physiological amounts are metabolized in the body, while large doses are excreted unchanged in urine. Modest amounts are stored in liver.

Physiological role and actions Nicotinic acid is readily converted to its amide which is a component of the coenzyme *Nicotinamide-adenine-dinucleotide* (NAD) and its *phosphate* (NADP) involved in oxidation-reduction reactions. These pyridine nucleotides act as hydrogen acceptors in the electron transport chain in tissue respiration, glycolysis and fat synthesis.

Nicotinic acid (but not nicotinamide) in large doses is a vasodilator, particularly of cutaneous vessels. It also lowers plasma lipids (*see* Ch. 17).

Deficiency symptoms Niacin deficiency produces 'Pellagra', cardinal manifestations of which are: *Dermatitis*—sun burn like dermal rash on hands, legs and face, *Diarrhoea*—with enteritis, stomatitis, glossitis, and *Dementia*—with hallucinations preceded by headache, insomnia, poor memory, motor and sensory disturbances.

Anaemia and hypoproteinaemia are common in pellagra. Chronic alcoholics are particularly at risk of developing pellagra.

Therapeutic uses
1. Prophylaxis and treatment of pellagra. Nicotinamide is preferred because it does not cause flushing and other side effects seen with nicotinic acid.
2. Hartnup's disease: in which tryptophan transport is impaired.
3. Nicotinic acid (not nicotinamide) has been used in peripheral vascular disease and as hypolipidaemic drug (*see* Ch. 17).

Adverse effects Nicotinic acid, in pharmacological doses, has many side effects and toxicities (*see* p. 293). Nicotinamide is innocuous.

Pyridoxine (Vit B_6)

Pyridoxine, Pyridoxal and *Pyridoxamine* are naturally occurring pyridine compounds that have vit B_6 activity. Dietary sources are—liver, meat, egg, soybean, vegetables and whole grain. All three forms of the vitamin are well absorbed from the intestine. They are oxidized in the body and excreted as pyridoxic acid. Little is stored.

Physiological role and actions Pyridoxine and pyridoxamine are readily oxidized to pyridoxal which is then phosphorylated to *pyridoxal phosphate*—the coenzyme form. Pyridoxal dependent enzymes include transaminases and decarboxylases involved in the synthesis and metabolism of amino acids, formation of 5-HT, dopamine, histamine, GABA and aminolevulinic acid (first step in synthesis of heme). High protein diet increases pyridoxine requirement.

Prolonged intake of large doses of pyridoxine can give rise to dependence, and has been linked with sensory neuropathy. In nonsuckling postpartal women, high doses of pyridoxine can suppress lactation. Otherwise, pyridoxine is free from pharmacological actions and side effects.

Drug interactions
1. Isoniazid reacts with pyridoxal to form a hydrazone, and thus interferes with generation of pyridoxal phosphate. Isoniazid also combines with pyridoxal phosphate, and this product cannot carryout the coenzyme function. Due to formation of hydrazones with isoniazid the renal excretion of pyridoxine compounds is increased. Thus, isoniazid therapy produces a pyridoxine deficiency state.

2. Hydralazine, cycloserine and penicillamine also interfere with pyridoxine utilization and action.

3. Pyridoxine, by promoting formation of dopamine from levodopa in peripheral tissues, reduces its availability in the brain, abolishing the therapeutic effect in parkinsonism.

Deficiency symptoms Deficiency of vit B_6 usually occurs in association with that of other B vitamins. Symptoms ascribed to pyridoxine deficiency are—seborrhoeic dermatitis, glossitis, growth retardation, mental confusion, lowered seizure threshold or convulsions, peripheral neuritis and anaemia.

Therapeutic uses
1. Prophylactically (2–5 mg daily) in alcoholics and patients with deficiency of other B vitamins.

2. To prevent and treat (10–100 mg/day) isoniazid, hydralazine and cycloserine induced neurological disturbances. Tubercular patients treated with isoniazid are often given pyridoxine concurrently.

3. Pyridoxine is combined with doxylamine for treating morning sickness.

4. Pyridoxine responsive anaemia (due to defective heme synthesis) and homocystinuria are rare genetic disorders that are benefited by large doses of pyridoxine.

VITAMIN C (ASCORBIC ACID)

Ascorbic acid is a 6 carbon organic acid with structural similarity to glucose. It is a potent reducing agent and the *l*-form is biologically active. Citrus fruits (lemons, oranges) and black currants are the richest sources; others are tomato, potato, green chilies, cabbage and other vegetables.

Ascorbic acid is nearly completely absorbed from the g.i.t. and widely distributed extra-and intracellularly. Increasing proportions are excreted in urine with higher intakes, because body is not able to store more than 2.5 g. It is partly oxidized to active (dehydroascorbic acid) and inactive (oxalic acid) metabolites.

Physiological role and actions Vit C plays a role in many oxidative and other metabolic reactions, e.g. hydroxylation of proline and lysine residues of protocollagen which is essential for formation and stabilization of collagen; conversion of folic acid to folinic acid, biosynthesis of adrenal steroids, catecholamines, oxytocin and vasopressin as well as metabolism of cyclic nucleotides and prostaglandins. Ascorbic acid is very important for maintenance of intercellular connective tissue.

Deficiency symptoms Severe vit C deficiency *Scurvy*, once prevalent among sailors is now seen only in malnourished infants, children, elderly, alcoholics and drug addicts. Symptoms stem primarily from connective tissue defect: increased capillary fragility—swollen and bleeding gums, petechial and subperiosteal haemorrhages, deformed teeth, brittle bones, impaired wound healing, anaemia and growth retardation.

Therapeutic uses

1. Prevention of ascorbic acid deficiency in individuals at risk (*see* above) and in infants: 50–100 mg/day.
2. Treatment of scurvy—0.5–1.5 g/day.
3. Postoperatively (500 mg daily): though vit C does not enhance normal healing, suboptimal healing can be guarded against.
4. Anaemia: Ascorbic acid enhances iron absorption and is frequently combined with ferrous salts. Anaemia of scurvy is corrected by ascorbic acid.
5. To acidify urine (1 g TDS-QID) in urinary tract infections.
6. Large doses (2–6 g/day) of ascorbic acid have been tried for a variety of purposes (common cold to cancer) with inconsistent results. Severity of common cold symptoms may be somewhat reduced, but not the duration of illness or its incidence.

Adverse effects Ascorbic acid is well tolerated in usual doses. Mega doses given for long periods can cause 'rebound scurvy' on stoppage. The risk of urinary oxalate stones may be increased.

CHAPTER 21

Anticancer and Immunosuppressant Drugs

ANTICANCER DRUGS

The anticancer drugs either kill cancer cells or modify their growth. However, selectivity of majority of drugs is limited and they are one of the most toxic drugs used in therapy. Cancer chemotherapy is now of established value and a highly specialized field to be handled by oncology specialists supported by a multidisciplinary team. Only the general principles and an outline along with the orodental implications will be presented here.

In addition to their prominent role in leukaemias and lymphomas, chemotherapeutic drugs are used in conjunction with surgery, radiotherapy and immunotherapy in the *combined modality approach* for many solid tumours, especially metastatic.

Depending on the type and stage of the malignancy, chemotherapy is employed for the following aims:

1. Cure or prolonged remission: as the primary treatment modality.
2. Palliation: Shrinkage of the tumour, alleviation of symptoms and/or prolongation of life.
3. Adjuvant chemotherapy: to mop up any residual malignant cells after surgery or radiotherapy.

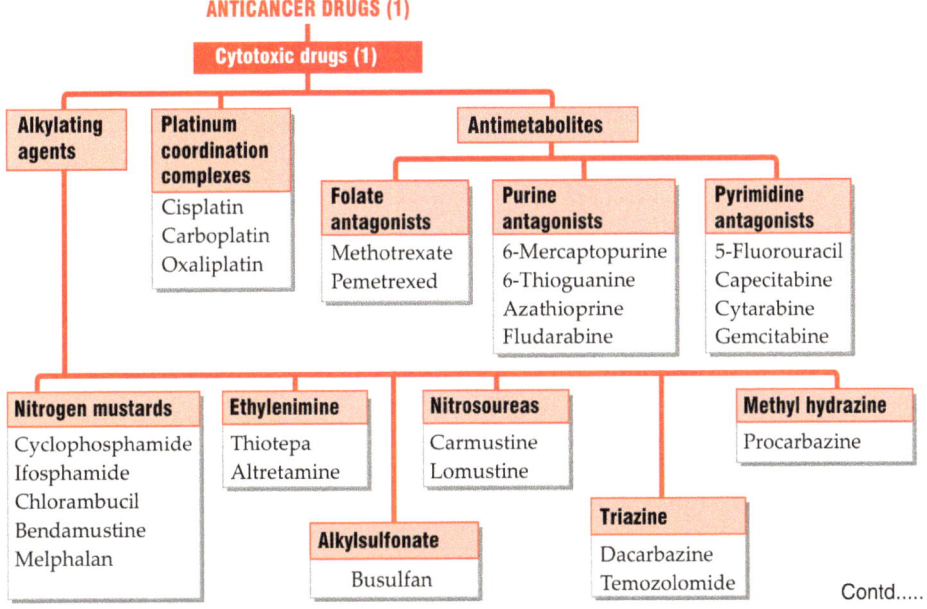

Contd.....

Chapter 21: Anticancer and Immunosuppressant Drugs

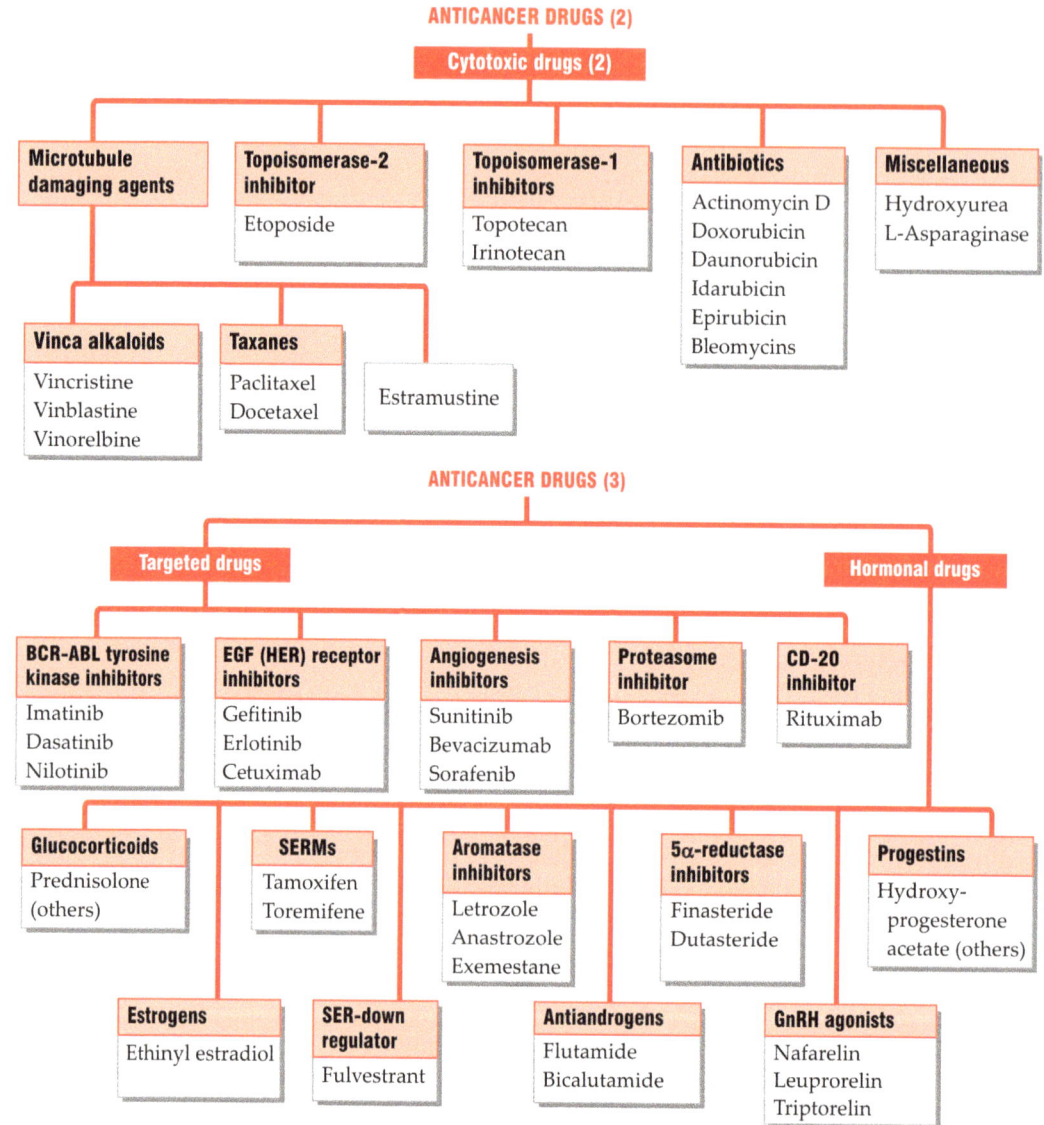

General toxicity of cytotoxic drugs

Majority of the cytotoxic drugs have more profound effect on rapidly multiplying cells, because the most important target of action are the nucleic acids or their precursors, and rapid nucleic acid synthesis occurs during cell division. Many cancers (especially large solid tumours) have a lower growth fraction (lower percentage of cells are in division) than normal bone marrow, epithelial linings, reticuloendothelial (RE) system and gonads. These tissues are particularly affected in a dose-dependent manner by majority of drugs; though there are differences in susceptibility to individual members.

1. Bone marrow Depression of bone marrow results in granulocytopenia, agranulocytosis, thrombocytopenia, aplastic anaemia.

This is the most serious toxicity; often limits the dose that can be employed. Infections and bleeding are the usual complications.

2. *Lymphoreticular tissue* Lymphocytopenia and inhibition of lymphocyte function results in suppression of cell mediated as well as humoral immunity.

Because of action (1) and (2) + damage to epithelial surfaces, the host defence mechanisms (specific as well as nonspecific) are broken down → susceptibility to all types of infections is increased. Of particular importance are the opportunistic infections caused by low pathogenicity organisms, e.g. *Candida*, *Pneumocystis jiroveci* and other fungi, *Herpes zoster*, cytomegalovirus, *Toxoplasma*.

3. *GIT* Stomatitis, diarrhoea, shedding of mucosa, haemorrhages occur due to decrease in the rate of renewal of the gastrointestinal mucous lining. Drugs that frequently cause mucositis are—bleomycin, actinomycin D, daunorubicin, doxorubicin, fluorouracil and methotrexate.

Nausea and vomiting are prominent with many cytotoxic drugs. This is due to direct stimulation of CTZ by the drug as well as generation of emetic impulses/mediators from the upper g.i.t. and other areas.

The emetogenic potential of cytotoxic drugs may be graded as:

High	Moderate	Mild
Cisplatin	Carboplatin	Bleomycin
Cyclophosphamide	Cytarabine	Chlorambucil
Actinomycin D	Procarbazine	Busulfan
Dacarbazine	Vinblastine	Fluorouracil
Lomustine	Doxorubicin	6-Thioguanine
	Daunorubicin	Hydroxyurea
	6-Mercapto-purine	Vincristine
		Methotrexate
		Etoposide
		l-Asparaginase

4. *Skin* Alopecia occurs due to damage to the cells in hair follicles. Dermatitis is another complication.

5. *Gonads* Inhibition of gonadal cells causes oligozoospermia and impotence in males; inhibition of ovulation and amenorrhoea are common in females.

6. *Foetus* Practically all cytotoxic drugs given to pregnant women profoundly damage the developing foetus → abortion, foetal death, teratogenesis.

7. *Carcinogenicity* Secondary cancers, especially leukaemias, lymphomas and histiocytic tumours appear with greater frequency many years after the use of cytotoxic drugs. This may be due to impairment of cell mediated and humoral *blocking factors* against neoplasia.

8. *Hyperuricaemia* This is secondary to massive cell destruction (uric acid is a product of purine metabolism). Gout and urate stones in the urinary tract may develop. Allopurinol is protective by decreasing uric acid synthesis.

In addition to these general toxicities, individual drugs may produce specific adverse effects, e.g. vincristine causes neuropathy, doxorubicin causes cardiomyopathy and cyclophosphamide produces alopecia and cystitis.

Oral complications of cancer chemotherapy

The oral mucosa is particularly susceptible to cytotoxic drugs, because epithelial cells have high rate of turnover. Many anticancer drugs produce oral lesions. *Oral mucositis* is often an early manifestation of toxicity. The gingival tissue and oral mucosa are regularly subjected to minor trauma during chewing and breaches are common. Oral microbial flora is large and can be the source of local (e.g. periodontal abscess) as well as bloodborne infection. Neutropenia and depression of immunity caused by the cytotoxic drugs indirectly increase the chances of *oral infections*, particularly those caused by low grade pathogens such as *Candida*, *Serratia*,

Pseudomonas, etc. Thrombocytopenia due to bone marrow depression may cause *gingival or mucosal bleeding*. Such bleeding may be checked by anti-fibrinolytic drugs like epsilon aminocaproic acid or tranexaemic acid. Platelet transfusion is required if the platelet count is very low. Chemotherapeutic drugs frequently produce *Xerostomia* which accelerates development of *dental caries* and *angular cheilitis*. Xerostomia may also cause *dysgeuesia* or *loss of taste sensation* by damaging taste buds. Administered to children during tooth development, cancer chemotherapy may cause *hypoplasia of tooth*, blunting of roots and even *tooth agenesis*.

Many of the oral/dental complications of chemotherapy can be minimized by a thorough dental check-up before starting the regimen. Any carious cavities, periodontal lesions, impacted last molars and other potential sources of infection should be appropriately treated. All sharp cusps or dentures should be smoothened to avoid injury. Good oral hygiene should be maintained throughout the course. Topical use of fluoride can retard caries development.

Stomatitis and oral ulcers can be treated with chlorhexidine mouthwash. Nystatin or clotrimazole lotion may be used for *Candida* infection. When the mucositis progresses, oral lesions become increasingly painful and may interfere with eating. Topical application of sucralfate and mesoprostol may afford some relief. Benzocaine lozenges or lidocaine gel can reduce pain, but may interfere with taste and increase the risk of injury to oral mucosa. Opioid analgesics may have to be prescribed. Systemic antibiotics to cover organisms like *Pseudomonas, Klebsiella, E.coli* are often needed in addition to those for common oral pathogens, *viz.* gram-positive cocci and anaerobes when chemotherapy related oral infections develop.

In a patient receiving chemotherapy, any dental procedure should be undertaken only after giving due regard to his/her immune and haemostatic status and in consultation with the patient's physician. Appropriate prophylactic antibiotic to eliminate the risk of infection is important, since infections can easily set in or get disseminated in subjects compromised by the chemotherapy.

NOTES ON ANTICANCER DRUGS

Alkylating agents

These compounds produce highly reactive carbonium ion intermediates which transfer alkyl groups to cellular macromolecules by forming covalent bonds. The position 7 of guanine residues in DNA is especially susceptible, but other molecular sites are also involved. This results in cross linking/abnormal base pairing/scission of DNA strand. Cross linking of nucleic acids with proteins can also take place.

Alkylating agents have cytotoxic and radiomimetic (like ionizing radiation) actions. Many are cell cycle non-specific, i.e. act on dividing as well as resting cells. Some have CNS stimulant and cholinergic properties.

Cyclophosphamide is the most commonly used alkylating agent, effective in a wide range of tumours, and has prominent immunosuppressant action. Alopecia and cystitis are the prominent toxicity. *Chlorambucil* is selective for lymphoid tissue and is used for maintenance therapy in chronic lymphocytic leukaemia and Hodgkin's disease. *Busulfan* is selective for myeloid elements and the drug of choice for chronic myeloid leukaemia. *Melphalan* is very effective in multiple myeloma. *Lomustine* is highly lipid soluble. It is especially valuable for brain tumours and meningeal leukaemia. The most important indication of *dacarbazine* is malignant melanoma. *Procarbazine* is an atypical alkylating agent which methylates and depolymerizes DNA causing DNA breaks. It is a component of the

MOPP regimen for Hodgkin's and related lymphomas. It is a weak MAO inhibitor—can interact with food and drugs.

Platinum coordination complexes

Cisplatin is a platinum complex that is hydrolysed intracellularly to release a highly reactive moiety which causes crosslinking of DNA and can react with SH groups of cellular proteins. Cisplatin has alkylating and radiomimetic properties and is commonly used for many solid tumours including those of lung, bladder, esophagaus, stomach, head and neck as well as metastatic testicular and ovarian carcinoma. Cisplatin needs to be infused i.v., and is highly emetogenic. Strong antiemetic pretreatment is required. *Carboplatin* is a less reactive second generation platinum complex that is better tolerated. Oxaliplatin is a third generation complex which is active against many tumours that have developed resistance to cisplatin.

Antimetabolites

These are analogues related to the normal components of DNA or of coenzymes involved in nucleic acid synthesis. The antimetabolites competitively inhibit utilization of normal substrate or get themselves incorporated forming dysfunctional macromolecules.

1. Folate antagonist

Methotrexate (Mtx) is one of the oldest and highly efficacious antineoplastic drugs. It inhibits dihydrofolate reductase (DHFRase)—blocking the conversion of dihydrofolic acid (DHFA) to tetrahydrofolic acid (THFA) which is an essential coenzyme required for one carbon transfer reactions in *de novo* purine synthesis and amino acid interconversions. The inhibition is pseudoirreversible because Mtx has 50,000 times higher affinity for the enzyme than the normal substrate. Methotrexate primarily inhibits DNA synthesis, but also affects RNA and protein synthesis. It exerts major toxicity on bone marrow.

Aspirin and sulfonamides decrease its renal tubular secretion—enhancing its toxicity.

The toxicity of Mtx cannot be overcome by folic acid, because it will not be converted to the active coenzyme form. However, *Folinic acid* (N5 formyl THFA or cirtrovorum factor) rapidly reverses the effects. High dose Mtx with 'folinic acid rescue' has been employed in many difficult-to-treat neoplasms. Mtx is used in choriocarcinoma, acute leukaemia, carcinoma of tongue/pharynx/lung, etc. and as immunosuppressant in rheumatoid arthritis, psoriasis, organ transplantation.

Pemetrexed This is a newer congener of methotrexate which primarily inhibits the enzyme thymidylate synthase in addition to DHFRase, and has found use in mesoepithelioma and non-small cell lung cancer.

2. Purine antagonists

Mercaptopurine (6-MP) and *thioguanine (6-TG)* are highly effective antineoplastic drugs. They are converted in the body to the corresponding monoribonucleotides which inhibit purine synthesis and utilization of purine nucleotides. They are especially useful in childhood acute leukaemia, choriocarcinoma and in some solid tumours.

Azathioprine is converted intracellularly into 6-MP and has marked effect on T-lymphocytes. It suppresses cell-mediated immunity (CMI) and is used primarily as immunosuppressant in organ transplantation, rheumatoid arthritis, etc.

Azathioprine and 6-MP are metabolized by xanthine oxidase; their metabolism is inhibited by allopurinol. Therefore, dose of azathioprine and 6-MP has to be reduced to ¼ to ½ if allopurinol is given concurrently. Thioguanine is not a substrate for xanthine oxidase; its dose need not be reduced if allopurinol is given.

Fludarabine is a newer antipurine that is active even in some slow growing and recurrent cancers.

The main toxicity of antipurines is bone marrow depression and mucositis. Jaundice and hyperuricaemia are also prominent.

3. Pyrimidine antagonists

Fluorouracil (5-FU) It is converted in the body to the corresponding nucleotide which blocks the conversion of deoxyuridilic acid to deoxythymidylic acid. Selective failure of DNA synthesis occurs. Concurrent i.v. infusion of leucovorin (folinic acid) enhances efficacy of 5-FU by facilitating its binding to the enzyme thymidylate synthese. Cisplatin is also synergistic. Most treatment protocols for 5-FU employ it alongwith leucovorin and cisplatin.

5-FU has been particularly used for many solid tumours—breast, colon, urinary bladder, liver, head and neck, etc. Topical application in cutaneous basal cell carcinoma has yielded gratifying results.

Capecitabine is an orally active prodrug of F.U., which is especially active against colorectal and breast cancers.

Cytarabine is phosphorylated in the body to the corresponding nucleotide which inhibits DNA synthesis by DNA polymerase. Its main use is to induce remission in acute leukaemia in children, also in adults. Other uses are—Hodgkin's disease and non-Hodgkin lymphoma.

Gemcitabine Administered by slow i.v. infusion, this pyrimidine antagonist is a reserve drug for nonresectable or metastatic carcinoma of pancreas, ovaries, bladder and non-small call lung cancer.

Microtubule damaging agents

Vinca alkaloids

These are mitotic inhibitors that bind to microtubular protein—'tubulin', thereby prevent its polymerization and assembly of microtubules. As a result, disruption of mitotic spindle occurs and cytoskeletal function is interfered. The chromosomes fail to move apart during mitosis: metaphase arrest occurs. These cytotoxic drugs are cell cycle specific and act in the mitotic phase.

Vincristine (oncovin) is very useful for inducing remission in childhood acute leukaemia. Other indications are lymphosarcoma, Hodgkin's disease, Wilms' tumour, Ewing's sarcoma and carcinoma lung. Prominent adverse effects are peripheral neuropathy and alopecia. Bone marrow depression is minimal.

Vinblastine is primarily employed along with other drugs in Hodgkin's disease and testicular carcinoma. Bone marrow depression is more prominent, while neurotoxicity and alopecia are less marked than with vincristine.

Vinorelbine is a semisynthetic vinblastine analogue which is primarily used in nonsmall cell lung cancer.

Taxanes

Paclitaxel is obtained from bark of the Western yew tree, which exerts cytotoxic action by a novel mechanism. It binds to β-tubulin and enhances its polymerization: a mechanism opposite to that of vinca alkaloids. This results in inhibition of normal dynamic reorganization of the microtubule network that is essential for interphase and mitotic functions.

The indications of paclitaxel are metastatic ovarian and breast carcinoma after failure of first line chemotherapy. It has also shown efficacy in advanced cases of head and neck cancer, small cell lung cancer, esophageal adenocarcinoma, etc. The major toxicity is reversible myelosuppression and 'stocking and glove' neuropathy.

Docetaxel is a more potent congener of paclitaxel found effective in breast and ovarian cancer refractory to first line drugs. Small cell cancer lung, pancreatic, gastric and head/neck carcinomas are the other indications. Major toxicity is neutropenia, but neuropathy is less frequent.

Estramustine This complex of estradiol with a nitrogen mustard has weak estrogenic, but no alkylating property. It binds to β-tubulin preventing its organization into microtubules and thus exerts antimitotic action. Because it is concentrated in prostate, the only indication is advanced or metastatic prostate cancer.

Topoisomerase-2 inhibitor

Etoposide is a semisynthetic derivative of podophyllotoxin, a plant glycoside. It is not a mitotic inhibitor, but arrests cells in the G_2 phase and causes DNA breaks by affecting DNA topoisomerase-2 function. Etoposide has been primarily used in testicular tumours, lung cancer, Hodgkin's and other lymphomas, carcinoma bladder.

Topoisomerase-1 inhibitors

Topotecan and *Irinotecan* are two semisynthetic analogues of camptothecin, an antitumour principle obtained from a Chinese tree. They act in a manner similar to etoposide, but interact with a different enzyme DNA topoisomerase-1.

Topotecan is used in metastatic carcinoma of ovary and small cell lung cancer after primary chemotherapy has failed. The major toxicity is bone marrow depression, especially neutropenia.

Irinotecan is a prodrug which is indicated in metastatic/advanced colorectal carcinoma, cancer lung/cervix/ovary, etc. Dose limiting toxicity is diarrhoea.

Antibiotics

These are products obtained from microorganisms and have prominent antitumour activity. Practically, all of them intercalate between DNA strands and interfere with its template function.

Actinomycin D (Dactinomycin) is highly efficacious in Wilms' tumour, rhabdomyosarcoma and a few other malignancies. Prominent adverse effects are vomiting, stomatitis, diarrhoea, desquamation of skin, alopecia and bone marrow depression.

Daunorubicin (Rubidomycin) and *Doxorubicin* are antitumour antibiotics with quite similar chemical structures. However, utility of daunorubicin is limited to acute leukaemia while doxorubicin, in addition, is effective in many solid tumours. They are capable of causing breaks in DNA strands by activating topoisomerase-2 and generating quinone-type free radicals.

Both these antibiotics produce cardiotoxicity (arrhythmias, cardiomyopathy—heart failure) as a unique adverse effect. Marrow depression, alopecia, stomatitis are the other toxic effects.

Bleomycin chelates copper or iron, produces superoxide ions and intercalates between DNA strands—causes chain scission and inhibits repair. It is highly effective in testicular tumour and squamous cell carcinoma of skin, oral cavity, head and neck, and esophagus; also useful in Hodgkin's lymphoma.

Mucocutaneous toxicity and pulmonary fibrosis, are the major toxicity, but myelosuppression is minimal.

Miscellaneous cytotoxic drugs

Hydroxyurea blocks the conversion of ribonucleotides to deoxyribonucleotides—thus interferes with DNA synthesis. It exerts S-phase specific action. Its primary therapeutic value is in chronic myeloid leukaemia, psoriasis, polycythaemia vera and in some solid tumours. Myelosuppression is the major toxicity.

L-Asparaginase is selectively toxic to childhood lymphoblastic leukaemia cells, because these cells are deficient in L-asparagine synthase and thus dependent on supply of L-asparagine from the medium. In combination with other drugs, it is used to induce remission in childhood lymphoblastic leukaemia, but response is short lasting.

It can cause liver damage and allergic reactions, but mucositis, bone marrow depression and alopecia do not occur.

TARGETED DRUGS

These are recently developed drugs which attack cancer-specific target biomolecules or processes. Targeted drugs can be devided in two major types:

A. Specific monoclonal antibodies that attack cell surface targets or tumour antigens, but need to be given parenterally.

B. Synthetic small molecular compounds which penetrate cells and affect cancer-specific enzymes or processes, and are active orally.

1. BCR-ABL tyrosine kinase inhibitors

Imatinib, Nilotinib and *Dasatinib* are synthetic compounds which inhibit a particular tyrosine protein kinase 'Bcr–Abl' expressed by chronic myeloid leukaemia cells and related tumours. These drugs are strickingly successful in such malignancies.

2. EGF receptor (HER) inhibitors

Epidermal growth factor (EGF) acts on a transmembrane receptor tyrosine kinase (*see* Fig. 3.7) to regulate growth and differentiation of epithelial cells. Certain epithelial cancers over-express EGF receptor and their growth is critically dependent upon activation of this receptor. *Gefitinib* and *Erlotinib* are orally active synthetic compounds which penetrate cells and bind to the tyrosine kinase domain of EGF receptor and prevent phosphorylation of regulatory proteins. They are effective in certain types of lung and pancreatic cancers.

Cetuximab is a chimeric monoclonal antibody directed to the extracellular domain of the EGF receptor. Its binding interferes with transmembrane signalling. Weekly i.v. infusion of cetuximab suppresses advanced/metastatic squamous carcinoma of head and neck and EGF positive colorectal cancer.

3. Angiogenesis inhibitors

Proliferation of new blood vessels (angiogenesis) is essential for growth and metastasis of cancers. The vascular endothelial growth factor (VEGF) is the most important stimulus for neovascularization. Tumours which overexpress VEGF receptor are susceptible to these drugs.

Bevacizumab is a monoclonal antibody that binds to the VEGF receptor interrupting angiogenic signalling. Combined with other drugs it is used in metastatic colorectal cancer and some other malignancies. *Sunitinib* is a synthetic VEGF receptor-2 inhibitor which is used orally for metastatic renal cell carcinoma and resistant g.i. stromal tumour.

Sorafenib is another orally active VEGF-receptor inhibitor, used as second-line drug for advanced renal cell cancer.

4. Proteasome inhibitor

Bortezomib is a unique boron containing compound that binds to and inhibits 'proteasomes', which are packaged complexes of proteolytic enzymes which control cell cycle by degrading intracellular signalling proteins. Bortezomib thus disrupts many intracellular signalling pathways, the most important of which involves the nuclear factor κB (NFκB). Multiple myeloma and few other neoplasms overexpress NF-κB and are suppressed by this drug.

5. CD20 inhibitor

Malignant cells express certain unique antigens on their surface to which monoclonal antibodies (MAbs) could be developed. The MAbs are sourced from hybridomas created by fusing a continuously proliferating cell line with antibody producing B-lymphocytes sensitized against a particular antigen. By cloning this hybridoma, antibody against that particular antigen can be obtained in large quantity for clinical use. CD20 is an antigen against which MAbs have been raised.

Rituximab It is a chimerized MAb that binds to the CD 20 B cell antigen which is expressed on the surface of B-lymphocytes and B cell lymphomas. Rituximab promotes apoptosis in B-cell lymphoma, non-Hodgkin lymphoma and chronic lyphocytic leukaemia which has yielded survival benefit to the patients with these malignancies.

HORMONAL DRUGS

These drugs are not cytotoxic, but modify the growth of hormone-dependent tumours. All hormonal drugs are only palliative.

Glucocorticoids have marked lympholytic action; they are primarily used in acute childhood leukaemia and lymphomas. They induce remission rapidly but relapses inevitably occur after variable intervals and gradually the responsiveness is lost. Considerable palliative effects are obtained in Hodgkin's disease and they have a secondary role in some hormone responsive breast cancers.

Corticosteroids are also valuable for the control of complications like hypercalcaemia, haemolysis and bleeding due to thrombocytopenia. Moreover, they afford symptomatic relief by antipyretic and mood elevating action and potentiate the antiemetic action of ondansetron/metoclopramide.

Estrogens produce symptomatic relief in carcinoma prostate, which is an androgen-dependent tumour. However, relapses eventually occur, but life is prolonged. Estrogens have now been superseded by GnRH agonists used along with an antiandrogen.

Many breast cancers have estrogen receptors in their cells. These tumours respond to estrogens/antiestrogens.

Selective estrogen receptor modulators (tamoxifen), *Selective estrogen receptor down regulator* (fulvestrant) and *Aromatase inhibitors* (letrozole, etc.) are the sheet anchor of adjuvant and palliative therapy of carcinoma breast, as well as for prevention of breast cancer. These drugs are described in Ch. 15.

Antiandrogen Flutamide and bicalutamide (*see* Ch. 15) antagonise androgen action on prostate carcinoma and have palliative effect in advanced/metastatic cases. Because they cause feedback increase in androgen secretion, combination with orchidectomy or superactive GnRH agonists is required to produce sustained therapeutic effect.

5-α reductase inhibitor Finasteride and dutasteride (*see* Ch. 15) inhibit conversion of testosterone to dihydrotestosterone in prostate and have been occasionally used for palliative effect in advanced carcinoma prostate.

GnRH agonists (*see* p. 231) Nafarelin and other superactive GnRH agonists indirectly inhibit estrogen/androgen secretion by suppressing FSH and LH release from pituitary, and have adjuvant/palliative effect in advanced estrogen/androgen dependent carcinoma breast/prostate.

Progestins bring about temporary remission in some cases of advanced, recurrent (after surgery/radiotherapy) and metastatic endometrial carcinoma.

GENERAL PRINCIPLES IN CHEMOTHERAPY OF CANCER

1. In cancer chemotherapy selectivity of drugs for the tumour cells is limited: toxicity is high. As such, measures to enhance selectivity need to be employed. Immunological defence against malignant cells is minimal or absent.

2. A single clonogenic malignant cell is capable of producing progeny that can kill the host. Survival time is related to the number of cells that escape chemotherapeutic attack.

3. In any cancer, subpopulations of cells differ in their rate of proliferation and susceptibility to cytotoxic drugs. These drugs kill cancer cells by first order kinetics, i.e. a certain fraction of cells present are killed by one treatment.

4. Drug regimens or treatment cycles which can effectively palliate large tumour burdens may be curative when applied to minute residual tumour cell population after surgery and/or irradiation. This is the basis of the combined modality approach (Fig. 21.1).

5. Whenever possible, complete remission should be the goal of cancer chemotherapy: drugs are often used at maximum tolerated doses. Intensive regimens used at an early stage in the disease yield better results.

6. Generally a combination of 2–5 drugs is given in intermittent pulses to achieve *total tumour cell kill*, giving time in between for normal cells to recover (Fig. 21.1).

Synergistic combinations and rational sequences are devised by utilizing:
- Drugs which are effective when used alone.
- Drugs with different mechanisms of action.
- Drugs with differing toxicities.
- Drugs with known synergistic biochemical interaction.

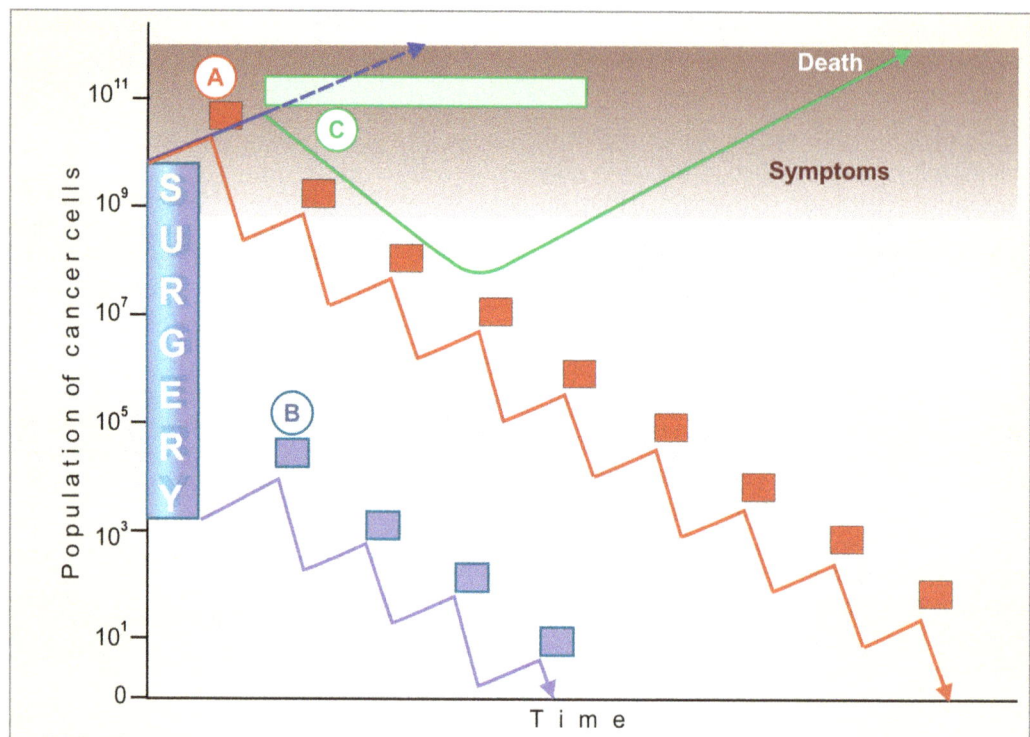

Fig. 21.1: Illustration of cancer cell dynamics with three chemotherapeutic approaches. The shaded area depicts symptoms, before which the cancer remains subclinical. The broken purple line indicates no treatment.
A. A rationally designed combination of 2–5 chemotherapeutic drugs (red bar) is given cyclically. Each cycle kills 99% tumour cells, reducing the tumour cell mass by 2 log units each time. Some regrowth occurs during the rest interval, but the rate of cell kill is more than regrowth and resistance does not develop. If the cycles are continued well beyond all symptoms disappear, cure may be achieved. Radiation may be used to supplement chemotherapy.
B. The cancer (in case of solid tumours) is resected surgically and the small number of residual cancer cells (at the primary site or in metastasis) are killed by relatively few cycles of adjuvant combination chemotherapy (blue bar). This may be supplemented by radiation (in case of radiosensitive tumours).
C. The chemotherapy is begun relatively late with a single but effective drug given continuously (green bar). It causes slower tumour cell kill, but symptom relief may occur. Resistance soon develops, and the tumour starts regrowing even with continued chemotherapy. Symptoms reappear and increase in severity. Ultimately failure of therapy and death occur.

- Empirically by trial and error; optimal schedules are mostly developed by this procedure.
- *Kinetic scheduling:* on the basis of cell cycle specificity/nonspecificity of drugs and the phase of cell cycle (*see* box) at which a drug exerts its toxicity.

Proliferating cells enter the cell cycle, phases of which are depicted in the box.

Cytotoxic drugs are either cell cycle specific or cell cycle nonspecific.

(a) *Cell cycle nonspecific* These drugs kill resting as well as dividing cells, e.g. cyclophosphamide, chlorambucil, carmustine, dacarbazine, L-asparaginase, cisplatin, procarbazine, actinomycin D, doxorubicin, daunorubicin.

(b) *Cell cycle specific* These drugs kill only actively dividing cells. Their toxicity is generally expressed in S phase. Some cell cycle specific cytotoxic drugs are— Methotrexate, cytarabine, 6-MP, azathioprine,

Phases of cell cycle	
G_1 phase	Pre (nucleic acid) synthesis interval.
S phase	Synthesis of DNA occurs.
G_2 phase	Post synthetic interval.
M phase	Mitosis occurs—two G_1 cells are produced, which either directly re-enter next cycle or pass into the nonproliferative (G_0) phase.
G_0 phase	Nonproliferating cells; a fraction of these are clonogenic—may remain quiescent for variable periods, but can be recruited in cell cycle if stimulated later.

6-TG, hydroxyurea, 5-FU, bleomycin, topotecan, vincristine, vinblastine, paclitaxel, etc. However, these drugs may show considerable phase selectivity.

The growth fraction of solid tumours is often low; it is logical to use cell cycle specific drugs in short courses (pulses) of treatment. This allows noncycling cells (which are generally less susceptible to drugs) to re-enter the cycle between drug courses.

7. Tumours often become resistant to the drug used repeatedly due to selection of less responsive cells.

8. Measures employed to ameliorate the toxicity of anticancer drugs are:
- Use of biological response modifiers like recombinant granulocyte colony stimulating factor (G-CSF) and granulocyte-macrophage colony stimulating factor (GM-CSF) viz. *molgramostim, filgrastim,* hasten recovery of neutrophil count following myelosuppressant chemotherapy.
- *Amifostine* provides free thiol radical and reduces renal toxicity of cisplatin as well as xerostomia due to radiotherapy.
- *Folinic acid* rescue can reduce methotrexate toxicity.
- Cystitis caused by cyclophosphamide can be blocked by *mesna* administered along with it.
- *Ondansetron* ± dexamethasone, lorazepam, aprepitant protect against cisplatin (and other emetic drugs) induced vomiting
- Hyperuricaemia due to destruction of bulky tumours can be reduced by *allopurinol*.

IMMUNOSUPPRESSANT DRUGS

Immunosuppressants are drugs which inhibit cellular or humoral or both immune response and have their major use in organ transplantation and autoimmune diseases. The drugs are classified in the chart:

The development of immune response and the sites of action of different immunosuppressant drugs is summarized in Fig. 21.2.

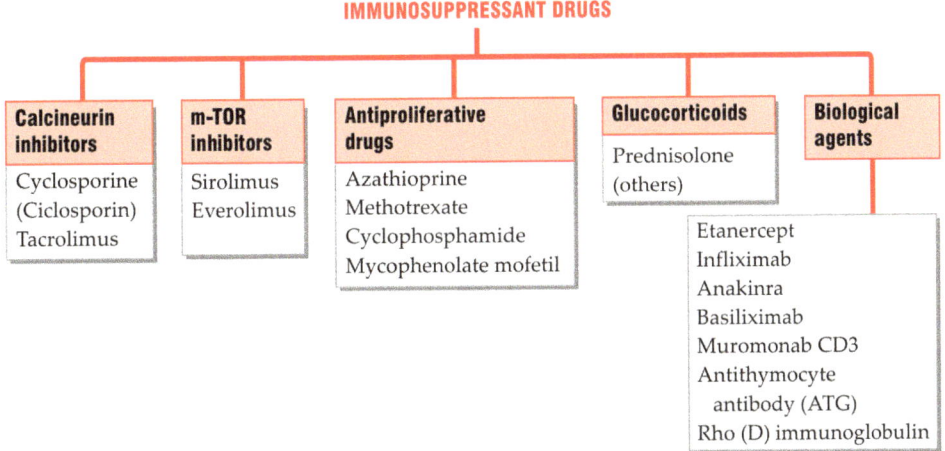

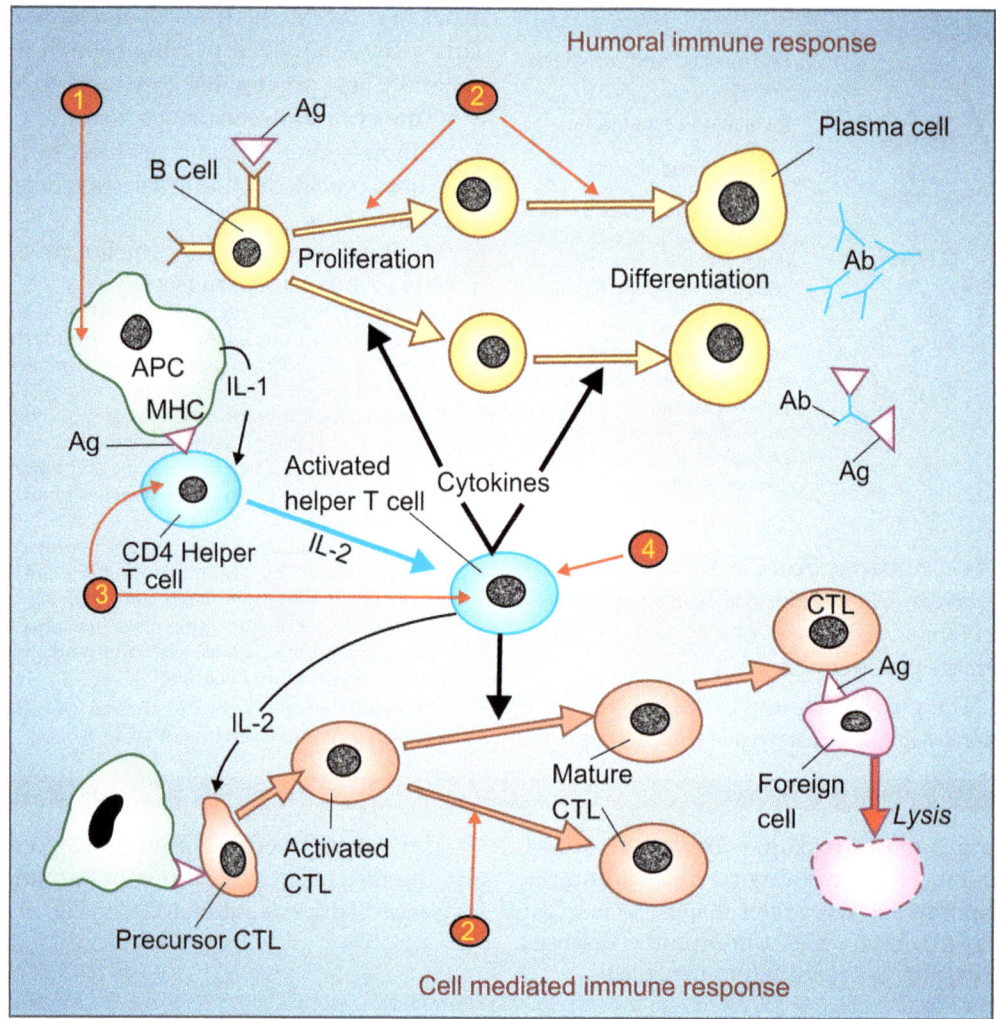

Fig. 21.2: Generation of humoral and cell-mediated immune response and sites of action of immunosuppressant drugs

The antigen (Ag) is processed by macrophages or other antigen presenting cells (APC), coupled with class II major histocompatibility complex (MHC) and presented to the CD4 helper T cell which are activated by interleukin-I (IL-1), proliferate and secrete cytokines—these in turn promote proliferation and differentiation of antigen activated B cells into antibody (Ab) secreting plasma cells. Antibodies finally bind and inactivate the antigen.

In cell-mediated immunity—foreign antigen is processed and presented to CD4 helper T cell which elaborate IL-2 and other cytokines that in turn stimulate proliferation and maturation of precursor cytotoxic lymphocytes (CTL) that have been activated by antigen presented with class I MHC. The mature CTL (Killer cells) recognize cells carrying the antigen and lyse them.

1. Glucocorticoids inhibit MHC expression and IL-1, IL-2, IL-6 production so that helper T-cells are not activated.
2. Cytotoxic drugs block proliferation and differentiation of T and B cells.
3. Cyclosporine, tacrolimus and sirolimus inhibit antigen stimulated activation and proliferation of helper T cells as well as expression of IL-2 and other cytokines by them.
4. Antibodies like muromonab CD3, antithymocyte globulin specifically bind to helper T cells, prevent their response and deplete them

Calcineurin inhibitors

Cyclosporine It is a cyclic polypeptide with 11 amino acids, obtained from a fungus and introduced in 1977 as a highly selective immunosuppressant which has markedly improved the success of organ transplantations. Cyclosporine profoundly and selectively inhibits T-lymphocyte proliferation, IL-2 and other cytokine production and response of inducer T-cells to IL-1 without any effect on suppressor T-cells.

Cyclosporine enters target cells and binds to a protein called *cyclophilin* (Fig. 21.3). The complex then binds to and inactivates the enzyme *calcineurin* which is involved in transcription of cytokine genes in the antigen activated helper T-cells. As a result, response of the helper T-cell to antigenic stimulation fails. T-cell proliferation and production of killer lymphocytes is attenuated.

Cyclosporine selectively suppresses cell-mediated immunity (CMI), prevents graft rejection and yet leaves the recipient with enough immune activity to combat bacterial infection. Unlike cytotoxic immunosuppressants, it is free of toxic effects on bone marrow and RE system. Humoral immunity remains intact. However, it is nephrotoxic (the major limitation), and impairs liver function.

The adverse effect of importance to dentists is that *cyclosporine causes gum hyperplasia in about 1/3rd recipients*. This can be minimized by good oral hygiene and plaque control. Other adverse effects are sustained rise in BP, precipitation of diabetes, hyperkalaemia, opportunistic infections, hirsutism, tremor and seizures.

Cyclosporine is a highly effective drug for prevention of graft rejection reaction. It is the standard drug for use in renal, bone marrow and other transplantations.

Cyclosporine is a second line drug in autoimmune diseases like severe rheumatoid arthritis, uveitis, dermatomyositis, etc. and in psoriasis.

Drug interactions: Cyclosporine can interact with a large number of drugs. All nephrotoxic drugs like aminoglycosides, vancomycin, amphotericin B and NSAIDs enhance its toxicity. By depressing renal function, it can reduce excretion of many drugs. Phenytoin, phenobarbitone, rifampin and other enzyme inducers lower its blood levels (transplant rejection may result). On the other hand, CYP3A4 inhibitors erythromycin, ketoconazole and related drugs inhibit cyclosporine metabolism to enhance its toxicity. K^+ supplements and K^+ sparing diuretics can produce marked hyperkalaemia in patients on cyclosporine.

Tacrolimus (FK506) This immunosuppressant is chemically different from cyclosporine but has the same mechanism of action and is ~100 times more potent. However, it binds to a different cytoplasmic protein labelled FKBP to inhibit calcineurin (Fig. 21.3). Gum hyperplasia due to tacrolimus is less marked. Therapeutic application, clinical efficacy, as well as toxicity profile are similar to cyclosporine.

mTOR inhibitor

Sirolimus This newer and potent immunosuppressant is a macrolide antibiotic which was earlier named *Rapamycin*. It binds to the same cytoplasmic protein FKBP as tacrolimus, but the sirolimus—FKBP complex inhibits a different kinase 'mTOR' and not calcineurin (Fig. 21.3). Inhibition of *mTOR* interrupts the signalling pathway that leads to proliferation and differentiation of T-cells. Sirolimus alone or in combination with other immunosuppressants is now an important drug to prevent and treat graft rejection reaction. Sirolimus coated stents are being used to reduce risk of restenosis

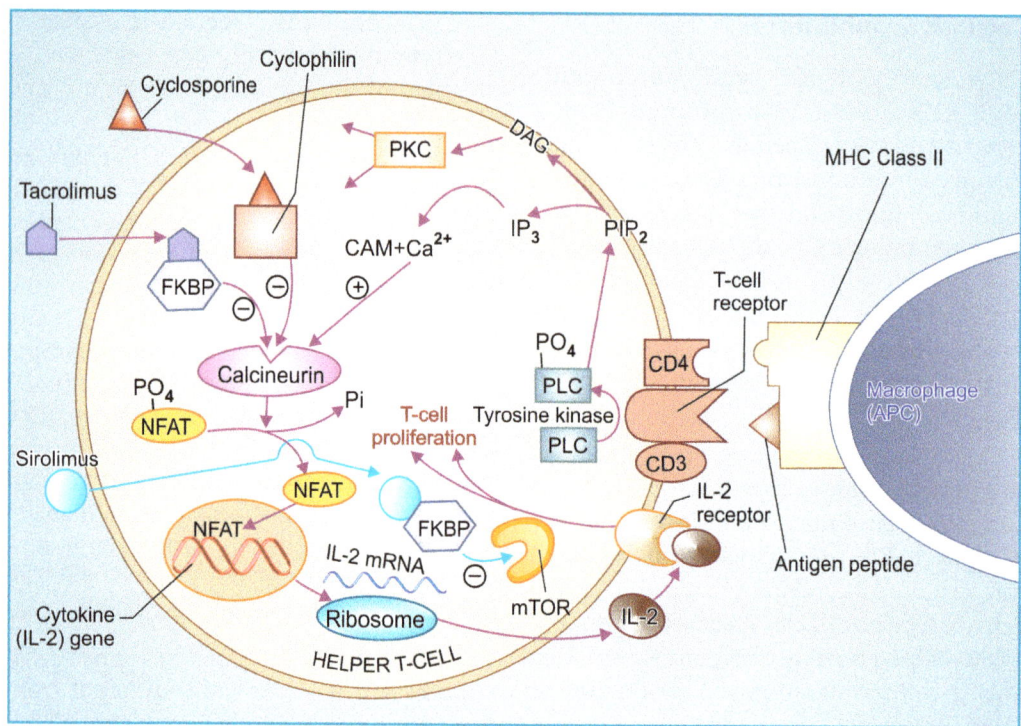

Fig. 21.3: Interaction between macrophage antigen presenting cell (APC) and helper T-cell in the immune response and mechanism of action of cyclosporine, tacrolimus and sirolimus.

Cyclosporine binds to an intracellular protein 'Cyclophilin' and this complex inhibits Ca^{2+}-Calmodulin (Ca^{2+}-CAM) activated phosphatase 'Calcineurin'. Tacrolimus also inhibits calcineurin, but after binding to a different protein FKBP (FK binding protein). Normally, after activation through T-cell receptor, calcineurin dephosphorylates a 'nuclear factor of activated T-cells' (NFAT) which translocates to the nucleus and triggers transcription of cytokine genes resulting in production of IL-2 and other cytokines. IL-2 diffuses out and acts on IL-2 receptor to stimulate T-cell proliferation and other processes, carrying forward the immune response.

Sirolimus also binds to FKBP, but this complex acts at a later stage, viz. it binds to and inhibits another kinase termed m-TOR (mammalian target of rapamycin) which is a key factor for progression of cell proliferation.

PLC—Phospholipase C; PIP_2—Phosphatidyl inositol bisphosphate; DAG—Diacyl glycerol; PKC—Protein kinase C.

after coronary angioplasty. Sirolimus (unlike cyclosporine) is not nephrotoxic and does not cause gum hyperplasia. However, it can cause thrombocytopenia, rise in serum lipids and liver damage.

Everolimus This newer congener of sirolimus has similar mechanism of action, immunosuppressant property and adverse effects, but has better oral bio-availability and shorter t½. In addition to use in organ transplantation, everolimus is indicated in some advanced cancers.

Antiproliferative drugs

Certain cytotoxic drugs used in cancer chemotherapy exhibit prominent immunosuppressant action, mainly by preventing clonal expansion of T and B lymphocytes (see Fig. 21.2).

Azathioprine (see p. 333) It is a purine antimetabolite which has more marked immunosuppressant than antitumour action. The basis for this difference is not clear, but may be due to its selective uptake into immune cells and intracellular conversion to the active metabolite 6-mercaptopurine. Azathioprine selectively affects differentiation and function of T cells and inhibits cytolytic lymphocytes; CMI is primarily depressed.

The most important application of azathioprine is prevention of renal and other graft rejection, but it is less effective than cyclosporine; generally combined with it or used in patients developing cyclosporine toxicity. It is a commonly used immunosuppressant for ulcerative colitis, progressive rheumatoid arthritis and some other autoimmune diseases.

Methotrexate This folate antagonist is a potent immunosuppressant which markedly depresses cytokine production and cellular immunity, and has anti-inflammatory property. Methotrexate has been used as a first line drug in many autoimmune diseases like rapidly progressing rheumatoid arthritis, severe psoriasis, pemphigus, myasthenia gravis, uveitis, chronic active hepatitis.

Cyclophosphamide This cytotoxic drug has more marked effect on B cells and humoral immunity compared to that on T cells and CMI. It has been particularly utilized in bone marrow transplantation. Low doses are occasionally used for maintenance therapy in pemphigus, systemic lupus erythematosus and idiopathic thrombocytopenic purpura.

Mycophenolate mofetil (MMF) It is a prodrug of mycophenolic acid which selectively inhibits inosine monophosphate dehydrogenase, an enzyme essential for *de novo* synthesis of guanosine nucleotides in the T and B cells (these cells, unlike others, do not have the purine salvage pathway). Lymphocyte proliferation, antibody production and CMI are inhibited. Sirolimus + glucocorticoid +MMF is a non-nephrotoxic combination utilized in renal transplantation. MMF is used in some autoimmune diseases as well.

Glucocorticoids (*see* Ch. 14)

Glucocorticoids have potent immunosuppressant and anti-inflammatory action, inhibit several components of the immune response. They particularly inhibit MHC expression and proliferation of T lymphocytes. Accordingly, they have a more marked effect on CMI.

Corticosteroids are widely employed as companion drug to cyclosporine in various organ transplants. They are the most effective drugs for suppressing graft *vs* host reaction. Glucocorticoids are used in practically all cases of severe autoimmune diseases, especially during exacerbation. Long-term complications are the greatest limitations of prolonged steroid use.

Biological agents

These are biotechnologically produced recombinant proteins or monoclonal/polyclonal antibodies directed against cytokines or lymphocyte surface antigens which play a key role in immune responses. Biological agents are mostly used as supplementary/reserve immunosuppressants.

1. Etanercept This fusion protein of human tumour necrosis factor (TNF) receptor and IgG$_1$ neutralizes TNF$_\alpha$ and TNF$_\beta$. TNF is secreted by activated macrophages and serves to amplify immune inflammation. Etanercept prevents activation of macrophages and T-cells. Combined with methotrexate, it is used in severe rheumatoid arthritis, plaque psoriasis, etc.

2. Infliximab It is a chimeral monoclonal antibody against TNF$_\alpha$ which is combined with methotrexate for refractory rheumatoid arthritis, Crohn's disease, psoriasis and some other severe autoimmune diseases.

3. Anakinra It is a recombinant human IL-1 receptor antagonist which prevents binding of IL-1 to its receptor, and is used in combination with methotrexate for rheumatoid arthritis.

4. Basiliximab It is a monoclonal antibody against CD-25 molecule which is expressed on the surface of activated T cells, and serves as a receptor for IL-2 through which cell proliferation and differentiation is promoted. Basiliximab acts as IL-2 antagonist and arrests the activated T-cells. It is used to supplement other immunosuppressants in renal transplantation.

5. Muromonab CD3 It is a murine monoclonal antibody against the CD3 glycoprotein located near to the T cell receptor on helper T cells. It inhibits participation of T cells in the immune response. T cells rapidly disappear from circulation leading to an immune blocked state.

Muromonab CD3 has been used as induction therapy together with corticosteroids and azathioprine for organ transplantation.

6. Antithymocyte globulin (ATG) It is a polyclonal antibody purified from horse or rabbits immunized with human thymic lymphocytes. It binds to T lymphocytes and depletes them, serving as a potent immunosuppressant. It has been used primarily to suppress acute allograft rejection episodes, but can also be used in induction regimens.

7. Anti-D immunoglobulin It is human IgG having a high titer of antibodies against Rh(D) antigens. It binds the Rho antigens and does not allow them to induce antibody formation in Rh negative individuals. It is used to prevent Rh haemolytic disease in Rh positive babies delivered by a Rh negative mother.

Adverse effects The two general untoward effects of immunosuppressant therapy are:

(a) Increased risk of bacterial, fungal, viral (especially CMV) as well as other opportunistic infections.
(b) Development of lymphomas and related malignancies after a long latency.

Section 3

Antimicrobials and Dental Therapeutics

Section Outline

22. Nonsteroidal Anti-inflammatory Drugs and Antipyretic-Analgesics
23. Opioid Analgesics and Antagonists
24. Local Anaesthetics
25. Antimicrobial Drugs: General Considerations
26. Sulfonamides, Cotrimoxazole, Quinolones and Nitroimidazoles
27. Beta-Lactam Antibiotics
28. Tetracyclines, Chloramphenicol and Aminoglycoside Antibiotics
29. Macrolide and Other Antibacterial Antibiotics
30. Antitubercular and Antileprotic Drugs
31. Antifungal Drugs
32. Antiviral Drugs (Non-retroviral)
33. Anti-retrovirus Drugs
34. Antiprotozoal Drugs
35. Antiseptics, Disinfectants and Other Locally Acting Drugs
36. Drugs and Aids with Specific Application in Dental Disorders
37. Management of Medical Emergencies in Dental Office
38. Drug Interactions

22 CHAPTER

Nonsteroidal Anti-inflammatory Drugs and Antipyretic-Analgesics

Pain (algesia) is an ill-defined, unpleasant sensation, usually evoked by an external or internal noxious stimulus. It is a warning signal and primarily protective in nature, but causes discomfort and suffering; may even be unbearable. *Dental pain is usually acute in nature* and is the most important symptom for which the patient comes to the dentist.

Analgesic is a drug that selectively relieves pain by acting in the CNS or on peripheral pain mechanisms, without significantly altering consciousness. Analgesics relieve pain as a symptom without affecting its cause. They are used when the noxious stimulus (evoking pain) cannot be removed, or as an adjuvant to more etiologic approach to pain, such as antibiotic treatment of apical tooth abscess.

Analgesics are divided into two groups, *viz.*

A. Opioid/narcotic/morphine like analgesics.

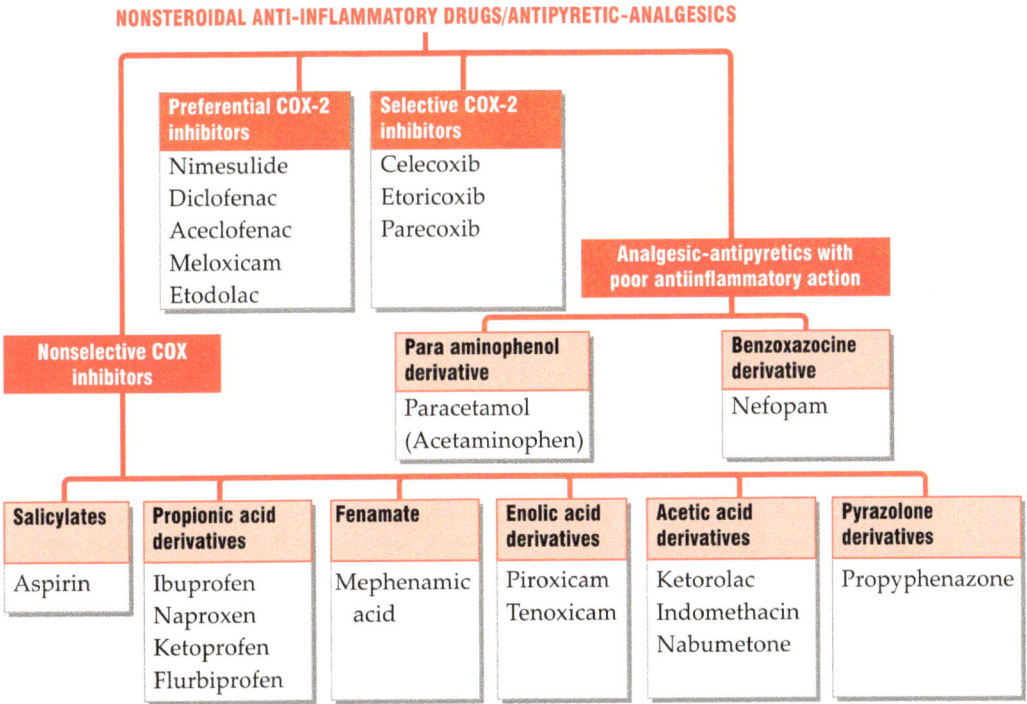

B. **Nonopioid/non-narcotic/antipyretic/ aspirin-like analgesics or nonsteroidal anti-inflammatory drugs (NSAIDs).**

The antipyretic-analgesics and NSAIDs are more commonly employed for dental pain, because tissue injury and inflammation due to tooth abscess, caries, gingivitis, tooth extraction, etc. is the major cause of acute dental pain.

The NSAIDs and antipyretic-analgesics are a class of drugs that have analgesic, antipyretic and anti-inflammatory actions in different measures. In contrast to morphine, they do not depress CNS, do not produce physical dependence, have no abuse liability and are particularly effective in inflammatory pain. They act primarily on peripheral pain mechanisms but also in the CNS to raise pain threshold. Many analgesics of this class are 'over-the-counter' or 'nonprescription' drugs.

NSAIDs and prostaglandin (PG) synthesis inhibition

In 1971, Vane and coworkers made the landmark observation that aspirin and some NSAIDs blocked prostaglandin (PG) generation. This is now considered to be the major mechanism of action of NSAIDs. Prostaglandins, prostacyclin (PG I_2) and thromboxane A_2 (TXA$_2$) are produced from arachidonic acid by the enzyme cyclooxygenase (*see* p. 122) which exists in a constitutive (COX-1) and an inducible (COX-2) isoforms; the former serves physiological 'house keeping' functions; while the latter, normally present in minute quantities, is induced by cytokines and other signal molecules at the site of inflammation → generation of large quantities of PGs locally which mediate many of the inflammatory changes. However, COX-2 is also constitutively present at some sites in the brain and in juxtaglomerular cells which may serve physiological role at these sites. Most NSAIDs inhibit COX-1 and COX-2 nonselectively, but there are some selective COX-2 inhibitors as well. Features of nonselective COX-1/COX-2 inhibitors (traditional NSAIDs) and selective COX-2 inhibitors are compared in Table 22.1.

Aspirin inhibits COX irreversibly by acetylating one of its serine residues; return of COX activity depends on synthesis of fresh enzyme.

Beneficial actions of NSAIDs due to PG synthesis inhibition

- Analgesia: prevention of pain nerve ending sensitization
- Antipyresis
- Antiinflammatory
- Antithrombotic
- Closure of ductus arteriosus in newborn

Other NSAIDs are competitive and reversible inhibitors of COX, return of activity depends on their dissociation from the enzyme which in turn is governed by the pharmacokinetic characteristics of the compound.

Table 22.1: Features of nonselective COX inhibitors and selective COX-2 inhibitors

Action	COX-1/COX-2 inhibitors	COX-2 inhibitors
1. Analgesic	+	+
2. Antipyretic	+	+
3. Antiinflammatory	+	+
4. Antiplatelet aggregatory	+	–
5. Gastric mucosal damage	+	–
6. Renal salt/water retention	+	+
7. Delay/prolongation of labour	+	+
8. Ductus arteriosus closure	+	?
9. Aspirin sensitive asthma precipitation	+	–

Analgesia PGs induce hyperalgesia (*see* p. 124 and Fig. 7.5) by affecting the transducing property of free nerve endings. As a result, stimuli that normally do not elicit pain are able to do so. NSAIDs do not affect the tenderness induced by direct application of PGs, but block the pain sensitizing mechanism triggered by bradykinin, TNFα, interleukins (ILs) and other algesic substances primarily by inhibiting COX-2. This constitutes the peripheral component of the analgesic action of NSAIDs. They are, therefore, more effective against inflammation associated pain, including acute dental/postextraction pain.

Antipyresis NSAIDs lower body temperature in fever, but do not cause hypothermia in normothermic individuals. Fever during infection/tissue injury is produced through the generation of pyrogen, ILs, TNFα, interferons, etc, which induce PG production in hypothalamus that raise its temperature set point. NSAIDs block the pyrogenic action of pyrogens but not that of PGE_2 injected into the hypothalamus. The COX isoform present at this site appears to be COX-2 (possibly COX-3 also: a splice variant of COX-1 that is inhibited by paracetamol). However, fever can occur through non-PG mediated mechanisms as well.

> **Shared toxicities of NSAIDs due to PG synthesis inhibition**
> - Gastric mucosal damage
> - Bleeding: inhibition of platelet function
> - Limitation of renal blood flow : Na^+ and water retention
> - Delay / prolongation of labour
> - Asthma and anaphylactoid reactions in susceptible individuals

Anti-inflammatory The most important mechanism of antiinflammatory action of NSAIDs is considered to be inhibition of COX-2 mediated enhanced PG synthesis at the site of injury. The anti-inflammatory potency of different compounds roughly corresponds with their potency to inhibit COX. However, nimesulide is a potent anti-inflammatory but relatively weak COX inhibitor. PGs are only one of the mediators of inflammation; inhibition of COX does not depress the production of other mediators like LTs, PAF, cytokines, etc. Inflammation is the result of concerted participation of a large number of vasoactive, chemotactic and proliferative factors at different stages, and there are many targets for anti-inflammatory action.

Activated endothelial cells express adhesion molecules (ELAM-1, ICAM-1) on their surface and play a key role in directing circulating leukocytes to the site of inflammation. Similarly, inflammatory cells express *selectins* and *integrins*. Certain NSAIDs may act by additional mechanisms including inhibition of expression and/or activity of some of these molecules and generation of superoxide or other free radicals. Growth factors like GM-CSF, IL-6 as well as lymphocyte transformation factors and TNFα may also be affected. Stabilization of lysosomal membrane of leucocytes and antagonism of certain actions of kinins may be contributing to the anti-imflammatory action of NSAIDs.

Dysmenorrhoea Involvement of PGs in dysmenorrhoea has been clearly demonstrated. Level of PGs in menstrual flow, endometrial biopsy and that of $PGF_{2\alpha}$ metabolite in circulation are raised in dysmenorrhoeic women. NSAIDs lower uterine PG levels and afford excellent relief in 60–70% dysmenorrhoeic women, as well as partial relief in the remaining.

Antiplatelet aggregatory NSAIDs inhibit synthesis of both proaggregatory (TXA_2) and antiaggregatory (PGI_2) prostanoids, but effect on platelet TXA_2 predominates. Therapeutic doses of most NSAIDs inhibit platelet aggregation, so that bleeding time is prolonged. *Aspirin is highly active*; acetylates platelet COX irreversibly in portal circulation before it is deacetylated by first pass metabolism in liver. Small doses are, therefore, able to exert antithrombotic effect for several days. *Risk of postextraction bleeding is enhanced.*

Ductus arteriosus closure During foetal circulation, ductus arteriosus is kept patent by local elaboration of PGE_2 by COX-2. Unknown mechanisms switch off this synthesis of PGs at birth and the ductus closes. When this fails to occur, small doses of indomethacin or aspirin bring about closure in majority of cases within a few hours by inhibiting PG production. Administration of NSAIDs in late pregnancy has been found to promote premature closure of ductus in some cases. *Dentists should avoid prescribing NSAIDs near term.*

Parturition Sudden spurt of PG synthesis by uterus occurs just before labour begins. This is believed to trigger labour and facilitate its progression. Accordingly, NSAIDs have the potential to delay and retard labour. However, labour can occur in the absence of PGs.

Gastric mucosal damage Gastric pain, mucosal erosion/ulceration and blood loss are produced by all NSAIDs to varying extents. Relative gastric toxicity is a major consideration in the choice of NSAIDs. Inhibition of synthesis of gastroprotective PGs (PGE_2, PGI_2) is clearly involved, though local action inducing back diffusion of H^+ ions in gastric mucosa also plays a role. Deficiency of PGs reduces mucus and HCO_3 secretion, tends to enhance acid secretion and may promote mucosal ischaemia. Thus, NSAIDs enhance aggressive factors and contain defensive factors in gastric mucosa. Therefore, they are ulcerogenic. Paracetamol, a very weak inhibitor of COX, is practically free of gastric toxicity and selective COX-2 inhibitors are relatively safer. Stable PG analogues (misoprostol) administered concurrently with NSAIDs counteract their gastric toxicity.

Renal effects Conditions leading to hypovolaemia, decreased renal perfusion and Na^+ loss induce renal PG synthesis which brings about intrarenal adjustments by promoting vasodilatation, inhibiting tubular Cl reabsorption (Na^+ and water accompany) and opposing ADH action.

NSAIDs produce renal effects by at least 3 mechanisms:
- COX-1 dependent impairment of renal blood flow and reduction of g.f.r.; this can worsen renal insufficiency.
- Juxtaglomerular COX-2 (probably COX-1 also) dependent Na^+ and water retention.
- Ability to cause papillary necrosis on habitual intake.

Renal effects of NSAIDs are not marked in normal individuals but become significant in those with CHF, hypovolaemia, hepatic cirrhosis, kidney disease and in patients receiving diuretics or antihypertensives. In such subjects, Na^+ retention and edema can occur; diuretic and antihypertensive drug effects are blunted.

Analgesic nephropathy occurs after years of heavy ingestion of analgesics. Such individuals probably have some personality defect. Pathological lesions are papillary necrosis, tubular atrophy followed by renal fibrosis. Urine concentrating ability is lost and the kidneys shrink. Because phenacetin was first implicated, it went into disrepute, though other analgesics are also liable to produce similar effects.

Anaphylactoid reactions Aspirin precipitates asthma, angioneurotic swellings, urticaria or rhinitis in certain susceptible individuals. These subjects react similarly to chemically diverse NSAIDs, ruling out immunological basis for the reaction. Inhibition of COX with consequent diversion of arachidonic acid to LTs and other products of lipoxygenase pathway may be instrumental, but there is no proof.

SALICYLATES

Aspirin

Aspirin is acetylsalicylic acid. It is rapidly converted in the body to salicylic acid which is responsible for most of the actions. Other actions are the result of acetylation of certain macromolecules including COX.

Aspirin is one of the oldest analgesic-anti-inflammatory drugs and has diverse uses.

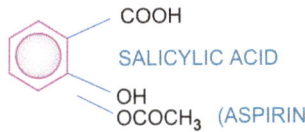

Pharmacological actions

1. Aspirin has analgesic, antipyretic and anti-inflammatory action. However, it is a weaker analgesic than morphine type drugs, but it effectively relieves inflammatory, tissue injury related, connective tissue and integumental pain. Aspirin is relatively ineffective in severe visceral and ischaemic pain. The analgesic action is mainly due to obtunding of peripheral pain receptors and prevention of PG-mediated sensitization of nerve endings. A central subcortical action raising threshold to pain perception also contributes to analgesia, but the morphine-like action on psychic processing or reaction component of the pain is missing. No sedation, subjective effects, tolerance or dependence is produced.

Aspirin resets the hypothalamic thermostat and rapidly reduces fever by promoting heat loss through sweating and cutaneous vasodilatation, but does not decrease heat production.

Anti-inflammatory action is exerted at high doses (3–5 g/day or 100 mg/kg/ day). Signs of inflammation like pain, tenderness, swelling, vasodilatation and leucocyte infiltration are suppressed. However, progression of the underlying disease in rheumatoid arthritis, rheumatic fever and osteoarthritis, etc. is not affected.

2. Aspirin as well as the salicylic acid released from it irritate gastric mucosa → cause epigastric distress, nausea and vomiting. At high doses it stimulates CTZ; the resulting vomiting has a central component as well.

Aspirin (pKa 3.5) remains unionized and diffusible in the acid gastric juice; but on entering the mucosal cell (pH 7.1), it ionizes and becomes indiffusible. This 'ion trapping' in the gastric mucosal cell enhances gastric toxicity. Moreover, aspirin particle coming in contact with gastric mucosa promotes local back diffusion of acid. This causes focal necrosis of mucosal cells and capillaries → acute ulcers, erosive gastritis, congestion and microscopic haemorrhages occur. The occult blood loss in stools is increased by even a single tablet of aspirin. Blood loss averages 5 ml/day at anti-inflammatory doses. Haematemesis occurs occasionally, which may be an idiosyncratic reaction.

Soluble aspirin tablets containing calcium carbonate + citric acid or other buffered preparations are less liable to cause gastric ulceration.

3. Aspirin, even in small doses, irreversibly inhibits TXA_2 synthesis by platelets. Thus, it interferes with platelet aggregation so that bleeding time is prolonged to nearly twice the normal value. This effect lasts for about a week (turnover time of platelets).

Long-term intake of large doses decreases synthesis of clotting factors in liver and predisposes to bleeding. This can be prevented by prophylactic vit K therapy.

4. The analgesic doses of aspirin (0.3–0.6 g) employed in dentistry or for headache, fever, etc. have practically no other action. However, high anti-inflammatory doses (3–5 g/day) produce several other effects:

- Cellular metabolism is enhanced, especially in skeletal muscles due to uncoupling of oxidative phosphorylation. Glucose utilization is increased resulting in fall in blood glucose level (especially in diabetics); liver glycogen is depleted. However, toxic doses may cause sympathetic stimulation and rise in blood sugar.
- Respiration is stimulated both by direct action on respiratory centre, as well as due to increased CO_2 production. Hyperventilation followed by respiratory depression occurs at toxic doses.
- Respiratory stimulation tends to washout CO_2 and produce respiratory alkalosis.

This is compensated by enhanced HCO$_3^-$ excretion by kidney. Most adults receiving 3–5 g/day stay in a state of *compensated respiratory alkalosis*. Still higher doses depress respiration while excess CO$_2$ production continues to cause *respiratory acidosis*. Increased production of metabolic acids (lactic, pyruvic, acetoacetic) may contribute to *metabolic acidosis*, since plasma HCO$_3^-$ is already low. Dehydration occurs due to excess water loss in urine, sweating and hyperventilation.

- Aspirin has no direct effect on heart or circulation, but doses which enhance metabolic rate, increase cardiac output indirectly. Toxic doses depress vasomotor centre, so that blood pressure may fall.
- Aspirin interferes with urate excretion and antagonises the uricosuric effect of probenecid. However, at high doses (≥ 5 g/day) it may block urate reabsorption and increase its excretion, but aspirin is not a reliable uricosuric.

Pharmacokinetics

Aspirin is absorbed from the stomach and small intestines. Its poor water solubility is the limiting factor in absorption: microfining the drug-particles and inclusion of a basic salt (solubility is more at higher pH) enhances absorption. However, higher pH also favours ionization, thus decreasing the diffusible form.

Aspirin is rapidly deacetylated in the gut wall, liver, plasma and other tissues to release salicylic acid which is the major circulating and active form. It is ~80% bound to plasma proteins and has a volume of distribution ~0.17 L/kg. Entry into brain is slow, but aspirin freely crosses placenta. Both aspirin and salicylic acid are conjugated in liver with glycine to form salicyluric acid (major pathway); and with glucuronic acid. The metabolites are excreted by glomerular filtration as well as tubular secretion. Only 1/10th is excreted as free salicylic acid.

The plasma t½ of aspirin as such is 15–20 min, but taken together with that of released salicylic acid, it is 3–5 hours. However, metabolic processes get saturated over the therapeutic range; t½ of anti-inflammatory doses may be 8–12 hours, while that during poisoning may be as long as 30 hours. Thus, elimination is dose dependent.

Adverse effects

(a) Side effects that occur at analgesic dose (0.3–0.6 g 6–8 hourly) are nausea, vomiting, epigastric distress, increased occult blood loss in stools. The most important adverse effect of aspirin is gastric mucosal damage and peptic ulceration.

(b) Hypersensitivity and idiosyncrasy Though infrequent, these reactions can be serious and include rashes, fixed drug eruption, urticaria, rhinorrhoea, angioedema, asthma, anaphylactoid reaction. Profuse gastric bleeding occurs in rare instances.

(c) Anti-inflammatory doses (3–5 g/day) produce the syndrome called salicylism— dizziness, tinnitus, vertigo, reversible impairment of hearing and vision, excitement, hyperventilation and electrolyte imbalance. Salt and water retention occurs in a dose-dependent manner.

An association between salicylate therapy and 'Reye's syndrome' (a rare form of hepatic encephalopathy seen in children having viral infection) has been noted. Long-term therapy with high dose aspirin can cause insidious onset hepatic injury.

(d) Acute salicylate poisoning It is more common in children. Manifestations are:

Vomiting, dehydration, electrolyte imbalance, acidotic breathing, hyper/hypoglycaemia, petechial haemorrhages, restlessness, delirium, hallucinations, hyperpyrexia, convulsions, coma and death due to respiratory failure + cardiovascular collapse.

Treatment is symptomatic and supportive. Most important is external cooling and i.v. fluid with Na^+, K^+, HCO_3 and glucose: according to need determined by repeated monitoring. Blood transfusion and vit K should be given if bleeding occurs.

Precautions and contraindications

- Aspirin is contraindicated in subjects who are sensitive to it, and in patients with peptic ulcer, bleeding tendencies, in children suffering from chicken-pox or influenza.
- In chronic liver disease aspirin can precipitate hepatic necrosis.
- Aspirin should be avoided in diabetics, in those with low cardiac reserve or frank CHF, and in juvenile rheumatoid arthritis.
- *Aspirin should be stopped 1 week before dental extraction and elective surgery.* In case this is not possible, adequate haemostasis must be ensured by packing the socket and use of local haemostatics if needed.
- Given repeatedly during pregnancy, it may be responsible for low birth weight babies. Delayed or prolonged labour, greater postpartum blood loss and premature closure of ductus arteriosus are possible if aspirin is taken at or near term.
- Aspirin should be avoided by breast-feeding mothers.
- Avoid high doses in G-6-PD deficient individuals—haemolysis can occur.

Interactions

1. Aspirin displaces warfarin, naproxen, sulfonylureas, phenytoin and methotrexate from binding sites on plasma proteins: toxicity of these drugs may occur. Antiplatelet action of aspirin increases the risk of bleeding in patients on oral anticoagulants.

2. Aspirin inhibits tubular secretion of uric acid (at analgesic doses) and antagonizes uricosuric action of probenecid. Tubular secretion of methotrexate is also interfered.

3. Aspirin blunts diuretic action of furosemide and thiazides. The K^+ conserving action of spironolactone is reduced due to competition between *aspirin* and *canrenone* (the active metabolite of spironolactone) for active transport in proximal tubules.

Uses

1. *As analgesic* For headache, toothache, backache, myalgia, joint pain, pulled muscle, neuralgias and dysmenorrhoea; it is effective in low doses (0.3–0.6 g) and analgesic effect is maximal at ~ 1000 mg. *Majority of painful dental conditions respond very well to these doses of aspirin repeated 6–8 hourly.*

2. *As antipyretic* It is effective in fever of any origin; dose is same as for analgesia. However, paracetamol, being safer, is generally preferred.

3. *Acute rheumatic fever* Aspirin is the first drug to be used in all cases; other drugs are added or substituted only when it fails or in severe cases (corticosteroids act faster).

4. *Rheumatoid arthritis* Aspirin in a dose of 3–5 g/day is effective in most cases. Since these doses of aspirin are poorly tolerated for long periods, the newer NSAIDs are preferred.

5. *Osteoarthritis* Aspirin affords symptomatic relief, but paracetamol is the first choice analgesic for most cases.

6. *Postmyocardial infarction and poststroke patients* By inhibiting platelet aggregation, aspirin lowers the incidence of reinfarction. Aspirin in low doses (75–150 mg/day) is now routinely prescribed to post-infarct patients. Aspirin reduces 'transient ischaemic attacks' and lowers incidence of stroke in such patients.

Adverse effects of NSAIDs

Gastrointestinal
Nausea, anorexia, gastric irritation, erosions, peptic ulceration, gastric bleeding/perforation, esophagitis

Renal
Na⁺ and water retention, edema, chronic renal failure, nephropathy, papillary necrosis (rare)

CVS
Rise in BP, risk of myocardial infarction (especially with COX-2 inhibitors), CHF

Hepatic
Raised transaminases, hepatic failure (rare)

CNS
Headache, tinnitus, mental confusion, vertigo, seizure precipitation

Haematological
Bleeding, thrombocytopenia, haemolytic anaemia, nutropenia

Others
Asthma exacerbation, nasal polyposis, skin rashes, pruritus, angioedema

---

ASPIRIN 350 mg tab, COLSPRIN 100, 325, 650 mg tabs, ECOSPRIN 75, 150, 325 mg tabs, DISPRIN 350 mg tab (with Cal. carbonate 105 mg + citric acid 35 mg) LOPRIN 75, 162.5 mg tabs.

An injectable preparation is also available: BIOSPIRIN: Lysine acetylsalicylate 900 mg + glycine 100 mg/vial for dissolving in 5 ml water and i.v. injection.

PROPIONIC ACID DERIVATIVES

Ibuprofen was the first member of this class to be introduced in 1969 as a better tolerated alternative to aspirin. Many others have followed. All have similar pharmacodynamic properties, but differ considerably in potency and to some extent in duration of action (Table 22.2).

All members inhibit PG synthesis, naproxen being the most potent; but their *in vitro* potency to inhibit COX does not closely parallel *in vivo* anti-inflammatory potency.

They inhibit platelet aggregation reversibly and cause short lasting prolongation of bleeding time.

Adverse effects Ibuprofen and all its congeners are better tolerated than aspirin. Side effects are milder and their incidence is lower.

Gastric discomfort, nausea and vomiting, though less than aspirin or indomethacin, are still the most common side effects. Gastric erosion and occult blood loss are rare.

CNS side effects include headache, dizziness, blurring of vision, tinnitus and depression.

Rashes, itching and other hypersensitivity phenomena are infrequent. However, these drugs can precipitate asthma in subjects sensitive to aspirin.

Fluid retention is less marked.

Table 22.2: Dosage and preparations of propionic acid derivatives

Drug	Plasma t½	Dosage	Preparations
1. Ibuprofen	2–4 hr	400–600 mg (5-10 mg/kg) TDS	BRUFEN, EMFLAM, IBUSYNTH 200, 400, 600 mg tab, IBUGESIC also 100 mg/5 ml susp.
2. Naproxen	12–16 hr	250 mg BD– TDS	NAPROSYN, NAXID, ARTAGEN, XENOBID 250 mg tab., NAPROSYN also 500 mg tab.
3. Ketoprofen	2–3 hr	50-100 mg BD–TDS	KETOFEN 50, 100 mg tab; OSTOFEN 50 mg cap. RHOFENID 100 mg tab, 200 mg SR tab; 100 mg/2 ml amp.
4. Flurbiprofen	4–6 hr	50–100 mg BD–QID	ARFLUR 50, 100 mg tab, 200 mg SR tab, FLUROFEN 100 mg tab

Drug interactions with NSAIDs

Pharmacodynamic		Pharmacokinetic	
Diuretics	: ↓ diuresis	Oral anticoagulants	Metabolism inhibited; Competition for plasma protein binding
β blocker	: ↓ antihypertensive effect	Sulfonylureas	
ACE inhibitors	: ↓ antihypertensive effect	Phenytoin	
Anticoagulants	: ↑ risk of g.i. bleed	Valproate	
Sulfonylureas	: ↑ risk of hypoglycaemia		
Alcohol	: ↑ risk of g.i. bleed	Digoxin	↓ Renal excretion of interacting drug
Cyclosporine	: ↑ nephrotoxicity	Lithium	
Corticosteroids	: ↑ risk of g.i. bleed	Aminoglycosides	
Selective serotonin reuptake inhibitors	: ↑ risk of g.i. bleed	Methotrexate	

Propionic acid NSAIDs are not to be prescribed to pregnant women and should be avoided in peptic ulcer patient.

Pharmacokinetics and interactions All propionic acid derivatives are well absorbed orally, highly bound to plasma proteins (90–99%), but displacement interactions are not clinically significant—dose of oral anticoagulants and oral hypoglycaemics need not be altered. Because they inhibit platelet function, use with anticoagulants should, nevertheless, be avoided.

Similar to other NSAIDs, they are likely to decrease diuretic and antihypertensive action of thiazides, furosemide and β blockers.

All propionic acid NSAIDs enter brain, synovial fluid and cross placenta. They are largely metabolized in liver by hydroxylation and glucuronide conjugation and excreted in urine as well as bile.

Uses

1. Ibuprofen, available as an 'over-the-counter' drug, is used as a simple analgesic and antipyretic in the same way as low dose of aspirin.
2. Ibuprofen and its congeners are widely used in rheumatoid arthritis, osteoarthritis and other musculoskeletal disorders, especially where pain is more prominent than inflammation.
3. These drugs are indicated in soft tissue injuries, *tooth extraction*, fractures, vasectomy, postpartum and postoperatively to suppress swelling and inflammation and are *very popular in dentistry*.

Ibuprofen It has been rated as the safest traditional NSAID by the spontaneous adverse drug reporting system in UK. Ibuprofen (400 mg) has been found equally or more efficacious than a combination of aspirin (650 mg) + codeine (60 mg) in relieving dental surgery pain, but is a weaker anti-inflammatory drug. Its antiplatelet action is short lasting, and it blocks the long-lasting antiplatelet effect of low-dose aspirin.

Naproxen The anti-inflammatory activity of naproxen is stronger, and it is indicated in acute gout, rheumatoid arthritis, ankylosing spondylitis, etc., but is infrequently used in dentistry.

Ketoprofen Though it has been shown to inhibit LOX as well, the anti-inflammatory effect of ketoprofen is similar to that of ibuprofen; side effects are more prominent.

Flurbiprofen The anti-inflammatory effect is stronger and may have some additional mechanisms. It is more commonly used in arthritis and topically in eye. Gastric tolerance is poorer than ibuprofen.

Choice among different members of this class is difficult; *naproxen* is probably more efficacious and better tolerated in antiinflammatory doses. However,

> **Comorbid conditions aggravated by NSAIDs**
> - Peptic ulcer
> - Hypertension
> - Congestive heart failure
> - Renal insufficiency
> - Haemostatic disorders

individuals vary in their preference for different members.

FENAMATE (Anthranilic acid derivative)

Mephenamic acid It is an analgesic, antipyretic and weaker anti-inflammatory drug, which inhibits COX as well as antagonises certain actions of PGs.

Oral absorption of mephenamic acid is slow but almost complete. It is highly bound to plasma proteins, partly metabolized and excreted in urine as well as bile. Plasma t½ is 2–4 hours.

Diarrhoea is the most important dose-related side effect. Epigastric distress is complained, but gut bleeding is not significant. Haemolytic anaemia is a rare but serious complication.

Mephenamic acid is indicated primarily as analgesic in muscle, joint and soft tissue pain where strong anti-inflammatory action is not needed. It may be used in dental pain, but has no distinct advantage.

Dose: 250–500 mg TDS; MEDOL 250, 500 mg cap; MEFTAL, 250, 500 mg tab, 100 mg/5 ml susp. PONSTAN 125, 250, 500 mg tab, 50 mg/ml syrup.

ENOLIC ACID DERIVATIVES

Piroxicam It is a long-acting NSAID with potent anti-inflammatory and good analgesic-antipyretic actions. It is a reversible inhibitor of COX. In addition, it decreases production of free radicals and IgM rheumatoid factor, and reduces leucocyte chemotaxis. Thus, piroxicam can inhibit inflammation in diverse ways.

Piroxicam is rapidly and completely absorbed: 99% plasma protein bound; largely metabolized in liver and excreted both in urine and bile. Plasma t½ is long—nearly 2 days. Single daily administration is sufficient.

Common side effects are heart burn, nausea and anorexia, but it is better tolerated and less ulcerogenic than indomethacin; causes less faecal blood loss than aspirin. Rashes and pruritus occur in < 1% patients. Edema and reversible azotaemia have been observed.

Piroxicam is suitable for use as long-term antiinflammatory drug in rheumatoid and osteoarthritis, ankylosing spondylitis, acute gout, as well as in dentistry, but is relatively more toxic.

Dose: 20 mg BD for two days followed by 20 mg OD: DOLONEX, PIROX 10, 20 mg cap, 20 mg dispersible tab, 20 mg/ml inj in 1 and 2 ml amps; PIRICAM 10, 20 mg cap.

Tenoxicam A congener of piroxicam with similar properties and uses.
TOBITIL 20 mg tab; dose 20 mg OD.

ACETIC ACID DERIVATIVES

Ketorolac This NSAID has potent analgesic and modest anti-inflammatory activity. In postoperative pain it has equalled the efficacy of morphine, but does not interact with opioid receptors and is free of opioid side effects. Like other NSAIDs, it inhibits PG synthesis and relieves pain primarily by a peripheral mechanism. In short-lasting pain, it has compared favourably with aspirin.

Ketorolac is rapidly absorbed after oral and i.m. administration. It is highly plasma protein bound and 60% excreted unchanged in urine. Major metabolic pathway is glucuronidation; plasma t½ is 5–7 hours.

Adverse effects Nausea, abdominal pain, dyspepsia, ulceration, loose stools, drowsiness, pain at injection site, rise in serum transaminase and fluid retention have been noted.

Use Ketorolac is frequently used in postoperative, dental and acute musculo-skeletal pain: 15–30 mg i.m. or i.v. is comparable to 10–12 mg morphine, and can be repeated every 4–6 hours (max. 90 mg/day).

Orally it is used in a dose of 10–20 mg 6 hourly for short-term management of moderate pain. In postoperative dental pain ketorolac has been rated superior to aspirin 650 mg, paracetamol 600 mg and equivalent to ibuprofen 400 mg. Continuous use for more than 5 days is not recommended.

KETOROL, ZOROVON, KETANOV, TOROLAC 10 mg tab, 30 mg in 1 ml amp.

Indomethacin This indole acetic acid derivative is a potent anti-inflammatory drug with prompt antipyretic action, and relieves inflammatory or tissue injury related pain. Indomethacin is a highly potent inhibitor of PG synthesis and suppresses neutrophil motility. Like aspirin, it uncouples oxidative phosphorylation at toxic doses.

Indomethacin is well absorbed orally. Rectal absorption is slow but dependable. It is 90% bound to plasma proteins, partly metabolized in liver to inactive products and excreted by kidney. Plasma t½ is 2–5 hours.

Adverse effects A high incidence (up to 50%) of gastrointestinal and CNS side effects is produced. Gastric irritation, nausea, anorexia, gastric bleeding and diarrhoea are prominent.
Frontal headache is common. Dizziness, ataxia, mental confusion, hallucination, depression and psychosis can occur.
Leukopenia, rashes and other hyper-sensitivity reactions are also reported.
Risk of bleeding is increased due to decreased platelet aggregability.
Indomethacin is contraindicated in machinery operators, drivers, psychiatric patients, epileptics, kidney disease, pregnant women and in children.

Dose: 25–50 mg BD-QID. Those not tolerating the drug orally may be given rectal suppository at night.

IDICIN, INDOCAP 25 mg cap, 75 mg SR cap, ARTICID 25, 50 mg cap, INDOFLAM 25, 75 mg caps, 1% eye drop. RECTICIN 50 mg suppository.

Uses Because of prominent adverse effects, indomethacin is used as a reserve drug in conditions requiring potent anti-inflammatory action like ankylosing spondylitis, acute exacerbations of destructive arthropathies, psoriatic arthritis and acute gout that are not responding to better tolerated NSAIDs. Use for dental pain is rarely justified.

Malignancy associated fever refractory to other antipyretics may respond to indomethacin.

Nabumetone It is a prodrug—generates an active metabolite (6-MNA) which inhibits both COX-1 and COX-2. It possesses analgesic, antipyretic and anti-inflammatory activities; effective in the treatment of rheumatoid and osteoarthritis as well as in soft tissue injury. Abdominal cramps, diarrhoea, rashes and photosensitivity can occur. However, nabumetone has failed to gain popularity in use.

NABUFLAM 500 mg tab; 1 tab OD

PYRAZOLONES

Antipyrine (phenazone) and amidopyrine (amino-pyrine) were introduced in 1884 as antipyretic and analgesic. Their use was associated with high incidence of agranulocytosis and they were banned globally. *Phenylbutazone* was introduced in 1949 and soon its active metabolite *oxyphenbutazone* was also marketed. These two potent anti-inflammatory drugs were also banned due to unacceptable risk of blood dyscrasias and other adverse effects.

Propyphenazone

This is the only pyrazolone still available in India, but is banned in many countries for risk similar to other drugs of this group. The FDC of propyphenazone (along with 327 other FDCs) was banned by the Govt. of India in 2018, but the ban has been lifted by the court till further order. Propyphenazone has fast onset short duration analgesic-antipyretic anti-inflammatory action, and is claimed not to produce agranulocytosis. Marketed only in combination with paracetamol as an 'over the counter drug', it is mostly taken by the laity for self medication of headache, toothache, bodyache, rheumatic pain, fever, etc.

Dose: 150–300 mg TDS;

in SARIDON: propyphenazone 150 mg + paracetamol 250 mg + caffeine 50 mg tab.

DART: propyphenazone 150 mg + paracetamol 300 mg + caffeine 50 mg tab.

PREFERENTIAL COX-2 INHIBITORS

Nimesulide This NSAID is a relatively weak inhibitor of PG synthesis and moderately COX-2 selective. Anti-inflammatory action may be exerted by other mechanisms as well, e.g. reduced generation of superoxide by neutrophils, inhibition of PAF synthesis and TNFα release, free radical scavanging. The analgesic, antipyretic and antiinflammatory activity of nimesulide has been rated comparable to other NSAIDs. It has been used primarily for short-lasting painful inflammatory conditions like sports injuries, sinusitis, dental surgery, bursitis, low backache, dysmenorrhoea, postoperative pain, osteoarthritis and for fever.

Nimesulide is almost completely absorbed orally, 99% plasma protein bound, extensively metabolized and excreted mainly in urine with a t½ of 2–5 hours.

Adverse effects of nimesulide are gastrointestinal (epigastralgia, heart burn, nausea, loose motions), dermatological (rash, pruritus) and central (somnolence, dizziness). Gastric tolerability of nimesulide is claimed to be better, but ulcer complications may be as prevalent as with other NSAIDs. Lately, several instances of fulminant hepatic failure have been associated with nimesulide and it has been withdrawn in several countries. Considering that it has not been marketed in the UK, USA, Australia and Canada, the overall safety of this drug, especially in children, has been questioned. However, aspirin sensitive patients do not cross-react with nimesulide.

Dose: 100 mg BD; NIMULID, NIMEGESIC, NIMODOL 100 mg tab, 50 mg/5 ml susp.

Diclofenac sodium An analgesic-antipyretic antiinflammatory drug, similar in efficacy to naproxen. It inhibits PG synthesis and is somewhat COX-2 selective. The antiplatelet action is weak due to relative sparing of COX-1, and it does not block the cardioprotective effect of low dose aspirin. Neutrophil chemotaxis and superoxide production at the inflammatory site are reduced.

Diclofenac is well absorbed orally, 99% protein bound, metabolized, and excreted both in urine and bile. The plasma t½ is ~ 2 hours. However, it has good tissue penetrability and action lasts 6–8 hours.

Adverse effects of diclofenac are generally mild: epigastric pain, nausea, headache, dizziness, rashes. Gastric ulceration and bleeding are less common. Some comparative trials have found its gastric toxicity to be similar to the selective COX-2 inhibitors celecoxib and etoricoxib. Reversible elevation of serum aminotransferases has been reported more frequently. Renal blood flow and g.f.r. may be reduced, especially at higher doses.

Diclofenac is among the most extensively used NSAIDs; employed in rheumatoid and osteoarthritis, ankylosing spondylitis, toothache, dysmenorrhoea and renal colic. It affords quick relief of pain and wound edema in post-traumatic and postoperative inflammatory conditions.

Dose: 50–75 mg TDS, then BD oral, 75 mg deep i.m. VOVERAN, DICLONAC, MOVONAC 50 mg enteric coated tab, 100 mg S.R. tab, 25 mg/ml in 3 ml amp. for i.m. inj. DICLOMAX 25, 50 mg tab, 75 mg/3 ml inj., DYNAPAR AQ: diclofenac sod. 75 mg in 1 ml inj. for i.m./i.v. injection.

Diclofenac potassium: VOLTAFLAM 25, 50 mg tab, ULTRA-K 50 mg tab; VOVERAN 1% topical gel.

Aceclofenac A moderately COX-2 selective congener of diclofenac having similar properties.

Dose: 100 mg BD; ACECLO, DOLOKIND 100 mg tab, 200 mg SR tab.

Meloxicam This newer congener of piroxicam has a COX-2 : COX-1 selectivity ratio of about 10. Since measurable inhibition of platelet TXA_2 production (a COX-1 function) occurs at therapeutic doses of meloxicam, it has been labelled 'preferential COX-2 inhibitor'. Gastric side effects of meloxicam are milder, but ulcer complications (bleeding, perforation) have been reported on long-term use. There is no convincing evidence that meloxicam is safer than other NSAIDs. Plasma t½ is 15–20 hours permiting single daily dose.

Dose: 7.5-15 mg OD; MELFLAM, MEL-OD, MUVIK, M-CAM 7.5 mg, 15 mg tabs.

Etodolac This newer indole-acetic acid NSAID is moderately COX-2 selective with properties similar to diclofenac. At lower doses, gastric tolerance is better than older NSAIDs. It is metabolized by hydroxylation and glucuronide conjugation, and excreted in urine with a t½ of 7 hours. Analgesia with etodolac lasts for 6–8 hours. Side effects are abdominal pain, rashes and dizziness.

Dose: 200–400 mg BD–TDS

ETOVA 200, 300, 400 mg tabs.

SELECTIVE COX-2 INHIBITORS (Coxibs)

Because of the theoretical advantage of inhibiting COX-2 which is induced at the sites of imflammation, without affecting the 'house keeping' COX-1 function, some highly selective COX-2 inhibitors have been introduced over the past 3 decades. They cause less gastric mucosal damage; occurrence of peptic ulcer and ulcer bleeds is clearly lower than with traditional NSAIDs. The selective COX-2 inhibitors do not depress TXA_2 production by platelets, because it is COX-1 dependent. They do not inhibit platelet aggregation or prolong bleeding time, but reduce PGI_2 production by vascular endothelium. Thus, these NSAIDs lack the cardioprotective property of aspirin.

Currently, 3 selective COX-2 inhibitors (also called coxibs) *Celecoxib*, *Etoricoxib* and *Parecoxib* are available, while *Rofecoxib* and *Valdecoxib* have been withdrawn globally for increasing cardiovascular (CV) risk.

The selective COX-2 inhibitors reduce endothelial PGI_2 (antiaggregatory) production without affecting TXA-2 (proaggregatory) synthesis by platelets. This disbalance appears to exert prothrombotic influence and enhance cardiovascular risk. Many large scale trials noted higher incidence of myocardial infarction (MI) among subjects receiving rofecoxib for several months. Later valdecoxib was also implicated. Accordingly, these drugs were withdrawn respectively in 2004 and 2005. However, no convincing evidence has emerged against celecoxib and etoricoxib. As such, these drugs continue to be used with a warning on the label.

It has been concluded that selective COX-2 inhibitors should be used in the lowest dose for the shortest period of time as per need. Moreover, they should be avoided in patients with history of ischaemic heart disease/hypertension/cardiac failure or cerebrovascular disease, who are predisposed to CV events.

Concerns, other than cardiovascular, have also been expressed about selective COX-2 inhibitors (*see* box).

> **Other concerns with selective COX-2 inhibitors**
> - COX-1 generated PGs may also play a role in inflammation: COX-2 inhibitors may not have as broad range of efficacy as traditional NSAIDs.
> - Ulcer injury and *H. pylori* induce COX-2 in gastric mucosa, which may contribute to gastroprotective PG synthesis; COX-2 inhibition may delay ulcer healing.
> - Juxtaglomerular COX-2 is constitutive; its inhibition can cause salt and water retention. Pedal edema, precipitation of CHF and rise in BP can occur with all coxibs.

Celecoxib The COX-2 selectivity of celecoxib is modest. It exerts anti-inflammatory, analgesic and antipyretic actions with low ulcerogenic potential. Platelet aggregation in response to collagen exposure remained unaffected in celecoxib recipients, and serum TXB_2 levels were not reduced. Though, tolerability of celecoxib is better than that of traditional NSAIDs, still abdominal pain, dyspepsia and mild diarrhoea are the usual side effects. Rashes, edema and a small rise in BP have also been noted.

Celecoxib is absorbed slowly, 97% plasma protein bound and metabolized primarily by CYP2C9 with a t½ of ~10 hours. It is approved for use in osteo- and rheumatoid arthritis in a dose of 100–200 mg BD.

CELACT, REVIBRA, COLCIBRA 100, 200 mg caps.

Etoricoxib This COX-2 inhibitor has the highest COX-2 selectivity. It is suitable for once-a-day treatment of osteoarthritis/rheumatoid arthritis, acute gouty arthritis, *acute dental surgery pain* and similar conditions, without affecting platelet function or damaging gastric mucosa. However, caution as stated above for any selective COX-2 inhibitor has to be applied. The t½ is ~ 24 hours. Side effects are *dry mouth, aphthous ulcers*, taste disturbance abdominal pain, pedal edema, rise in BP and paresthesias.

Dose: 60–120 mg OD; ETOSHINE, TOROCOXIA, ETOXIB, NUCOXIA 60, 90, 120 mg tabs.

Parecoxib It is a prodrug of valdecoxib suitable for injection, and to be used in postoperative or similar short-term pain, with efficacy similar to ketorolac. Like valdecoxib, it carries the risk of producing serious cutaneous reaction; should be stopped at the first appearance of a rash.

Dose: 40 mg oral/i.m./i.v., repeated after 6–12 hours.
REVALDO, VALTO-P 40 mg/vial inj, PAROXIB 40 mg tab.

PARA-AMINO PHENOL DERIVATIVES

Phenacetin introduced in 1887 phenacetin was extensively used as analgesic-antipyretic, but was banned because it was implicated in analgesic abuse nephropathy (*see* p. ?).

$NH-CO-CH_3$

PARACETAMOL

OH $O-C_2H_5$ PHENACETIN

Paracetamol (acetaminophen) It is the deethylated active metabolite of phenacetin which was also introduced in the last century but has come into common use only since 1950.

Actions The central analgesic action of paracetamol is like that of aspirin, i.e. it raises pain threshold, but has weak peripheral anti-inflammatory component. Analgesic action of aspirin and paracetamol is additive. Paracetamol is a good and promptly acting antipyretic.

Paracetamol has negligible anti-inflammatory action. It is a poor inhibitor of PG synthesis in peripheral tissues, but is more active on COX in the brain. One explanation offered for the discrepancy between its analgesic-antipyretic and anti-inflammatory actions is its poor ability to inhibit COX in the presence of peroxides which are generated at sites of inflammation but are not present in brain. The ability of paracetamol to inhibit

COX-3 (*see* p. 349) could also account for its analgesic-antipyretic action.

In contrast to aspirin, paracetamol does not stimulate respiration or affect acid-base balance, because it does not accelerate cellular metabolism. It has no effect on CVS. Gastric irritation is insignificant—mucosal erosion and bleeding occur rarely only in overdose. Paracetamol does not affect platelet function or clotting factors, and is not uricosuric.

Pharmacokinetics Paracetamol is well absorbed orally; only about 1/4th is protein bound in plasma; distribution in the body is quite uniform. It is conjugated with glucuronic acid and sulfate and is excreted rapidly in urine. Plasma t½ is 2–3 hours. Effects after an oral dose last for 3–5 hours.

Adverse effects In isolated antipyretic doses paracetamol is safe and well tolerated. Nausea and rashes occur occasionally, leukopenia is rare.

Acute paracetamol poisoning It occurs specially in small children who have low hepatic glucuronide conjugating ability. If a large dose (> 150 mg/kg or > 10 g in an adult) is taken, serious toxicity can occur.

Early manifestations are just nausea, vomiting, abdominal pain and liver tenderness with no impairment of consciousness. After 12–18 hours centrilobular hepatic necrosis occurs which may be accompanied by renal tubular necrosis and hypoglycaemia that may progress to coma. Fulminating hepatic failure and death are likely if the plasma levels are high. If the levels are lower—recovery with supportive treatment is the rule.

Mechanism of toxicity N-acetyl-p-benzoquinoneimine (NABQI) is a highly reactive arylating minor metabolite of paracetamol which is detoxified by conjugation with glutathione. When a very large dose of paracetamol is taken, glucuronidation capacity is saturated, more of minor metabolite is formed—hepatic glutathione is depleted and this metabolite binds covalently to proteins in liver cells (and renal tubules) causing necrosis. Toxicity shows a threshold effect; manifesting only when glutathione is depleted to a critical point.

In chronic alcoholics even 5–6 g/day taken for a few days can result in hepatotoxicity because alcoholism induces CYP2E1 that metabolises paracetamol to NABQI.

Treatment
Apart from supportive measures, the specific antidote is N-acetylcysteine infused i.v. or given orally. It replenishes hepatic glutathione and prevents binding of the toxic metabolite to other cellular constituents. This antidote is practically ineffective if started 12–16 hours or more after paracetamol ingestion.

Uses Paracetamol is one of the most commonly used 'over-the-counter' analgesic for headache, musculoskeletal pain, toothache, etc. where antiinflammatory action is not required. It is relatively ineffective when inflammation is prominent (as in rheumatoid arthritis). It is one of the best drugs to be used as antipyretic.

Dose to dose paracetamol is equally efficacious as aspirin for noninflammatory conditions. Clinical studies have found *paracetamol and aspirin to be equieffective in relieving pain after the extraction of third molars.* However, it is much safer than aspirin in terms of gastric irritation, ulceration and bleeding (can be given to ulcer patients). Because it does not prolong bleeding time, risk of tooth extraction haemorrhage is not accentuated. Paracetamol can be used in all age groups (infants to elderly), pregnant/lactating women, in presence of other disease states and in patients in whom aspirin is contraindicated. It does not have significant drug interactions. Thus, it may be preferred over aspirin for most minor conditions.

Dose: Adults 325–650 mg, children 10–15 mg/kg, 3–4 times a day.

CROCIN 0.5, 1.0 g tabs; METACIN, PARACIN 500 mg tab, 125 mg/5 ml syrup, 150 mg/ml paed. drops, ULTRAGIN, PYRIGESIC, CALPOL 500 mg tab, 125 mg/5ml syrup, NEOMOL, FEVASTIN, FEBRINIL 300 mg/2 ml inj. CROCIN PAIN RELIEF: Paracetamol 650 mg + Caffeine 50 mg tab.

BENZOXAZOCINE DERIVATIVE

Nefopam It is a nonopioid analgesic which does not inhibit PG synthesis, but relieves traumatic, dental, postoperative and short-lasting musculoskeletal pain.

Nefopam produces anticholinergic (dry mouth, urinary retention, blurred vision) and sympathomimetic (tachycardia, nervousness) side effects. Nausea is often dose limiting. It is contraindicated in epileptics. It may be used occasionally as a reserve analgesic.

Dose: 30–60 mg TDS oral, 20 mg i.m. 6 hourly.
NEFOMAX 30 mg tab, 20 mg in 1 ml amp.

Analgesics/NSAIDs in dentistry

The antipyretic-analgesics/NSAIDs are the mainstay for management of acute dental pain. While pain during an invasive dental procedure is allayed by a local anaesthetic, that before and after it is treated mostly with analgesics and NSAIDs. There is ample evidence of their efficacy in most types of pain encountered in dentistry. The cause and nature of pain (mild, moderate or severe; acute or chronic; ratio of pain: inflammation) along with consideration of the risk factors in the particular patient govern selection of the analgesic. Also to be considered are the past experience of the patient, acceptability and individual preference. Though NSAIDs have a common spectrum of adverse effects, they differ quantitatively among themselves in producing various side effects. Moreover, patients differ in their analgesic response to different NSAIDs. If one NSAID is unsatisfactory in a patient, it does not mean that other NSAIDs will also be unsatisfactory. Some subjects 'feel better' on a particular drug, but not on a closely related one. Thus, no single drug is superior to all others for every patient. It is in this context that availability of such a wide range of NSAIDs may be welcome. Some guidelines are:

1. Mild-to-moderate pain with little inflammation—*paracetamol* or low-dose *ibuprofen*.
2. Postextraction or similar acute but short-lasting pain—*ketorolac*, or *diclofenac sod.* by i.m. or i.v. injection.
3. Gastric intolerance to conventional NSAIDs or predisposed patients—*etoricoxib* or *paracetamol*.
4. Patients with history of asthma or anaphylactoid reaction to aspirin/other NSAIDs—*nimesulide, etoricoxib*.
5. Paediatric patients—only *paracetamol, aspirin, ibuprofen* and *naproxen* have been adequately evaluated in children—should be preferred in them. Due to risk of Reye's syndrome, aspirin should be avoided unless viral infection can be ruled out.
6. Pregnancy—*paracetamol* is the safest; *low-dose aspirin* is probably the second best.
7. Hypertensive, diabetic, ischaemic heart disease, epileptic and other patients receiving long-term regular medication—possibility of drug interaction with NSAIDs should be considered and the physician consulted.
8. Patients with risk factors for cardiovascular diseases, stroke—avoid etoricoxib/celecoxib; *ibuprofen* or low-dose *aspirin* may be used.

Analgesic combinations

Combination of aspirin and paracetamol is additive (not supra-additive) and a ceiling analgesic effect is obtained when the total amount of aspirin + paracetamol is ~ 1000 mg. The same is true of combinations of paracetamol with other NSAIDs like ibuprofen, diclofenac, etc. There is no convincing evidence that such combinations are superior to single agents either in efficacy or in safety. If at all used, such combinations should be limited to short periods.

Combination of codeine (an opioid analgesic) with aspirin or paracetamol is also additive, but in this case combination provides additional analgesia beyond the ceiling effect of aspirin/paracetamol, provided each is given at its full dose, which will produce opioid side effects (nausea, constipation, drowsiness) as well. The mechanisms of pain relief by these two classes of drugs are different. Such combination should be considered only for pain refractory to a single agent.

23
CHAPTER

Opioid Analgesics and Antagonists

OPIOID ANALGESICS

Opium The dark brown, resinous material obtained from poppy (*Papaver somniferum*) capsule is called 'Opium'. It contains two types of alkaloids.

Phenanthrene derivatives
Morphine (10% in opium)
Codeine (0.5% in opium)

Benzoisoquinoline derivatives
Papaverine (1%) ⎫
                 ⎬ Nonanalgesic
Noscapine (6%)   ⎭

Opium has been known from the earliest times. Galen (2nd century AD) introduced tincture of opium. Serturner, a pharmacist, isolated the active principle of opium in 1806 and named it *'morphine'* after the Greek god of dreams *Morpheus*. In the last century a large number of semisynthetic and synthetic compounds have been developed with morphine-like, antagonistic and mixed agonistic-antagonistic properties of this class of drugs.

MORPHINE

Morphine is the principal alkaloid in opium and is described as prototype of this class of drugs.

Pharmacological actions

1. CNS Morphine has site specific depressant and stimulant actions in the CNS produced primarily through interaction with μ opioid receptor as a full agonist. The depressant effects are:

(a) *Analgesia* Morphine is a strong analgesic. Though dull, poorly localized visceral pain is relieved better than sharply defined somatic pain; higher doses can mitigate even severe pain—degree of analgesia increasing with the dose. Nociceptive pain arising from stimulation of peripheral pain receptors is relieved better than neuretic pain (such as trigeminal neuralgia) due to inflammation of or damage to neural structures. The associated reactions to intense pain (apprehension, fear, autonomic effects) are also dampened. Suppression of pain perception is selective, without affecting other sensations or producing proportionate generalized CNS depression (contrast general anaesthetics).

Perception of pain and its emotional or suffering component are both altered so that pain is no longer as unpleasant or distressing, i.e. the patient tolerates pain better. The analgesic action of morphine has a spinal and a supraspinal component. Intrathecal injection has been shown to cause segmental analgesia without affecting other modalities. The action appears to be exerted through interneurones which are involved in the 'gating' of pain impulses. Release of glutamate from the primary pain afferents in the spinal cord and its postsynaptic action on dorsal horn neurones is inhibited by morphine. Action at supraspinal sites in the medulla, periaqueductal gray matter, limbic and cortical areas may alter processing and interpretation of pain impulses. In addition, the supraspinal action of morphine augments the inhibitory impulses through descending pathways to the spinal cord. Several aminergic (5-HT, NA), GABAergic and other neuronal systems appear to be involved. Simultaneous action at spinal and supraspinal sites greatly amplifies the analgesic action.

(b) *Sedation* The character of sedation caused by morphine is different from that produced by hypnotics. Drowsiness, indifference to surroundings and to own body occurs without motor incoordination and ataxia. Higher doses progressively produce sleep and coma. Morphine has no anticonvulsant action, rather, fits may be precipitated.

(c) *Mood and subjective effects* Morphine produces prominent subjective effects. It has a calming influence; there is loss of apprehension, feeling of detachment, lack of initiative, limbs feel heavy and body warm, mental clouding and inability to concentrate occurs. In the absence of pain or apprehension, these effects are generally perceived to be unpleasant by normal people. However, patients in pain or anxiety; especially addicts, perceive it as pleasurable: refer it as 'high'. Rapid i.v. injection by addicts gives them a 'kick' or 'rush' which is intensely pleasurable—akin to orgasm. Thus, one has to learn to perceive the *euphoric* effect of morphine.

(d) *Respiratory depression* Morphine depresses respiratory centre in a dose-dependent manner; rate and tidal volume are both decreased. However, analgesic dose in an otherwise healthy individual produces no cognizable respiratory depression. But the same may be marked in sedated patients or those with pulmonary/cardiac/hepatic or renal disease. The cause of death in morphine poisoning is respiratory failure. Neurogenic, hypercapnoeic and later hypoxic drives to the respiratory centre are suppressed in succession. In addition, there is indifference to breathing: apnoeic patient may breath if commanded.

(e) *Cough suppression* The cough centre is depressed. It is more sensitive to morphine than respiratory centre.

(f) *Temperature regulation* The hypothalamic thermostatic centre is depressed; hypothermia occurs in cold surroundings.

(g) *Vasomotor centre* It is depressed at relatively higher doses and contributes to the fall in BP.

Morphine stimulates:

(a) *CTZ* Nausea and vomiting occur as side effects. Morphine appears to sensitize the CTZ to vestibular and other impulses. Larger doses depress vomiting centre directly: emetics should not be tried in morphine poisoning.

(b) *Edinger Westphal nucleus* of III nerve is stimulated producing miosis. No miosis occurs on topical application of morphine to the eye because it is a central action exerted in the brain.

(c) *Vagal centre* It is stimulated; morphine can cause bradycardia.

(d) *Certain cortical areas and hippocampal cells* are stimulated. Truncal rigidity and immobility is consistently manifested at high doses. This resembles catalepsy seen in rats and mice. Convulsions may occur in morphine poisoning. The proconvulsant action has been ascribed to inhibition of GABA release by hippocampal interneurones. Species like the cat, lion, horse, sheep and cow are uniformly excited and develop hyperthermia.

2. Neuroendocrine actions Morphine weakens hypothalamic influence on pituitary.

As a result ACTH, FSH and LH levels tend to fall, while GH and prolactin release tends to increase (because they are under predominant inhibitory control). Heavy abusers of morphine may suffer from impotence, menstrual irregularities, and infertility. Morphine enhances ADH release and can reduce urine volume.

3. *CVS* Morphine causes vasodilatation due to:
(a) histamine release.
(b) depression of vasomotor centre.
(c) direct action decreasing tone of blood vessels.

There is a shift of blood from pulmonary to systemic circuit due to greater vasodilatation in the latter. Therapeutic doses cause little change in BP of recumbent normovolaemic patient. Postural hypotension and fainting can occur due to vasodilatation and impairment of vascular reflexes. Morphine has little direct effect on heart. Cardiac work is consistently reduced due to decrease in peripheral resistance imparting antiischaemic property. Intracranial tension tends to rise as a consequence of CO_2 retention leading to cerebral vasodilatation.

4. *GIT* Constipation is a prominent feature of morphine action. Several factors contribute:
(a) Action directly on intestines and in CNS increases tone and segmentation, but decreases propulsive movements. Tone of duodenum and colon may be increased to the level of spasm.
(b) Spasm of pyloric, ileocaecal and anal sphincters.
(c) Decrease in all gastrointestinal secretions.
(d) Central action causing inattention to defecation reflex.

No tolerance develops to this action, so that addicts remain chronically constipated.

5. *Other smooth muscles*
(a) *Biliary tract* Morphine causes spasm of sphincter of Oddi → intrabiliary pressure is increased → may cause biliary colic.
(b) *Urinary bladder* Tone of both detrusor and sphincter is increased → urinary urgency and difficulty in micturition.
(c) *Bronchi* Morphine releases histamine which can cause bronchoconstriction. This is of no consequence in normal individuals, but can be dangerous in asthmatics.

Pharmacokinetics

The oral absorption of morphine is unreliable because of high and variable first pass metabolism; oral bioavailability is 1/6 to 1/4th of parenterally administered drug. About 30% is bound to plasma proteins. Only a small fraction enters brain rather slowly. Morphine freely crosses placenta and can affect the foetus more than the mother. It is primarily metabolized in liver by glucuronide conjugation. Morphine-6-glucuronide is an active metabolite which accumulates during chronic dosing and contributes to the analgesia despite its restricted passage across blood-brain barrier. Glucuronides of morphine are readily excreted by the kidney and to some extent in bile. Plasma t½ of morphine averages 2–3 hours. Effect of a parenteral dose lasts 4–6 hours. Elimination is almost complete in 24 hours and morphine is noncumulative. Small amounts may persist due to enterohepatic circulation.

Adverse Effects

Side effects of morphine are sedation, mental clouding, lethargy and other subjective effects which may even be dysphoric in some subjects; vomiting is occasional in recumbent patients; constipation is common. Respiratory depression, blurring of vision, urinary retention (especially in elderly males) are the other side effects. BP may fall, especially in hypovolaemic patient and if he/she walks about.

Urticaria, itch, swelling of lips may develop due to histamine release.

Acute morphine poisoning In the nontolerant adult, 50 mg of morphine i.m. produces serious toxicity. Manifestations are extensions of pharmacological action, Viz., stupor or coma, flaccidity, shallow and occasional breathing, cyanosis, pinpoint pupil, fall in BP and shock, convulsions may be seen in few, pulmonary edema occurs at terminal stages, death is due to respiratory failure.

Treatment: Consists of respiratory support and maintenance of BP by i.v. fluids, vasoconstrictors. Gastric lavage should be done with pot. permanganate to remove unabsorbed drug.

Naloxone 0.4–0.8 mg i.v. repeated every 2–3 minutes till respiration picks up, is the specific antidote. It has a short duration of action. Injection should be repeated every 1–4 hours, according to response.

Tolerance and dependence High degree of tolerance can be developed to morphine and related opioids if the drug is taken repeatedly. Tolerance is partly pharmacokinetic (enhanced rate of metabolism) but mainly pharmacodynamic (cellular tolerance). Addicts tolerate morphine in grams: lethal dose is markedly increased, but no tolerance develops to constipating, miotic and proconvulsant actions of morphine. Cross tolerance among opioids is of high degree. Morphine tolerant subjects are partially cross tolerant to other CNS depressants as well.

Morphine produces pronounced addiction and dependence, its abuse liability is rated high. Concern about abuse has been a major limitation in the use of morphine, but appropriate medical use of morphine seldom progresses to dependence and abuse.

Withdrawal of morphine in dependent subjects is associated with marked drug seeking behaviour. Physical manifestations of abstinence are—lacrimation, sweating, yawning, anxiety, fear, restlessness, gooseflesh, mydriasis, tremor, insomnia, abdominal colic, diarrhoea, dehydration, rise in BP, palpitation and rapid weight loss. Delirium and convulsions are seen only occasionally.

Treatment: consists of withdrawal of morphine and substitution with oral methadone which is long acting and orally effective, followed by gradual withdrawal of methadone. However, craving for the opioid may persist for long time, and relapse rate among postaddicts is high. Long-term methadone maintenance and other techniques using agonist-antagonistic drugs are also employed.

Precautions, Contraindications and Interactions

Morphine is a drug of emergency, but due care has to be taken in its use.

1. Infants and the elderly are more susceptible to the respiratory depressant action of morphine.

2. Morphine is risky in patients with respiratory insufficiency (emphysema, pulmonary fibrosis, cor pulmonale), sudden deaths have occurred.

3. Bronchial asthma: Morphine can precipitate an attack by its histamine releasing action.

4. Head injury: morphine is contraindicated in patients with head injury. Reasons are—
- By retaining CO_2, it increases intracranial tension which will add to that caused by head injury itself.
- Even therapeutic doses can cause marked respiratory depression in these patients.
- Vomiting, miosis and altered mentation produced by morphine interfere with assessment of progress in head injury cases.

(A head injury case may have orofacial injury as well, and a dentist may be part of the management team).

5. Hypotensive states and hypovolaemia exaggerate fall in BP due to morphine.
6. Elderly male: chances of urinary retention are high.
7. Hypothyroidism, liver and kidney disease patients are more sensitive to morphine.
8. Unstable personalities: are liable to continue with its use and become addicted.

Phenothiazines and tricyclic antidepressants potentiate morphine and other opioids, either by retarding its metabolism or by a pharmacodynamic interaction.

Dose 10–50 mg oral, 10–15 mg i.m. or s.c. or 2–6 mg i.v.; children 0.1–0.2 mg/kg i.m. or s.c.
MORPHINE SULPHATE 10 mg/ml inj; MORCONTIN 10, 30, 60, 100 mg continuous release tabs; 30–100 mg BD; RILIMORF 10,20 mg tabs, 60 mg SR tab.

CODEINE

It is methyl-morphine; occurs naturally in opium, and is partly converted in the body to morphine. Codeine is less potent than morphine (1/10th as analgesic), also less efficacious, i.e. cannot relieve severe pain, because it acts as a partial agonist at μ opioid receptor with low ceiling effect. The degree of analgesia is comparable to aspirin (60 mg codeine ~ 600 mg aspirin).

However, codeine is a more selective cough suppressant (1/3rd as potent as morphine); subanalgesic doses (10–30 mg) suppress cough. Because codeine has very low affinity for the opioid receptors, its analgesic action has been ascribed to morphine generated on its demethylation by CYP2D6.

Codeine has good activity by oral route (oral: parenteral ratio 1:2). A single oral dose acts for 4–6 hours. Constipation is prominent, but other side effects are mild. It has been used to control diarrhoea. The abuse liability of codeine is low. Though codeine phosphate is water soluble and can be injected, parenteral preparation is not available.

SEMISYNTHETIC AND SYNTHETIC OPIOIDS

Semisynthetic	Synthetic
Heroin	Pethidine
(Diacetyl morphine)	Fentanyl
Pholcodine	Methadone
	Tramadol
	Tapentadol

1. Heroin (Diamorphine, Diacetylmorphine) It is about 3 times more potent than morphine; more lipid soluble: enters brain more rapidly but duration of action is similar. It is considered to be more euphorient (especially on i.v. injection) and highly addicting. Therefore, it has been banned in most countries.

2. Pholcodine It has codeine-like properties and has been used mainly as antitussive; claimed to be less constipating.

3. Pethidine (Meperidine)

Though chemically unrelated to morphine, pethidine interacts with μ opioid receptors, and its actions are blocked by the opioid antagonist naloxone. Important differences between morphine and pethidine are:
1. Dose to dose 1/10th in analgesic potency; however, analgesic efficacy approaches near to that of morphine, and is higher than that of codeine.
2. After i.m. injection, the onset of action is more rapid but duration is shorter (3–4 hours).
3. It does not effectively suppress cough.
4. Spasmogenic action on smooth muscles is less marked—miosis, constipation and urinary retention are less prominent.
5. Tachycardia (due to antimuscarinic action) occurs instead of bradycardia.
6. It is better absorbed; oral: parenteral activity ratio is higher than morphine (1/3–1/2). Pethidine is nearly completely metabolized in liver, mainly by hydrolysis producing *mepiridinic acid* as the major metabolite. A small fraction is demethylated to *norpethidine*, which has excitatory effects. The plasma t½ of pethidine is 2–3 hours.

Side effects These are similar to morphine, but constipation, urinary retention and miosis

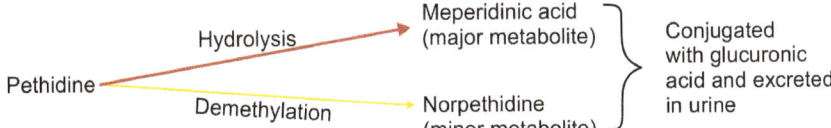

are less prominent. Some atropinic effects (dry mouth, blurred vision, tachycardia) may be noted in addition.

Overdose of pethidine produces many excitatory effects—tremors, mydriasis, hyperreflexia, delirium, myoclonus and convulsions due to accumulation of the minor metabolite *norpethidine*.

Pethidine injected in patients receiving a selective serotonin reuptake inhibitor (SSRI) may produce 'Serotonin syndrome' manifesting as agitation, rigidity, hyperthermia, delirium, muscle twitchings by enhancing 5-HT release.

Use Pethidine is primarily used as an analgesic (substitute of morphine) and in preanaesthetic medication, but not for cough or diarrhoea. Potential adverse effects due to accumulation of norpethidine limit its utility in patients who require repeated dosing.
Dose: 50–100 mg i.m., s.c. (may cause irritation, local fibrosis on repeated injection), occasionally given orally or i.v.
PETHIDINE HCL 100 mg/2 ml inj; 50, 100 mg tab.

4. Fentanyl A pethidine congener, 80–100 times more potent than morphine in producing both analgesia and respiratory depression. At analgesic doses it produces few cardiovascular effects and has little propensity to release histamine. Because of high lipid solubility, it enters brain rapidly and produces peak analgesia in 5 min after i.v. injection. The duration of action is short: starts wearing off after 30–40 min due to redistribution, while elimination t½ is ~4 hr. In the injectable form it is almost exclusively used in anaesthesia (*see* p. 135). Transdermal fentanyl has become a frequently used opioid analgesic for cancer or other types of chronic pain.

DUROGESIC transdermal patch delivering 25 µg/hr, 50 µg/hr, 75 µg per hour, 100 µg/hr. The patch is changed every 2 to 3 days.

5. Methadone A synthetic opioid, chemically dissimilar but pharmacologically very similar to morphine. It has analgesic, respiratory depressant, emetic, antitussive, constipating and biliary actions similar to morphine.

The most important feature of methadone is high oral: parenteral activity ratio (1 : 2) and its firm binding to tissue proteins. It cumulates in tissues on repeated administration—duration of action is progressively lengthened due to gradual release from these sites; plasma t½ on chronic use is 24–36 hours. It is metabolized in liver, primarily by demethylation and cyclization.

Because of slow and persistent action, the sedative and subjective effects are less intense. It is probably incapable of inducing the 'kick' in abusers. The abuse potential is rated lower than morphine. Tolerance develops more slowly. Withdrawal syndrome is of gradual onset, taking 1–2 days after discontinuation, is prolonged and less severe.

Methadone has been used primarily as substitution therapy of opioid dependence. Another technique is *methadone maintenance* therapy in opioid addicts— sufficient dose of methadone is given orally to produce high degree of tolerance so that pleasurable effects of i.v. doses of morphine or heroin are not perceived and the subject gives up the habit.

Methadone can also be used as an analgesic for the same conditions as morphine; dose 2.5–10 mg oral or i.m. but not s.c.

6. Tramadol This centrally acting analgesic is an atypical opioid which relieves pain by opioid as well as additional mechanisms. Its affinity for µ opioid receptor is moderate while that for κ and δ is weak. Unlike other opioids, it inhibits reuptake of NA and 5-HT, and thus activates monoaminergic spinal inhibition of pain. Its analgesic action is only partially reversed by the opioid antagonist naloxone.

Injected i.v. 100 mg tramadol is equianalgesic to 10 mg i.m. morphine; oral bioavailability is good (oral: parenteral dose ratio 1.4 : 1). The t½ is 3–5 hours and effects last for 4–6 hrs. Tramadol causes less respiratory depression, sedation, constipation, urinary retention and rise in intrabiliary pressure than morphine. It is well tolerated; side effects are dizziness, nausea, sleepiness, dry mouth and sweating. Haemodynamic effects are minimal.

Tramadol is indicated for mild-to-medium intensity short-lasting pain due to dental afflictions, diagnostic procedures, injury, surgery, visceral illness, etc. as well as for chronic pain including cancer pain, but is not effective in severe pain. Little tendency to dose escalation is seen and abuse potential is low.

Dose: 50–100 mg oral/i.m./slow i.v. infusion (children 1–2 mg/kg) 4–6 hourly.
CONTRAMAL, DOMADOL, TRAMAZAC 50 mg cap, 100 mg SR tab; 50 mg/ml inj in 1 and 2 ml amps
ULTRACET: tramadol 75 mg + paracetamol 325 mg tab.

7. Tapentadol
It is a newer atypical opioid similar to tramadol in structure and mechanism of action. It acts mainly via monoaminergic pain mechanisms. Binding to μ opioid receptor is weak. Compared to tramadol, it primarily activates central noradrenergic pain pathways to elicit analgesia. Tapentadol is well absorbed orally, largely glucuronide conjugated and metabolite is excreted in urine. Like tramadol, it is useful in relieving moderately severe pain. Side effects are also similar to those of tramadol, but nausea and vomiting is less prominent. It can precipitate 'serotonin syndrome' in patients receiving SSRIs, and seizures in predisposed patients. Thus, tapentadol is an alternative to tramadol for mild-to-moderate pain.

Dose: 50–100 mg 2–4 times a day.
TAPOSER, DUOVOLT, TAPCYNTA 50, 75, 100 mg tabs.
TAPOSER-P: tapentadol 50 mg + paracetamol 325 mg tab.

Uses (of morphine and its congeners)

1. As analgesic Opioid analgesics are indicated in severe pain of any type. However, *their use in dentistry is very limited*. They only provide symptomatic relief without affecting the cause.

Important features of analgesics with agonist, partial agonist and agonist-antagonist action on opioid receptors are compared in Table 23.1.

Morphine and its parenteral congeners are indicated in traumatic, visceral, ischaemic (myocardial infarction), postoperative, burn, cancer pain and the like. It should be

Table 23.1: Comparative features of opioid analgesics, partial agonist analgesics and agonist-antagonist analgesics

Drug	Nature of analgesia	Ceiling efficacy	Oral-parenteral ratio	Equivalent analgesic dose	Duration of analgesia
1. Morphine	μ agonist	++++	Low	10 mg	4–6 hr
2. Codeine	Partial μ agonist	+	High	60 mg	4–6 hr
3. Pethidine	μ agonist	++++	Medium	60–100 mg	2–4 hr
4. Methadone	μ agonist	++++	High	6–10 mg	4–6 hr $
5. Fentanyl	μ agonist	++++	Low	0.1 mg	1–1.5 hr
6. Tramadol	μ agonist (low affinity)	++	High	50–100 mg	4–6 hr
7. Pentazocine	κ agonist	++	Medium	30–60 mg	3–5 hr
8. Butorphanol	κ agonist	+++	— #	2.0 mg	4–6 hr
9. Nalbuphine	κ agonist	+++	— #	10 mg	3–6 hr
10. Buprenorphine	Partial μ agonist	+++	Low	0.3 mg	6–8 hr

+ to ++++ Low to high (full) analgesic efficacy.
# Parenteral use only; no oral preparation.
$ Duration of action increases after repeated dosing.

given promptly in myocardial infarction to allay apprehension and reflex sympathetic stimulation.

Adequate use of morphine (even i.v.) is indicated in an emergency. Patients in severe pain require higher doses of opioids, and tolerate them without manifesting toxicity. Morphine may prevent neurogenic shock and other autonomic effects of excruciating pain such as that of crush injuries, fracture mandible/maxilla, etc. Neuropathic pain responds less predictably to opioid analgesics.

Transdermal fentanyl is a suitable option for chronic cancer and other terminal illness pain.

For milder pain, e.g. toothache, headache, neuralgias, etc., aspirin-like analgesics are preferred. When they are not effective alone, codeine or tramadol/tapentadol may be added. The combination enhances the ceiling analgesia. For more severe and longer lasting pain, one of the NSAIDs may be combined with the opioid.

2. Preanaesthetic medication Morphine and pethidine are used in selected patients.

3. Balanced anaesthesia and surgical analgesia Fentanyl or morphine are an important component of anaesthetic techniques (*see* p. 135, 136).

4. Relief of anxiety and apprehension Specially in myocardial infarction, internal bleeding (haematemesis, threatened abortion, etc.) morphine has been employed.

5. Acute left ventricular failure (cardiac asthma) Morphine (i.v.) affords dramatic relief by:
(a) Reducing preload on heart due to vasodilatation.
(b) Tending to shift blood from pulmonary to systemic circuit; relieves pulmonary congestion and edema.
(c) Allays air hunger by depressing respiratory centre.
(d) Cuts down sympathetic stimulation by calming the patient, reduces cardiac work.

6. Cough Codeine or its substitutes are widely used for suppressing dry, irritating cough.

7. Diarrhoea The constipating action of codeine, loperamide and diphenoxylate has been used to check diarrhoea.

OPIOID RECEPTORS

Morphine and other opioids exert their actions by interacting with specific receptors present on neurones in the CNS and in peripheral tissues. Chemical modification of the morphine structure has yielded a number of compounds which have a complex pattern of morphine-like and other agonistic and antagonistic actions that cannot be explained on the basis of a single opioid receptor. Radioligand binding studies have divided the opioid receptors into three types (μ, κ, δ); and these receptors have been cloned. Each type of opioid receptor has a specific pharmacological profile and pattern of anatomical distribution in the brain, spinal cord and peripheral tissues. Subtypes of μ and κ receptor have been identified. The actions mediated by the 3 types of opioid receptors are listed in Table 23.2.

Opioid ligands can interact with different types of opioid receptors as agonists, partial agonists or competitive antagonists. The overall pattern of effect of a particular agent depends not only on the nature of its interaction with different opioid receptors but also on its relative affinity for these, e.g. morphine is an agonist on μ, κ and δ receptors, but its affinity for μ receptors is much higher than that for the other two. The effects, therefore, are primarily the result of μ receptor activation.

The nature and intensity of action of agonist-antagonist opioids, opioid peptides and opioid antagonists are summarized in Table 23.3.

Chapter 23: Opioid Analgesics and Antagonists

Table 23.2: Actions ascribed to different types of opioid receptors

μ (mu)	κ (kappa)	δ (delta)
Analgesia (supraspinal μ₁ + spinal μ₂)	Analgesia (spinal κ₁) (Supraspinal-κ₃)	Analgesia (Spinal + Affective component of supraspinal)
Respiratory depression (μ₂)	Respiratory depression (lower ceiling)	Respiratory depression
Sedation	Dysphoria, hallucinations	Affective behaviour
Euphoria	Miosis (lower ceiling)	Reinforcing actions
Miosis	Sedation	Reduced g.i. motility
Muscular rigidity	Physical dependence (nalorphine type)	Proconvulsant
Reduced g.i. motility (μ₂)		
Physical dependence (morphine type)		

Table 23.3: Nature of interaction of opioid ligands with the three types of opioid receptors

Ligand	μ (mu)	κ (kappa)	δ (delta)
1. Morphine	Ago. (St)	Ago. (W)	Ago. (W)
2. Nalorphine	Anta. (St)	Ago. (M)	—
3. Pentazocine	P.Ago., Anta. (W)	Ago. (M)	—
4. Butorphanol	P.Ago (W)	Ago. (St)	—
5. Nalbuphine	Anta. (W)	Ago. (St)	—
6. Buprenorphine	P.Ago	Anta. (M)	—
7. Naloxone	Anta. (St)	Anta. (M)	Anta. (W)
8. Met/Leu Enkephalin	Ago. (M)	—	Ago. (St)
9. β-Endorphin	Ago. (St)	—	Ago. (St)
10. Dynorphin A, B	Ago. (W)	Ago. (St)	Ago. (W)

P. Ago—Partial agonist: have lower efficacy, though affinity (potency) may be high.
St—Strong action; M—Moderate action; W—Weak action (low affinity).

μ receptor The μ receptor is characterized by its high affinity for morphine. It is the major receptor mediating actions of morphine and its congeners. Endogenous ligands for μ receptor are peptides called *Endomorphins 1 and 2*. These have now been found in mammalian brain, and produce biological effects ascribed to this receptor. High density of μ receptors has been detected in periaqueductal grey, thalamus, nucleus tractus solitarious, nucleus ambiguus and area postrema.

κ receptor This receptor is defined by its high affinity for ketocyclazocine and dynorphin A; the latter is considered to be its endogenous ligand. Analgesia caused by κ agonists is primarily spinal, but lower ceiling supraspinal analgesia is also produced.

δ receptor This receptor has high affinity for Leu/Met enkephalins which are its endogenous ligands. The δ mediated analgesia is again mainly spinal (δ receptors are present in dorsal horn of spinal cord). The limbic areas are rich in δ receptors, suggesting role of these receptors in the affective component of supraspinal analgesia, as well as in the reinforcing actions and dependence. Myenteric plexus neurones express high density of δ receptors which mediate reduced g.i. motility.

Opioid receptor transducer mechanisms

All 3 types of opioid receptors (μ, κ, δ) have been cloned; all are G-protein coupled receptors (GPCRs) located mostly on prejunctional neurones. They generally exercise inhibitory modulation by decreasing release of the junctional transmitter (Fig. 23.1). As such, various monoaminergic (NA, DA, 5-HT), GABA, glutamate (NMDA) pathways are intricately involved in opioid actions.

Opioid receptor activation reduces intracellular cAMP formation and opens K⁺ channels (mainly through μ and δ receptors) or suppresses voltage gated N type Ca^{2+} channels (mainly κ receptor). These actions result in neuronal hyperpolarization and reduced availability of intracellular Ca^{2+} which translates into decreased neurotransmitter release by neurones in the brain, spinal cord and myenteric plexus.

COMPLEX ACTION OPIOIDS

Clinically, the agonist-antagonist (agonist at one opioid receptor, antagonist at another) and partial/weak agonist (low intrinsic activity) opioids are analgesics of limited efficacy comparable to low doses of morphine. They cause low ceiling respiratory depression and are less addicting. However, in only few situations they have proven to be advantageous over the full μ agonists.

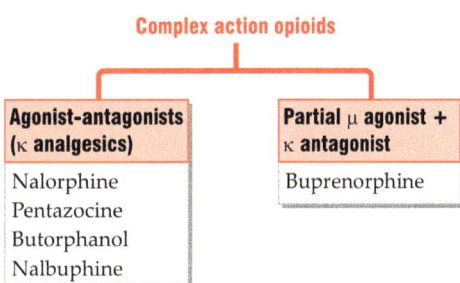

Complex action opioids

Agonist-antagonists (κ analgesics)	Partial μ agonist + κ antagonist
Nalorphine	Buprenorphine
Pentazocine	
Butorphanol	
Nalbuphine	

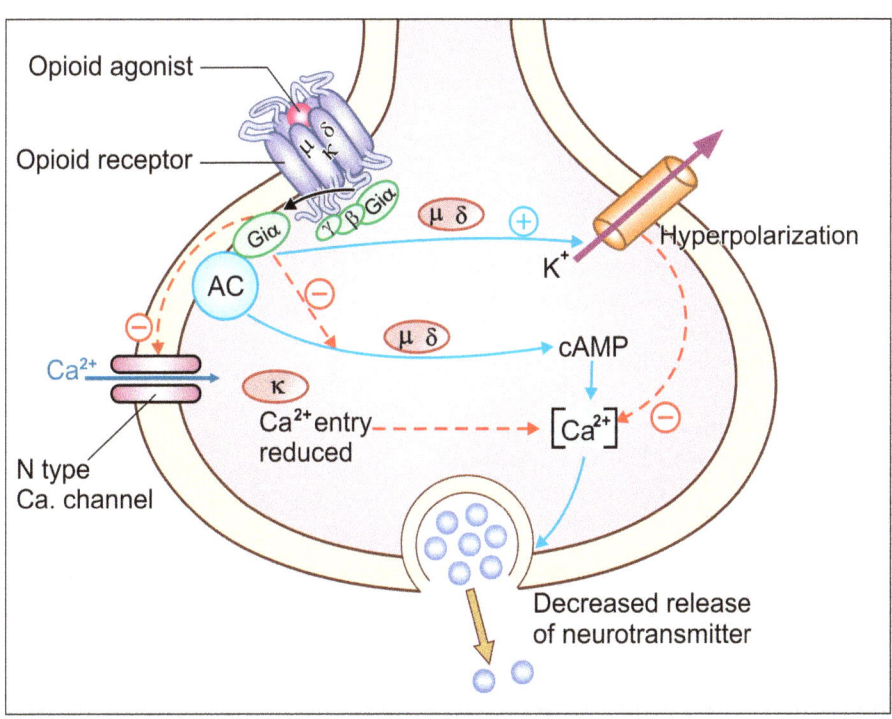

Fig. 23.1: Opioid receptor transducer mechanisms
AC—Adenylyl cyclase; Gi—coupling protein; cAMP—Cyclic AMP

1. **Nalorphine** It is a κ agonist and μ antagonist; has analgesic action, but not used clinically because of dysphoric and psychotomimetic effects. Naloxone has replaced it as a morphine antidote.

2. **Pentazocine** It is the first agonist-antagonist to be used as an analgesic. Pentazocine has more marked κ agonistic and weak μ antagonistic action. Its distinctive features are:

- Analgesia caused by pentazocine is primarily spinal ($κ_1$) and has a different character than that caused by morphine.
- Sedation and respiratory depression is 1/3 to 1/2 of morphine at lower doses, and has a lower ceiling, does not increase much beyond 60 mg dose.
- Tachycardia and rise in BP are produced due to sympathetic stimulation.
- Biliary spasm and constipation are less marked.
- Vomiting is uncommon. Other side effects are sweating and lightheadedness.
- Subjective effects are pleasurable (morphine like) at lower doses. Pentazocine is recognised by post-addicts as an opiate. However, as dose is increased, subjective effects become unpleasant, and psychotomimetic effects appear.

Tolerance, psychological and physical dependence to pentazocine develops on repeated use. Withdrawal syndrome has features of both morphine and nalorphine abstinence, but is milder in intensity. 'Drug seeking' occurs. Abuse liability is rated lower than morphine.

Injected in morphine dependent subjects, it precipitates withdrawal. The antagonistic action is not enough to be useful in morphine poisoning.

Pharmacokinetics and use Pentazocine is effective orally, though considerable first pass metabolism occurs; oral: parenteral ratio is 1 : 3. It is oxidized and glucuronide conjugated in liver and excreted in urine. Plasma t½ is 3–4 hours, duration of action of a single dose is 4–6 hours.

Oral dose: 50–100 mg, efficacy like codeine.
Parenteral dose: 30–60 mg i.m., s.c., may cause local fibrosis on repeated injection due to irritant property.
FORTWIN 25 mg tab., 30 mg/ml inj., SUSEVIN 30 mg/ml inj.; FORTAGESIC: Pentazocine 15 mg + paracetamol 500 mg tab.

Pentazocine is indicated for postoperative and moderately severe pain in burns, trauma, fracture, cancer, etc., but is not a favoured analgesic.

3. **Butorphanol** It is a κ analgesic, similar to but more potent than pentazocine (butorphanol 2 mg = pentazocine 30 mg). Sedation, nausea, cardiac stimulation and other side effects are similar to pentazocine, but subjective effects are less dysphoric and less psychotomimetic. BP is not increased.

The abuse potential of butorphanol is low. The most outstanding feature is that butorphanol can neither substitute for nor antagonize morphine. This shows its very weak interaction with μ receptors.

Butorphanol has been used in a dose of 1–4 mg i.m. or i.v. for postoperative and other short-lasting painful conditions, but should be avoided in patients with cardiac ischaemia.
BUTRUM 1 mg/ml, 2 mg/ml inj.

4. **Nalbuphine** Structurally related to naloxone, this is another κ agonist which has weak μ receptor antagonistic activity, so that it can precipitate morphine withdrawal in dependent subjects. Nalbuphine is a more potent analgesic than pentazocine, and produces few dysphoric/psychotomimetic effects. However, no greater analgesia or respiratory depression occurs beyond 30 mg i.m. dose. Unlike pentazocine it does not cause sympathetic stimulation or any cardiovascular effects. Dependence, withdrawal symptoms and abuse potential are low (like pentazocine). Nalbuphine is indicated in postoperative and other moderately severe pain requiring a parenteral opioid. Cardiac ischaemia is no restriction to its use.

Dose: 10 mg i.m. or s.c. or slow i.v. injection every 4–6 hours.
NALFY, RUFFY 10 mg in 1 ml and 20 mg in 1 ml inj.

Buprenorphine It is a highly lipid-soluble μ analgesic that is 25 times more potent than morphine, but has lower ceiling effect. Onset of action is slower and duration longer. After a single dose, analgesia lasts for 6–8 hours; but with repeated intake, duration of action increases to ~24 hours due to accumulation of the drug in tissues.

Sedation, vomiting, miosis, subjective and cardiovascular effects are similar to morphine, but constipation is less marked. Postural hypotension is prominent. Respiratory depression and analgesia exhibit ceiling effect. It substitutes for morphine at low levels of dependence but precipitates withdrawal in highly dependent subjects, reflecting its partial agonistic action at μ receptors.

Lower degree of tolerance and dependence (psychic as well as physical) develops with buprenorphine on chronic use. Its withdrawal syndrome resembles that of morphine but is delayed for several days, is milder and longer lasting. 'Drug seeking' is present. Abuse liability is rated lower than morphine.

Naloxone (even high dose) only partially reverses buprenorphine effects and is unable to precipitate its withdrawal, probably due to very tight binding of buprenorphine to the opioid receptor.

Buprenorphine has good efficacy by the sublingual route, is highly plasma protein bound and remains in tissues for several days; t½ is 40 hours. It is mostly excreted unchanged in bile.
Dose: 0.3–0.6 mg i.m., s.c. or slow i.v., also sublingual 0.2–0.4 mg 6–8 hourly.
NORPHIN, TIDIGESIC 0.3 mg/ml inj. 1 and 2 ml amps. 0.2 mg sublingual tab; BUPRIGESIC, PENTOREL 0.3 mg/ml inj in 1, 2 ml amp.

Use: Buprenorphine is indicated for long-lasting painful conditions requiring an opioid analgesic, e.g. cancer pain. It may also be used for postoperative pain and in myocardial infarction, but *seldom for dental pain.*

PURE OPIOID ANTAGONISTS

1. Naloxone It is N-alylnor-oxymorphone and a competitive antagonist for all types of opioid receptors. However, it blocks μ receptors at much lower doses than those needed to block κ or δ receptors. It is devoid of any kind of agonistic activity even at high doses. No subjective or autonomic effects or dependence are produced.

Injected intravenously (0.4–0.8 mg) it promptly antagonizes all actions of morphine—analgesia is gone, respiration is not only normalized but even stimulated, and pupils dilate.

At 4–10 mg dose, it also antagonizes the agonistic actions of κ analgesics (pentazocine).

Naloxone 0.4 mg i.v. precipitates morphine withdrawal in dependent subjects: the syndrome lasts for 2–3 hours.

Naloxone is inactive orally because of high first pass metabolism in liver. Injected i.v. it acts in 2–3 min. Plasma t½ is 1 hour in adults and 3 hours in newborns.
NARCOTAN 0.4 mg in 1 ml (adult) and 0.04 mg in 2 ml (infant) amps; NALOX, NEX 0.4 mg inj.

Use Naloxone is the drug of choice for morphine poisoning (0.4–0.8 mg i.v. every 2–3 min: max 10 mg) and for reversing neonatal asphyxia due to opioid use during labour.

2. Naltrexone It is chemically related to naloxone and is another pure opioid antagonist devoid of subjective and other agonistic effects. Naltrexone differs from naloxone in being orally active, more potent and having a long duration of action (1–2 days) which makes it suitable for 'opioid blockade' therapy of postaddicts. Alcohol craving is also reduced by naltrexone, and it is being used to prevent relapse of heavy drinking.

NALTIMA, NALTROX 50 mg tab.

ENDOGENOUS OPIOID PEPTIDES

In the mid 1970s, with herculean efforts, a number of peptides having morphine-like actions were isolated from mammalian brain, pituitary, spinal cord and g.i.t. These are active in very small amounts, their actions are blocked by naloxone, and they bind with high affinity to the opioid receptors. There are 3 major families of opioid peptides. Each is derived from a specific large precursor polypeptide.

1. Endorphins β-endorphin (β-END) having 31 amino acids is the most important. It is derived from *Pro-opiomelanocortin* (POMC) which also gives rise to γ-MSH, ACTH and two lipotropins. β-END is primarily a μ agonist but also has δ action.

2. Enkephalins Methionine-enkephalin (met-ENK) and leucine-enkephalin (leu-ENK) are the most important. Both are pentapeptides derived from the larger peptide *proenkephalin*. The two ENKs have a slightly different spectrum of activity; while met-ENK has equal affinity for μ and δ sites, leu-ENK prefers δ receptors.

3. Dynorphins Dynorphin A and B (DYN-A, DYN-B) are 8–17 amino acid peptides derived from *prodynorphin* which contains 3 leu-ENK residues also. DYNs are more potent on κ receptors, but also activate μ and δ receptors.

The opioid peptides constitute an endogenous opioid system which normally modulates pain perception, mood, hedonic (pleasure related) and motor behaviour, emesis, pituitary hormone release and g.i.t. motility, etc.

β-END injected directly into brain is 20–40 times more potent analgesic than morphine. Its primary localization in hypothalamus and pituitary and its long t½ ascribes it a *neurohormone* function which modulates the release of other hormones.

The wide distribution of ENKs and DYNs and their short t½ suggests function as *neuromodulator* or *neurotransmitter*. They appear to regulate pain responsiveness at spinal and supraspinal levels. Opioid peptides also appear to participate in regulation of affective behaviour and autonomic function.

Morphine and other opioids act as exogenous agonists on some of the receptors for these peptides. This has given an explanation for the existence of specific receptors in the body for exogenous substances like morphine.

Opioids in dental pain

Dental pain is mostly either due to or associated with inflammation. As such, the anti-inflammatory analgesics or NSAIDs are more effective and more suitable than opioid analgesics. The latter are occasionally employed as additional drugs with aspirin, paracetamol, ibuprofen or the like to boost the analgesic effect. When an opioid has to be given, an oral drug like codeine / tramadol is most suited, because dental patients are mostly ambulatory and suffer from dull, continuous, short-lasting pain. Oral tapentadol or pentazocine are the alternatives. Risk of producing dependence is negligible with such use. Role of injected opioids like morphine, pethidine or fentanyl in dentistry is limited to occasional intraoperative or perioperative use to supplement the local anaesthetic and to allay apprehension.

Clearly, the place of analgesics in dental pain is secondary to treatment of the cause of pain by appropriate local (antiseptics, cavity filling, root canal therapy, etc.) and systemic (antibiotics) measures. Short-term use of opioids, as is made in dentistry, has no significant drug interactions and does not require modification of other concurrent medication.

24
CHAPTER

Local Anaesthetics

Local anaesthetics (LAs) are drugs which upon topical application or local injection cause reversible loss of sensory perception, especially of pain, in a restricted area of the body. They block generation and conduction of nerve impulse at any part of the neurone with which they come in contact, without causing any structural damage. Thus, not only sensory but also motor impulses are interrupted when a LA is applied to a mixed nerve, resulting in muscular paralysis and loss of autonomic control as well.

Local anaesthetics are employed routinely by dentists; so much so that current practice of dentistry is inconceivable without local anaesthesia. Important differences between general and local anaesthesia are listed in Table 24.1.

Chemistry

The clinically useful LAs are weak bases with amphiphilic property. A hydrophilic secondary or tertiary amine on one side and a lipophilic aromatic residue on the other are joined by an alkyl chain through an ester or amide linkage.

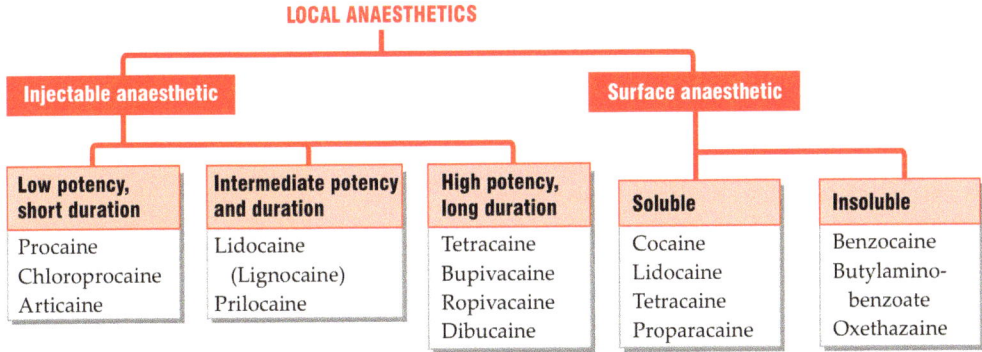

PROCAINE (ester)

LIDOCAINE (amide)

LOCAL ANAESTHETICS

Injectable anaesthetic

Low potency, short duration	Intermediate potency and duration	High potency, long duration
Procaine	Lidocaine	Tetracaine
Chloroprocaine	(Lignocaine)	Bupivacaine
Articaine	Prilocaine	Ropivacaine
		Dibucaine

Surface anaesthetic

Soluble	Insoluble
Cocaine	Benzocaine
Lidocaine	Butylamino-
Tetracaine	benzoate
Proparacaine	Oxethazaine

Table 24.1: Comparative features of general and local anaesthesia

	General anaesthesia	Local anaesthesia
1. Site of action	CNS	Peripheral nerves
2. Area of body involved	Whole body	Restricted area
3. Consciousness	Lost	Unaltered
4. Care of vital functions	Essential	Usually not needed
5. Physiological trespass	High	Low
6. Poor health patient	Risky	Safer
7. Use in non-cooperative patient	Possible	Not possible
8. Major surgery	Preferred	Cannot be used
9. Minor surgery	Not preferred	Preferred

Ester linked LAs Cocaine, procaine, chloroprocaine, tetracaine, benzocaine, proparacaine.

Amide linked LAs Lidocaine, bupivacaine, dibucaine, prilocaine, ropivacaine.

Features of amide LAs (compared to ester LAs)
- Produce more intense and longer lasting anaesthesia
- Bind to α_1 acid glycoprotein in plasma
- Not hydrolysed by plasma esterases
- Rarely cause hypersensitivity reactions; no cross sensitivity with ester LAs

Because of their short duration, less intense analgesia and higher risk of hypersensitivity, the ester linked LAs are rarely used for infiltration or nerve block, but are still used topically on mucous membranes.

Mechanism of action

The LAs block nerve conduction by restricting the entry of Na^+ ions during upstroke of action potential (AP). As the concentration of the LA is increased, the rate of rise of AP and maximum depolarization decreases (Fig. 24.1) causing slowing of conduction. Finally, local depolarization fails to reach the threshold potential and conduction block ensues.

The LAs interact with a receptor situated within the voltage sensitive Na^+ channel and raise the threshold of channel opening: Na^+ permeability fails to increase in response to an impulse or stimulus. The details are explained in Fig. 24.2. At physiological pH, the LA molecule is partly ionized. The equilibrium between the unionized base form (B) and the ionized cationic form (BH^+) depends on the pKa of the LA.

The LA penetrates the axonal membrane in the unionized base (B) form, but the active species is the cationic (BH^+) form. This form is able to approach its receptor easily when the channel is open at the inner face, and it binds more avidly to the activated as well as inactivated state of the channel compared to the resting state. Thus, a resting nerve is rather resistant to blockade. Blockade develops rapidly when the nerve is stimulated repeatedly. The degree of blockade is frequency dependent, i.e. greater

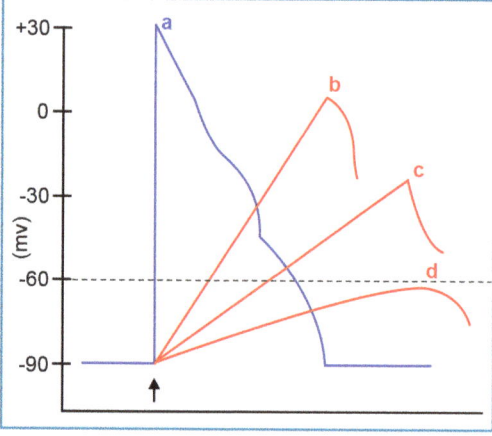

Fig. 24.1: Effect of progressively increasing concentrations (b, c, d) of a local anaesthetic on the generation of an action potential in a nerve fibre, (a) Untreated nerve fibre

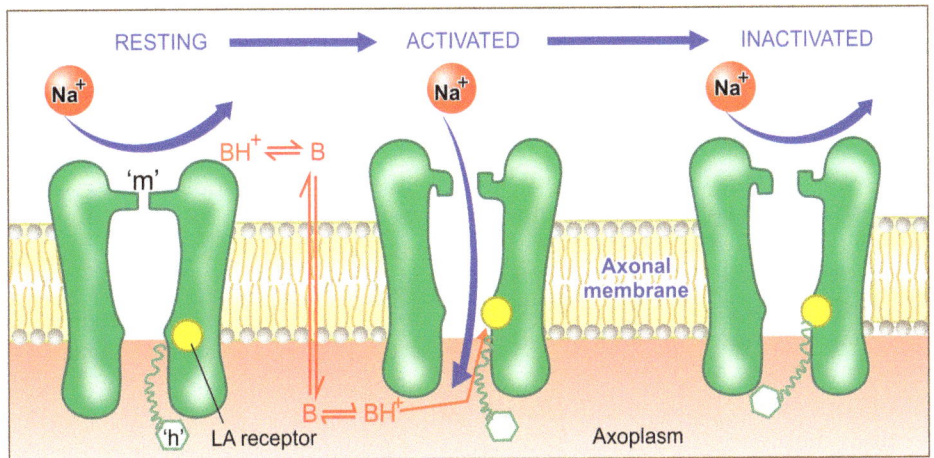

Fig. 24.2: A model of the axonal Na⁺channel depicting the site and mechanism of action of local anaesthetics
The Na⁺ channel has an activation gate (make or 'm' gate) near its extracellular mouth and an inactivation gate (halt or 'h' gate) at the intracellular mouth. In the resting state the activation gate is closed. Threshold depolarization of the membrane opens the activation gate allowing Na⁺ ions to flow in along the concentration gradient, thereby depolarizing the membrane. Within a few msec, the inactivation gate closes and ion flow ceases. The channel recovers to the resting state in a time-dependent manner.

The local anaesthetic (LA) receptor is located within the channel in its intracellular half. The LA traverses the membrane in its lipophilic form (B), reionizes in the axoplasm and approaches the LA receptor through the intracellular mouth of the channel. It is the cationic form (BH⁺) of the LA which primarily binds to the receptor. The receptor has higher affinity or is more accessible to the LA in the activated as well as inactivated state compared to resting state. Binding of the LA to its receptor stabilizes the channel in the inactivated state and thus reduces the probability of channel opening.

blockade at higher frequency of stimulation. Blockade of conduction by LA is not due to hyperpolarization. In fact, resting membrane potential is unaltered because K⁺ channels are blocked only at higher concentrations of the LA.

The onset time of blockade is related primarily to the pKa of the LA. Those LAs with lower pKa (7.6–7.8), e.g. lidocaine, are fast acting, because 30–40% LA is in the base form at pH 7.4 and it is this form which penetrates the axon. Procaine, tetracaine, bupivacaine have higher pKa (8.1–8.9), only 15% or less is unionized at pH 7.4; these LAs are slow acting. Chloroprocaine is an exception, having rapid onset despite high pKa (9.1).

Local actions

The clinically used LAs have no/minimal local irritant action and block sensory nerve endings, nerve trunks, neuromuscular junction, ganglionic synapse and receptors (non-selectively), i.e. those structures which function through increased Na⁺ permeability. They also reduce release of acetylcholine from motor nerve endings. Injected around a mixed nerve they cause anaesthesia of skin and paralysis of voluntary muscle supplied by that nerve.

Sensory and motor fibres are inherently equally sensitive, but some LAs exhibit unequal ability to block them, e.g. epidural bupivacaine produces sensory block at much lower concentration than that needed for motor block. Sensitivity to LA is determined by diameter of the fibres as well as by fibre type. In general smaller fibres are more sensitive than larger fibres. Diameter remaining the same, myelinated nerves are blocked earlier than nonmyelinated. Fibres differ in the critical length of the axon that must be exposed to the LA for effective blockade. Smaller fibres tend to have shorter critical lengths because in them voltage changes propagate passively for shorter distances. Also, more slender axons have shorter internodal distances and LAs easily enter the axon at the nodes of Ranvier. The density of Na^+ channels is much higher at these nodes. Moreover, frequency dependence of blockade makes smaller sensory fibres more vulnerable since they generate high frequency longer lasting action potentials than the motor fibres.

Autonomic fibres are generally more susceptible than somatic fibres. Among the somatic afferents order of blockade is: pain—temperature sense—touch—deep pressure sense. Since pain is generally carried by smaller diameter fibres than those carrying other sensations or motor impulses, pain is the first modality to be affected by LAs. Applied to the tongue, bitter taste is lost first followed by sweet and sour, and salty taste last of all.

In general, fibres that are more susceptible to LA are the first to be blocked and the last to recover. Also, location of the fibre within a nerve trunk determines the latency, duration and often the depth of local anaesthesia. Nerve sheaths restrict diffusion of the LA into the nerve trunk so that fibres in the outer layers are blocked earlier than the inner or core fibres. As a result, the more proximal areas supplied by a nerve are affected earlier because axons supplying them are located more peripherally in the nerve than those supplying distal areas. The differential arrangement of various types of sensory and motor fibres in a mixed nerve may partly account for the differential blockade.

The LA often fails to afford adequate pain control in inflamed tissues (like infected tooth). The likely reasons are:
a. Inflammation lowers pH of the tissue—greater fraction of the LA is in the ionized form hindering diffusion into the axolemma.
b. Blood flow to the inflamed area is increased — the LA is removed more rapidly from the site.
c. Effectiveness of Adr injected with the LA is reduced at the inflamed site.
d. Inflammatory products may oppose LA action.

Addition of a vasoconstrictor, e.g. adrenaline (1:50,000 to 1:200,000):
- prolongs duration of action of the LA by decreasing its rate of removal from the local site into the circulation.
- enhances the intensity of nerve block.
- reduces systemic toxicity of LAs: rate of absorption is reduced and metabolism keeps the plasma concentration lower.
- provides a more bloodless field for surgery.
- increases the chances of subsequent local tissue edema and necrosis as well as delays wound healing by reducing oxygen supply and enhancing oxygen consumption in the affected area.
- may raise BP and promote arrhythmia in susceptible individuals.

Systemic actions

Any LA injected or applied locally is ultimately absorbed and can produce systemic effects depending on the concentration attained in the plasma and the tissues.

C.N.S. All LAs are capable of producing a sequence of CNS stimulation followed by depression. *Cocaine* is a powerful CNS stimulant causing in sequence euphoria—excitement—mental confusion—restlessness—tremor and twitching of muscles—convulsions—unconsciousness—respiratory depression—death, in a dose-dependent manner.

The synthetic LAs are much less potent in this regard. At safe clinical doses, they produce little apparent CNS effects. The early neurological symptoms of overdose with *lidocaine* and other clinically used LAs are—circumoral numbness, abnormal sensation in the tongue, dizziness, blurred vision, tinnitus followed by drowsiness, dysphoria and lethargy. Still higher doses produce excitation, restlessness, agitation, muscle twitching, seizures and finally unconsciousness.

The basic action of all LAs is neuronal inhibition; the apparent stimulation seen initially is due to inhibition of inhibitory neurones. At high doses, all neurones are depressed, and flattening of waves in the EEG is seen.

CVS

Heart LAs are cardiac depressants, but no significant effects are observed at conventional doses. At high doses or on inadvertent i.v. injection, they decrease automaticity, excitability, contractility, conductivity and prolong refractory period (RP). They have a quinidine-like antiarrhythmic action. *Procaine* is not used clinically as antiarrhythmic because of short duration of action and propensity to produce CNS effects, but its amide derivative *procainamide* is a class IA antiarrhythmic. Electrophysiological properties of the heart may be markedly altered at high plasma cocentrations; QTc interval is prolonged and LAs can themselves induce cardiac arrhythmias. *Bupivacaine* is relatively more cardiotoxic and has produced ventricular tachycardia or fibrillation. *Lidocaine* has little effect on contractility and conductivity. It abbreviates RP and has little proarrhythmic potential. It is used as an antiarrhythmic (*see* Ch. 12).

Blood vessels Systemically LAs tend to produce fall in BP. This is primarily due to sympathetic blockade. Locally at the site of injection, LAs cause direct relaxation of arteriolar smooth muscle. Bupivacaine is more vasodilatory than lidocaine, while prilocaine is the least vasodilatory. Toxic doses of LAs produce cardiovascular collapse. *Cocaine* has sympathomimetic property; causes local vasoconstriction, marked rise in BP and tachycardia.

Pharmacokinetics

Because LAs act at or near their site of administration, pharmacokinetic characteristics are not important determinants of their local anaesthetic efficacy, but markedly influence their systemic effects and toxicity.

Soluble surface anaesthetics (lidocaine, tetracaine) are rapidly absorbed from mucous membranes and abraded areas, but absorption from intact skin is minimal. Rate of absorption depends on the blood flow to the area of application or injection; faster absorption occurring from more vascular tissues. Thus, intra-oral injection results in quicker and higher blood levels than s.c. injection on limbs or trunk. The entry into blood after injection of LA within an alveolar bone (maxilla) is very rapid. Once absorbed, the LA being lipophilic, rapidly enters highly perfused organs, *viz.* brain, heart, liver and kidney.

Procaine is negligibly bound to plasma proteins, but amide LAs are bound to plasma α_1 acid glycoprotein. LAs are rapidly but transiently bound to tissues, especially nerves, at the site of injection. Ester-linked LAs (procaine, etc.) are rapidly hydrolysed by plasma pseudocholinesterase and the remaining by esterases in the liver. Amide linked LAs (lidocaine, etc.) are degraded only in the liver microsomes by dealkylation and hydrolysis. Metabolism of lidocaine is hepatic blood flow dependent. The maximal safe dose of LAs is lower in patients with hepatic disease and in the elderly who have decreased liver function.

The LAs are ineffective after oral ingestion, due to high first pass metabolism in the liver.

Adverse effects

Systemic toxicity on rapid i.v. injection is related to the intrinsic anaesthetic potency of the LA. However, toxicity after topical application or regional injection is influenced by the relative rates of absorption and metabolism. Those rapidly absorbed but slowly metabolized are more toxic.

1. CNS effects are light-headedness, dizziness, auditory and visual disturbances, mental confusion, disorientation, shivering, twitchings, involuntary movements, finally convulsions and respiratory arrest. This can be prevented and treated by diazepam/midazolam.
2. Cardiovascular toxicity of LAs is manifested as bradycardia, hypotension, cardiac arrhythmias and vascular collapse.
3. Injection of LAs may be painful, but local tissue toxicity of LAs is low. However, wound healing may be sometimes delayed. Addition of vasoconstrictors enhances the local tissue damage. Localized mucosal sloughing and necrosis are rare complications. Vasoconstrictors should not be added for ring block of hands, feet, fingers, toes, penis and in pinna. Bupivacaine has the highest local tissue irritancy.
4. Hypersensitivity reactions like rashes, angioedema, dermatitis, contact sensitivity, asthma and rarely anaphylaxis occur. Allergic reactions are more common with ester linked LAs, but rare with lidocaine or its congeners. Cross reactivity is frequent among ester compounds, but not with amide linked LAs.

Often, methylparaben added as a preservative in certain LA solutions is responsible for the allergic reaction.

Precautions and interactions

1. Before injecting the LA, aspirate lightly to avoid intravascular injection.
2. Inject the LA slowly and take care not to exceed the maximum safe dose, especially in children.
3. Propranolol (probably other β blockers also) may reduce metabolism of lidocaine and other amide LAs by reducing hepatic blood flow.
4. Vasoconstrictor (adrenaline) containing LA should be avoided for patients with ischaemic heart disease, cardiac arrhythmia, thyrotoxicosis, uncontrolled hypertension, and in those receiving β blockers (rise in BP can occur due to unopposed α action) or tricyclic antidepressants (uptake blockade and potentiation of Adr).

INDIVIDUAL LOCAL ANAESTHETICS

Important features of frequently used local anaesthetics are presented in Table 24.2.

Cocaine It is a natural alkaloid from the leaves of *Erythroxylon coca*, a south American plant growing on the foothills of the Andes. The natives of Peru and Bolivia habitually chew these leaves. Cocaine is a good surface anaesthetic and is rapidly absorbed from buccal mucous membrane. It was first used for ocular anaesthesia in 1884. Cocaine should never be injected; it is a protoplasmic poison and causes tissue necrosis. Cocaine produces prominent CNS stimulation with marked effect on mood and behaviour. It induces a sense of wellbeing, delays fatigue and increases power

Table 24.2: Comparative features of commonly used local anaesthetics

Drug	Surface anaesthesia	Relative potency	Conc. used (%)	Nerve block Max. dose*	Onset	Duration (Min)	Cardio-toxicity
Lidocaine	+	1	0.5–2.0	300 mg	Fast	60–120	+
Bupivacaine	–	4–5	0.25–0.5	150 mg	Interm.	120–360	+++
Ropivacaine	–	3–4	0.25–0.75	200 mg	Slow	120–300	++

* Maximal injectable dose without adrenaline; addition of adrenaline may increase safe limit by up to 50%.

of endurance. In susceptible individuals it produces a state referred to as 'high' leading to strong psychological but little physical dependence. Cocaine is unique among drugs of abuse in not producing significant tolerance on repeated use. Sometimes reverse tolerance is seen (behavioural effects are experienced at lower doses).

In the periphery, it blocks uptake of NA and Adr into adrenergic nerve endings, resulting in higher concentration of the transmitter around the receptors. This produces sympathomimetic effects, and causes potentiation of NA and Adr. Local vasoconstriction, tachycardia, rise in BP and mydriasis are the reflection of its sympathomimetic action.

Because of these central and peripheral effects as well as local tissue toxicity, cocaine is not used clinically.

Procaine It is the first synthetic local anaesthetic introduced in 1905. Its popularity declined after the introduction of lidocaine. Procaine is not used now. It is not a surface anaesthetic.

Lidocaine (Lignocaine) Introduced in 1948, it is currently the most widely used LA. It is a versatile LA, good both for surface application as well as for injection, and is available in a variety of formulations. Lidocaine is the standard LA in dentistry (*see* p. 386). Injected around a nerve, it blocks conduction within 3 min, whereas procaine may take 15 min. Moreover, anaesthesia is more intense and longer lasting. Vasodilatation occurs at the injected area. Lidocaine is used for surface application, infiltration, nerve block, epidural and spinal anaesthesia. Cross sensitivity with ester LAs is not seen. Overdose of lidocaine causes muscle twitching, convulsions, cardiac arrhythmias, fall in BP, coma and respiratory arrest like other LAs. Lidocaine is also used as an antiarrhythmic (*see* Ch. 12).

XYLOCAINE, GESICAIN 4% topical solution, 2% jelly, 2% viscous, 5% ointment, 1% and 2% injection (with or without adrenaline), 5% heavy (for spinal anaesthesia); 100 mg/ml spray (10 mg per puff).

For dental anaesthesia: 1.5 ml cartridge or prefilled syringe containing lidocaine 2% with or without adrenaline 1:80000 is mostly used. The cartridge formulation is preservative free. This formulation is particularly indicated in patients who are allergic to the preservative and not to lidocaine.

Prilocaine It is similar to lidocaine but does not cause vasodilatation at the site of infiltration and has lower CNS toxicity due to larger volume of distribution.

Eutectic lidocaine/prilocaine This is a unique preparation which can anaesthetise intact skin after surface application. *Eutectic mixture* refers to lowering of melting point of two solids when they are mixed. This happens when lidocaine and prilocaine are mixed in equal proportion at 25 C. The resulting oily liquid is emulsified into water to form a cream that is applied under occlusive dressing for 1 hr before i.v. cannulation, split skin graft harvesting and other superficial procedures. Numbness up to a depth of 5 mm lasts for 1–2 hr after removal. It can be used as an alternative to lidocaine infiltration.

PRILOX 5% cream.

In dentistry, this formulation has been tried for obtunding pain of intrapalatal injection and as alternative to infiltration anaesthesia for some procedures.

Tetracaine (Amethocaine) A highly lipid-soluble PABA ester, more potent and more toxic due to slow hydrolysis by plasma pseudocholinesterase. It is both surface and conduction block anaesthetic, but its use is restricted to topical application to the eye, nose, throat and tracheobronchial tree. Because of rapid mucosal absorption and high systemic toxicity, its use for surface anaesthesia in the mouth is restricted.

ANETHANE powder for solution, 1% ointment.

Bupivacaine A more potent and long-acting highly lipid soluble amide linked LA: used for infiltration, nerve block, epidural and spinal anaesthesia of long duration. However, due to slow onset of action, bupivacaine is not preferred for peripheral nerve block. A 0.25% solution injected epidurally produces adequate analgesia without significant motor blockade. As a result, it has become very popular in obstetrics and for postoperative pain relief by continuous epidural infusion. Because of high lipid solubility, systemically absorbed bupivacaine distributes more in tissues than in blood. It is more prone to prolong QTc interval and induce ventricular tachycardia or cardiac depression. Cardiotoxicity is the primary concern which limits the total dose of bupivacaine. Its use in dentistry is described on p. 387.

MARCAIN 0.5%, inj for nerve block; 0.5% hyperbaric for spinal anaesthesia.
SENSORCAINE 0.25%, 0.5% inj, 0.5% heavy inj.

Levobupivacaine is the S(–) enantiomer of bupivacaine; equally potent LA as the racemic drug, but less cardiotoxic and less prone to cause seizures in overdose.

Ropivacaine A newer bupivacaine congener, equally long acting but less cardiotoxic. It blocks A δ and C fibres (involved in pain transmission) more completely than A β fibres which control motor function. Equieffective concentrations of ropivacaine are higher than those of bupivacaine. Continuous epidural ropivacaine is being used for relief of postoperative and labour pain. It can also be employed for nerve blocks.
ROPIN 0.2% inj.

Dibucaine (Cinchocaine) It is the most potent, most toxic and longest acting LA. It is used as a surface anaesthetic on less delicate mucous membranes (anal canal).
NUPERCAINAL 1% ointment, in OTOGESIC 1% ear drops.

Articaine This injectable LA is approved only for use in dentistry. Administered by infiltration, 4% articaine produces short lasting anaesthesia for dental procedures. It is not advocated for nerve block, because of higher risk of nerve damage and long lasting paresthesias.

Proparacaine It is a fast acting surface anaesthetic used exclusively in the eye. Ocular irritation is minimal and allergic reactions are rare compared to tetracaine.
PARACAINE 0.5% eye drops.

Benzocaine and Butylaminobenzoate (Butamben) Because of very low aqueous solubility, these LAs are not significantly absorbed from mucous membranes or from abraded skin. They produce long-lasting numbness without systemic toxicity. They are used as lozenges for stomatitis, sore throat; as dusting powder/ointment on wounds/ulcerated surfaces and for anorectal lesions.
PROCTOSEDYL-M: Butylaminobenzoate 1% oint with framycetin and hydrocortisone acetate: for piles.
PROCTOQUINOL 5% ointment of benzocaine.
ZOKEN 20% gel.

Oxethazaine A potent topical anaesthetic, unique in ionizing to a very small extent even at low pH values. It is, therefore, effective in anaesthetising gastric mucosa despite acidity of the medium. Swallowed along with antacids it affords symptomatic relief in gastritis, drug induced gastric irritation, gastroesophageal reflux and heartburn.
MUCAINE 0.2% in alumina gel + magnesium hydroxide suspension; 5-10 ml orally.

USES AND TECHNIQUES OF LOCAL ANAESTHESIA

1. Surface anaesthesia This is produced by topical application of a surface anaesthetic to mucous membranes or to abraded skin. Only the superficial layer of skin is anaesthetised. Onset and duration of anaesthesia depends on the site, the drug, its concentration and form, e.g. lidocaine (10%) sprayed in the mouth or throat acts in 2–5 min and produces anaesthesia for 30–45 min. Addition of Adr does not affect duration of topical anaesthesia. Absorption of soluble LAs from mucous membranes is rapid; blood concentrations of lidocaine and tetracaine sprayed in throat/tracheobronchial tree approach those attained on i.v. injection—toxicity can occur. Except for eutectic lidocaine/prilocaine, no other LA is capable of anaesthetizing intact skin. Surface anaesthesia is extensively used in the eye, throat, urethra, and anal canal. Topical LA is occasionally applied in the mouth for stomatitis/oral ulcers, and in nose/ear for painful lesions. Use of surface anaesthesia for painful mucosal lesions in the mouth is restricted by the attendant oral numbness, loss of taste and increased risk of bite/thermal injuries.

2. Infiltration anaesthesia Dilute solution of the LA is infiltrated under the skin in the area of operation so that it blocks the sensory nerve endings. Onset of action is almost immediate and duration is shorter than that after nerve block, e.g. infiltration anaesthesia lasts for 30–60 min after lidocaine, and for 90–180 min after bupivacaine. This technique is used for minor operations, e.g. incisions, excisions, some dental procedures, hydrocele, herniorrhaphy, etc., when the area to be anaesthetized is small. Relatively larger amount of the LA is required compared to the area anaesthetised, but motor function is not affected.

3. Conduction block The LA is injected around nerve trunks so that the area distal to injection is anaesthetised and paralysed.

(a) Field block It is produced by injecting the LA subcutaneously in a manner that all nerves coming to a particular field are blocked—as is done for dental procedures, herniorrhaphy, appendicectomy, scalp stitching, operations on forearms and legs, etc. Larger area can be anaesthetised with lesser drug compared to infiltration. The same concentration of LA as for infiltration is used for field block.

(b) Nerve block It is produced by injection of the LA around the appropriate nerve trunks or plexuses. The area of resulting anaesthesia is larger compared to the amount of drug used. Muscles supplied by the injected nerve/plexus are paralysed. The latency of anaesthesia depends on the drug and the area to be covered by diffusion, e.g. lidocaine anaesthetises intercostal nerves within 3 min, but brachial plexus block may take 15 min. For plexus block a 'flooding' technique is used and larger volumes are needed. Nerve block lasts longer than field block or infiltration anaesthesia. Frequently performed nerve blocks are—lingual, intercostal, ulnar, sciatic, femoral, brachial plexus, trigeminal, facial, phrenic, etc. Nerve block is used for many dental procedures including tooth extraction, operations on the eye, limbs, abdominal wall, fracture setting, trauma to the ribs, neuralgias, persistent hiccup, etc.

4. Spinal anaesthesia The LA is injected in the subarachnoid space between L2–3 or L3–4, i.e. below the lower end of spinal cord. The primary site of action is the nerve roots in the cauda equina rather than the spinal cord. Lower abdomen and lower limbs are anaesthetised and paralysed. The level of anaesthesia depends on the volume and speed of injection, specific gravity of the drug solution and posture of the patient. The drug solution could be hyperbaric (in 10% glucose) or isobaric with CSF.

Nerve roots rapidly take up and retain the LA. Since autonomic preganglionic fibres are more sensitive and somatic motor fibres less sensitive than somatic sensory fibres, the level of sympathetic block is about 2 segments higher and the level of motor paralysis about 2 segments lower than the level of cutaneous analgesia.

The duration of spinal anaesthesia depends on the drug used and its concentration. Lidocaine, bupivacaine and ropivacaine are the LAs used for spinal as well as epidural anaesthesia. The later two are longer acting than lidocaine. Addition of 0.2–0.4 mg of adrenaline to the LA prolongs spinal anaesthesia by about 1/3rd.

Spinal anaesthesia is used for operations on the lower limbs, pelvis, lower abdomen, prostatectomy, fracture setting, obstetric procedures, caesarean section, etc.

Possible complications of spinal anaesthesia are fall in BP, respiratory paralysis, headache nausea/vomiting, cauda equina syndrome (loss of control over bladder and bowel sphincter) and rarely meningitis.

5. Epidural anaesthesia The spinal dural space is filled with semiliquid fat through which nerve roots travel. The LA injected in this space—acts primarily on nerve roots (in the epidural as well as subarachnoid spaces to which it diffuses) and a small amount permeates through intervertebral foramina to produce multiple paravertebral blocks. Epidural injection can be made in the thoracic, lumbar or sacral region according to the area of desired anaesthesia.

Cardiovascular complications are similar to that after spinal anaesthesia, but headache and neurological complications are less likely, because intrathecal space is not entered. The zone of differential sympathetic blockade is not evident after epidural injection, but motor paralysis is 4–5 segments caudal. Continuous epidural anaesthesia (for prolonged postoperative pain control) can be instituted by inserting a catheter and making repeated injections.

Local anaesthesia in dentistry

In the practice of dentistry LAs are mainly used by nerve block (for branches of lingual nerve) or by infiltration/regional block techniques to carry out various restorative/operative procedures. Less commonly, they are applied topically to painful oral ulcers and other superficial lesions.

The total amount of LA injected for dental anaesthesia is generally much smaller (e.g. 20 – 80 mg of lidocaine) than that used for other purposes like brachial plexus block, multiple nerve blocks or epidural anaesthesia. As such, systemic toxicity of dental anaesthesia is usually not a major concern. Reports of serious adverse effects are rare. Many side effects that have been described (like palpitation, pallor, sweating, uneasiness, giddiness, fainting, nausea, tremor) in fact have their origin in the apprehension of the patient to the injection given in the mouth. However, because the volume of LA needed for dental anaesthesia in children is only marginally less than that in adults, a higher per kg dose is injected and the safety margin is reduced; systemic toxicity is more likely. It is, therefore, desirable to use Adr containing LA in children, though the longer duration of resulting soft tissue anaesthesia is apprehended to cause more postoperative biting injuries.

Because of greater vascularity in the upper jaw, soft tissue anaesthesia after maxillary infiltration of the LA is shorter lasting than the same drug injected into the lower jaw. This difference in duration of action is more marked for plain LA solutions than for those containing a vasoconstrictor. After nerve block, the duration of dental pulp anaesthesia is generally 1/5th to 1/3rd that of soft tissue anaesthesia. The plain solution may be preferred when a shorter duration of soft tissue anaesthesia without complete pulpal anaesthesia is required or when operative haemorrhage is not a concern, and when a vasoconstrictor is contraindicated. Plain LA has been considered appropriate for short maxillary arch procedures.

Lidocaine (2%) with adrenaline (1:80,000) is the standard LA preparation used in dental practice. It produces good soft tissue as well as pulpal anaesthesia and reduces postextraction bleeding. After injection, pulpal anaesthesia is obtained in 2–3 min and lasts for 40–60 min, whereas soft tissues remain anaesthetised for 2–3 hours. However, complete pain relief may not be achieved in few patients with very sensitive teeth or marked inflammation. In comparison, plain lidocaine (2%) provides soft tissue anaesthesia for 45–90 min, while pulpal anaesthesia is brief (10–20 min) and unreliable. Moreover, haemorrhage control is poor due to vasodilatory action of lidocaine. Use of plain lidocaine in dentistry is limited to superficial and brief procedures or when a vasoconstrictor is contraindicated. After intraoral injection, systemic absorption of lidocaine is relatively rapid due to high lipid solubility.

Topically, lidocaine may be applied on painful oral ulcers and prior to intraoral injection of the LA in apprehensive patients.

The 10% spray formulation produces widespread oral mucosal anaesthesia which may be utilized before taking impressions or dental X-ray in fussy patients.

Bupivacaine (0.5%) with adrenaline (1:200,000) is less frequently used in dentistry. Because of very high lipid solubility, it is largely taken up by periodontal soft tissues while penetration into bone is poorer. The onset of pulpal anaesthesia is slower, may take > 5 min to start, is less intense and relatively short-lasting (<2 hr), while soft tissues may remain anaesthetized for up to 8 hours. Long-lasting oral surgery or procedures which require extended postoperative pain control, such as removal of impacted third molars are the indications for use of bupivacaine.

Articaine Because of rapid onset, short duration (~ 1 hour) anaesthesia produced on infiltration, articaine is being used for many periodontal and some dental procedures. However, it is not available in India.

Ropivacaine is occasionally used in dentistry, and there is no specific indication for it.

Antimicrobial Drugs: General Considerations

Antimicrobial drugs are the greatest contribution of the 20th century to therapeutics. Their advent changed the outlook of the physician about the power drugs can have on diseases. They are one of the few class of drugs which can cure rather than just palliate diseases. As a class, they are one of the most frequently used as well as misused drugs. Apart from analgesics, they are the commonest drugs that dentists routinely prescribe.

Drugs in this class differ from all others in that they are designed to inhibit/kill the infecting organism and to have no/minimal effect on the recipient. This type of therapy is generally called *chemotherapy* which has come to mean 'treatment of systemic infections with specific drugs that selectively suppress/kill the infecting microorganism without significantly affecting the host.' The basis of selective microbial toxicity is the action of the drug on a component of the microbe (e.g. bacterial cell wall) or metabolic process (e.g. folate synthesis) that is not found in the host, or a high affinity for certain microbial biomolecules. Due to analogy between the malignant cell and the pathogenic microbes, treatment of neoplastic diseases with drugs is also called chemotherapy.

Antibiotics These are substances produced by microorganisms, which selectively suppress the growth of or kill other microorganisms at very low concentrations. This definition excludes other natural substances which also inhibit microorganisms but are produced by higher forms (e.g. antibodies) or even those produced by microbes but are needed in high concentrations (ethanol, lactic acid, H_2O_2).

Chemotherapeutic agent Initially, this term was restricted to synthetic compounds, but now since many antibiotics and their analogues have been synthesized, this criterion has become irrelevant; both synthetic and microbiologically produced drugs need to be included together. However, it would be more meaningful to use the term *antimicrobial agent* (AMA) to designate synthetic as well as naturally obtained drugs that attenuate microorganisms.

The *history* of antimicrobial therapy may be divided into 3 phases.
(a) The period of empirical use: of 'mouldy curd' by Chinese on boils, chaulmoogra oil by the Hindus in leprosy, chenopodium by Aztecs for intestinal worms, mercury by Paracelsus (16th century AD) for syphilis, cinchona bark (17th century AD) for fevers.
(b) Ehrlich's phase of dyes and organometallic compounds (1890–1935): With the discovery of microbes in the later half of the 19th century and that they are the cause of many diseases: Ehrlich toyed with the idea that if certain dyes could selectively stain microbes, they could also be selectively toxic to these organisms, and tried methylene blue, trypan red, etc. He developed the arsenicals—*atoxyl* for sleeping sickness, *arsphenamine* in 1906 and neoarsphenamine in 1909 for syphilis. He coined the term 'chemotherapy' because he used drugs of known chemical structure (that of most other drugs in use at that time was not known) and showed that selective attenuation of infecting parasite was a practical proposition.

(c) The modern era of antimicrobial therapy was ushered by Domagk in 1935 by demonstrating the therapeutic effect of *Prontosil*, a sulfonamide dye, in pyogenic infection. It was soon realized that the active moiety was paraamino benzene sulfonamide, and the dye part was not essential. Sulfapyridine (M & B 693) was the first sulfonamide to be marketed in 1938.

The phenomenon of *antibiosis* was demonstrated by Pasteur in 1877, when he observed that growth of anthrax bacilli in urine was inhibited by air-borne bacteria. Fleming (1929) found that a diffusible substance was elaborated by *Penicillium* mould which could destroy *Staphylococcus* on the culture plate. He named this substance *penicillin* but could not purify it. Chain and Florey followed up this observation in 1939 which culminated in the clinical use of penicillin in 1941. Because of the great potential of this discovery in treating war wounds, commercial manufacture of penicillin soon started.

In the 1940s, Waksman and his colleagues undertook a systematic search of Actinomycetes as source of antibiotics and discovered *streptomycin* in 1944. This group of soil microbes proved to be a treasure-house of antibiotics and soon tetracyclines, chloramphenicol, erythromycin and many others followed. All three groups of scientists Domagk, Fleming-Chain-Florey and Waksman were awarded the Nobel Prize for their discoveries.

In the past 50 years emphasis has shifted from searching new antibiotic producing organisms to developing semisynthetic derivatives of older antibiotics which have more desirable properties or have differing spectrum of activity. Few novel synthetic AMAs (e.g. fluoroquinolones, oxazolidinones) have also been produced.

CLASSIFICATION

Antimicrobial drugs can be classified on several criteria:

A. Chemical structure
1. *Sulfonamides and related drugs:* Sulfadiazine and others, Dapsone (DDS), Paraaminosalicylic acid (PAS).
2. *Diaminopyrimidines:* Trimethoprim, Pyrimethamine.
3. *Quinolones:* Nalidixic acid, Norfloxacin, Ciprofloxacin, Moxifloxacin, etc.
4. *β-lactam antibiotics:* Penicillins, Cephalosporins, Monobactams, Carbapenems.
5. *Tetracyclines:* Oxytetracycline, Doxycycline, etc.
6. *Glycylcycline:* Tigecycline.
7. *Nitrobenzene derivative:* Chloramphenicol.
8. *Aminoglycosides:* Streptomycin, Gentamicin, Neomycin, etc.
9. *Macrolide antibiotics:* Erythromycin, Clarithromycin, Azithromycin, etc.
10. *Lincosamide antibiotics:* Lincomycin, Clindamycin.
11. *Polypeptide antibiotics:* Polymyxin-B, Colistin, Bacitracin, Tyrothricin.
12. *Glycopeptides:* Vancomycin, Teicoplanin
13. *Oxazolidinone:* Linezolid.
14. *Nitrofuran derivatives:* Nitrofurantoin, Furazolidone.
15. *Nitroimidazoles:* Metronidazole, Tinidazole.
16. *Nicotinic acid derivatives:* Isoniazid, Pyrazinamide, Ethionamide.
17. *Polyene antibiotics:* Nystatin, Amphotericin-B, Hamycin.
18. *Azole derivatives:* Miconazole, Clotrimazole, Ketoconazole, Fluconazole.
19. *Others:* Rifampin, Spectinomycin, Sod. fusidate, Cycloserine, Viomycin, Ethambutol, Clofazimine, Griseofulvin.

B. Type of organisms against which primarily active
1. *Antibacterial:* Penicillins, Aminoglycosides, Erythromycin, Fluoroquinolones etc.
2. *Antifungal:* Griseofulvin, Amphotericin B, Ketoconazole, etc.
3. *Antiviral:* Acyclovir, Amantadine, Zidovudine, etc.
4. *Antiprotozoal:* Chloroquine, Pyrimethamine, Metronidazole, Diloxanide, etc.
5. *Anthelmintic:* Mebendazole, Pyrantel, Niclosamide, Diethyl carbamazine, etc.

Chapter 25: Antimicrobial Drugs: General Considerations

C. Spectrum of activity

Narrow spectrum
Penicillin G
Streptomycin
Erythromycin

Broad spectrum
Tetracyclines
Chloramphenicol

The initial distinction between narrow and broad-spectrum antibiotics is no longer clearcut. Drugs with all ranges of intermediate band width, e.g. extended spectrum penicillins, newer cephalosporins, aminoglycosides, fluoroquinolones are now available. However, the terms 'narrow spectrum' and 'broad spectrum' are still applied.

D. Type of action

Primarily bacteriostatic

Sulfonamides
Tetracyclines
Chloramphenicol
Erythromycin
Clindamycin
Linezolid
Ethambutol

Primarily bactericidal

Penicillins
Aminoglycosides
Polypeptides
Cephalosporins
Vancomycin
Fluoroquinolones
Rifampin
Cotrimoxazole
Metronidazole

Some primarily static drugs may become cidal at higher concentrations (as attained in the urinary tract), e.g. sulfonamides, erythromycin, nitrofurantoin. On the other hand, some cidal drugs, e.g. cotrimoxazole, streptomycin may only be static under certain circumstances.

E. Natural sources of antibiotics:

Fungi
Penicillin
Cephalosporin
Griseofulvin

Bacteria
Polymyxin B
Colistin
Bacitracin
Tyrothricin
Aztreonam

Actinomycetes
Aminoglycosides
Tetracyclines
Chloramphenicol
Macrolides
Polyenes

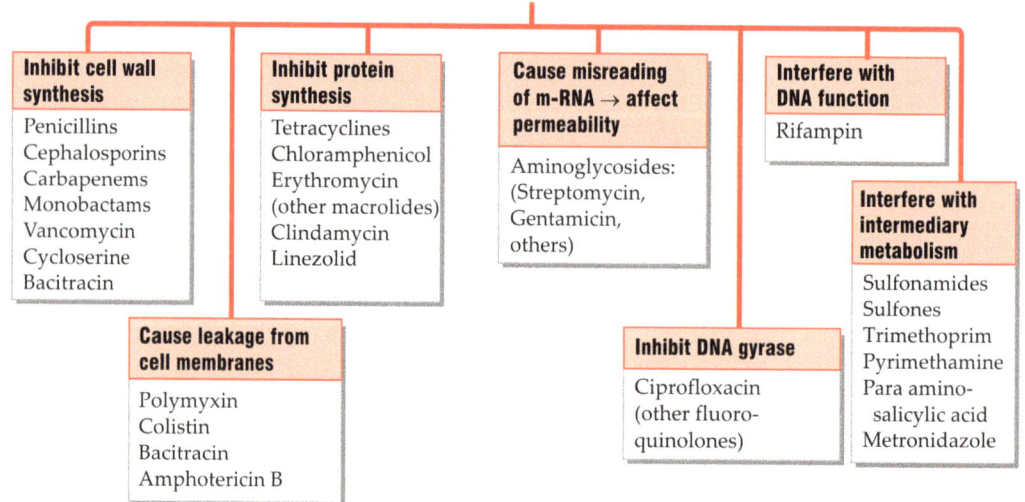

MECHANISM OF ACITON OF ANTIBACTERIAL DRUGS

Inhibit cell wall synthesis
Penicillins
Cephalosporins
Carbapenems
Monobactams
Vancomycin
Cycloserine
Bacitracin

Inhibit protein synthesis
Tetracyclines
Chloramphenicol
Erythromycin
(other macrolides)
Clindamycin
Linezolid

Cause misreading of m-RNA → affect permeability
Aminoglycosides:
(Streptomycin, Gentamicin, others)

Interfere with DNA function
Rifampin

Cause leakage from cell membranes
Polymyxin
Colistin
Bacitracin
Amphotericin B

Inhibit DNA gyrase
Ciprofloxacin
(other fluoro-quinolones)

Interfere with intermediary metabolism
Sulfonamides
Sulfones
Trimethoprim
Pyrimethamine
Para amino-salicylic acid
Metronidazole

PROBLEMS THAT ARISE WITH THE USE OF AMAs

1. Toxicity

(a) Local irritancy: This is exerted at the site of administration. Gastric irritation on oral ingestion, pain and abscess formation at the site of i.m. injection, thrombophlebitis of the injected vein are the complications. Practically all AMAs are irritants, especially erythromycin, tetracyclines, certain cephalosporins and chloramphenicol.

(b) Systemic toxicity: Practically all AMAs produce dose related and predictable organ toxicities. Characteristic toxicities are exhibited by different AMAs.
Some have a *high therapeutic index*—doses up to 100-fold range may be given without apparent damage to host cells. These include penicillins, some cephalosporins and erythromycin.
Others have a *lower therapeutic index*—doses have to be individualized and toxicity watched for, e.g.:

Aminoglycosides	: 8th cranial nerve and kidney toxicity.
Tetracyclines	: liver and kidney damage.
Vancomycin	: hearing loss, kidney damage.
Chloramphenicol	: bone marrow depression.

Still others have a *very low therapeutic index*—use is highly restricted to conditions where no suitable alternative is available, e.g. :

Polymyxin B	: neurological and renal toxicity.
Amphotericin B	: kidney, bone marrow and neurological toxicity.

2. Hypersensitivity reactions

Practically all AMAs are capable of causing hypersensitivity reactions. These are unpredictable and unrelated to dose. The whole range of reactions from rashes to anaphylactic shock can be produced. The more commonly involved AMAs in hypersensitivity reactions are—penicillins, cephalosporins, sulfonamides, fluoroquinolones.

3. Drug resistance

It refers to unresponsiveness of a microorganism to an AMA and is akin to the phenomenon of tolerance seen in higher organisms.

Natural resistance Some microbes have always been resistant to certain AMAs. They lack the metabolic process or the target site which is affected by the particular drug. This is generally a group or species characteristic, e.g. gram-negative bacilli are normally unaffected by penicillin G, aerobic organisms are not affected by metronidazole, while anaerobic bacteria are not inhibited by aminoglycoside antibiotics, or *M. tuberculosis* is insensitive to tetracyclines. This type of resistance does not pose a significant clinical problem.

Acquired resistance The development of resistance by an organism (which was sensitive earlier) due to the use of an AMA over a period of time is called acquired resistance. This can happen with any microbe and is a major clinical problem. However, development of resistance is dependent on the microorganism as well as on the drug. Some bacteria are notorious for rapid acquisition of resistance, e.g. staphylococci, coliforms, tubercle bacilli. Others like *Strep. pyogenes* and spirochetes have not developed significant resistance to penicillin despite its widespread use for > 50 years.

Resistance may be developed by mutation or gene transfer.

Mutation It is a stable and heritable genetic change that occurs spontaneously and randomly among microorganisms.

Mutation is not induced by the AMA. Any sensitive population of a microbe contains a few mutant cells which require higher concentration of the AMA for inhibition. These cells are selectively preserved and get a chance to proliferate when the sensitive cells are eliminated by the AMA. Thus, in time it would appear that a sensitive strain has been replaced by a resistant one, as happens when a single antitubercular drug is used. Mutation and resistance may be:

(i) Single step: A single gene mutation may confer high degree of resistance which emerges rapidly, e.g. enterococci to streptomycin, *E. coli* and *Staphylococci* to rifampin.

(ii) Multistep: A number of gene modifications are involved; sensitivity decreases gradually in a stepwise manner. Resistance to erythromycin, tetracyclines and chloramphenicol is developed by many organisms in this manner.

Gene transfer (infectious resistance) The resistance causing gene is passed from one organism to another. Rapid spread of resistance can occur by this mechanism, and high level resistance to several antibiotics (multi drug resistance) can be acquired concurrently. Gene transfer can occur in the following 3 ways:

(i) Conjugation This refers to sexual contact through the formation of a bridge or sex pilus, and is common among gram-negative bacilli of the same or another species. This may involve chromosomal or extrachromosomal (plasmid) DNA. The gene carrying the 'resistance' or 'R' factor is transferred only if another 'resistance transfer factor' (RTF) is also present. Conjugation frequently occurs in the colon where a large variety of gram-negative bacilli come in close contact. Even nonpathogenic organisms may transfer R factor to pathogenic organisms, which may become widespread by contamination of food or water. Chloramphenicol resistance of typhoid bacilli, streptomycin resistance of *E. coli*, and many others have been traced to this mechanism.

(ii) Transduction It is the transfer of gene carrying resistance through the agency of a bacteriophage. The R factor is taken up by the phage and delivered to another bacterium which it infects.

(iii) Transformation A resistant bacterium may release the resistance carrying DNA into the medium and this may be imbibed by another sensitive organism—becoming unresponsive to the drug. This mechanism is probably not clinically significant.

Resistance once acquired by any of the above mechanisms becomes prevalent due to the *selection pressure* of a widely used AMA, i.e. presence of the AMA provides opportunity for the resistant subpopulation to thrive in preference to the sensitive population.

Resistant organisms can be drug tolerant or drug destroying or drug impermeable.

(a) Drug tolerant The target biomolecule of the microorganism loses affinity for a particular AMA, e.g. resistant *Staph. aureus* and *E. coli* develop a RNA polymerase that does not bind rifampin, certain penicillin-resistant pneumococcal strains have altered penicillin binding proteins. Mutational target site modification is often responsible for fluoroquinolone and macrolide resistance. Another mechanism is acquisition of an alternative metabolic pathway, e.g. certain sulfonamide-resistant bacteria switch over to utilizing preformed folic acid in place of synthesizing it from PABA taken up from the medium.

(b) Drug destroying The resistant microbe elaborates an enzyme which inactivates the drug, e.g.
- β-lactamases are produced by staphylococci, *Haemophilus*, gonococci, etc. which inactivate penicillin G. The β-lactamases may be present in low quantity but strategically located periplasmically (as in gram-negative bacteria) so that the drug is inactivated soon after entry, or may be elaborated in large quantities (by gram-positive bacteria) to diffuse into the medium and destroy the drug before entry.
- Chloramphenicol acetyl transferase is acquired by resistant *E. coli*, *H. influenzae* and *S. typhi*.

- Many of the aminoglycoside-resistant coliforms produce enzymes which adenylate/acetylate/phosphorylate specific aminoglycoside antibiotics.

(c) Drug impermeable Many hydrophilic antibiotics gain access into the bacterial cell through specific channels formed by proteins called 'porins', or need specific transport mechanisms. These channels/transporters may be lost by the resistant strains, e.g. concentration of some aminoglycosides and tetracyclines in the resistant gram-negative bacterial strains has been found to be much lower than that in their sensitive counterparts when both were exposed to equal concentrations of the drugs. Similarly, the low degree penicillin-resistant gonococci are less permeable to penicillin G; chloroquine-resistant *P. falciparum* accumulates less chloroquine. The bacteria may also acquire plasmid directed inducible energy dependent efflux proteins in their cell membrane which pump out tetracyclines. Active efflux-based resistance has been detected for erythromycin and fluoroquinolones as well.

Cross resistance Acquisition of resistance to one AMA conferring resistance to another AMA, to which the organism has not been exposed, is called cross resistance. This is more commonly seen between chemically or mechanistically related drugs, e.g. resistance to one sulfonamide means resistance to all others, and resistance to one tetracycline means insensitivity to all others. Such cross resistance is often complete. However, resistance to one aminoglycoside may not extend to another, e.g. gentamicin-resistant strains may respond to amikacin. Sometimes unrelated drugs show partial cross resistance, e.g. between tetracyclines and chloramphenicol, between erythromycin and lincomycin.

Prevention of drug resistance It is of utmost clinical importance to curb development of drug resistance. Measures are:
(a) No indiscriminate and inadequate or unduly prolonged use of AMAs should be made. This would minimize the selection pressure and resistant strains will get less chance to preferentially propagate. Symptom-determined shorter courses of AMAs are advocated for acute localized infections in otherwise healthy patients.
(b) Prefer rapidly acting and selective (narrow spectrum) AMAs whenever possible; broad-spectrum drugs should be used only when a specific one cannot be determined or is not suitable.
(c) Use combination of AMAs whenever prolonged therapy is undertaken, e.g. in tuberculosis, SABE and for HIV-AIDS.
(d) Infection by organisms notorious for developing resistance, e.g. *Staph. aureus, E. coli, M. tuberculosis, Proteus*, etc. must be treated intensively.

4. Superinfection (Suprainfection)

This refers to the appearance of a new infection as a result of antimicrobial therapy.

Use of most AMAs causes some alteration in the normal microbial flora of the body. The normal flora contributes to host defence by elaborating substances called *bacteriocins* which inhibit pathogenic organisms. Further, ordinarily, the pathogen has to compete with the normal flora for nutrients, etc. to establish itself. Lack of competition may allow even a normally nonpathogenic component of the flora (e.g. *Candida*), which is not inhibited by the drug to predominate and invade. More complete the suppression of body flora, greater are the chances of developing superinfection. Thus, superinfection is commonly associated with the use of broad/extended spectrum antibiotics, such as tetracyclines, chloramphenicol, ampicillin, newer cephalosporins; especially when combinations of these are employed. Tetracyclines are more liable than chloramphenicol and ampicillin is more liable than amoxicillin to cause superinfection diarrhoeas because of incomplete absorption in the ileum; higher amounts reach the lower bowel and cause greater suppression of colonic bacteria.

Superinfections are more common when host defence is compromised.

Conditions predisposing to superinfections
- Corticosteroid therapy
- Leukaemias and other malignancies, especially when treated with anticancer drugs (these drugs are immunosuppressant as well, and decrease WBC count)
- Acquired immunodeficiency syndrome (AIDS)
- Agranulocytosis
- Diabetes, disseminated lupus erythematosus

Sites involved in superinfection are those that normally harbour commensals, i.e. oropharynx; intestinal, respiratory and genitourinary tracts; occasionally skin.

Superinfections are generally more difficult to treat. The organisms frequently involved in superinfections, diseases caused and drugs for treating them are:

(a) *Candida albicans*: thrush, monilial diarrhoea, vulvovaginitis; treat with nystatin or clotrimazole.
(b) Resistant staphylococci: enteritis; treat with cloxacillin/vancomycin/linezolid.
(c) *Clostridium difficile*: pseudomembranous enterocolitis associated with the use of clindamycin, tetracyclines, aminoglycosides, ampicillin, etc. It is more common after colorectal surgery. The organism produces an enterotoxin which damages gut mucosa forming plaques. Metronidazole and vancomycin are the drugs of choice.
(d) *Proteus*: Urinary tract infection, enteritis; treat with a cephalosporin or gentamicin.
(e) *Pseudomonas*: Urinary tract infection, enteritis; treat with carbenicillin, piperacillin, ceftazidime, cefoperazone or gentamicin.

To minimize superinfections:
- Use specific (narrow-spectrum) AMA whenever possible.
- Do not use antimicrobials to treat trivial, self-limiting or untreatable (viral) infections.
- Do not unnecessarily prolong antimicrobial therapy.

5. Nutritional deficiencies

Some of the B complex group of vitamins and vit K synthesized by the intestinal flora is utilized by man. Prolonged use of antimicrobials which alter this flora may result in vitamin deficiencies.

Neomycin causes morphological abnormalities in the intestinal mucosa which can produce steatorrhoea and malabsorption syndrome.

6. Masking of an infection

A short course of an AMA may be sufficient to treat one infection but only briefly suppress another one contacted concurrently. The other infection will be masked initially, only to manifest later in a severe form. Examples are:
(i) Syphilis masked by the use of a single dose of penicillin which is sufficient to cure gonorrhoea.
(ii) Tuberculosis masked by a short course of streptomycin given for a minor respiratory infection.

CHOICE OF AN ANTIMICROBIAL AGENT

After having established the need for using a systemic AMA in a patient by ascertaining that the condition is due to a treatable (mostly bacterial) infection, and that it is not likely to resolve by itself or by the use of local measures (antiseptics, drainage of pus, etc.), one has to choose an appropriate AMA from the large number available. The choice depends on the particulars of the patient, the infecting organism and the drug.

Patient factors

1. *Age* may affect kinetics of many AMAs. The t½ of aminoglycosides is prolonged in the elderly and they are more prone to develop VIII nerve toxicity. Tetracyclines accumulate in the developing teeth and bone —discolour and weaken teeth. As such, tetracyclines are contraindicated below the age of 6 years.

2. *Renal and hepatic function* Cautious use and modification of the dose of an AMA (with low safety margin) becomes necessary when the organ of its disposal is impaired (*see* box).

Antimicrobials needing dose reduction/avoidance in renal failure	
Reduce dose even in mild failure	
Aminoglycosides	Amphotericin B
Cephalosporins	Ethambutol
Vancomycin	Flucytosine
Reduce dose only in moderate-severe failure	
Metronidazole	Carbenicillin
Cotrimoxazole	Fluoroquinolones
Aztreonam	Clarithromycin
Meropenem	Imipenem
Drugs to be avoided	
Nalidixic acid	Tetracyclines (except doxycycline)
Nitrofurantoin	

Antimicrobials to be avoided or used at lower dose *in liver disease* are:

Antimicrobials in liver disease	
Drugs to be avoided	
Erythromycin estolate	Tetracyclines
Pyrazinamide	Nalidixic acid
	Pefloxacin
Dose reduction needed	
Chloramphenicol	Isoniazid
Metronidazole	Rifampin
Clindamycin	

3. *Local factors* The conditions prevailing at the site of infection greatly affect the action of AMAs.

(a) Presence of pus and secretions decrease the efficacy of most AMAs, especially sulfonamides and aminoglycosides. Antibiotics cannot cure periodontal or periapical abscesses, unless the pus is surgically drained. Drainage of the abscess reduces the population of causative bacteria, suppresses anaerobic bacteria by exposure to oxygen, and improves diffusion of the antibiotic into the abscess cavity. Adequate drainage of pus and exudates is very important for the cure of orofacial infections.

(b) Presence of necrotic material or foreign body, including implants and prosthesis, makes eradication of infection practically impossible. Bacteria adhering to foreign surfaces create a biofilm around them and grow very slowly, rendering them difficult to reach and less vulnerable to the antibiotic.

(c) Haematomas foster bacterial growth; tetracyclines, penicillins and cephalosporins get bound to the degraded haemoglobin in the haematoma.

(d) Lowering of pH at site of infection reduces activity of macrolide and aminoglycoside antibiotics.

(e) Anaerobic environment in the centre of an abscess impairs bacterial transport processes which concentrate aminoglycosides in the bacterial cell, rendering them less susceptible.

(f) Penetration barriers at certain sites may hamper the access of the AMA to the site, such as in subacute bacterial endocarditis (SABE), endophthalmitis, root canal of teeth, etc.

4. *Drug allergy* History of previous exposure to an AMA should be obtained. If a drug has caused allergic reaction—it has to be avoided in that patient, e.g. erythromycin or clindamycin are the alternative drugs for dental infection in patients allergic to penicillin. β-lactams, sulfonamides and fluoroquinolones frequently cause drug allergy.

5. Impaired host defence Integrity of host defence plays a crucial role in overcoming an infection. Pyogenic infections occur readily in neutropenic patients. If cell-mediated immunity is impaired (e.g. AIDS), infections by low-grade pathogens and intracellular organisms abound. In an individual with normal host defence, a bacteriostatic AMA may achieve cure; while intensive therapy with cidal drugs is imperative in those with impaired host defence (*see* box on p. 394) or when the organisms are protected by a barrier, e.g. intraosseous infections, SABE. Even with cidal drugs complete eradication of the organism may not occur.

6. Pregnancy All AMAs should be avoided in the pregnant because of risk to the foetus. Penicillins, many cephalosporins and erythromycin are safe, while safety data on most others is not available. Therefore, manufacturers label 'contraindicated during pregnancy'. Tetracyclines are clearly contraindicated. They carry risk of acute yellow atrophy of liver, pancreatitis and kidney damage in the mother. They also cause teeth and bone deformities in the offspring. Aminoglycosides can cause foetal ear damage. Animal studies indicate increased risk to the foetus especially with fluoroquinolones, cotrimoxazole, chloramphenicol, sulfonamides and nitrofurantoin. Though metronidazole has not been found to be teratogenic, its mutagenic potential warrants caution in use during pregnancy.

7. Genetic factors Primaquine, sulfonamides, chloramphenicol and fluoroquinolones carry the risk of producing haemolysis in G-6PD deficient patient.

Organism-related considerations

Each AMA has a specific effect on a limited number of microbes. Chemotherapy must be rational and demands a diagnosis to be successful. A clinical diagnosis should first be made, at least tentatively, and the likely pathogen guessed.

Oro-dental infections Ideally, the identity and antimicrobial sensitivity of the infecting bacteria should be determined before instituting systemic antibacterial therapy. However, being time consuming (at least 48 hours) and expensive, this is impractical for most dental infections which are acute in nature and treatment cannot be delayed. Moreover, it is not always possible to obtain appropriate samples of the infected material for bacteriological testing. Nevertheless, a good guess can generally be made from the clinical features and local experience. The causative organisms of common orodental infections, *viz.* alveolar abscesses, periodontal abscesses, dental pulp infections, chronic periodontitis, acute necrotizing ulcerative gingivitis (ANUG) are usually *Bacteroides* and other anaerobes like *Fusobacterium, Porphyromonas, Prevotella, Veillonella, Peptostreptococci* (mostly gram-negative and a few gram-positive), aerobic gram-positive cocci, chiefly viridans group *Streptococci* and spirochetes. The anaerobes predominate, more so in abscesses than in cellulitis.

Orodental infections are often mixed bacterial infections. Therefore, the drugs mostly selected are from penicillin/amoxicillin (with or without clavulanic acid), some cephalosporins like cefuroxime or cefaclor which are active on anaerobes, erythromycin, azithromycin, clindamycin, vancomycin, doxycycline, ofloxacin and metronidazole/tinidazole. Most dentists initiate empirical therapy with amoxicillin + metronidazole. Further therapy is modified on the basis of clinical response, but hasty and arbitrary changes in antibiotic therapy are not advisable. If possible (especially in serious infections), specimen for bacteriological examination should be collected before initiating empirical therapy, so that in case of failure of the initially chosen drug, alternative AMA could be selected in the light of bacteriological findings.

In a few situations like ANUG and oral thrush the clinical diagnosis itself indicates the infecting organism and directs the choice of drug (amoxicillin or doxycycline + metronidazole for ANUG; nystatin or clotrimazole for thrush).

Bacteriological sensitivity testing This is generally done by disk-agar diffusion method using standardized concentrations of antibiotics based on clinically attained plasma concentrations of these. As such, they provide only qualitative results; may serve as indicators, but not definitive measures of sensitivity. Broth cultures with *break-point* concentration (concentration that demarcates between sensitive and resistant bacteria) of antibiotics generally yield more reliable results. Break-point concentrations are based on clinically attainable serum concentrations of the antibiotic.

Minimum inhibitory concentration (MIC), i.e. the lowest concentration of an antibiotic which prevents visible growth of a bacterium determined in microwell culture plates using serial dilutions of the antibiotic is more informative, but not estimated routinely.

Minimum bactericidal concentration (MBC) of the antibiotic is determined by subculturing from tubes with no visible growth. If the organism is killed, no growth will occur; but if it was only inhibited in the parent culture—it will grow on subculturing in antibiotic-free medium. MBC is the concentration of the antibiotic which kills 99.9% of the bacteria. A small difference between MIC and MBC indicates that the antibiotic is primarily bactericidal, while a large difference indicates bacteriostatic action. MBC is not used to guide selection of antibiotics in clinical practice.

Postantibiotic effect (PAE) After a brief exposure if the organism is placed in antibiotic-free medium, it starts multiplying again, but after a lag period which depends on the antibiotic as well as the organism. This lag period in growth resumption is known as 'postantibiotic effect'. A long postantibiotic effect has been noted with fluoroquinolones, aminoglycosides and rifampin.

Drug factors

When any one of a number of AMAs could be used to treat an infection, choice among them is based upon specific properties of these AMAs:

1. *Spectrum of activity:* For definitive therapy, a narrow spectrum drug which selectively affects the concerned organism is preferred, because it is generally more effective than a broad-spectrum AMA and is less likely to disturb the normal microbial flora. However, for empirical therapy, often a broad-spectrum drug has to be used to cover all likely pathogens.

2. *Type of activity:* A bactericidal antibiotic may be preferred over bacteriostatic because it directly reduces the number of bacteria at the site of infection, while bacteriostatic drug only prevents increase in their number. This is specially important while treating patients with impaired host defence, life-threatening infections, infections at less accessible sites (endodontic infections, osteomyelitis, SABE) or when carrier state is possible (typhoid). Further, acute infections generally resolve faster with bactericidal than with bacteriostatic drugs, and some bactericidal drugs exert prolonged postantibiotic effect (PAE), so that maintenance of drug level continuously above MIC is not essential. With bacteriostatic AMAs, the bacteria start multiplying again when drug level falls below MIC, which may result in relapse of infection.

3. *Sensitivity of the organism:* This is assessed on the basis of MIC values (seldom determined for dental infections) and consideration of PAE.

4. *Relative toxicity:* Obviously, a less toxic antibiotic is preferred, e.g. a β-lactam over an aminoglycoside or erythromycin over clindamycin.

5. *Pharmacokinetic profile:* For optimum action, the antibiotic has to be present at the site of infection in sufficient concentration for an adequate length of time. This depends on their pharmacokinetic characteristics. Most antibiotics are given at 2–4 half-life intervals—thus attaining therapeutic concentrations

only intermittently. For many organisms, aminoglycosides, fluoroquinolones and metronidazole produce *'concentration-dependent killing'*—inhibitory effect depends on the ratio of peak concentration to the MIC. The same daily dose of gentamicin produces better action when given as a single dose than if it is divided into 2–3 portions. On the other hand, β-lactams, vancomycin and macrolides produce *'time-dependent killing'*—antimicrobial action depends on the length of time the concentration remains above the MIC; division of daily dose improves the effect. However, the doses should be so spaced that the surviving organisms again start multiplying and a cidal action is exerted.

Penetration into the site of infection also depends on the pharmacokinetic properties of the drug. A drug, which penetrates better and attains higher concentration at the site of infection is likely to be more effective. Penetration of AMAs into bone is generally poor, but clindamycin penetrates very well and is a good choice for purulent osteitis and certain other tooth infections. The fluoroquinolones have excellent tissue penetration—attain high concentrations in soft tissues, lungs, prostate, joints, etc. Ciprofloxacin and rifampin have very good intracellular penetration. Cefuroxime, ceftriaxone, chloramphenicol, ciprofloxacin attain high CSF concentration. Ampicillin, cephalosporins and erythromycin attain high biliary concentration.

6. *Route of administration:* Many AMAs can be given orally as well as parenterally, but aminoglycosides, penicillin G, ticarcillin, many cephalosporins, vancomycin, etc. have to be given by injection only. For less severe infections, an oral antibiotic is preferable; but for serious infections, e.g. spreading cellulitis, meningitis, septicaemias, a parenteral antibiotic would be more reliable.

7. *Evidence of clinical efficacy:* Relative value of different AMAs in treating an infection is decided on the basis of comparative clinical trials. Optimum dosage regimens and duration of treatment are also determined on the basis of such trials. Reliable clinical trial data, if available, is the final guide for choice of the antibiotic.

8. *Cost:* Less expensive drugs are to be preferred.

COMBINED USE OF ANTIMICROBIALS

More than one AMAs are frequently used concurrently. This should be done only with a specific purpose and not blindly in the hope that if one is good, two should be better and three should cure almost any infection. The objectives of using antimicrobial combinations are:

1. **To achieve synergism** Every AMA has a specific effect on selected microorganisms. Depending on the drug pair as well as the organism involved, either synergism (supra-additive effect), additive action, indifference or antagonism may be observed when two AMAs belonging to different classes are used together.

Synergism may manifest in terms of decrease in the MIC of one AMA in the presence of another, or the MICs of both may be lowered. If the MIC of each AMA is reduced to 25% or less, the pair is considered synergistic, 25–50% of each is considered *additive* and more than 50% of each indicates *antagonism*. Thus, a synergistic drug sensitizes the organisms to the action of the other member of the pair. This may also manifest as a more rapid lethal action of the combination than either of the individual members resulting in faster cure of the infection. Synergistic prolongation of PAE has also been demonstrated for combinations of β-lactams with an aminoglycoside and by the addition of rifampin to a variety of antibiotics.

Every combination is unique; the same drugs may be synergistic for one organism but antagonistic for another. However, general principles are:

(a) Two bacteriostatic agents are often additive, but rarely synergistic, i.e. combination of tetracyclines, chloramphenicol, erythromycin, etc. A sulfonamide used with trimethoprim is a special case where supra-additive effect is obtained because of sequential block in folate metabolism (Ch. 26). The combination often exerts cidal action which is curative in some infections while the individual components are only static or ineffective in these.

(b) Two bactericidal drugs are frequently additive and sometimes synergistic if the organism is sensitive to both, e.g.:
- Penicillin/ampicillin + streptomycin/gentamicin for enterococcal SABE
- Ticarcillin + gentamicin for *Pseudomonas* infection, especially in neutropenic patients
- Rifampin + isoniazid in tuberculosis.

In the above cases, the combination produces faster cure and reduces the chances of relapse by more complete eradication of the pathogen.

(c) Combination of a bactericidal with a bacteriostatic drug may be synergistic or antagonistic depending on the organism. Antagonism is possible because cidal drugs act primarily on rapidly multiplying bacteria, while the static drug retards multiplication. On the other hand, synergism has been observed in case of:
- Penicillin + sulfonamide for actinomycosis
- Streptomycin + chloramphenicol for *K. pneumoniae* infection

Thus, wherever possible, synergistic combinations may be used to treat infections that are normally difficult to cure. Full doses of individual drugs are given for this purpose.

2. To prevent emergence of resistance Mutation conferring resistance to one AMA is independent of that conferring resistance to another. If the incidence of resistant mutants of a bacillus infecting an individual for drug P is 10^{-5} and for drug Q is 10^{-7}, then only one out of 10^{12} bacilli will be resistant to both. The chances of its surviving host defence and causing a relapse would be meagre.

This principle of using two or more AMAs together is valid primarily for chronic infections needing prolonged therapy. It has been widely employed in tuberculosis, leprosy and now adopted for malaria, *H. pylori*, HIV as well. It is of little value in most acute and short-lived infections.

3. To broaden the spectrum of antimicrobial action This is needed in:

(a) Treatment of mixed infection Many orodental infections are mixed infections, as are bronchiectasis, peritonitis, certain urinary tract infections, brain abscesses, diabetic foot infection, bedsores, and gynaecological infections. In these infections often both aerobic and anaerobic organisms sensitive to different drugs are involved. Obviously, two or more AMAs have to be used to cover the pathogens. Drugs should be chosen preferably on the basis of bacteriological diagnosis and sensitivity pattern, and should be employed in full doses. Clindamycin or metronidazole are generally included to cover anaerobes. It may sometimes be possible to find a single agent effective against all the causative organisms.

(b) Initial treatment of severe infections Where bacterial diagnosis is not known; drugs covering both gram-positive and gram-negative (in certain situations anaerobes as well), e.g. ampicillin + gentamicin; cephalosporin or erythromycin + an aminoglycoside ± metronidazole or clindamycin, may be given together. Rational combinations increase the certainty of curing the infection in the first attempt, but should be continued only till bacteriological data become available. When the organism and its sensitivity has been determined, severity

of infection is in itself not an indication for combination therapy. Combinations should not be used as a substitute for accurate diagnosis.

(c) Topically Generally, AMAs which are not used systemically, are poorly absorbed from the local site and cover a broad range of gram-positive and gram-negative bacteria are combined for topical application, e.g. bacitracin, neomycin, polymyxin B, fusidic acid.

Disadvantages of antimicrobial combinations

1. They foster a casual rather than rational outlook in the diagnosis of infections and choice of AMA.
2. Increased incidence and variety of adverse effects. Toxicity of one agent may be enhanced by another, e.g. vancomycin + tobramycin may produce exaggerated kidney damage.
3. Increased risk of superinfections.
4. If inadequate doses of nonsynergistic drugs are used — emergence of resistance may be promoted.
5. Higher cost of therapy.

PROPHYLACTIC USE OF ANTIMICROBIALS

This refers to the use of AMAs for preventing the setting in of an infection or suppressing contacted infection before it becomes clinically manifest. AMAs are frequently given prophylactically; but in a number of circumstances, this is at best wasteful if not harmful. The difference between treating an infection and preventing it is that treatment is directed against a specific organism infecting an individual patient, while prophylaxis is often against all organisms capable of causing infection.

Antimicrobial prophylaxis is highly successful when it is directed against specific organisms, e.g. use of benzathine penicillin to prevent streptococcal infection responsible for rheumatic fever, or isoniazid ± rifampicin to prevent tuberculosis in contacts, or mefloquine/doxycycline to prevent malaria in travellers to endemic areas. On the other hand, when it is intended to prevent infection in general, antibiotic prophylaxis often serves no purpose, may even be deleterious by increasing the likelihood of resistant infections. It is not possible to prevent all infections at all times in all individuals. Use of antibiotics in patients of viral upper respiratory infections to prevent secondary bacterial invasion, or to cover clean elective surgery or normal labour, or to prevent chest infection in unconscious patients falls in this category.

Though the merit of antibiotic prophylaxis in certain high-risk situations has been questioned, it is frequently given in case of:
(a) Dirty contaminated wounds (e.g. from roadside accidents).
(b) Catheterization/instrumentation of urinary tract, endoscopies.
(c) Chronic obstructive lung disease: to prevent acute exacerbation.
(d) Immunocompromised patients.
(e) Surgical wound infection.

Antimicrobial prophylaxis in dentistry

This is warranted for two distinct purposes, *viz.*
- Prevention of local wound infection, and
- Prevention of distant infection (e.g. bacterial endocarditis) in predisposed patients following dental procedures.

Prophylaxis of dental wound infection

Wound infection occurs due to microbial contamination of the surgical site. It is important for the dental surgeon to see that the wound left after tooth extraction or other surgery does not get infected. Use of sterile instruments, cross-infection control measures (antiseptic/disinfectant, etc.) and good surgical technique to minimise tissue damage, haematoma formation, and local devascularization are the primary, and often the only measures needed. In addition, systemic antimicrobial prophylaxis is advocated in selected situations.

Prophylaxis should be employed only when there is a clear risk of wound infection that outweighs the possible drawbacks of antibiotic use. In general, antibiotic prophylaxis is not required for routine dental surgery, except in patients at special risk. Simple extractions and minor periodontal procedures in otherwise healthy subjects are associated with very low risk of wound infection. Incidence of postoperative infection is quite low even after difficult surgery such as removal of impacted third molar, and antimicrobial prophylaxis is not required. However, it may be given when surgery involves extensive instrumentation, bone cutting or is prolonged. It has been found that the incidence of postoperative infection is higher when oral surgery had lasted 2 hours or more. Prophylaxis should also be given for procedures in which a prosthesis is inserted into the bone or soft tissue, such as dental implants. Extensive reconstructive surgery of upper or lower jaw also warrants antibiotic prophylaxis.

All orodental procedures which disturb/damage mucosa including extractions, scaling, etc. need to be covered by prophylaxis in diabetics, corticosteroid recipients and in other immunocompromised subjects.

The selection of drug, dose, timing and duration of prophylactic medication is crucial. It is important that the antibiotic is not started prematurely and is not continued beyond the time when bacteria have access to the surgical wound. Administration of the AMA has to be so timed that peak blood levels occur when the clot is forming in the surgical wound. Thus, most of the oral drugs are given 1 hour before tooth extraction or other short procedures, while i.v. or i.m. drugs are given just prior to it. Most of the AMAs do not penetrate the clot once it is formed and is older than 3 hours. Thus, late and prolonged presence of the antibiotic in circulation serves no purpose, but can foster resistant organisms. However, when the surgery has been performed in the presence of local infection, continuation of the prophylactic AMA beyond 4 hours after the dental procedure may be justified. In case of prolonged dental surgery, the antibiotic may be repeated i.v. during the procedure.

To be maximally effective, a relatively high dose of the AMA is selected which yields peak blood levels several times higher than MIC for the common oral pathogens. Because the resident oral flora is generally the source of the infecting organism for dental surgery wounds, the prophylactic AMA should be active against gram-positive cocci and oral anaerobes. Being bactericidal and safe, amoxicillin is generally the first choice drug. The commonly employed antibiotics for prevention of wound infection in dentistry are listed in the box.

Oral (single dose given 1 hour before procedure)

1. Amoxicillin 2 g (50 mg/kg)
2. Cephalexin   2 g (50 mg/kg)
3. Cefadroxil   2 g (50 mg/kg)
4. Clindamycin 600 mg (20 mg/kg) } For patients allergic to penicillin
5. Azithromycin 500 mg (15 mg/kg)

Parenteral (single injection just before procedure)

1. Ampicillin 2 g (50 mg/kg) i.m/i.v
2. Cefazolin   1 g (25 mg/kg) i.v.
3. Clindamycin 600 mg (20 mg/kg) i.v. for penicillin allergic patients

Prophylaxis of distant infection

Injury (dental procedure) to a mucosa that is laden with bacteria introduces some of these into the bloodstream. Transient bacteraemia occurs regularly during dental extraction, scaling, intraligamentary local anaesthetic injection, root canal treatment, placement of dental implant or any other procedure in which the gingival margin is manipulated. The blood-borne bacteria can cause life-threatening endocarditis in subjects with postrheumatic or congenital endocardial abnormalities such as mitral stenosis and other valvular defects, artificial heart valves or previous history of bacterial endocarditis. As such, it is imperative that the above-mentioned orodental procedures are covered with antibiotic prophylaxis in susceptible individuals.

Though prophylaxis has also been advocated by some experts for subjects with hip/knee joint replacement and other orthopedic prosthesis, this is considered unnecessary by others because of lack of evidence that prosthetic joint gets infected following dental procedures. However, due to serious nature of infection at these sites, prophylaxis may be given to patients at special risk such as recent joint replacement, past history of prosthetic joint infection and patients with rheumatoid arthritis.

The same antibiotics and regimens listed above for prevention of dental wound infection can be employed for prophylaxis of distant infections. However, since patients with prosthetic heart valves, those with history of bacterial endocarditis in the past and those to be operated under general anaesthesia are considered to be at greater risk and have a poorer prognosis if they develop bacterial endocarditis, it has been advocated that gentamicin 120 mg (2 mg/kg) i.m./i.v. may be given just before the dental procedure in addition to amoxicillin (or its substitute) and another dose of amoxicillin 500 mg (12.5 mg/kg) be repeated 6 hours after the procedure.

An alternative regimen used in patients allergic to penicillin is vancomycin 1 g (20 mg/kg) i.v. over 2 hours + gentamicin 120 mg (2 mg/kg) i.m./i.v. just before the procedure.

Antiseptic rinse with chlorhexidine (0.2%) held in the mouth for 1 minute just before dental treatment has been advocated as an adjuvant measure because it has been shown to reduce the severity of bacteraemia following dental extraction.

FAILURE OF ANTIMICROBIAL THERAPY

Antimicrobials may fail to cure an infection/fever, or there may be relapses. This is rare when antimicrobial therapy was begun, in the first place, on sound clinical and/or bacteriological basis. When a real or apparent failure of the antimicrobial regimen occurs, the diagnosis and therapy should be reviewed. One of the following causes will usually be identified:
1. Improper selection of drug, dose, route or duration of treatment.
2. Treatment begun too late.
3. Failure to take necessary adjuvant measures, e.g. drainage of abscesses, empyema, etc.; removal of renal stones, other foreign bodies; cavity closure; control of diabetes, etc.
4. Poor host defence—as in leukaemias, neutropenia and other causes; especially if bacteriostatic AMA is used.
5. Infecting organism present behind barriers, such as vegetation on heart valves (in SABE), inside the eyeball, blood-brain barrier.

Sulfonamides, Cotrimoxazole, Quinolones and Nitroimidazoles

SULFONAMIDES

Sulfonamides were the first antimicrobial agents (AMAs) effective against pyogenic bacterial infections. Sulfonamido-chrysoidine (Prontosil Red) was one of the dyes included by Domagk to treat experimental streptococcal infection in mice and found it to be highly effective. Subsequently an infant was cured of staphylococcal septicaemia (which was 100% fatal at that time) by prontosil. By 1937, it became clear that prontosil was broken down in the body to release *sulfanilamide* which was the active antibacterial agent. A large number of sulfonamides were produced and used extensively, but because of rapid emergence of bacterial resistance and the availability of many safer and more effective antibiotics, they are currently used only in combination with trimethoprim (as cotrimoxazole) or pyrimethamine (for malaria).

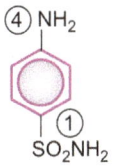

SULFANILAMIDE

Chemistry All sulfonamides may be considered to be derivatives of sulfanilamide (p-aminobenzene sulfonamide). Individual members differ in the nature of N ① (Sulfonamido N) substitution, which governs solubility, potency and pharmacokinetic property. A free amino group in the para position N ④ is required for antibacterial activity.

Sulfonamides that are still of clinical interest are listed below:

Antibacterial spectrum

Sulfonamides are primarily bacteriostatic against many gram-positive and gram-negative bacteria. However, bactericidal

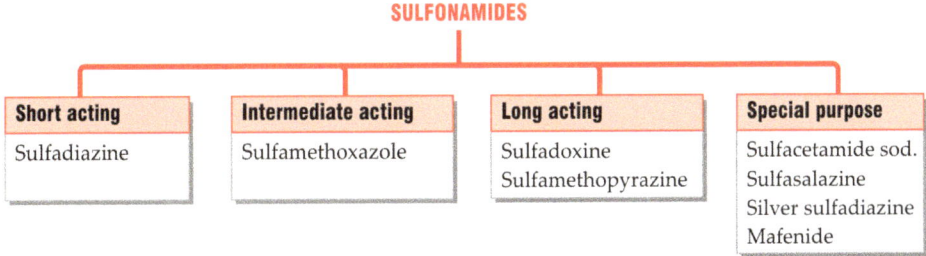

concentrations may be attained in urine. Sensitivity patterns among microorganisms have changed from time to time and place to place. Those still sensitive are:

many *Strepto. pyogenes, Haemophilus influenzae, H. ducreyi, Calymmatobacterium granulomatis, Vibrio cholerae.* Only a few gonococci, meningococci, pneumococci, *Escherichia coli,* and *Shigella* respond, but majority are resistant. Anaerobic bacteria are not susceptible.

Chlamydiae: trachoma, lymphogranuloma venereum, inclusion conjunctivitis, and *Actinomyces, Nocardia* and *Toxoplasma* are sensitive.

Mechanism of action
Many bacteria synthesize their own folic acid (FA) of which p-aminobenzoic acid (PABA) is a constituent, and is taken up from the medium. Sulfonamides being structural analogues of PABA, competitively inhibit bacterial folate synthase, so that FA is not formed and a number of essential metabolic reactions suffer.

Host cells also require FA, but they utilize preformed FA supplied in diet and are unaffected by sulfonamides. Evidences in favour of this mechanism of action of sulfonamides are:

(a) PABA, in small quantities, antagonizes the antibacterial action of sulfonamides.
(b) Only those microbes which synthesize their own FA, and cannot take it from the medium are susceptible to sulfonamides.

Pus and tissue extracts contain purines and thymidine which decrease bacterial requirement for FA and antagonize sulfonamide action. Pus is also rich in PABA.

Resistance to sulfonamides
Most bacteria are capable of developing resistance to sulfonamides. Prominent among these are gonococci, pneumococci, *Staph. aureus,* meningococci, *E. coli, Shigella, Strep. pyogenes, Strep. viridans* and anaerobes. The resistant mutants either:

(a) produce increased amounts of PABA, or
(b) their folate synthase enzyme has low affinity for sulfonamides, or
(c) adopt an alternative pathway in folate metabolism.

When an organism is resistant to one sulfonamide, it is resistant to them all. No cross resistance between sulfonamides and other class of AMAs has been noted. Development of resistance has markedly limited the clinical usefulness of this class of compounds.

Pharmacokinetics
Sulfonamides are nearly completely absorbed from g.i.t. Extent of plasma protein binding differs considerably (10–95%) among different members. The highly protein bound members are longer acting. Sulfonamides are widely distributed in the body. They enter CSF and cross placenta.

The primary pathway of metabolism of sulfonamides is acetylation at N^4 by nonmicrosomal N-acetyl transferase, primarily in liver. The acetylated derivative is inactive, but can contribute to the adverse effects. It is generally less soluble in acidic urine—may precipitate and cause crystalluria.

Sulfonamides are excreted mainly by the kidney. The more lipid-soluble members are highly reabsorbed in the tubule, therefore are longer acting.

Sulfamethoxazole Due to slower oral absorption and urinary excretion it has intermediate duration of action. The t½ in adults averages 10 hours. It is the preferred compound for combining with trimethoprim because the t½ of both is similar.

Sulfadoxine, Sulfamethopyrazine These are ultralong acting compounds, action lasting > 1 week because of high plasma protein binding and slow renal excretion (t½ 5–9 days). They attain low plasma concentration (of free form) and are not suitable for treatment of acute pyogenic infections. They are used in combination with pyrimethamine in the treatment of malaria, *Pneumocystis jiroveci* pneumonia in AIDS patients and in toxoplasmosis. They have caused serious cutaneous reactions.

Sulfacetamide sod. It is a highly soluble compound yielding neutral solution which is only mildly irritating to the eye in concentrations up to 30%. It is used topically for ocular infections caused by susceptible bacteria and chlamydia.

Sulfasalazine It is used in ulcerative colitis and rheumatoid arthritis (see p. 312).

Mafenide It is not a typical sulfonamide, because a —CH_2— bridge separates the benzene ring and the amino group. It is used only topically for infections caused by *Pseudomonas,* clostridia and for burn dressing to prevent infection.

Silver sulfadiazine Used topically as 1% cream for burn dressing. It is active against a large number of bacteria and fungi, even those resistant to other sulfonamides, e.g. *Pseudomonas*. It slowly releases silver ions which appear to be largely responsible for the antimicrobial action.

Adverse effects

Adverse effects to sulfonamides are relatively common. Sulfonamides can cause nausea, vomiting epigastric pain, crystalluria due to precipitation of the drug or its metabolite in urine, rashes and hepatitis. Stevens-Johnson syndrome and other severe cutaneous reactions have been reported, especially with long acting sulfonamides. Haemolysis can occur in G-6PD deficient subjects.

Uses

Systemic use of sulfonamides alone (not combined with trimethoprim or pyrimethamine) is rare now.

Ocular sulfacetamide sod. (10–30%) is a cheap alternative in trachoma/inclusion conjunctivitis. Topical silver sulfadiazine or mafenide are used for preventing infection on burn surfaces.

COTRIMOXAZOLE

The fixed dose combination of trimethoprim and sulfamethoxazole is called *cotrimoxazole*. Trimethoprim is a diaminopyrimidine related to the antimalarial drug pyrimethamine which selectively inhibits *bacterial dihydrofolate reductase* (DHFRase). Cotrimoxazole introduced in 1969 causes sequential block of folate metabolism as depicted in Fig. 26.1. Trimethoprim is >50,000 times more active against bacterial DHFRase than against the mammalian enzyme. Thus, human folate metabolism is not interfered at antibacterial concentrations of trimethoprim. Individually, both sulfonamide and trimethoprim are bacteriostatic, but the combination becomes cidal against many organisms.

Sulfamethoxazole was selected for combining with trimethoprim because both have nearly the same t½ (~ 10 hr). Optimal synergy in case of most organisms is exhibited at a concentration ratio of sulfamethoxazole 20 : trimethoprim 1, and the MIC of each component may be reduced by 3–6 times. The 20:1 ratio is obtained in the plasma when sulfamathoxazole and trimethoprim are given in a dose ratio of 5 : 1, because trimethoprim enters many tissues, has a larger volume of distribution than sulfamethoxazole and attains lower plasma concentration. However, the concentration ratio in many tissues is less than 20 : 1. Trimethoprim adequately crosses blood-brain barrier and placenta, while sulfamethoxazole has a poorer entry. Moreover, trimethoprim is more rapidly absorbed than sulfamethoxazole, so that their concentration ratios may vary with time. Trimethoprim is 40% plasma protein bound, while sulfamethoxazole is 65% bound. Trimethoprim is partly metabolized in liver and excreted in urine.

Spectrum of action Antibacterial spectra of trimethoprim and sulfonamides overlap considerably. Additional organisms covered by the combination are—*Salmonella typhi, Serratia, Klebsiella, Enterobacter, Yersinia enterocolitica, Pneumocystis jiroveci* and many sulfonamide-resistant strains of *Staph. aureus, Strep. pyogenes, Shigella,*

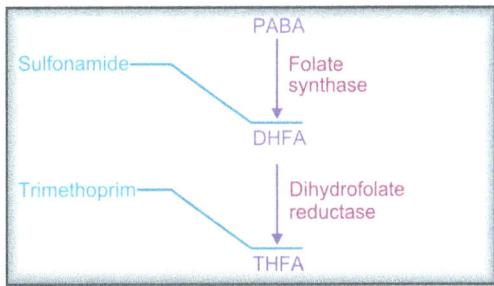

Fig. 26.1: Sequential block in bacterial folate metabolism
PABA—Paraaminobenzoic acid; DHFA—Dihydrofolic acid; THFA—Tetrahydrofolic acid

enteropathogenic *E. coli, H.influenzae*, gonococci and meningococci.

Resistance Bacteria are capable of acquiring resistance to trimethoprim mostly through mutational or plasmid mediated acquisition of a DHFRase having lower affinity for the inhibitor. Resistance to the combination has been slow to develop compared to either drug alone. Widespread use of the combination has resulted in reduced responsiveness of many originally sensitive strains.

Adverse effects All adverse effects seen with sulfonamides can be produced by cotrimoxazole.
- Nausea, vomiting, stomatitis, headache and rashes are the usual manifestations.
- Folate deficiency (megaloblastic anaemia) is infrequent, occurs only in patients with marginal folate levels.
- Blood dyscrasias occur rarely.

Cotrimoxazole should not be given during pregnancy. Trimethoprim being an antifolate, there is theoretical teratogenic risk. Neonatal haemolysis and methaemoglobinaemia can occur if it is given to the mother near term.

Patients with renal disease may develop uraemia. Dose should be reduced in moderately severe renal impairment.

Preparations SEPMAX, CIPLIN, ORIPRIM, SUPRISTOL, FORTRIM

Trimethoprim		Sulfamethoxazole
80 mg	+	400 mg tab: 2 BD for 2 days then 1 BD.
160 mg	+	800 mg tab: double strength (DS); 1 BD.
20 mg	+	100 mg pediatric tab.
40 mg	+	200 mg per 5 ml susp; infant 2.5 ml (not to be used in newborns), children 1–5 yr 5 ml, 6–12 year 10 ml (all BD).

Uses

The popularity of cotrimoxazole for treatment of systemic infections has declined. It is still useful in tonsillitis, pharyngitis, sinusitis, otitis media, chronic bronchitis, etc. but is *only occasionally employed for orodental infections; possibly as an alternative drug for patients allergic to β-lactam antibiotics.* Urinary tract infections, both acute as well as recurrent cases and those with prostatitis are its major indications now. Many cases of bacterial diarrhoeas and dysentery respond to cotrimoxazole. Used in high doses, it is a first line drug for *Pneumocystis jiroveci* pneumonia in AIDS patients.

QUINOLONES

These are synthetic antimicrobials having a quinolone structure. They are active primarily against gram-negative bacteria, though the newer fluorinated compounds also inhibit gram-positive ones. The first member *Nalidixic acid* introduced in mid-1960s had usefulness restricted to urinary and g.i. tract infections because of low potency, modest blood and tissue levels, limited spectrum of activity, and high frequency of bacterial resistance. A breakthrough was achieved in the early 1980s by fluorination of the quinolone structure at position 6 and introduction of a piperazine substitution at position 7 resulting in derivatives called *fluoroquinolones (FQs)* with high potency, expanded spectrum, slow development of

NALIDIXIC ACID

CIPROFLOXACIN

resistance, better tissue penetration and good tolerability.

Nalidixic acid

It is active against gram-negative bacteria, especially coliforms: *E. coli, Proteus, Klebsiella, Enterobacter, Shigella* but not *Pseudomonas*. It acts by inhibiting bacterial DNA gyrase and is bactericidal. Resistance to nalidixic acid develops rather rapidly.

Nalidixic acid is absorbed orally, partly metabolized in liver and excreted in urine with a plasma t½ ~8 hrs. Concentration of the free drug in plasma and most tissues is nontherapeutic for systemic infections. However, high concentration attained in urine (20–50 times than in plasma) is lethal to the common urinary pathogens.

Adverse effects
Side effects are g.i. upset and rashes. Most important toxicity is neurological—headache, drowsiness, vertigo, visual disturbances, occasionally seizures.
Dose: 0.5–1 g TDS or QID; GRAMONEG, DIARLOP, 0.5 g tab, 0.3 g/5 ml susp.

Use: Nalidixic acid has poor activity against oral pathogens and has no utility in dentistry. It is occasionally used as a urinary antiseptic and in diarrhoea.

FLUOROQUINOLONES

These are quinolone antimicrobials having one or more fluorine substitutions. The 'first generation' fluoroquinolones (FQs) introduced in 1980s have one fluoro substitution. In the 1990s, compounds with additional fluoro and other substitutions have been developed—further extending antimicrobial activity to gram-positive cocci and anaerobes, and/or confering metabolic stability (longer t½). These are referred to as 'second generation' FQs.

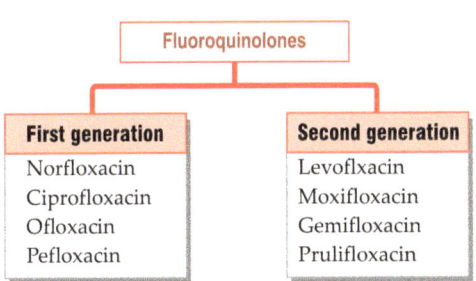

Mechanism of action The FQs inhibit the enzyme *bacterial DNA gyrase* (found in gram negative bacteria) which nicks double-stranded DNA, introduces negative supercoils and then reseals the nicked ends. This is necessary to prevent excessive positive supercoiling of the strands when they separate to permit replication or transcription. The DNA gyrase consists of two A and two B subunits; the A subunit carries out nicking of DNA, B subunit introduces negative supercoils and then A subunit reseals the strands. FQs bind to A subunit with high affinity and interfere with its strand cutting and resealing function.

In gram-positive bacteria the major target of FQ action is a similar enzyme called *topoisomerase IV* which nicks and separates daughter DNA strands after DNA replication. Greater affinity for topoisomerase IV may confer higher potency against gram-positive bacteria. The bactericidal action probably results from digestion of the DNA by exonucleases whose production is signalled by the damaged DNA.

In place of DNA gyrase or topoisomerase IV, the mammalian cells possess an enzyme topoisomerase II (that also removes positive supercoils) which has very low affinity for FQs—hence the low toxicity to host cells.

Mechanism of resistance Because of the unique mechanism of action, plasmid mediated transferable resistance is less likely. Resistance noted so far is due to chromosomal mutation producing a DNA gyrase or topoisomerase IV with reduced affinity for FQs, or due to reduced permeability/increased efflux of these drugs across bacterial membranes. In contrast to nalidixic acid, the FQ-resistant mutants are not easily selected. Therefore, resistance to FQs has been slow to develop. However, increasing resistance has been reported among *Salmonella, Pseudomonas,* staphylococci, gonococci and pneumococci.

Ciprofloxacin (prototype)

It is the most potent first generation FQ active against a broad range of bacteria; the most susceptible ones are the aerobic gram-negative bacilli, especially the Enterobacteriaceae and *Neisseria*. The MIC of ciprofloxacin against these bacteria is usually < 0.1 µg/ml, while gram-positive bacteria are inhibited at relatively higher concentrations. The spectrum of action is summarized below:

Highly susceptible

E. coli	Neisseria gonorrhoeae
K. pneumoniae	N. meningitidis
Enterobacter	H. influenzae
Salmonella typhi	H. ducreyi
Nontyphoid Salmonella	Campylobacter jejuni
Shigella	Yersinia enterocolitica
Proteus	Vibrio cholerae

Moderately susceptible

Pseudomonas aeruginosa	Legionella
Mycoplasma	Brucella
Chlamydia pneumophila	Listeria
Staph. epidermidis	Bacillus anthracis
Branhamella catarrhalis	Mycobact. tuberculosis

Organisms which have shown low/variable susceptibility are: *Strep. pyogenes, Strep. faecalis, Strep. pneumoniae, MRSA, Mycobact. kansasii, Mycobact. avium.*

Notable resistant bacteria are: *Bacteroides fragilis, Clostridia,* anaerobic cocci. As such, majority of oral pathogens are not covered by ciprofloxacin (and other FQs).

The distinctive microbiological features of ciprofloxacin (also other FQs) are:
- Bactericidal activity and high potency.
- Relatively long postantibiotic effect on Enterobacteriaceae, *Pseudomonas* and *Staph*.
- Low frequency of mutational resistance.
- Low propensity to select plasmid type resistant mutants.
- Protective intestinal streptococci and anaerobes are spared.
- Less active at acidic pH.

Pharmacokinetics Ciprofloxacin is rapidly absorbed orally, but food delays absorption, and first pass metabolism occurs. The pharmacokinetic parameters are given in Table 26.1. Ciprofloxacin (and other FQs except norfloxacin) attain bactericidal levels in blood, and have good tissue penetrability. Concentration in lung, sputum, muscle, prostate and phagocytes exceeds that in plasma, but CSF and aqueous levels are lower. It is excreted primarily in urine, both by glomerular filtration and tubular secretion. Urinary and biliary concentrations are 10–50-fold higher than plasma.

Adverse effects Ciprofloxacin has good safety record: side effects occur in ~10% patients, but are generally mild; discontinuation is needed only in 1.5%.
- Gastrointestinal: nausea, vomiting, bad taste, anorexia. Because gut anaerobes are not affected—diarrhoea is infrequent.
- CNS: dizziness, headache, restlessness, anxiety, insomnia, impairment of concentration. Tremor and seizures are rare, occur only at high doses.
- Skin/hypersensitivity: rash, pruritus, photosensitivity, urticaria, swelling of lips, etc.
- Tendonitis and tendon rupture: few cases are reported; risk is higher after 60 years age.

Ciprofloxacin and other FQs are contraindicated during pregnancy. Use in children requires caution due to fear of damage to weight bearing joints.

Interactions

- Plasma concentration of theophylline is increased by ciprofloxacin due to inhibition of metabolism. CNS toxicity can occur. Warfarin levels are also increased.

Table 26.1: Pharmacokinetic characteristics and doses of fluoroquinolones

	CIPROFL	NORFL	PEFL	OFL	LEVOFL	GEMI	PRULI	MOXI
1. Oral bioavailability (%)	60–80	35–45	90–100	85–95	~100	70	90	85
2. Plasma protein binding (%)	20–35	15	20–30	25	25	55–73	45	40
3. Vol. of distribution (L/kg)	3–4	2	2	1.5	1.3	–	–	2
4. Percent metabolized	20	25	85	5–10	5	–	>90	70–80
5. Elimination t½ (hr)	3–5	4–6	8–14	5–8	8	7	10–12	10–15
6. Routes of administration	oral, i.v.	oral	oral, i.v.	oral, i.v.	oral, i.v.	oral	oral	oral, i.v.
7. Dose (mg) : oral	250–750 (BD)	400 (BD)	400 (BD)	200–400 (BD)	500 (OD)	320 (OD)	600 (OD)	400 (OD)
: i.v.	100–200	—	400	200	500	—	—	400

- NSAIDs may enhance the CNS toxicity of FQs; seizures are reported.
- Antacids, sucralfate and iron salts given concurrently reduce absorption of FQs.

CIFRAN, CIPLOX, CIPROBID, QUINTOR, CIPROLET 250, 500, 750 mg tab, 200 mg/100 ml i.v. infusion, 3 mg/ml eye drops.

Uses Ciprofloxacin is effective in a broad range of infections including some difficult to treat ones. Because of wide spectrum bactericidal activity, oral efficacy and good tolerability, it is being extensively employed for blind therapy of any infection, but should not be used for minor cases or where gram-positive organisms and/or anaerobes are primarily causative. As such, it is *not a suitable drug for majority of orodental infections*. The only specific indication is infection caused by susceptible *Pseudomonas*, but such infection are rare in dental practice. Because ofloxacin and moxifloxacin are more active against gram-positive bacteria and anaerobes, these FQs *have greater potential utility in dentistry*. Ciprofloxacin may be combined with metronidazole for some refractory mixed infections like periodontitis.

Ciprofloxacin is a very popular drug for many systemic infections, *viz.* urinary tract infection, bacterial gastroenteritis, gonorrhoea caused by penicillinase producing as well as nonpenicillinase producing gonococci, chancroid, skin and soft tissue infections, wound and gynaecological infections, skeletal infections, etc. It is not a primary drug for respiratory tract infections. In combination with other antibiotics, ciprofloxacin has been used for serious infections like gram-negative septicaemias, meningitis, etc. Initially, ciprofloxacin was effective in treating typhoid, but has become relatively unreliable now.

Norfloxacin It is less potent than ciprofloxacin. Gram-positive organisms and many *Pseudomonas* are not inhibited. Moreover, it attains lower and nontherapeutic concentration in tissues.

Norfloxacin is primarily used for urinary and genital tract infections. It is also good for bacterial diarrhoeas.

NORBACTIN, NORFLOX 200, 400, 800 mg tab, 3 mg/ml eye drops; UROFLOX, NORILET 200, 400 mg tab. BACIGYL 400 mg tab, 100 mg/5 ml susp.

Pefloxacin It is the methyl derivative of norfloxacin; more lipid soluble, completely absorbed orally, penetrates tissues better and attains higher plasma concentrations. It is highly metabolized—partly to norfloxacin which contributes to its activity. Pefloxacin has longer t½: cumulates on repeated dosing achieving plasma concentrations twice as high as after a single dose. Because of this, it is effective in some systemic infections in addition to those of the urinary and g.i. tract.

PELOX, 200, 400 mg tab, to be taken with meals; 400 mg/5 ml inj (to be diluted in 100–250 ml of glucose solution but not saline since it precipitates in presence of Cl ions), PERTI, 400 mg tab.

Ofloxacin This FQ is some what less active than ciprofloxacin against gram-negative bacteria, but equally or more potent than ciprofloxacin for gram-positive organisms and certain anaerobes. Thus, it is better suited for orodental infections. It also inhibits *M. tuberculosis*; and is highly active against *M. leprae*. For leprosy, it is being used in alternative multidrug therapy regimens.

Ofloxacin is relatively lipid soluble; oral bioavailability is high: attains higher plasma concentrations. It is excreted largely unchanged in urine; dose needs to be reduced in renal failure.

Ofloxacin is comparable to ciprofloxacin in the therapy of systemic and mixed infections. It is particularly suitable for chronic bronchitis and other respiratory or ENT infections.

ZANOCIN, TARIVID 100, 200, 400 mg tab; 200 mg/100 ml i.v. infusion, ZENFLOX also 50 mg/5 ml susp.

Levofloxacin It is the active levoisomer of ofloxacin having improved activity against *Strep. pneumoniae* and some other gram-positive and gram-negative bacteria. Anaerobes are moderately susceptible. Oral bioavailability of levofloxacin is nearly 100%; oral and i.v. doses are similar. It is mainly excreted unchanged and a single daily dose is sufficient. Pharmacokinetic interactions with other drugs are not significant.

The primary indication of levofloxacin is community-acquired pneumonia and exacerbations of chronic bronchitis, but can be used for some dental infections as well. High cure rates have been noted in sinusitis, pyelonephritis and skin/soft tissue infections. Levofloxacin is a component of the standard treatment regimen for multidrug resistant tuberculosis (MDR-TB).

LEVOFLOX, GLEVO, LEVODAY 250, 500, 750 mg tabs, 500 mg/100 ml inj.

Moxifloxacin Another long-acting 2nd generation FQ having high activity against *Str. pneumoniae*, other gram-positive bacteria including β-lactam/macrolide resistant ones and some anaerobes. It is the most active FQ against *M. tuberculosis*, and is used for MDR-TB Bacterial topoisomerase IV is the major target of action. Moxifloxacin is primarily used for pneumonias, bronchitis, sinusitis, otitis media, etc. and has been tried in orodental infections as an alternative drug. Excitation, irritability and insomnia are prominent side effects. It should not be given to patients predisposed to seizures and to those receiving proarrhythmic drugs, because it can prolong Q-T interval. Phototoxicity occurs rarely.

Dose: 400 mg OD; MOXIF, MOXICIP 400 mg tab., 400 mg/100 ml inj. VIGAMOX 0.5% eye drops.

Gemifloxacin This potent second generation FQ has enhanced activity against aerobic gram positive bacteria, including some resistant strains and certain anaerobes. Gemifloxacin is primarily indicated in pneumonia and exacerbations of chronic bronchitis. A higher incidence of skin rashes has been reported. It can enhance warfarin effect, and carries the risk of additive Q-T prolongation with other drugs.

Dose: 320 mg OD for 5-7 days.

GAMETOP, GEMBAX, TOPGEM 320 mg tab.

Prulifloxacin It is the prodrug of ulifloxacin, a broad spectrum FQ active against many gram negative and some gram positive bacteria, including *Staph. aureus* and *Strep. pneumoniae*. It is rapidly absorbed orally and converted to ulifloxacin by first pass metabolism. Ulifloxacin is excreted unchanged in urine. A single daily dose of 600 mg is effective in urinary tract as well as in respiratory tract infections. Tolerability profile is similar to ciprofloxacin. Photosensitivity is rare and it is claimed not to prolong Q-Tc interval.

ALPRULI, PRULIFACT PRULIFLOX 600 mg tab.

NITROIMIDAZOLES

Metronidazole

Metronidazole, the prototype member of this class was introduced in 1959 for trichomonas vaginitis and later found to be an effective antiprotozoal drug against *Entamoeba histolytica* and *Giardia lamblia* as well. Its efficacy in anaerobic bacterial infection was a chance discovery, and it is now extensively used to treat oral and other anaerobic bacterial infections. Several congeners of metronidazole have been subsequently produced, of which *Tinidazole*, *Secnidazole*, *Ornidazole* and *Satranidazole* are in clinical use.

Many anaerobic bacteria, such as *Bact. fragilis*, *Bact. melaninogenicus*, *Fusobacterium*, *Clostridium perfringens*, *Cl. difficile*, *Peptococcus*, *Peptostreptococcus*, *Prevotella*, *Veillonella*, *Campylobacter*, *Helicobacter pylori* and spirochetes are susceptible to metronidazole. Metronidazole does not affect aerobic bacteria. Clinically significant resistance has not developed among *E. histolytica*, but decreased responsiveness of *T. vaginalis* has been observed in some areas. Anaerobic bacteria can also develop metronidazole resistance, but this is not a clinical problem except in case of *H. pylori*.

Metronidazole is selectively toxic to anaerobic and microaerophilic microorganisms. After entering the cell by diffusion, its nitro group is reduced by certain redox proteins operative only in anaerobic microbes to a highly reactive nitro radical which exerts cytotoxicity. The nitro radical of metronidazole acts as an electron sink which competes with the biological electron acceptors of the anaerobic organism for the electrons generated by the pyruvate: ferredoxin oxidoreductase (PFOR) enzyme pathway of pyruvate oxidation. The energy metabolism of anaerobes is, thus, disrupted. Aerobic environment attenuates cytotoxicity of metronidazole by inhibiting its reductive activation. Anaerobes which develop metronidazole resistance have been found deficient in the mechanism that generates the reactive nitro radical from it or have lower levels of PFOR.

Metronidazole, in addition, has been found to inhibit cell-mediated immunity, to induce mutagenesis and to cause radiosensitization.

Pharmacokinetics Metronidazole is almost completely absorbed from the small intestines: little unabsorbed drug reaches the colon. It is widely distributed in the body, attaining therapeutic concentration in saliva vaginal secretion, semen, and CSF. Metabolism occurs in liver primarily by oxidation and glucuronide conjugation followed by excretion in urine. Plasma t½ is 8 hrs.

Adverse effects Side effects of metronidazole are relatively frequent and unpleasant, but mostly nonserious.

- Anorexia, nausea, bitter or metallic taste and abdominal cramps are the most common. Looseness of stool is occasional.
- Urticaria, flushing, heat, itching and erruptions occur in allergic subjects. This reaction warrants immediate stoppage of the drug and precludes future use of nitroimidazoles by such subjects.
- Less frequent side effects are—headache, glossitis, dryness of mouth and impairment of concentration.
- Prolonged administration may cause peripheral neuropathy and CNS effects. Seizures have followed very high doses. Leucopenia is likely with repeated courses.
- On i.v. injection, thrombophlebitis of injected vein occurs if the solution is not well diluted.

Metronidazole is contraindicated in neurological disease, blood dyscrasias, first trimester of pregnancy (though no teratogenic effect has yet been demonstrated, its mutagenic potential warrants caution) and chronic alcoholism.

Interactions A disulfiram-like intolerance to alcohol occurs in some patients taking metronidazole, while majority of people can take alcohol during metronidazole therapy without any reaction. Patients should be advised to exercise caution when metronidazole is prescribed.

Enzyme inducers (phenobarbitone, rifampin) may lower metronidazole levels and reduce its efficacy.

Cimetidine can retard metronidazole metabolism: its dose may need to be decreased.

Metronidazole enhances warfarin action by inhibiting its metabolism; prothrombin time of patients taking warfarin should be monitored when metronidazole is prescribed.

Metronidazole can decrease renal elimination of lithium and precipitate its toxicity.

Preparations

FLAGYL, METROGYL, METRON, ARISTOGYL 200, 400 mg tab, 200 mg/5 ml susp. (as benzoyl metronidazole: tasteless); 500 mg/100 ml i.v. infusion; UNIMEZOL 200, 400 mg tabs, 200 mg/5 ml susp. METROGYL GEL: 1% gel for vaginal/topical use on mucosa.

Uses

Oro-dental infections Metronidazole in a dose of 200–400 mg TDS (15–30 mg/kg/day) is extensively used to treat orodental infections, because anaerobic bacteria are frequently involved. Certain oral anaerobes not inhibited by penicillin/amoxicillin are susceptible to metronidazole.

It is the drug of choice for acute necrotizing ulcerative gingivitis (ANUG), also called 'trench mouth', which is caused by a mixed flora of anaerobes like fusobacteria, spirochetes and bacteroides. Amoxicillin, erythromycin or tetracycline are often combined with metronidazole for ANUG. The response is rapid with disappearance of the causative spirochete-fusobacterium complex from the lesions and resolution of pain, bleeding, ulceration and bad breath within 2 to 3 days. A 5-day course is often sufficient.

Periodontitis, pericoronitis, acute apical infections and some endodontic infections also respond well to metronidazole given for 5–7 days. Because it is not active against aerobic and facultative bacteria, metronidazole is mostly combined with a penicillin, cephalosporin or macrolide antibiotic.

Other bacterial infections Metronidazole is an effective drug for anaerobic bacterial infections that occur at sites other than oral cavity as well, e.g. following colorectal/pelvic surgery, appendicectomy, brain abscesses, endocarditis, etc. Because these are serious and often mixed infections, metronidazole is generally given i.v. (15 mg/kg over 1 hr) and combined with gentamicin or a 2nd/3rd generation cephalosporin. Oral metronidazole is the drug of choice for antibiotic associated pseudomembranous enterocolitis caused by *Cl. difficile*. Used along with clarithromycin/amoxicillin and a proton pump inhibitor, metronidazole is a component of triple drug therapy for eradication of *H. pylori* in patients with peptic ulcer/nonulcer dyspepsia. In combination with cefuroxime or gentamicin, metronidazole is given before gut and biliary tract surgery.

Protozoal infections The most important clinical use of metronidazole is to treat protozoal infections. It is the drug of choice for all forms of *amoebiasis*, including acute dysentery, chronic intestinal amoebiasis and liver abscess. It is also a first line drug for *intestinal giardiasis* and *trichomonas vaginitis*. Nonspecific bacterial vaginosis also responds to oral metronidazole.

Tinidazole It is an equally efficacious congener of metronidazole, similar to it in every way except:
- Metabolism is slower; t½ is ~12 hours; duration of action is longer; thus, it is

more suited for single dose or once daily therapy of amoebiasis, giardiasis and trichomoniasis.
- Some comparative trails in amoebiasis have reported higher cure rates.
- It is claimed to be better tolerated; the incidence of side effects is lower: metallic taste (2%), nausea (1%), rash (0.2%).

TINIBA 300, 500, 1000 mg tabs; 800 mg/400 ml i.v. infusion; TRIDAZOLE, 300, 500 mg tab; FASIGYN 0.5 g and 1 g tab.

For *orodental infections*, tinidazole is used in a dose of 0.5 g (10 mg/kg) BD for 5 days. In other serious anaerobic infections the recommended dose is 2 g orally followed by 0.5 g BD for 5 days. In case oral treatment is not possible, 800 mg can be infused slowly i.v. daily till oral therapy is instituted. A single 2 g (oral) or 0.8 g (i.v.) dose is given for prophylaxis of anaerobic infection before colorectal surgery.

Secnidazole A congener of metronidazole with the same spectrum of activity and potency. Absorption after oral administration is rapid and complete, but metabolism is slower resulting in a plasma t½ of 17–29 hours. In intestinal amoebiasis, a single 2 g dose has been found to yield cure rates equal to multiple doses of metronidazole and tinidazole. Side effect profile is similar to metronidazole and the reported incidence is 2–10%. Secnidazole can be used as an alternative to metronidazole in dentistry, but has not gained popularity.

SECNIL, SECZOL 0.5, 1.0 g tabs; NOAMEBA-DS 1.0 g tab.

Ornidazole It has activity similar to metronidazole, but it is slowly metabolized—has longer t½ (12–14 hr). Dose and duration of regimens for amoebiasis, giardiasis, trichomoniasis, anaerobic infections and bacterial vaginosis resemble those for tinidazole. Side effect profile is also similar.

DAZOLIC 500 mg tab, 500 mg/100 ml vial for i.v. infusion. ORNIDA 500 mg tab, 125 mg/5 ml susp.

Satranidazole Another nitroimidazole having longer t½ (14 hr) and greater potency. It is claimed to be better tolerated; nausea, vomiting, metallic taste are absent or milder. Neurological and disulfiram-like reactions are less likely. It does not produce the acetamide metabolite which is a weak carcinogen. However, its role in dental infections has not been defined.

SATROGYL 300 mg tab.

Beta-Lactam Antibiotics

These are antibiotics having a β-lactam ring. The two major groups are penicillins and cephalosporins, which are the most commonly used antibiotics in dentistry. Monobactams and carbapenems are the later additions.

PENICILLINS

Penicillin was the first antibiotic to be used clinically in 1941. It is a miracle that the least toxic drug of its kind was the first to be discovered. It was originally obtained from the fungus *Penicillium notatum*, but the present source is a high yielding mutant of *P. chrysogenum*.

Chemistry and properties The penicillin nucleus consists of fused thiazolidine and β-lactam rings to which side chains are attached through an amide linkage (Fig. 27.1). Penicillin G (PnG), having a benzyl side chain (at R), is the original penicillin used clinically.

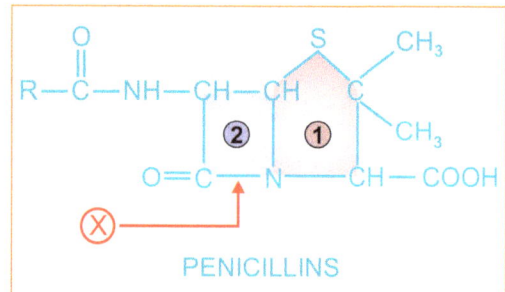

Fig. 27.1: Chemical structure of penicillins. (1) Thiazolidine ring; (2) Beta-lactam ring; (X) Bond which is broken by penicillinase (a β-lactamase).

The side chain of natural penicillin can be split off by an amidase to produce 6-amino-penicillanic acid. Other side chains can then be attached to it resulting in different semisynthetic penicillins with unique antibacterial activities and different pharmacokinetic properties.

At the carboxyl group attached to the thiazolidine ring, salt formation occurs with Na^+ and K^+. These salts are more stable than the parent acid. Sod. PnG is highly water soluble. It is stable in the dry state, but solution deteriorates rapidly at room temperature, though remains stable at 4° C for 3 days. Therefore, PnG solutions are always prepared freshly. PnG is also thermolabile and acid labile.

Unitage 1 U of crystalline sod. benzyl penicillin = 0.6 µg of the standard preparation. Accordingly 1 g = 1.6 million units or 1 MU = 0.6 g.

Mechanism of action

All β-lactam antibiotics interfere with the synthesis of bacterial cell wall. The bacteria synthesize UDP-N-acetyl muramic acid pentapeptide, called 'Park nucleotide' (because Park in 1957 found it to accumulate when susceptible *Staphylococcus* was grown in the presence of penicillin) and UDP-N-acetyl glucosamine. The peptidoglycan residues are linked together forming long strands and UDP is split off. The final step is cleavage of the terminal D-alanine of the peptide chains by transpeptidases; the energy so released is utilized for establishment of cross linkages between peptide chains of the neighbouring strands (Fig. 27.2). This cross linking provides stability and rigidity to the cell wall.

The β-lactam antibiotics inhibit the transpeptidases so that cross linking (which maintains the close knit structure of the cell wall) does not take place. These enzymes and related proteins constitute the *penicillin binding proteins (PBPs)* which have been located in the bacterial cell membrane. Each organism has several PBPs and PBPs obtained from different species differ in their affinity towards different β-lactam antibiotics. This fact probably explains their differing sensitivity to the various β-lactam antibiotics.

When bacteria divide in the presence of a β-lactam antibiotic—cell wall deficient (CWD) forms are produced. Because the interior of the bacterium is hyperosmotic, the CWD forms swell and burst; bacterial lysis occurs. This is how β-lactam antibiotics exert bactericidal action. Lytic effect of these antibiotics may also be due to derepression of some bacterial autolysins which normally function during cell division.

Rapid cell wall synthesis occurs when the organisms are actively multiplying; β-lactam antibiotics are more lethal in this phase.

The peptidoglycan cell wall is unique to bacteria. No such substance is synthesized (particularly, D-alanine is not utilized) by higher animals. This is why penicillin is practically nontoxic to man.

In gram-positive bacteria, the cell wall is almost entirely made of peptidoglycan, which is >50 layers thick and extensively cross linked, so that it may be regarded as a single giant mucopeptide molecule. In gram-

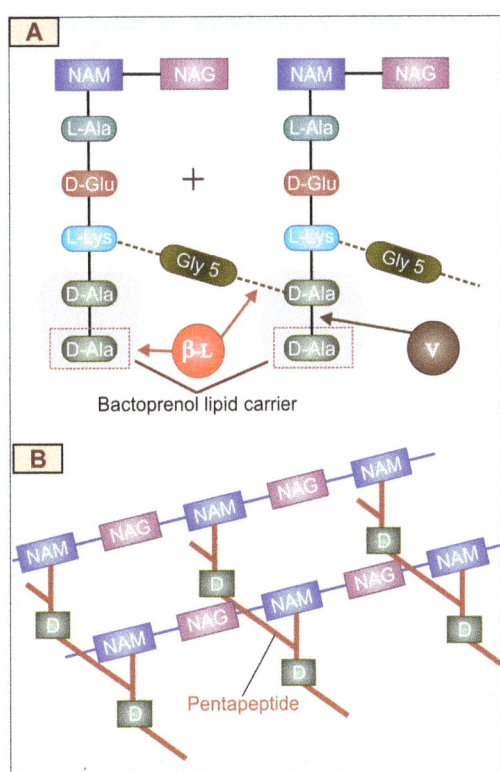

Fig. 27.2: Key features of bacterial cell wall synthesis and cell wall structure, depicting the site of action of β-lactam antibiotics and vancomycin
A. Cross linking of peptidoglycan residues of neighbouring strands by cleavage of terminal D-alanine (D-Ala) and transpeptidation with the chain of 5 glycine (Gly5) residues. The β-lactam antibiotics (β-L) block cleavage of terminal D-Ala and transpeptidation. The peptidoglycan units are synthesized within the bacterial cell and are transported across the cell membrane by attachment to a bactoprenol lipid carrier for assembly into strands. Vancomycin (V) binds tightly to the terminal D-Ala-D-Ala sequence and prevents its release from the carrier, so that further transpeptidation cannot take place.
B. The highly cross linked peptidoglycan strands in bacterial cell wall
NAM—N-acetyl muramic acid;
NAG—N-acetylglucosamine; L-Ala—L-alanine; D-Glu—D-glutamic acid; L-Lys—L-Lysine

negative bacteria, it consists of alternating layers of lipoprotein and peptidoglycan (each layer 1–2 molecule thick with little cross linking). This may be the reason for higher susceptibility of the gram-positive bacteria to PnG.

Blood, pus, and tissue fluids do not interfere with the antibacterial action of β-lactam antibiotics.

PENICILLIN-G (BENZYL PENICILLIN)

Antibacterial spectrum PnG is a narrow spectrum antibiotic; activity is limited primarily to gram-positive bacteria and few others.

Cocci: *Streptococci* (except *viridans*, group D or enterococci) are highly sensitive, so are many pneumococci. *Staph. aureus*, though originally very sensitive, has acquired resistance to such an extent that it must be counted out of PnG spectrum. Gram-negative cocci—*Neisseria gonorrhoeae* and *N. meningitidis* are susceptible to PnG, though increasing number of gonococci have developed partial to high degree resistance.

Bacilli: Gram-positive bacilli—majority of *B. anthracis, Corynebacterium diphtheriae*, and practically all *Clostridia* (*tetani* and others), *Listeria* are highly sensitive, so are spirochetes (*Treponema pallidum* and others), but *Bacteroides fragilis* is largely resistant, though *Bact. melaninogenicus* is susceptible. Other anaerobes involved in orodental infections such as fusobacteria, peptostreptococci, *Eubacterium, Campylobacter, Prevotella* and *Porphyromonas* are responsive to PnG.

Actinomyces israelii is only moderately sensitive. Majority of aerobic gram-negative bacilli, *Mycobacterium tuberculosis*, rickettsiae, chlamydiae, protozoa, fungi and viruses are totally insensitive to PnG.

Bacterial resistance Many bacteria are inherently insensitive to PnG because in them the target enzymes and PBPs are located deeper under lipoprotein barrier where PnG is unable to penetrate or they have low affinity for PnG. The primary mechanism of acquired resistance is production of penicillinase.

Penicillinase It is a narrow spectrum β-lactamase which opens the β-lactam ring to inactivate PnG and some closely related congeners. Majority of *Staphylococci*, some strains of gonococci, *B. subtilis, E. coli, H. influenzae* and few other bacteria produce penicillinase. The gram-positive penicillinase producers elaborate large quantities of the enzyme which diffuses into the surroundings and can protect other inherently sensitive bacteria as well. In gram-negative bacteria, penicillinase is found in small quantity, but is strategically located in between the lipoprotein and peptidoglycan layers of the cell wall. Staphylococcal penicillinase is inducible, and methicillin is an important inducer; while in gram-negative organisms, it is mostly a constitutive enzyme.

Some resistant bacteria become *penicillin tolerant* and not penicillin destroying. Their target enzymes are altered to have low affinity for penicillin, e.g. highly resistant pneumococci isolated in some areas have altered PBPs. The methicillin-resistant *Staph. aureus* (MRSA) have acquired a PBP which has very low affinity for β-lactam antibiotics. The low level penicillin-resistant gonococci become less permeable to the drug, while high degree resistant ones produce penicillinase, as do highly resistant *H. influenzae*. Both these organisms appear to have acquired the penicillinase plasmid by conjugation or transduction and then propagated it by selection.

The gram-negative bacteria have 'porin' channels formed by specific proteins located in their outer membrane. Permeability of various β-lactam antibiotics through these channels differs: ampicillin and other members, which are active against gram-negative bacteria, cross the porin channels much better than PnG. Some gram-negative bacteria become resistant by loss of, or alteration of porin channels.

Pharmacokinetics

Penicillin G is acid labile. It is destroyed by gastric acid. As such, less than 1/3rd of an oral dose is absorbed in the active form. Absorption of sod. PnG from i.m. site is rapid and complete; peak plasma level is attained in 30 min. PnG is distributed mainly extracellularly; reaches most body fluids, but penetration in serous cavities and CSF is poor. About 60% is plasma protein bound. Because of rapid excretion, very little PnG is metabolized.

The pharmacokinetics of PnG is dominated by very rapid renal excretion; about 10% by glomerular filtration and the rest by tubular secretion. The plasma t½ of PnG in healthy adult is 30 min. Neonates have slow tubular secretion—t½ of PnG is longer. Aged people and those with renal failure excrete penicillin slowly. Tubular secretion of penicillins is blocked by probenecid—higher and longer lasting plasma concentrations are achieved. In addition, probenecid decreases the volume of distribution of penicillins.

Preparations and dose

1. *Sod. penicillin G (crystalline penicillin) injection*: 0.5–5 MU i.m./i.v. 6–12 hourly. It is available as dry powder in vials to be dissolved in sterile water at the time of injection.
BENZYL PENICILLIN 0.5, 1 MU inj.

Repository penicillin G injections These are insoluble salts of PnG which must be given by deep i.m. (never i.v.) injection. They release PnG slowly at the site of injection, which then meets the same fate as soluble PnG.
1. *Procaine penicillin G inj.* 0.5–1 MU i.m. 12–24 hourly as aqueous suspension. Plasma concentrations attained are lower, but are sustained for 1–2 days; PROCAINE PENICILLIN-G 0.5, 1 MU dry powder in vial.
Fortified procaine penicillin G inj: contains 3 lac U procaine penicillin and 1 lac U sod. penicillin G to provide rapid as well as sustained blood levels. FORTIFIED P.P. INJ 3+1 lac U vial, BISTREPEN 6 + 4 lac U/vial.
2. *Benzathine penicillin G* 0.6–2.4 MU i.m. every 2–4 weeks as aqueous suspension. It releases penicillin extremely slowly—plasma concentrations are very low but remain effective for prophylactic purposes for up to 4 weeks.
PENDURE-LA (long acting), LONGACILLIN, 0.6, 1.2, 2.4 MU as dry powder in vial.

Adverse effects

PenicillinG is one of the most nontoxic antibiotics.

Local irritancy and toxicity Pain at i.m. injection site, nausea on oral ingestion and thrombophlebitis of injected vein are dose-related expressions of irritancy.

Hypersensitivity These reactions are the major problem in the use of penicillins. Individuals with an allergic diathesis are more prone to develop penicillin reactions. PnG is the most common drug implicated in drug allergy. This scare has eliminated it from general use.

Manifestations of penicillin allergy are—rash, itching, urticaria and fever. Wheezing, angioneurotic edema, serum sickness and exfoliative dermatitis are less common. Anaphylaxis is rare (1 to 4 per 10,000 patients) but may be fatal. Fear of causing anaphylactic shock has severely restricted the use of injected PnG.

All forms of natural and semisynthetic penicillins can cause allergy, but it is more commonly seen after parenteral than oral administration. Incidence is highest with procaine penicillin: procaine is itself allergenic. The course of penicillin hypersensitivity is unpredictable, i.e. an individual who tolerated penicillin earlier may show allergy on subsequent administration and *vice versa*.

There is partial cross sensitivity between different types of penicillins; an individual who has exhibited immediate type of hypersensitivity, i.e. urticaria, angioedema, bronchospasm, anaphylaxis or serum sickness with one penicillin should not be given any other type of penicillin. However, if the earlier reaction had been only a rash, penicillin may be given cautiously—often no untoward effect is seen. History of penicillin allergy must be elicited before injecting it. A scratch test or intradermal test (with 2–10 U) may be performed first. On occasions, this itself has caused fatal anaphylaxis. Testing with benzylpenicilloyl-polylysine is safer. However, a negative intradermal test does not rule out delayed hypersensitivity.

Topical use of penicillin is highly sensitizing (contact dermatitis and other reactions).

If a patient is allergic to penicillin, it is best to use an alternative antibiotic.

Uses

Penicillin G is the drug of choice for infections caused by organisms susceptible to it, unless the patient is allergic to this antibiotic. However, in practice it is hardly used due to fear of causing anaphylaxis.

1. *Dental infections* Parenteral PnG remains effective in majority of common infections encountered in dentistry, particularly those arising as a sequelae of carious lesions and are caused by both aerobic and anaerobic bacteria such as *Streptococci, Peptostreptococci, Eubacterium, Prevotella, Porphyromonas, Fusobacterium*. PnG can be used for periodontal abscess, periapical abscess, pericoronitis, acute suppurative pulpitis, oral cellulitis, etc. For *trench mouth* or acute necrotizing ulcerative gingivitis (ANUG) which is a mixed infection caused by spirochetes and fusobacteria, PnG (i.m.) or amoxicillin (oral) are generally combined with metronidazole. Penicillin G can also be employed prophylactically to cover dental procedures in patients at risk. However, many originally susceptible oral pathogens have acquired penicillin resistance and dental (as well as medical) practitioners are too scared to inject PnG unless there is no other choice. Therefore, *in dental practice, use of PnG is rare.*

2. *General medical uses* Other medical conditions treated with PnG are:
- Streptococcal infections: pharyngitis, tonsillitis, otitis media, scarlet fever, rheumatic fever, bacterial endocarditis caused by viridans *streptococci*.
- Pneumococcal infections (pneumonia, meningitis) only if the infecting strain is sensitive to PnG.
- Meningococcal meningitis and other meningococcal infections.
- Gonorrhoea caused by nonpenicillinase producing *N. gonorrhoeae* that are still sensitive to PnG.
- Syphilis: benzathine penicillin is the drug of choice for all stages of syphilis, because *T. pallidum* has not developed penicillin resistance.
- Diphtheria, tetanus and other rare infections like gas gangrene, anthrax, actinomycosis.

Prophylactic uses of PnG are:
- To prevent recurrence of rheumatic fever: benzathine penicillin is the preparation of choice.
- Surgical prophylaxis (in combination with gentamicin).
- To protect agranulocytosis patients (an aminoglycoside may be given in combination).

SEMISYNTHETIC PENICILLINS

Semisynthetic penicillins are produced by chemically combining specific side chains (in place of benzyl side chain of PnG) or by incorporating specific precursors in the mould cultures. Thus, procaine penicillin and benzathine penicillin are salts of PnG and *not* semisynthetic penicillins. The aim of producing semisynthetic penicillins is to overcome the shortcomings of PnG, which are:

1. Poor oral efficacy.
2. Susceptibility to penicillinase.
3. Narrow spectrum of activity.
4. Hypersensitivity reactions (this has not been overcome in any preparation).

In addition, some β-lactamase inhibitors have been developed which themselves are not antibacterial but augment the activity of penicillins against β-lactamase producing organisms.

Acid-resistant alternative to penicillin-G

Phenoxymethyl penicillin (Penicillin V)

It differs from PnG only in that it is acid stable; oral absorption is better; peak blood

Penicillins

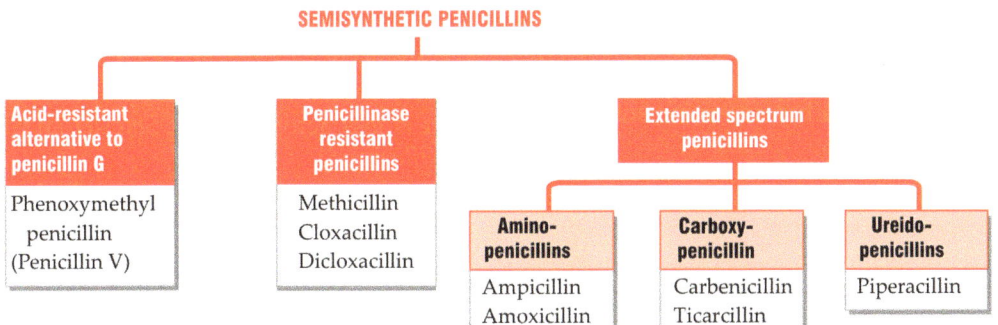

level is reached in 1 hour and plasma t½ is 30–60 min.

The antibacterial spectrum of penicillin V is identical to that of PnG, but it is less active against *Neisseria*, other gram-negative bacteria and anaerobes. Oral penicillin V may be used to treat some nonserious dental infections and trench mouth (ANUG), but it cannot be depended upon for more serious infections. Other conditions occasionally treated with penicillin V are streptococcal pharyngitis, sinusitis, otitis media and minor pneumococcal infections.

Dose: 250–500 mg, children 125–250 mg; given 6 hourly (250 mg = 4 lac U). CRYSTAPEN-V, KAYPEN, 125, 250 mg tab, 125 mg/5 ml dry syr—for reconstitution, PENIVORAL 65, 130 mg tab.

Penicillinase-resistant penicillins

These congeners have side chains that protect the β-lactam ring from attack by staphylococcal penicillinase. However, nonpenicillinase producing organisms are less sensitive to these drugs than to PnG. Their only indication is infections caused by penicillinase producing *Staphylococci*, but not methicillin-resistant *Staph. aureus* (MRSA). Clinical utility of these penicillins has markedly declined because MRSA have become universally prevalent.

Methicillin It is penicillinase resistant but not acid resistant. Methicillin is no longer clinically used, because it caused haematuria, interstitial nephritis and albuminuria. Moreover, MRSA are widespread now.

The MRSA are insensitive to cloxacillin and to other β-lactams, erythromycin, aminoglycosides and tetracyclines. The MRSA have altered PBPs which do not bind penicillins. The drug of choice for these organisms is vancomycin/linezolid.

Dicloxacillin/Cloxacillin It is highly penicillinase as well as acid resistant, but less active against PnG sensitive organisms: should not be used as substitute of PnG. It is more active than methicillin against penicillinase producing *Staph*, but not against MRSA. Because staphylococcal infections are rare in the oral cavity, *cloxacillin is infrequently used in dentistry*.

Cloxacillin is incompletely but dependably absorbed from oral route, especially if taken in empty stomach. It is > 90% plasma protein bound. Elimination occurs primarily by kidney, also partly by liver. Plasma t½ is about 1 hour.

Dose: 0.25–0.5 g orally every 6 hours; for severe infections 0.25–1 g may be injected i.m. or i.v.—higher blood levels are produced.

KLOX, BIOCLOX, 0.25, 0.5 g cap; 0.25, 0.5 g/vial inj. CLOPEN 0.25, 0.5 g cap.

Extended spectrum penicillins

These semisynthetic penicillins are in addition active against a variety of gram-negative bacilli, because of improved ability to penetrate through their cell membrane, but are susceptible to certain β-lactamases. They can be grouped according to the nature of the side chain substitution and spectrum of activity into amino-penicillins and carboxy/ureido-penicillins.

1. Aminopenicillins

This group, includes ampicillin and amoxicillin, and has an amino substitution in the side chain.

Ampicillin It is active against all organisms sensitive to PnG. In addition, several gram-negative bacilli, e.g. *H. influenzae, E. coli, Proteus, Salmonella, Shigella* and *Helicobacter pylori* are inhibited. However, due to widespread use, many of these bacteria have developed resistance; usefulness of this antibiotic has decreased considerably.

Ampicillin is more active than PnG for *Strep. viridans*, enterococci and *Listeria* (therefore better suited for dental infections), equally active for pneumococci, gonococci and meningococci, but penicillin-resistant strains are resistant to ampicillin as well. It is less active against other gram-positive cocci. Penicillinase producing *Staph.* are not affected, as are other gram-negative bacilli, such as *Pseudomonas, Klebsiella*, indole positive *Proteus* and anaerobes like *Bacteroides fragilis*.

Pharmacokinetics Ampicillin is not degraded by gastric acid; oral absorption is incomplete but adequate. Food interferes with absorption. It is partly excreted in bile and reabsorbed—enterohepatic circulation occurs. However, primary channel of excretion is kidney, but tubular secretion is slower than for PnG; plasma t½ is 1 hour.

Dose: 0.5–2 g oral/i.m./i.v. depending on severity of infection, every 6 hours; children 25–50 mg/kg/day. AMPILIN, ROSCILLIN, BIOCILIN 250, 500 mg cap; 125, 250 mg/5 ml dry syr; 100 mg/ml pediatric drops; 250, 500 mg and 1.0 g per vial inj.

Amoxicillin It is a close congener of ampicillin; similar to it in all respects except:
- Oral absorption is better; food does not interfere with absorption; higher and more sustained blood levels are produced.
- Incidence of diarrhoea is lesser.
- It is less active against *Shigella* and *H. influenzae*.
- It is more active against relatively penicillin resistant *Strep. pneumoniae*.

Many physicians prefer it over ampicillin. *Amoxicillin is one of the most frequently used antibiotics for treatment of dental infections, since majority of cases resolve with 250–500 mg TDS given for 5 days. It is also the first choice drug for prophylaxis of postextraction local wound infection as well as for distant infection (endocarditis) following dental surgery in susceptible patients (see p. 401, 402).*

Dose: 0.25–1 g TDS oral/i.m. or slow i.v. injection; children 25–50 mg/kg/day; AMOXYLIN, NOVAMOX, SYNAMOX 250, 500 mg cap, 125 mg/5 ml dry syr. AMOXIL, MOX 250, 500 mg caps; 125 mg/5 ml dry syr; 250, 500 mg/vial inj. MOXYLONG: Amoxicillin 250 mg + probenecid 500 mg tab (also 500 mg + 500 mg DS tab).

Uses of ampicillin and amoxicillin

Because of their broader spectrum of action covering both gram-positive and gram-negative aerobic as well as anaerobic bacteria that are mostly causative agents of dental infections, *aminopenicillins are one of the commonest antibiotics used in dentistry.* Amoxicillin is generally preferred over ampicillin because it produces higher and more sustained blood levels. Diarrhoea is less common with amoxicillin. Any of the two is combined with metronidazole for treating ANUG.

The general medical indications of aminopenicillins are:
1. Urinary tract infections: response rate has declined now due to emergence of resistant strains.
2. Respiratory tract infections: bronchitis, sinusitis, otitis media, etc.

3. Gonorrhoea caused by nonpenicillinase producing *N. gonorrhoeae* can be treated with a single oral dose 3.5 g + 1 g probenecid.
4. Bacillary dysentery due to *Shigella*: ampicillin is preferred over amoxicillin, but fewer cases respond now.
5. Typhoid fever: seldom effective now due to widespread resistance.
6. Cholecystitis: responds well.
7. Subacute bacterial endocarditis: preferred over PnG and combined with gentamicin.
8. Septicaemias: combined with gentamicin or 3rd generation cephalosporin.
9. *H. pylori* eradication: as a component of triple drug regimen.

Adverse effects Diarrhoea is frequent after oral administration of ampicillin, because it is incompletely absorbed, and the unabsorbed drug irritates the lower intestines as well as causes marked alteration of bacterial flora. Amoxicillin is less likely to cause diarrhoea.

Aminopenicillins produce a high incidence (up to 10%) of rashes, especially in patients with AIDS, EB virus infections or lymphatic leukaemia. Concurrent administration of allopurinol also increases the incidence of rashes. Sometimes, the rashes may not be allergic but toxic in nature.

Patients with a history of immediate type of hypersensitivity to PnG should not be given ampicillin or amoxicillin.

Interactions Hydrocortisone inactivates ampicillin / amoxicillin if mixed in the i.v. solution.
By inhibiting colonic flora, it may interfere with deconjugation and enterohepatic cycling of oral contraceptives; may result in failure of oral contraception.
Probenecid retards renal excretion of ampicillin / amoxicillin.

2. Carboxypenicillins

Carbenicillin The special feature of this penicillin congener is its activity against *Pseudomonas aeruginosa* and indole positive *Proteus* which are not inhibited by PnG or aminopenicillins. However, *Pseudomonas* strains less sensitive to carbenicillin have developed, and utility of this penicillin has declined.

Carbenicillin is inactive orally; has to be administered i.m. or i.v. The t½ is 1 hour. High doses have caused bleeding by interfering with platelet function. This appears to result from perturbation of agonist receptors on platelet surface.
CARBELIN 1 g, 5 g, per vial inj.

The indications for carbenicillin are—serious infections caused by *Pseudomonas* or *Proteus*, e.g. burns, urinary tract infection, septicaemia. Orodental infections are rarely caused by *Pseudomonas*; if at all, they occur in immunocompromised patients. These may be treated with ticarcillin or piperacillin.

Ticarcillin It is similar in properties to carbenicillin, but is more active and produces fewer adverse effects. Ticarcillin has therefore, replaced carbenicillin for treating *Pseudomonas* and *Proteus* infections. Its combination with clavulanic acids extends efficacy to cover β-lactamase producing strains. Gentamicin is often combined with it for treating serious *Pseudomonas* infections.

Dose: 3 g i.m./i.v. 6 hourly.
TIMENTIN inj: Ticarcillin disod. + clavulanate pot. 3.1 g/ vial inj., dry powder for reconstitution before injection.

3. Ureidopenicillins

Piperacillin This antipseudomonal penicillin is about 8 times more active than carbenicillin. In addition, it has good activity against *Klebsiella* and some *Bacteroides*. Piperacillin is mostly used for serious gram negative infections in neutropenic/immunocompromised patients and in burn cases. It is combined with tazobactam to

cover β-lactamase producing strains (*see* p. 423). Elimination t½ is 1 hour. Concurrent use of gentamicin or tobramycin is advised.
Dose: 100–150 mg/kg/day in 3 divided doses.
PIPRAPEN 1 g, 2 g vials; PIPRACIL 2 g, 4 g vials for inj; contains 2 mEq Na⁺ per g.

BETA-LACTAMASE INHIBITORS

β-lactamases are a family of enzymes produced by many gram-positive and gram-negative bacteria that inactivate β-lactam antibiotics by opening the β-lactam ring. Different β-lactamases differ in their substrate affinities. Three inhibitors of this enzyme *clavulanic acid, sulbactam* and *tazobactam* are available for clinical use only in combination with specific penicillins or cephalosporins.

Clavulanic acid Obtained from *Streptomyces clavuligerus*, it has a β-lactam ring but no antibacterial activity of its own. It inhibits a wide variety (class II to class V) of β-lactamases (but not class I cephalosporinase) produced by both gram-positive and gram-negative bacteria.

Clavulanic acid is a 'progressive' inhibitor because binding with β-lactamase is reversible initially, but becomes covalent later—inhibition increasing with time. Called a 'suicide' inhibitor, it gets inactivated after binding to the enzyme. Clavulanate permeates the outer layers of the cell wall of gram-negative bacteria and inhibits the periplasmically located β-lactamase.

Pharmacokinetics Clavulanic acid has rapid oral absorption and a bioavailability of 60%; can also be injected. Its elimination t½ of 1 hr and tissue distribution matches amoxicillin with which it is combined (called coamoxiclav). However, it is eliminated mainly by glomerular filtration and its excretion is not affected by probenecid. Moreover, it is largely hydrolysed and decarboxylated before excretion, while amoxicillin is primarily excreted unchanged by tubular secretion.

Uses Addition of clavulanic acid re-establishes the activity of amoxicillin against β-lactamase producing resistant *Staph. aureus* (but not MRSA that have altered PBPs), *Peptococcus, H. influenzae, N. gonorrhoeae, E. coli, Proteus, Klebsiella, Salmonella, Shigella* and *Bact. fragilis*. Clavulanic acid does not potentiate the action of amoxicillin against strains that are already sensitive to it. Coamoxiclav is indicated for:
- Skin and soft tissue infections, intra-abdominal and gynaecological sepsis, urinary, biliary and respiratory tract infections: especially for hospital-acquired infections.
- *Dental infections caused by β-lactamase producing bacteria.*
- Gonorrhoea (including PPNG).

AUGMENTIN, ENHANCIN, AMONATE: Amoxicillin 250 mg + clavulanic acid 125 mg tab; 500 mg +125 mg tab; 125 mg + 31.5 mg per 5 ml dry syrup; CLAVAM 250 mg + 125 mg tab, 500 mg + 125 mg tab, 875 mg + 125 mg tab, 125 mg + 32 mg per 5 ml syr.
Also AUGMENTIN, CLAVAM inj. Amoxicillin 1 g + clavulanic acid 0.2 g vial and 0.5 g + 0.1 g vial; inject 1 vial deep i.m. or i.v. 6–8 hourly for severe infections. It is more expensive than amoxicillin alone.

Adverse effects Side effects are the same as for amoxicillin alone, but g.i. tolerance is poorer—especially in children. Other adverse effects are *Candida* stomatitis/vaginitis and rashes. Some cases of hepatic injury have been reported with the combination.

Sulbactam It is a semisynthetic β-lactamase inhibitor, related chemically as well as in activity to clavulanic acid. Sulbactam also is a progressive inhibitor, highly active against class II to V but poorly active against class I β-lactamase. On weight basis, it is 2–3 times less potent than clavulanic acid for most types of the enzyme, but the same level of inhibition can be obtained at the higher concentrations achieved clinically. Sulbactam does not induce chromosomal β-lactamases, while clavulanic acid can induce some of them.

Oral absorption of sulbactam is inconsistent. Therefore, it is preferably given parenterally. It has been combined with ampicillin for use against β-lactamase producing resistant strains. Absorption of its complex salt with ampicillin—*sultamicillin tosylate* is better, which is given orally. Indications of ampicillin-sulbactam combination are:

- PPNG gonorrhoea; sulbactam *per se* as well inhibits *N. gonorrhoeae*.
- Mixed aerobic-anaerobic infections, tooth abscess, intra-abdominal, gynaecological, surgical and skin/soft tissue infections, especially those acquired in the hospital.

SULBACIN, AMPITUM: Ampicillin 1 g + sulbactam 0.5 g per vial inj; 1–2 vial deep i.m. or i.v. injection 6–8 hourly. Sultamicillin tosylate: BETAMPORAL, SULBACIN 375 mg tab.

Sulbactam has been combined with cefoperazone and ceftriaxone as well.

Pain at the site of injection, thrombophlebitis of injected vein, rash and diarrhoea are the main adverse effects.

Tazobactam is another β-lactamase inhibitor, similar to sulbactam whose pharmacokinetics matches with that of piperacillin, with which it is combined for use in severe infections like peritonitis, pelvic/urinary/respiratory infections caused by β-lactamase producing bacilli. However, the combination is not active against piperacillin-resistant *Pseudomonas*, and against *Pseudomonas* that develop resistance by losing permeability to piperacillin.

Dose: 0.5 g combined with piperacillin 4 g injected i.v. over 30 min 8 hourly.

PYBACTUM, TAZACT, TAZOBID, TAZAR 4 g + 0.5 g vial for inj., also 2.0 g + 250 mg and 1.0 g + 125 mg vials. Tazobactam has been combined with ceftriaxone as well.

CEPHALOSPORINS

These are a group of semisynthetic antibiotics derived from 'cephalosporin-C' obtained from a fungus *Cephalosporium*. They are chemically related to penicillins; the nucleus consists of a β-lactam ring fused to a dihydrothiazine ring, (7-aminocephalosporanic acid). By addition of different side chains at position 7 of β-lactam ring (altering spectrum of activity) and at position 3 of dihydrothiazine ring (affecting pharmacokinetics), a large number of semisynthetic compounds have been produced. Cephalosporins have been conventionally divided into 4 generations, and some lately developed members have been designated '5th generation'. This division has a chronological sequence of development, but more importantly, takes into consideration the overall antibacterial spectrum as well as potency.

CEPHALOSPORIN

All cephalosporins are bactericidal and have the same mechanism of action as penicillin, i.e. inhibition of bacterial cell wall synthesis. However, they bind to different proteins than those which bind penicillins. This may explain differences in spectrum, potency and lack of cross resistance.

Acquired resistance to cephalosporins could have the same basis as for penicillins, i.e.:

(a) alteration in target proteins (PBPs) reducing affinity for the antibiotic.

Chapter 27: Beta-Lactam Antibiotics

First generation cephalosporins

Parenteral	Oral
Cefazolin	Cephalexin
	Cefadroxil

Second generation cephalosporins

Parenteral	Oral
Cefuroxime	Cefaclor
	Cefuroxime axetil
	Cefprozil

Third generation cephalosporins

Parenteral	Oral
Cefotaxime	Cefixime
Ceftizoxime	Cefpodoxime proxetil
Ceftriaxone	Cefdinir
Ceftazidime	Ceftibuten
Cefoperazone	

Fourth generation cephalosporins

Parenteral
Cefepime
Cefpirome

Fifth generation cephalosporins

Parenteral
Ceftaroline fosamil
Ceftobiprole medocaril

(b) impermeability to the antibiotic or its efflux, so that it does not reach its site of action.

(c) elaboration of β-lactamases which destroy specific cephalosporins (cephalosporinases). This is the most important mechanism of resistance.

Though the incidence is low, resistance has been developed by some organisms, even against the third generation compounds. Individual cephalosporins differ in their:

- Antibacterial spectrum and relative potency against specific organisms.
- Susceptibility to β-lactamases from different organisms.
- Pharmacokinetic properties—many have to be injected, some are oral; majority are not metabolized but are excreted rapidly by the kidney and have short t½s, probenecid inhibits their tubular secretion.

FIRST GENERATION CEPHALOSPORINS

These were developed in the 1960s, have high activity against gram-positive but weaker against gram-negative bacteria.

Cefazolin It is active against most PnG sensitive organisms, i.e. streptococci (*pyogenes* as well *viridans*), gonococci, meningococci, *C. diphtheriae*, *H.influenzae*, clostridia, and *Actinomyces*. While *Klebsiella* and *E. coli* are sensitive, cefazolin is susceptible to staphylococcal β-lactamase. It can be given i.m. as well as i.v. and has a longer t½ (2 hours) due to slower tubular secretion; attains higher concentration in plasma and in bile. It is the preferred cephalosporin for surgical prophylaxis.

Dose: 0.5 g 8 hourly (mild cases), 1 g 6 hourly (severe cases) i.m. or i.v; surgical prophylaxis 1.0 g ½ hour before surgery.
ALCIZON, ORIZOLIN, REFLIN 0.25 g, 0.5 g, 1 g per vial inj.

Cephalexin It is an orally effective first generation cephalosporin, similar in spectrum to cefazolin, but less active against *H. influenzae*. It is little bound to plasma proteins, attains high concentration in bile and is excreted unchanged in urine; t½ ~60 min. *It finds place in dentistry as an alternative to amoxicillin.*

Dose: 0.25–1 g 6–8 hourly (children 25–100 mg/kg/day).
CEPHACILLIN 250, 500 mg cap; SPORIDEX, ALCEPHIN, CEPHAXIN 250, 500 mg cap, 125 mg/5 ml dry syr., 100 mg/ml pediatric drops.
ALCEPHIN-LA: Cephalexin + probenecid (250 + 250 mg and 500 + 500 mg) tabs.

Cefadroxil A close congener of cephalexin; has good tissue penetration including that in alveolar bone (tooth socket). It exerts more sustained action at the site of infection and can be given 12 hourly despite a t½ of 1 hr. It is excreted unchanged in urine, but dose needs to be reduced only if creatinine clearance is < 50 ml/min. The antibacterial activity of cefadroxil and indications are similar to those of cephalexin. It is *frequently selected for dental infections.*

Dose: 0.5–1 g BD. DROXYL 0.5, 1 g tab, 250 mg/5 ml syr; CEFADROX 0.5 g cap, 125 mg/5 ml syr and 250 mg kid tab; KEFLOXIN 0.5 g cap, 0.25 g Distab, 125 mg/5 ml susp.

SECOND GENERATION CEPHALOSPORINS

These were developed subsequent to the first generation compounds and are more active against gram-negative organisms, with wider coverage, including some strains resistant to first generation compounds. Few members are active against anaerobes as well. Utility of 2nd generation compounds has declined in favour of 3rd generation cephalosporins.

Cefuroxime It is resistant to gram-negative β-lactamases: has high activity against PPNG and ampicillin-resistant *H. influenzae*, while retaining significant activity on gram-positive cocci and certain anaerobes. It is well tolerated by i.m. route and has been used in some mixed infections as well.
CEFOGEN, SUPACEF, FUROXIL 250 mg and 750 mg/vial inj; 0.75–1.5 g i.m. or i.v. 8 hourly, children 30–100 mg/kg/day.

Cefuroxime axetil This ester of cefuroxime is effective orally, though absorption is incomplete. The activity depends on *in vivo* hydrolysis and release of cefuroxime. Because of activity on anaerobes, *it is frequently chosen for dental infections*.
Dose: 250–500 mg BD, children half-dose; CEFTUM, SPIZEF 125, 250, 500 mg cap, tab and 125 mg/5 ml susp.

Cefaclor It can be given orally and is more active than the first generation compounds against *H. influenzae*, *E. coli*, *Pr. mirabilis* and anaerobes found in oral cavity. Susceptibility to β-lactamases limits its utility.
KEFLOR, VERCEF, DISTACLOR 250 mg cap, 125 and 250 mg distab, 125 mg/5 ml dry syr, 50 mg/ml ped. drops.

Cefprozil Oral absorption of this cephalosporin is good (> 90%) and it has augmented activity against *Strep. pyogenes*, *Strep. pneumoniae*, *H. influenzae*, *Moraxella* and *Klebsiella*, but not MRSA. The primary indications are bronchitis, ENT and skin infections.
Dose: 250–500 mg BD; child 20 mg/kg/day: ORPROZIL, ZEMETRIL 250, 500 mg tabs; REFZIL 125 mg/5 ml and 250 mg/ 5 ml syr.

THIRD GENERATION CEPHALOSPORINS

These compounds introduced in the 1980s have highly augmented activity against gram-negative Enterobacteriaceae and few members inhibit *Pseudomonas* as well. All are highly resistant to β-lactamases from gram-negative bacteria. However, they are less active on gram-positive cocci and anaerobes. As such, they are less suitable for dental infections.

Cefotaxime It is the prototype of the third generation cephalosporins; exerts potent action on aerobic gram-negative as well as some gram-positive bacteria, but is not so active on anaerobes, *Staph. aureus* and *Ps. aeruginosa*. Prominent indications are meningitis caused by gram-negative bacilli (attains relatively high CSF levels), life-threatening resistant/hospital-acquired infections, septicaemias and infections in immunocompromised patients. It is rarely used in dentistry.

Cefotaxime is deacetylated in the body; the metabolite exerts weaker but synergistic action with the parent drug. The plasma t½ of cefotaxime is 1 hr.
Dose: 1–2 g i.m. or i.v. 6–12 hourly.
OMNATAX, ORITAXIM, CLAFORAN 0.25, 0.5, 1.0 g per vial inj.

Ceftizoxime It is similar in antibacterial activity and indications to cefotaxime, but is not metabolized—excreted by the kidney at a slower rate; t½ 1.5–2 hr.
Dose 0.5–1 g i.m./i.v. 8 or 12 hourly.
CEFIZOX, EPOCELIN 0.5 and 1 g per vial inj.

Ceftriaxone The distinguishing feature of this cephalosporin is its longer duration of action (t½ 8 hr), permitting once or at the most twice daily dosing. Penetration into

CSF is good, and it is eliminated equally in urine and bile.

Ceftriaxone has shown high efficacy in a wide range of serious infections including bacterial meningitis, multiresistant typhoid fever, abdominal sepsis and septicaemias; also useful in gonorrhoea and syphilis.

Hypoprothrombinaemia and bleeding are the specific adverse effects. Haemolysis is reported.

OFRAMAX, MONOCEF, MONOTAX 0.25, 0.5, 1.0 g per vial inj;1–2 g i.v. or i.m./day.

Ceftazidime The most prominent feature of this third generation cephalosporin is its high activity against *Pseudomonas aeruginosa*, and the specific indications are febrile neutropenic patients, burn, etc. Its activity against Enterobacteriaceae is similar to that of cefotaxime, but it is less active on *Staph. aureus*, other gram-positive cocci and anaerobes like *Bact. fragilis*. Its plasma t½ is 1.5–1.8 hr.

Neutropenia, thrombocytopenia, rise in plasma transaminases and blood urea have been reported.

Dose: 0.5–2 g i.m. or i.v. every 8 hr, children 30 mg/kg/day. Resistant typhoid 30 mg/kg/day.

FORTUM, CEFAZID, ORZID 0.25, 0.5 and 1 g per vial inj. COMBITAZ: Ceftazidime 1 g + tazobactum 125 mg/vial inj.

Cefoperazone Like ceftazidime, it differs from other third generation compounds in having stronger activity on *Pseudomonas* and weaker activity on other organisms. It is good for *S. typhi* and *B. fragilis* also, but more susceptible to β-lactamases. The indications are—severe urinary, biliary, respiratory, skin-soft tissue infections, and septicaemias. It is primarily excreted in bile; t½ is 2 hr. Cefoperazone has hypoprothrombinaemic action but does not affect platelet function. A disulfiram-like reaction with alcohol has been reported.

Dose: 1-2 g i.m./i.v. 12 hourly.

MAGNAMYCIN 0.25 g, 1 g, 2 g inj; CEFOMYCIN, NEGAPLUS 1 g inj.

Cefixime It is an orally active third generation cephalosporin, highly active against Enterobacteriaceae, *H. influenzae*, *Strep. pyogenes*, *Strep. pneumoniae* and is resistant to many β-lactamases. However, it is not active on *Staph. aureus* and *Pseudomonas*. It is longer acting (t½ 3 hr) and has been used in a dose of 200–400 mg BD for respiratory, urinary and biliary infections. Stool changes and diarrhoea are the most prominent side effects.

TOPCEF, ORFIX 100, 200 mg tab/cap, TAXIM-O 100 mg, 200 mg tabs, 50 mg/5 ml dry syr.

Cefpodoxime proxetil It is the orally active ester prodrug of 3rd generation cephalosporin cefpodoxime. In addition to being highly active against Enterobacteriaceae and streptococci, it inhibits *Staph. aureus*. It is used mainly for respiratory, urinary, skin and soft tissue infections.

Dose: 200 mg BD (max 800 mg/day)

CEFOPROX, CEPODEM, DOXCEF 100, 200 mg tab, 100 mg/5 ml dry syr.

Cefdinir This orally active 3rd generation cephalosporin has good activity against many β-lactamase producing organisms. Most respiratory pathogens including gram-positive cocci are susceptible. Its indications are pneumonia, acute exacerbations of chronic bronchitis, ENT and skin infections.

Dose: 300 mg BD

SEFDIN, ADCEF 300 mg cap, 125 mg/5 ml susp.

Ceftibuten Another oral 3rd generation cephalosporin, active against gram-positive and few gram-negative bacteria but not *Staph. aureus*. It is indicated in respiratory, ENT and orodental infections.

Dose: 200 mg BD or 400 mg OD.

PROCADAX 400 mg cap, 90 mg/5 ml powder for oral suspension.

FOURTH GENERATION CEPHALOSPORINS

This subgroup of cephalosporins is characterized by non-susceptibility to inducible chromosomal β-lactamases

Cephalosporins

produced by certain resistant bacteria, while retaining high activity against Enterobacteriaceae.

Cefepime Developed in 1990s, it has antibacterial spectrum similar to that of 3rd generation compounds, but is highly resistant to β-lactamases, hence active against many bacteria resistant to the earlier drugs. *Ps. aeruginosa*, *Strep. pneumoniae*, *H. influenzae* and *Staph. aureus* are also inhibited but not MRSA. Due to high potency and extended spectrum, it is effective in many serious infections like hospital-acquired pneumonia, febrile neutropenia, bacteraemia, septicaemia, etc.

Dose: 1–2 g i.v. 8–12 hourly; KEFAGE, CEPIME 0.5, 1.0 g inj.

Cefpirome This 4th generation cephalosporin has become available for the treatment of serious and resistant hospital-acquired infections including septicaemias, lower respiratory tract infections, etc. Its zwitterion character permits better penetration through porin channels of gram-negative bacteria. It is resistant to many β-lactamases and is more potent; than the 3rd generation compounds.

Dose: 1–2 g i.m./i.v. 12 hourly;
CEFROM, CEFORTH 1 g inj. BACIROM, CEFOR 0.25, 0.5 and 1.0 g inj.

FIFTH GENERATION CEPHALOSPORINS

These recently introduced cephalosporins are distinguished by their ability to kill MRSA and some other bacteria which have developed β-lactam resistance by producing altered PBPs. Accordingly, they are effective in many resistant and hospital-acquired infections.

Ceftaroline fosamil It is a prodrug; after i.v. infusion, it is rapidly converted by phosphatases to the active moiety 'ceftaroline' which exerts cidal action on MRSA, penicillin resistant *Strep. pneumoniae*, *Enterococcus faecalis* and some other gram +ive and gram –ive bacteria. It has high affinity for PBP2a found in MRSA and PBP2b, PBP2x occurring in penicillin resistant *Strep. pneumoniae*, thereby interfering with transpeptidation step of bacterial cell wall synthesis. However, it is susceptible to several β-lactamases. Ceftaroline fosamil is approved for use in skin/soft tissue infections and for community-acquired pneumonia (CAP) caused by MRSA and resistant *Strep. pneumoniae* respectively. It is mainly excreted by kidney with a t½ of 2.6 hours. Adverse effects are headache, itching, rashes, diarrhoea and irritation of the injected vein.

ZINFORO, TEFLARO 600 mg/vial inj; 600 mg is infused i.v. over 1 hour every 12 hours.

Ceftobiprole medocaril Another 5th generation cephalosporin active against MRSA, and several other gram +ive and gram –ive bacteria associated with CAP as well as hospital-acquired pneumonia (HAP). It is also a prodrug; rapidly hydrolysed by type A esterases in human body to active 'ceftobiprole', which is mostly excreted unchanged by glomerular filtration with a t½ of 3 hours. Ceftobiprole binds to PBP2a in MRSA, to PBP2b and PBP2x in penicillin resistant *Strep. pneumoniae* and to PBP5 in resistant *Enterococcus faecails* to exert bactericidal activity. It is approved for treatment of HAP, severe cases of CAP and for resistant skin/soft tissue infections.

Adverse effects

Cephalosporins are generally well tolerated but are more toxic than penicillin.

1. *Pain* after i.m. injection occurs with some cephalosporins. Thrombophlebitis can occur on i.v. injection.
2. *Diarrhoea* due to alteration of gut ecology or irritative effect is more common with oral cephalexin, cefixime and parenteral cefoperazone which is largely excreted in bile.

3. *Hypersensitivity reactions* are the most important adverse effects of cephalosporins. The manifestations are similar to those with penicillin, but incidence is lower. Rashes are the most frequent reactions, while anaphylaxis, angioedema, asthma and urticaria are occasional. About 10% patients allergic to penicillin show cross reactivity with cephalosporins. Those with a history of immediate type of reactions to penicillin should better not be given a cephalosporin. Skin tests for sensitivity to cephalosporins are unreliable.

A positive Coombs' test occurs in many but haemolysis is rare.

4. *Nephrotoxicity* Some cephalosporins have low-grade nephrotoxicity which may be accentuated by pre-existing renal disease and concurrent administration of an aminoglycoside or loop diuretic.

5. *Bleeding* occurs with cephalosporins having a methylthiotetrazole or similar substitution at position 3 (cefoperazone, ceftriaxone). This is due to hypoprothrombinaemia caused by the same mechanism as warfarin.

6. Neutropenia and thrombocytopenia are rare adverse effects reported with ceftazidime and some others.

7. A disulfiram-like interaction with alcohol has been reported with cefoperazone.

Uses

A. *Dental infections:* There are no compelling indications for cephalosporins in dentistry except as alternative to penicillin/amoxicillin, especially in patients who develop rashes or other milder allergic reactions (but not immediate type of hypersensitivity), and in cases with penicillin/amoxicillin-resistant infection. As such, they are used to a lesser extent than penicillins. Only oral antibiotics are routinely employed in dentistry, while parenteral ones are reserved for serious and fulminating infections. Therefore, when used, *one of the orally active 1st or 2nd generation cephalosporin is mostly selected for orodental infections*. The first generation agents like *cephalexin* or *cephadroxil* are used because of their high activity against gram-positive aerobic bacteria and their good penetration into alveolar bone (like tooth socket). Though they do not directly kill anaerobes, removal of aerobic organisms improves oxygen availability at the local site, especially in alveolar bone, and indirectly checks growth of anaerobes.

The 2nd generation compounds like *cefuroxime axetil* and *cefaclor* are the only ones with good activity against oral anaerobes, and are the preferred cephalosporins for dental indications. Cephalosporins are especially valuable for orodental infections caused by *Klebsiella*, which though rare, may infect neutropenic patients. Anaerobes are less prominent in acute gingival cellulitis which often responds rapidly to cephalosporins. *Cephalexin* and *cephadroxil* are alternatives to amoxicillin for prophylaxis of local wound infection as well as for preventing bacterial endocarditis following dental surgery in predisposed patients.

B. *General medical uses:* Cephalosporins are now extensively used in medicine.

1. As alternatives to PnG in allergic patients (other than immediate hypersensitivity), one of the first generation compounds may be used.

2. Respiratory, urinary and soft tissue infections caused by gram-negative organisms, especially *Klebsiella, Proteus, Enterobacter, Serratia*. The 5th generation cephalosporins, ceftaroline fosamil and ceftobiprole medocaril are reserve drugs for resistant cases of CAP, HAP and soft-tissue infections.

3. Penicillinase producing staphylococcal infections. Ceftaroline fosamil is an alternative drug for MRSA.

4. Septicaemias caused by gram-negative organisms: an aminoglycoside may be combined with a cephalosporin.

5. Surgical prophylaxis: Cefazolin is employed for most types of surgeries.

6. Meningitis caused by *H. influenzae*, Enterobacteriaceae: cefuroxime, cefotaxime and ceftriaxone are specially used. Ceftazidime + gentamicin is the most effective therapy for *Pseudomonas* meningitis.

7. Gonorrhoea caused by penicillinase producing organisms: ceftriaxone is a first choice drug for single dose therapy. For chancroid also, a single dose is as effective as cotrimoxazole or erythromycin given for 7 days.

8. Typhoid: ceftriaxone and cefoperazone are the fastest acting drugs.

9. Mixed aerobic-anaerobic infections seen in cancer patients, those undergoing colorectal surgery, obstetric complications: cefuroxime, cefaclor or one of the third generation compounds is used.

10. Hospital-acquired infections, especially of respiratory tract, resistant to commonly used antibiotics: cefotaxime, ceftizoxime or a fourth generation drug may work.

11. Prophylaxis and treatment of infections, especially of respiratory tract, in neutropenic patients: ceftazidime or another third generation compound, alone or in combination with an aminoglycoside.

MONOBACTAM

Aztreonam It is an atypical β-lactam antibiotic in which the other ring is missing (hence monobactam), but acts by binding to specific PBPs. The spectrum of action is narrow; it inhibits gram-negative enteric bacilli and *H. influenzae* at very low concentrations and *Pseudomonas* at moderate concentrations, but does not affect gram-positive cocci or faecal anaerobes. It is resistant to gram-negative β-lactamases. The main indications of aztreonam are hospital-acquired infections originating from urinary, biliary, gastrointestinal and female genital tracts.

Lack of cross sensitivity with other β-lactam antibiotics appears to be the most promising feature of aztreonam: permiting its use in patients allergic to penicillins or cephalosporins. There is no specific indication of aztreonam in dentistry. It is eliminated in urine with a t½ of 1.8 hours.
Dose: 0.5–2 g i.m. or i.v. 6–12 hourly.
AZENAM, TREZAM 0.5 g, 1 g, 2 g per vial inj.

CARBAPENEMS

Imipenem It is a potent and broad spectrum β-lactam antibiotic whose range of activity includes gram-positive cocci, Enterobacteriaceae, *Ps. aeruginosa*, *Listeria* as well as anaerobes like *Bact. fragilis* and *Cl. difficile*. It is resistant to most β-lactamases and inhibits penicillinase producing staphylococci, but is not reliable for MRSA.

A limiting feature of imipenem is its rapid hydrolysis by the enzyme dehydropeptidase I located on the brush border of renal tubular cells. An innovative solution to this problem is its combination with *cilastatin*, a reversible inhibitor of dehydropeptidase I, which has matched pharmacokinetics with imipenem (t½ of both is 1 hr) and protects it. All carbapenems are eliminated by kidney.

Imipenem-cilastatin 0.5 g i.v. 6 hourly (max 4 g/day) has proved effective in a wide range of serious hospital-acquired infections, including those in neutropenic, cancer and AIDS patients, but has been overtaken by meropenem and other newer congeners.

Imipenem has propensity to induce seizures at higher doses and in predisposed patients. Diarrhoea, vomiting and rashes are the other side effects.
IMINEM, LASTINEM 250 mg + 250 mg/vial and 500 mg + 500 mg/vial inj.

Meropenem This newer carbapenem is not hydrolysed by renal peptidase; does not need to be protected by cilastatin. Like imipenem, it is active against both gram-positive and gram-negative bacteria, aerobes as well as anaerobes and is not destroyed by many β-lactamases.

Meropenem is a reserve drug for the treatment of serious nosocomial infections like septicaemia, febrile neutropenia, intra-abdominal and pelvic infections, etc. caused by cephalosporin-resistant bacteria. It can also be employed for serious/ difficult to treat orodental infections. The adverse effects of meropenem are similar to imipenem, but it is less likely to cause seizures, and is preferred over imipenem.

Dose: 0.5-2.0 g (10-40 mg/kg) by slow i.v. injection 8 hourly.

MERONEM, MENEN, UBPENEM 0.5, 1.0 g/vial inj.

Faropenem Another carbapenem β-lactam antibiotic that is orally active against many gram-positive as well as gram-negative bacteria, including some anaerobes. *Strep. pneumoniae, H. influenzae* and *Moraxella catarrhalis* are highly susceptible. It has been mainly used in respiratory, ENT and genitourinary infections. Usual side effects are diarrhoea, abdominal pain, nausea and rashes.

Dose: 150-300 mg TDS oral;

FARONEM, FAROZET 150 mg, 200 mg tab.

Doripenem This carbapenem has antimicrobial activity similar to meropenem, and is more active against some resistant *Pseudomonas*. Other properties, including nonsusceptibility to renal peptidase, and clinical indications are also similar to meropenem. Adverse effects are nausea, diarrhoea, superinfections and phlebitis of the injected vein.

Dose: 500 mg by slow i.v. infusion over 1 hour, every 8 hours.

SUDOPEN 250 mg, 500 mg/vial inj; DORIGLEN 500 mg/vial inj.

Ertapenem It is a new, relatively narrow spectrum carbapenem that is highly active against *E. coli, H. influenzae, K. pneumoniae, Morexella catarrhalis; Proteus* and several anaerobes, but has little action on *Pseudomonas, Acinetobacter*, MRSA, penicillin resistant *Strep. pneumoniae*, etc. Bacteria develop ertapenem resistance mainly by upregulating antibiotic efflux and by losing porin channels. Indications of ertapenem include resistant skin and skin structure infection, complicated urinary tract infection, diabetic foot, CAP, intra-abdominal/pelvic infections and colo-rectal surgery. Another important feature is its longer half-life of 4 hours, permitting once daily i.v. infusion. It is excreted mainly in urine. Adverse effects are—headache, diarrhoea, thrombophlebitis of injected vein, but risk of seizures is low.

Dose: 1 mg infused i.v. over 60 min daily for 7–14 days.

ERTACRIT, ZIVATOR 1 g per vial inj; to be reconstituted before infusion.

28
CHAPTER

Tetracyclines, Chloramphenicol and Aminoglycoside Antibiotics

TETRACYCLINES

These are a class of antibiotics having a nucleus of four cyclic rings.

TETRACYCLINE

All tetracyclines are obtained from soil actinomycetes. The first to be introduced was *chlortetracycline* in 1948. It contrasted markedly from penicillin and streptomycin (the other two antibiotics generally available at that time) in being active orally and in affecting a wide range of microorganisms—hence called '*broad-spectrum antibiotic*'. Other tetracyclines were produced later, either from mutant strains or semisynthetically. A new synthetic subclass 'glycylcyclines' represented by Tigecycline has been added recently.

All tetracyclines are mildly bitter solids which are slightly water soluble, but their hydrochlorides are more soluble. Aqueous solutions are unstable. All have practically the same antimicrobial activity (with minor differences). The subsequently developed members (doxycycline, minocycline) have high lipid solubility, greater potency and some distinctive features. The clinically relevant tetracyclines and glycylcycline are:

Tetracycline	Doxycycline
Oxytetracycline	Minocycline
Demeclocycline	

Glycylcycline: Tigecycline

Mechanism of action The tetracyclines are primarily bacteriostatic. They inhibit protein synthesis by binding to 30S ribosomes in susceptible organisms. Subsequent to such binding, attachment of aminoacyl-t-RNA to the acceptor (A) site of mRNA-ribosome complex is interfered with (Fig. 28.1). As a result, the peptide chain fails to grow.

The sensitive organisms have an energy dependent active transport process which concentrates tetracyclines intracellularly. In gram-negative bacteria tetracyclines diffuse through the porin channels as well. The more lipid-soluble members (doxycycline, minocycline) enter by passive diffusion also (this is partly responsible for their higher potency). The carrier involved in active transport of tetracyclines is absent in the host cells. Moreover, protein synthesizing apparatus of host cells is less susceptible to tetracyclines. These two factors are responsible for the selective toxicity of tetracyclines for the microbes.

Antimicrobial spectrum When originally introduced, tetracyclines inhibited practically all types of pathogenic microorganisms except fungi and viruses; hence the name 'broad-spectrum antibiotic'. However, promiscous and often indiscriminate use has gradually narrowed the field of their usefulness.

1. Cocci: All gram-positive and gram-negative cocci were originally sensitive, but now only few *Strep. pyogenes, Staph. aureus* and enterococci respond. Responsiveness of *Strep. pneumoniae* has decreased.

Chapter 28: Tetracyclines, Chloramphenicol and Aminoglycoside Antibiotics

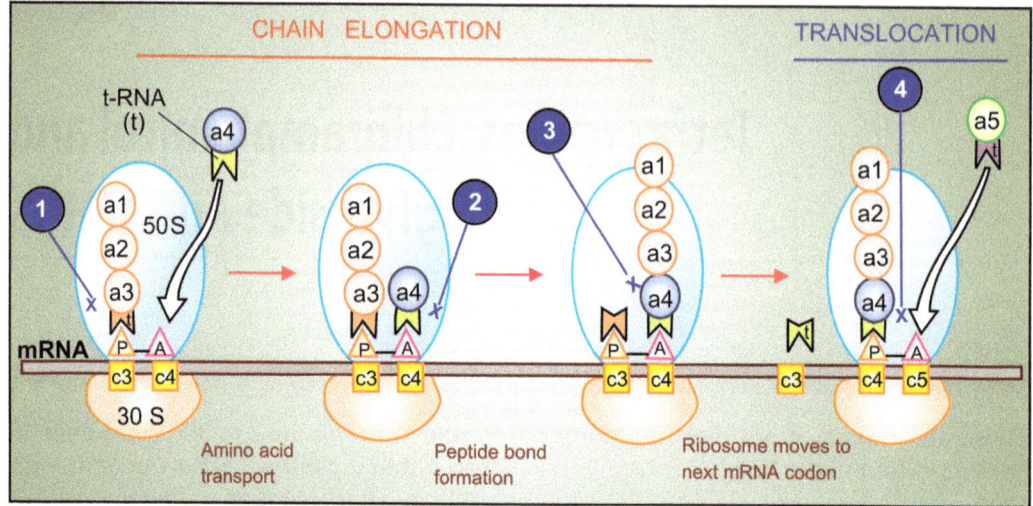

Fig. 28.1: Bacterial protein synthesis and the site of action of antibiotics
The messenger RNA (mRNA) attaches to the 30S ribosome. The initiation complex of mRNA starts protein synthesis and polysome formation. The nacent peptide chain is attached to the peptidyl (P) site of the 50S ribosome. The next amino acid (a) is transported to the acceptor (A) site of the ribosome by its specific tRNA which is complementary to the base sequence of the next mRNA codon (C). The nacent peptide chain is transferred to the newly attached amino acid by peptide bond formation. The elongated peptide chain is shifted back from the 'A' to the 'P' site and the ribosome moves along the mRNA to expose the next codon for amino acid attachment. Finally, the process is terminated by the termination complex and the protein is released.
(1) Aminoglycosides bind to several sites at 30S and 50S subunits as well as to their interface—freeze initiation, interfere with polysome formation and cause misreading of mRNA code.
(2) Tetracyclines bind to 30S ribosome and inhibit aminoacyl tRNA attachment to the 'A' site.
(3) Chloramphenicol binds to 50S subunit—interferes with peptide bond formation and transfer of peptide chain from 'P' site.
(4) Erythromycin and clindamycin also bind to 50S ribosome and hinder translocation of the elongated peptide chain back from 'A' site to 'P' site and the ribosome does not move along the mRNA to expose the next codon. Peptide synthesis may be prematurely terminated.

Tetracyclines (especially minocycline) are now active against only few *N. gonorrhoeae* and *N. meningitidis*.
2. Most gram-positive bacilli, e.g. *Clostridia* and other anaerobes, *Listeria, Corynebacteria, Propionibacterium acnes, B. anthracis* are inhibited but not *Mycobacteria*, except *M. leprae* (to minocycline) and some atypical ones.
3. Sensitive gram-negative bacilli are—*H. ducreyi, Calymmatobacterium granulomatis, V. cholerae, Yersinia pestis, Y. enterocolitica, Campylobacter, Helicobacter pylori, Brucella, Pasteurella multocida, F. tularensis* and many anaerobes; some *H. influenzae* have become insensitive.
    Enterobacteriaceae are now largely resistant. Notable bacilli that are not inhibited are *Pseudomonas aeruginosa, Proteus, Klebsiella, Salmonella typhi* and many *Bact. fragilis*. MIC against anaerobes is relatively higher.
4. Spirochetes, including *T. pallidum* and *Borrelia* are quite sensitive.
5. All rickettsiae (typhus, etc.) and chlamydiae are highly sensitive.
6. *Mycoplasma* and *Actinomyces* are moderately sensitive.
7. *Entamoeba histolytica* and *Plasmodia* are inhibited at high concentrations.

Resistance Resistance to tetracyclines develops slowly in a graded manner. Usually, the tetracycline concentrating mechanism becomes less efficient in resistant bacteria, or the bacteria acquire capacity to pump it out. However, doxycycline and minocycline are not efficiently effluxed. Therefore, these agents may be active even in bacteria resistant to other tetracyclines. Another mechanism is plasmid mediated synthesis of a 'protection' protein which protects the ribosomal binding site from the tetracycline. Due to widespread use, tetracycline resistance has become common among gram positive cocci, *E. coli, Enterobacter* and some other bacteria. Nearly complete cross-resistance is seen among different tetracyclines.

Partial cross resistance between tetracyclines and chloramphenicol has been noted.

Pharmacokinetics

The pharmacokinetic features of various tetracyclines are compared in Table 28.1. The older tetracyclines are incompletely absorbed from g.i.t.; absorption is better if taken in empty stomach. Doxycycline and minocycline are completely absorbed irrespective of food. Tetracyclines have chelating property—form insoluble and unabsorbable complexes with calcium and other metals. Milk, iron preparations, nonsystemic antacids and sucralfate reduce their absorption. Administration of these substances and tetracyclines should be staggered, if they cannot be avoided altogether.

Tetracyclines are widely distributed in the body (volume of distribution > 1 L/kg). *They are concentrated in liver, spleen, gingival tissue and bind to the connective tissue in bone and teeth.* Highly lipid soluble minocycline accumulates in body fat.

Most tetracyclines are primarily excreted in urine by glomerular filtration; dose has to be reduced in renal failure; doxycycline is an exception to this. Tetracyclines are

Table 28.1: Comparative features of tetracyclines

	Tetracycline (T) Oxytetracycline (OxyT)	Demeclocycline (Deme)	Doxycycline (Doxy) Minocycline (Mino)
1. Source	Oxy T: *S. rimosus* T: semisynthetic	*S. aureofaciens* (mutant)	Doxy: semisynthetic Mino: semisynthetic
2. Potency	Low	Intermediate	High (Doxy < Mino)
3. Intestinal absorption	60–80%	60–80%	95–100% No interference by food
4. Plasma protein binding	OxyT: Low T: Intermediate	High	High
5. Elimination	T: Rapid renal excretion Oxy T	Partial metabolism, slower renal excretion	Doxy: Primarily excreted in faeces as conjugate Mino: Primarily metabolized, excreted in urine and bile
6. Plasma t½	6–10 hr.	12–18 hr.	18–24 hr.
7. Dosage	250–500 mg QID or TDS	300 mg BD	200 mg initially, then 100–200 mg OD
8. Alteration of intestinal flora	Marked	Moderate	Least
9. Incidence of diarrhoea	High	Intermediate	Low
10. Phototoxicity	Low	Highest	Doxy: High
11. Specific toxicity	OxyT: less tooth discolouration	More phototoxic, diabetes insipidus	Doxy: low renal toxicity. Mino: Vestibular toxicity

partly metabolized and significant amounts enter bile—some degree of enterohepatic circulation occurs. They are secreted in milk in amounts sufficient to affect the suckling infant.

Enzyme inducers like phenobarbitone, carbamazepine and phenytoin enhance metabolism and shorten the t½ of doxycycline.

Administration Oral capsule is the dosage form in which tetracyclines are most commonly administered. The capsule should be taken ½ hr before or 2 hr after food.

Tetracyclines are not recommended by i.m. route because it is painful and absorption from the injection site is poor. Slow i.v. injection may be given in severe cases, but is rarely required now. Doxycycline 100 mg once or twice daily is the most commonly used tetracycline. Topical application of tetracyclines is not advised, except in the eye.

Preparations

1. Oxytetracycline: TERRAMYCIN 250, 500 mg cap, 50 mg/ml in 10 ml vials inj; 3% skin oint, 1% eye/ear oint.
2. Tetracycline: ACHROMYCIN, HOSTACYCLINE, RESTECLIN 250, 500 mg cap. 3% skin oint, 1% eye/ear drops and oint.
3. Demeclocycline (Demethylchlortetracycline): LEDERMYCIN 150, 300 mg cap/tab.
4. Doxycycline: TETRADOX, DOXICIP, DOXT, NOVADOX, 100 mg cap.
5. Minocycline: CYANOMYCIN, DIVAINE 50, 100 mg caps.

Adverse effects

Irritative effects Tetracyclines have irritant property: can cause epigastric pain, nausea, vomiting and diarrhoea on oral intake. The irritative diarrhoea is to be distinguished from that due to superinfection. Esophageal ulceration has occurred by release of the material from capsules in the esophagus during swallowing, especially with doxycycline. Thrombophlebitis of the injected vein can occur on i.v. injection.

Organ toxicity

1. *Liver damage* Fatty infiltration of liver and jaundice occurs occasionally. Tetracyclines are risky in pregnant women, can precipitate acute hepatic necrosis which may be fatal.

2. *Kidney damage* Patients with kidney disease run the risk of tetracycline induced kidney damage. Tetracyclines, except doxycycline, accumulate and worsen renal failure. A reversible *Fanconi syndrome* like condition is produced by outdated tetracyclines. This is caused by degradation products—epitetracycline, anhydrotetracycline and epianhydrotetracycline.

3. *Phototoxicity* A sun burn-like or other severe skin reaction on exposed parts is seen in some individuals. A higher incidence has been noted with demeclocycline and doxycycline. Distortion of nails occurs occasionally.

4. *Teeth and bones* Tetracyclines have chelating property. Calcium-tetracycline chelate gets deposited in developing teeth and bone. Given from midpregnancy to 5 months of extrauterine life, tetracyclines affect the deciduous teeth. Brown discolouration, ill-formed teeth which are more susceptible to caries are produced. Tetracyclines given between 3 months and 6 years of age affect the crown of permanent anterior dentition. Repeated courses are more damaging.

Given during late pregnancy or childhood, tetracyclines can temporarily suppress bone growth. Deformities and reduction in height are a possibility with prolonged use.

5. *Antianabolic effect* Tetracyclines reduce protein synthesis, induce negative nitrogen balance and tend to increase blood urea.

6. **Diabetes insipidus** Demeclocycline antagonizes ADH action and reduces urine concentrating ability of the kidney.

7. **Vestibular toxicity** Minocycline can cause ataxia, vertigo and nystagmus which subside when the drug is discontinued.

Hypersensitivity Allergic reactions are infrequent with tetracyclines. However, skin rashes, urticaria, glossitis, pruritus ani and vulvae, even exfoliative dermatitis have been reported.

Superinfection Tetracyclines are frequently responsible for superinfections, because they cause marked suppression of the resident flora.

Though mouth, skin or vagina may be involved, intestinal superinfection by *Candida albicans* is most prominent with tetracyclines. Pseudomembranous enterocolitis is rare but serious. *Pseudomonas* and *Proteus* may also overgrow in the bowel. Higher doses suppress the flora more completely, increasing the chance of superinfection. The tetracycline should be discontinued at the first sign of superinfection and appropriate therapy instituted.

Doxycycline and minocycline are less liable to cause diarrhoea, because only small amounts reach the lower bowel in the active form.

Precautions

1. Tetracyclines are contraindicated during pregnancy, lactation and in children.
2. They should be avoided in patients taking diuretics, because blood urea may rise in such patients.
3. Tetracyclines should be used cautiously in renal or hepatic insufficiency.
4. Preparations should never be used beyond their expiry date.

Uses

Orodental conditions Tetracyclines are of limited usefulness in treating acute dental infections and are seldom selected for this purpose. However, they benefit certain forms of periodontal disease, probably by virtue of their broad-spectrum antimicrobial action as well as by suppressing the activity of matrix metalloproteinases derived from neutrophils and fibroblasts that contribute to the gingival inflammation. These enzymes are Ca^{2+} dependent, and tetracyclines chelate Ca^{2+}. Moreover, tetracyclines may benefit periodontal inflammation by scavenging free (oxygen) radicals.

Tetracyclines have an important adjuvant role in the management of chronic periodontitis refractory to conventional therapy with local hygienic and surgical measures, and in juvenile periodontitis. In refractory periodontal disease 2-week tetracycline (1 g/day) or doxycycline (0.1–0.2 g/day) therapy controls gingival inflammation and helps to normalise the periodontal microflora from a mixture of anaerobic gram-negative bacilli + spirochetes to the usual one in which gram-positive bacteria predominate. Tetracyclines are highly active against *Actinobacillus sp.* that is held responsible for destruction of gums and bone loss in juvenile periodontitis. Appropriate surgical treatment combined with 2 to 4-week tetracycline therapy halts progression of this disease.

General medical uses Although tetracyclines are broad-spectrum antibiotics, they are employed only for those infections for which a more selective and less toxic AMA is not available. Clinical use of tetracyclines has declined due to availability of fluoroquinolones and other efficacious AMAs.

1. Tetracyclines may be employed for empirical therapy of nonserious infections when the nature and sensitivity of the

infecting organism is not clear. However, they are not dependable for empirical treatment of serious/life-threatening infections. They may also be used for initial treatment of *mixed infections*.

2. Tetracyclines are still the drug of **first choice** in:
(a) Venereal diseases: Lymphogranuloma venereum, granuloma inguinale, nonspecific urethritis caused by *Chlamydia trachomatis*.
(b) Atypical pneumonia due to *Mycoplasma pneumoniae* and psittacosis.
(c) Cholera: Tetracyclines have adjuvant value by reducing stool volume and limiting the duration of diarrhoea.
(d) Plague: Tetracyclines are preferred for mass treatment of suspected cases during an epidemic, though streptomycin often acts faster.
(e) Rickettsial infections: typhus, rocky mountain spotted fever, Q fever, etc.

3. Tetracyclines are **second choice** drugs:
(a) To penicillin/ampicillin for tetanus, anthrax, actinomycosis and *Listeria* infections.
(b) To ceftriaxone for gonorrhoea and syphilis in patients allergic to penicillin.
(c) To azithromycin for trachoma due to *Ch. trachomatis* and pneumonia due to *Ch. pneumoniae*.

4. Other situations in which tetracyclines may be used are:
- Community-acquired pneumonia (CAP).
- Amoebiasis: along with other amoebicides for chronic intestinal amoebiasis.
- As adjuvant to quinine or sulfadoxine-pyrimethamine for chloroquine-resistant *P. falciparum* malaria.
- Acne: prolonged therapy with low doses may be used in severe cases.
- Chronic obstructive lung disease: prophylactic use may reduce the frequency of exacerbations.

Tigecycline

It is the first member of a new class of synthetic tetracycline analogue (glycylcyclines) which is active against bacteria that have developed resistance to tetracyclines. Most gram positive and gram negative cocci including anaerobes and resistant strains, Enterobacteriaceae, but not *Pseudomonas* and *Proteus* are inhibited by tigecycline. The tetracycline sensitive organisms like *Rickettsia, Chlamydia, Mycoplasma, Legionella,* etc. are responsive to tigecycline as well. Though tigecycline acts in the same manner as tetracyclines, there is no cross resistance among these two groups because:
- Tetracycline efflux pumps acquired by resistant bacteria have low affinity for tigecycline.
- The ribosomal protection protein against tetracycline found in some resistant bacteria does not protect the ribosomal site from tigecycline.

Tigecycline is not absorbed orally, and is administered only by slow i.v. infusion. Its t½ is long (36–60 hours). Adverse effects are similar to those of tetracyclines. Tigecycline is approved only for treatment of serious infections in hospitalized patients, like pneumonia, complicated skin/intra-abdominal infection, etc.

At present, there is no indication for tigecycline in dentistry.

Dose: 100 mg (loading dose), followed by 50 mg 12 hourly i.v. over 30–60 min.
TYGACIL, TIGIMAX 50 mg powder/vial for reconstitution.

CHLORAMPHENICOL

Chloramphenicol was initially obtained from *Streptomyces venezuelae* in 1947. It was soon synthesized chemically and the commercial product now is all synthetic.

$$O_2N-\bigcirc-\underset{OH}{\underset{|}{CH}}\underset{}{CH}-NH-\underset{}{\overset{O}{\overset{\|}{C}}}-CHCl_2 \quad (CH_2OH)$$

CHLORAMPHENICOL

It is a yellowish white crystalline solid, aqueous solution is quite stable, stands boiling, but needs protection from light. The nitrobenzene moiety of chloramphenicol is probably responsible for the antibacterial activity and its intensely bitter taste.

Mechanism of action Chloramphenicol inhibits bacterial protein synthesis by interferring with 'transfer' of the elongating peptide chain to the newly attached aminoacyl-tRNA at the ribosome-mRNA complex. It specifically attaches to the 50S ribosome near the acceptor (A) site and prevents peptide bond formation between the newly attached amino acid and the nascent peptide chain (*see* Fig. 28.1).

At high doses, it can inhibit mammalian mitochondrial protein synthesis as well. Bone marrow cells are specially susceptible.

Antimicrobial spectrum Chloramphenicol is primarily bacteriostatic, though high concentrations have been shown to exert cidal effect on some bacteria, e.g. *H. influenzae* and *N. meningitidis*. It is a broad-spectrum antibiotic, active against the same range of organisms (gram-positive and negative cocci and bacilli, rickettsiae, chlamydia, mycoplasma) as tetracyclines. Notable differences between these two are:

- Chloramphenicol is highly active against *Salmonella* including *S. typhi*, but resistant strains are now rampant.
- It is more active than tetracyclines against *H. influenzae* (though some have now developed resistance), *B. pertussis*, *Klebsiella* and anaerobes including *Bact. fragilis*.
- It is less active against gram-positive cocci and spirochetes, while *Chlamydia*, *Entamoeba* and *Plasmodia* are not inhibited.

Like tetracyclines, it is ineffective against *Mycobacteria*, *Pseudomonas*, many *Proteus*, viruses and fungi.

Resistance Most bacteria are capable of developing resistance to chloramphenicol, which generally emerges in a graded manner, similar to tetracyclines. Being orally active, broad spectrum and relatively cheap, chloramphenicol was extensively and often indiscriminately used, especially in developing countries, resulting in high incidence of resistance among many gram-positive and gram-negative bacteria.

In many areas, highly chloramphenicol resistant *S. typhi* have emerged due to transfer of R factor by conjugation. Resistance among gram-negative bacteria is generally due to acquisition of R plasmid encoded for an acetyl transferase—an enzyme which inactivates chloramphenicol. In many cases, this plasmid has also carried resistance to ampicillin and tetracycline. Multidrug-resistant *S. typhi* have arisen.

Decreased permeability into the resistant bacterial cells and lowered affinity of bacterial ribosome for chloramphenicol are other mechanisms of resistance. Partial cross resistance between chloramphenicol and erythromycin/clindamycin has been noted. Some cross resistance with tetracyclines also occurs.

Pharmacokinetics Chloramphenicol is rapidly and completely absorbed after oral ingestion, 50–60% bound to plasma proteins and very widely distributed: volume of distribution 1 L/kg. It freely penetrates serous cavities and blood-brain barrier, as well as crosses placenta and is secreted in bile and milk.

Chloramphenicol is primarily conjugated with glucuronic acid in the liver and little is excreted unchanged in urine. Cirrhotics and neonates, who have low conjugating ability, require lower doses. The metabolite is excreted mainly in urine. Plasma t½ of chloramphenicol is 3–5 hours in adults.

Administration The commonest route of administration of chloramphenicol is oral—as capsules; 250–500 mg 6 hourly, children 25–50 mg/kg/day. It is also available for application to eye/ear, but topical use at other sites is not recommended.
CHLOROMYCETIN, ENTEROMYCETIN, PARAXIN, 250 mg, 500 mg cap, 1% eye oint, 0.5% eye drops, 5% ear drops, 1% applicaps.

Chloramphenicol palmitate (CHLOROMYCETIN PALMITATE, ENTEROMYCETIN, PARAXIN 125 mg/5 ml oral susp) is an insoluble tasteless ester of chloramphenicol, which is inactive as such. It is nearly completely hydrolysed in the intestine by pancreatic lipase and absorbed as free chloramphenicol, but produces lower plasma concentration.

Adverse effects

1. *Bone marrow depression* Of all drugs, chloramphenicol is the most prominent cause of aplastic anaemia, agranulocytosis, thrombocytopenia or pancytopenia. Two forms are recognized:
   (a) Non-dose related idiosyncratic reaction: This is rare (1 in 40,000), unpredictable, but serious, often fatal, probably has a genetic basis and is more common after repeated courses. Aplastic anaemia is the most common manifestation.
   (b) Dose and duration of therapy related myelosuppression. This is a direct toxic effect, predictable and probably due to inhibition of mitochondrial enzyme synthesis. This is often reversible without long-term sequelae.
2. *Hypersensitivity reactions* These are infrequent; produce rashes, fever, atrophic glossitis, angioedema.
3. *Irritative effects* Nausea, vomiting, diarrhoea, pain on injection.
4. *Superinfections* These are similar to tetracyclines, but less common.
5. *Gray baby syndrome* It occurred when high doses (~100 mg/kg) were given prophylactically to neonates, especially premature. An ashen gray cyanosis develops, followed by cardiovascular collapse and death.
   It occurs because of inability of the newborn to adequately metabolize and excrete chloramphenicol.

Interactions
Chloramphenicol inhibits warfarin, cyclophosphamide and phenytoin metabolism. Toxicity of these drugs can occur if dose adjustments are not done. Phenobarbitone, phenytoin, rifampin enhance chloramphenicol metabolism by enzyme induction → reduce its concentration → failure of therapy may occur.

Being bacteriostatic, chloramphenicol can antagonize cidal action of β-lactams and aminoglycosides certain bacteria.

Uses

Because of risk of serious (though rare) bone marrow aplasia:

(a) Never use chloramphenicol for minor infections or those of undefined etiology.
(b) Do not use chloramphenicol for infections treatable by other safer antimicrobials.
(c) Avoid repeated courses.
(d) Daily dose not to exceed 2–3 g; duration of therapy to be < 2–3 weeks, total dose in a course < 28 g.
(e) Regular blood counts (especially reticulocyte count) may detect dose-related bone marrow toxicity but not the idiosyncratic type.

In view of the above considerations, *there is hardly any indication in dentistry that warrants use of chloramphenicol* despite its broad-spectrum antimicrobial action. In general medicine also systemic use of chloramphenicol is restricted to a few conditions.

1. *H. influenzae meningitis* Chloramphenicol has excellent penetrability into CSF and is highly efficacious, but the 3rd generation cephalosporins are mostly used now.
2. *Anaerobic infections* caused by *Bact. fragilis* and others respond well to chloramphenicol. However, clindamycin or metronidazole are preferred for these infections.
3. *Intraocular infections* Chloramphenicol is the preferred drug for endophthalmitis caused by sensitive bacteria, because it attains high concentrations in ocular fluids.
4. *Typhoid fever:* Chloramphenicol was the drug of choice, but is not used now due to spread of resistant *S. typhi*.
5. Chloramphenicol may be used as a second line drug in brucellosis, cholera, rickettsial/chlamydial infections, whooping cough and urinary tract infections.
6. Topically, it is used in conjunctivitis and otitis externa. Risk of sensitization prohibits topical use at other sites.

AMINOGLYCOSIDE ANTIBIOTICS

These are a group of natural and semisynthetic antibiotics having polybasic amino groups linked glycosidically to two or more aminosugar residues. While they are extensively used to treat medical, surgical, gynaecological and other systemic infections, aminoglycosides are seldom employed in dentistry.

Unlike penicillin, which was a chance discovery, aminoglycosides are products of deliberate search for drugs effective against gram-negative bacteria. Streptomycin was the first member discovered in 1944 by Waksman and his colleagues. It assumed great importance because it was active against tubercle bacilli. Others were produced later. All aminoglycosides are produced by soil actinomycetes and have many common properties (*See box*).

Common properties of aminoglycoside antibiotics

1. All are used as sulfate salts, which are highly water soluble; solutions are stable for months.
2. They ionize in solution; are not absorbed orally; distribute only extracellularly; do not penetrate brain or CSF.
3. All are excreted unchanged in urine by glomerular filtration.
4. All are bactericidal and more active at alkaline pH.
5. They act by interfering with bacterial protein synthesis.
6. All are active primarily against aerobic gram-negative bacilli; do not inhibit anaerobes.
7. There is only partial cross resistance among them.
8. They have relatively narrow margin of safety.
9. All exhibit ototoxicity and nephrotoxicity.

Systemic aminoglycosides

Streptomycin	Amikacin
Gentamicin	Netilmicin
Kanamycin	Paromomycin
Tobramycin	

Topical aminoglycosides

Neomycin	Framycetin

Mechanism of action

The aminoglycosides are bactericidal antibiotics, all having the same general pattern of action which may be described in two main steps:

(a) Transport of the aminoglycoside through the bacterial cell wall and cytoplasmic membrane.

(b) Binding to ribosomes resulting in inhibition of protein synthesis.

Transport of aminoglycoside into the bacterial cell is a multistep process. They diffuse across the outer coat of gram-negative bacteria through porin channels. Entry from the periplasmic space across the cytoplasmic membrane is carrier mediated which is linked to the electron transport chain. Thus, penetration is dependent upon maintenance of a polarized membrane and on energy-dependent phase 1 (EDP_1) transport needing oxygen. This is inactivated under anaerobic conditions; therefore, anaerobes are not sensitive. Penetration is also favoured by high pH; aminoglycosides are ~20 times more active in alkaline than in acidic medium.

Once inside the bacterial cell, aminoglycosides bind to several sites on 30S and 50S subunits as well as to 30S-50S interface. They freeze initiation of protein synthesis (*see* Fig. 28.1), prevent polysome formation and promote their disaggregation to nonfunctional monosomes so that only one ribosome is attached to each strand of mRNA. Binding of aminoglycoside to 30S-50S juncture causes distortion of mRNA codon recognition resulting in misreading of the code, so that one or more wrong amino acids are entered in the peptide chain and/or peptides of abnormal lengths are produced. Different aminoglycosides cause misreading at different levels depending upon their selective affinity for specific ribosomal proteins.

The cidal action of these drugs appears to be based on secondary changes in the integrity of bacterial cell membrane, because other antibiotics which inhibit protein synthesis (tetracyclines, chloramphenicol, erythromycin) are only static. After exposure to aminoglycosides, sensitive bacteria become more permeable; ions, amino acids and even proteins leak out followed by cell death. This probably results from incorporation of the defective proteins into the cell membrane. One of the consequences of aminoglycoside induced alteration of cell membrane is augmentation of the carrier-mediated energy-dependent phase II (EDP_2) entry of the antibiotic, which reinforces the lethal action.

The cidal action of aminoglycosides is concentration dependent, i.e. rate of bacterial cell killing is directly related to the ratio of the peak antibiotic concentration to the MIC value. They also exert a long and concentration dependent 'postantibiotic effect'.

Mechanism of resistance

Resistance to aminoglycosides is acquired by one of the following mechanisms:
- Acquisition of cell membrane bound modifying enzymes which phosphorylate/adenylate or acetylate the antibiotic. The conjugated aminoglycosides do not bind to the target ribosomes and are incapable of enhancing active transport (EDP_2). These enzymes are acquired mainly by conjugation and transfer of plasmids. Nosocomial microbes have become rich in such plasmids, some of which encode for multidrug resistance. This is the most important mechanism of development of resistance to aminoglycosides. Susceptibility of different aminoglycosides to these enzymes differs. Thus, cross resistance among different members is partial or absent.
- Mutation decreasing the affinity of ribosomal proteins that normally bind the aminoglycoside: this mechanism can confer high degree resistance, but operates to a limited extent.
- Decreased efficiency of the aminoglycoside transporting mechanism: either the pores in the outer coat become less permeable or the active transport is interfered. This again is not frequently encountered in the clinical setting.

Shared toxicities

The aminoglycosides produce toxic effects which are common to all members, but the relative propensity differs (Table 28.2). The toxic effects depend on the dose as well as duration of exposure.

1. Ototoxicity This is the most important adverse effect. The vestibular or the cochlear part may be primarily affected by a particular aminoglycoside. Aminoglycosides are concentrated in the labyrinthine fluid and are slowly removed from it when the plasma concentration falls. Ototoxicity is greater when plasma concentration of the drug is persistently high and above a threshold value. The vestibular/cochlear sensory cells and hairs undergo concentration dependent destructive changes.

Table 28.2: Comparative toxicity of aminoglycoside antibiotics (tentative)

Systemic aminoglyco-side	Ototoxicity		Nephro-toxicity
	Vestibular	Cochlear	
1. Streptomycin	++	±	+
2. Gentamicin	++	+	++
3. Kanamycin	+	++	++
4. Tobramycin	+±	+	+±
5. Amikacin	+	+±	+±
6. Netilmicin	+±	+	+±

Cochlear damage It starts from the base and spreads to the apex; hearing loss affects the high frequency sound first, then progressively encompasses the lower frequencies. Tinnitus heralds hearing loss. No regeneration of the sensory cells occurs; auditory nerve fibres degenerate in retrograde manner—deafness is permanent, but tinnitus often disappears on stopping the drug. Older patients and those with pre-existing hearing defect are more susceptible.

Vestibular damage Headache is usually first to appear, followed by nausea, vomiting, dizziness, nystagmus, vertigo and ataxia. When the drug is stopped at this stage, it passes into a chronic phase lasting 6 to 10 weeks in which the patient is asymptomatic while in bed and has difficulty only during walking. Recovery (often incomplete) occurs over 1–2 years. Permanency of changes depends on the extent of initial damage and the age of the patient (elderly have poor recovery).

2. *Nephrotoxicity* It manifests as tubular damage resulting in loss of urinary concentrating power, low g.f.r., nitrogen retention, albuminuria and casts. Amino-glycoside toxicity is related to the total amount of the drug received by the patient. It is more in the elderly and in those with pre-existing kidney disease. Provided the drug is promptly discontinued, renal damage caused by aminoglycosides is totally reversible. An important implication of aminoglycoside induced nephrotoxicity is reduced clearance of the antibiotic resulting in higher blood levels which causes enhanced ototoxicity.

3. *Neuromuscular blockade* All aminoglycosides reduce ACh release from the motor nerve endings. Effect of this action is not manifested ordinarily in the clinical use of these drugs. However, apnoea and fatalities have occurred when these antibiotics were put into peritonial or pleural cavities after an operation, especially if a curare-like muscle relaxant had been used during surgery.

Precautions and interactions

1. Avoid aminoglycosides during pregnancy due to risk of foetal ototoxicity.
2. Avoid concurrent use of other nephrotoxic drugs, e.g. NSAIDs, amphotericin B, vancomycin, cyclosporine and cisplatin.
3. Cautious use in patients >60 years age and in those with kidney damage.
4. Do not mix aminoglycoside with any drug in the same syringe/infusion bottle.

Pharmacokinetics

All systemically administered amino-glycosides have similar pharmacokinetic features. They are highly ionized, and are neither absorbed nor destroyed in the g.i.t. However, absorption from i.m. injection site is rapid: peak plasma levels are attained in 30–60 minutes. Aminoglycosides are distributed only extracellularly, so that volume of distribution (~ 0.3 L/kg) is nearly equal to the extracellular fluid volume. Relatively higher concentrations are present in endolymph and renal cortex, which are responsible for ototoxicity and nephrotoxicity. Aminoglycosides enter CSF poorly, but cross placenta and can be found in foetal blood and in amniotic fluid. Their use during pregnancy can cause hearing loss in the offspring.

Aminoglycosides are not metabolized in the body, and are excreted unchanged by glomerular filtration. The plasma t½ ranges between 2–4 hours. Renal clearance of aminoglycosides parallels creatinine clearance (CLcr). The t½ is prolonged and accumulation occurs in patients with renal insufficiency and in the elderly. Reduction in dose or increase in dose-interval is essential in these situations. This should be done according to the measured CLcr. A simple guide to dose calculation in renal insufficiency is given in the box.

Chapter 28: Tetracyclines, Chloramphenicol and Aminoglycoside Antibiotics

Guideline for dose adjustment of gentamicin in renal insufficiency	
CLcr (ml/min)	% of daily dose
70	70% daily
50	50% daily
30	30% daily
20–30	80% alternate day
10–20	60% alternate day
<10	40% alternate day

Dosing regimens

Because of low safety margin, the daily dose of aminoglycosides must be precisely calculated accordingly to body weight and the level of renal function. For an average adult with normal renal function (CLcr > 70 ml/min), the usual doses are:

Gentamicin/tobramycin/netilmicin } 3–5 mg/kg/day

Streptomycin/kanamycin/amikacin } 7.5–15 mg/kg/day

Considering the short t½ (2–4 hr) of aminoglycosides, the daily doses are conventionally divided into 3 equal parts and injected i.m. (or i.v. slowly over 60 min) every 8 hours. However, most authorities now recommend a single total daily dose regimen for patients with normal renal function. This is based on the considerations that:
- Aminoglycosides exert concentration dependent bactericidal action and a long post-antibiotic effect (*see* p. 397), therefore higher plasma concentrations attained after the single daily dose will be equally or more effective than the divided doses.
- With the single daily dose, the plasma concentration will remain subthreshold for ototoxicity and nephrotoxicity for a longer period each day allowing washout of the drug from the endolymph and the renal cortex.

In comparative studies the single daily dose regimen has been found to be less nephrotoxic, but both regimens appear to be equally ototoxic and equally effective. Single daily doses are also more convenient.

Gentamicin

It was the 3rd systemically administered aminoglycoside antibiotic to be introduced for clinical use in 1964, but it quickly surpassed streptomycin because of higther potency and broader spectrum of activity. Currently, it is the most commonly used aminoglycoside for acute infections and may be considered prototype of the class. Gentamicin is active mainly against aerobic gram-negative bacilli, including *E. coli, Klebsiella pneumoniae, Enterobacter, H. influenzae, Proteus, Serratia* and *Pseudomonas aeruginosa*. Limited number of gram-positive bacteria are susceptible, especially *Staph. aureus, Strep. faecalis* and some *Listeria*, but *Strep. pyogenes, Strep. pneumoniae* and enterococci are usually unaffected.

Gentamicin is ineffective against *Mycobacterium tuberculosis* and other mycobacteria. It is more potent (its MIC are lower) than streptomycin, kanamycin and amikacin, but equally potent as tobramycin, sisomicin and netilmicin. It synergises with β-lactam antibiotics.

Dose: 3–5 mg/kg/day (single dose or divided in 3 doses) i.m. or in i.v. line over 30–60 min.
GARAMYCIN, GENTASPORIN, GENTICYN 20, 60, 80, 240 mg per vial inj; also 0.3% eye/ear drops, 0.1% skin cream.

Use in dentistry Because of its predominantly gram-negative spectrum of activity, inefficacy against anaerobes and need for parenteral administration, gentamicin (other aminoglycosides as well) is not employed to treat dental infections. The only application in dentistry is to combine gentamicin 2 mg/kg i.m./i.v. (single dose) with amoxicillin or vancomycin for prophylaxis of bacterial endocarditis following dental surgery in patients with prosthetic heart valves, or in those having past history of bacterial endocarditis, or those to be operated under general anaesthesia.

General medical uses Gentamicin is the cheapest (other than streptomycin) and the first line aminoglycoside antibiotic.

However, because of low therapeutic index, its use should be restricted to serious gram-negative bacillary infections.

1. Gentamicin is very valuable for preventing and treating respiratory infections in critically ill patients, such as those in resuscitation wards and in intensive care units. It is often combined with a penicillin/cephalosporin or another antibiotic in these situations. However, resistant strains have emerged in many hospitals and nosocomial infections are less amenable to gentamicin now.
2. *Pseudomonas, Proteus* or *Klebsiella* infections in burns, urinary tract infection, pneumonia, lung abscesses, osteomyelitis, septicaemia, etc.
3. Meningitis caused by gram negative bacilli.
4. Subacute bacterial endocarditis (SABE): it is generally combined with penicillin/ampicillin/vancomycin.

Streptomycin

It is the first aminoglycoside antibiotic obtained from *Streptomyces griseus*; which was used extensively in the past, but is now practically restricted to treatment of tuberculosis. It is less potent (MICs are higher) than many other aminoglycosides. The antimicrobial spectrum of streptomycin is relatively narrow: primarily covers aerobic gram-negative bacilli. Sensitive organisms are—*H. ducreyi, Brucella, Yersinia pestis, Francisella tularensis, Nocardia, Calym. granulomatis, M. tuberculosis*. Only few strains of *E. coli, H. influenzae, Klebsiella*, enterococci and some gram-positive cocci are now inhibited.

Many organisms rapidly develop resistance to streptomycin, either by one-step mutation or by acquisition of a plasmid which codes for modifying enzymes. If it is used alone, *M. tuberculosis* also become resistant.

Only partial and often unidirectional cross resistance occurs between streptomycin and other aminoglycosides.

Adverse effects About 1/5 patients given streptomycin 1 g BD i.m. experience vestibular disturbances, but only few given 0.75–1.0 g/day. Auditory disturbances are less common.

Streptomycin has the lowest nephrotoxicity among aminoglycosides; probably because it is not concentrated in the renal cortex. Hypersensitivity reactions are rare. Superinfections are not significant. Pain at injection site is common. Streptomycin is contraindicated during pregnancy due to risk of foetal ototoxicity.

AMBISTRYN-S 0.75, 1 g dry powder per vial for inj.
Acute infections: 1 g (0.75 g in those above 50 yr age) i.m. OD or BD for 7–10 days.

Uses Streptomycin is not used in dentistry. In general medicine, use of streptomycin is largely restricted to tuberculosis, as a reserve or supplemental 1st line drug. Rare indications are plague and tularaemia. In most other conditions it has been replaced by gentamicin or other aminoglycosides.

Kanamycin

Obtained from *S. kanamyceticus* (in 1957), it was the second systemically used aminoglycoside. It is similar to streptomycin in all respects including lack of activity against *Pseudomonas*. However, it is more toxic, both to the cochlea and to kidney. Hearing loss is more common than vestibular disturbance.

Because of toxicity and narrow spectrum of activity, it has been largely replaced by other aminoglycosides. It is occasionally used in urinary tract infection, and as a second line drug in resistant tuberculosis.

Dose: 0.5 g i.m. BD-TDS: KANAMYCIN, KANCIN, KANAMAC 0.5, 1 g inj.

Tobramycin

It was obtained from *S. tenebrarius* in the 1970s. The antibacterial and pharmacokinetic properties, as well as dosage are almost identical to gentamicin, but it is 2–4 times more active against *Pseudomonas* and *Proteus*. Tobramycin is be used only as a reserve alternative to gentamicin. Ototoxicity and nephrotoxicity is probably lower than gentamicin.

Dose: 3–5 mg/kg day in 1–3 doses.
TOBACIN 20, 60, 80 mg in 2 ml inj. 0.3% eye drops.
TOBRANEG 20, 40, 80 mg per 2 ml inj.

Amikacin

It is a semisynthetic derivative of kanamycin to which it resembles in pharmacokinetics, dose and toxicity. The outstanding feature of amikacin is its resistance to bacterial aminoglycoside modifying enzymes. Thus, it has the widest spectrum of activity, including many organisms resistant to other aminoglycosides.

The range of conditions in which amikacin can be used is the same as for gentamicin. It is recommended as a reserve drug for hospital acquired gram-negative bacillary infections and in multidrug resistant tuberculosis. More hearing loss than vestibular disturbance occurs in toxicity.

Dose: 15 mg/kg/day in 1–3 doses; urinary tract infection 7.5 mg/kg/day.
AMICIN, MIKACIN, MIKAJECT 100 mg, 250 mg, 500 mg in 2 ml inj.

Netilmicin

This semisynthetic aminoglycoside has a broader spectrum of activity than gentamicin. It is relatively resistant to aminoglycoside modifying enzymes and thus effective against some gentamicin-resistant strains. It is more active against *Klebsiella, Enterobacter* and *Staphylococci,* but less active against *Ps. aeruginosa.*

Pharmacokinetic characteristics and dosage of netilmicin are similar to gentamicin, but toxicity may be lower.
Dose: 4–6 mg/kg/day in 1–3 doses; NETROMYCIN 10, 25, 50 mg in 1 ml, 200 mg in 2 ml and 300 mg in 3 ml inj.

Neomycin

Obtained from *S. fradiae,* it is a wide spectrum aminoglycoside, active against most gram-negative bacilli and some gram-positive cocci. However, *Pseudomonas* and *Strep. pyogenes* are not sensitive. Neomycin is highly toxic to the internal ear (mainly auditory) and to kidney. It is, therefore, not used systemically. It is poorly absorbed from the g.i.t. Oral and topical administration does not ordinarily cause systemic toxicity.

Dose: 0.25–1 g QID oral, 0.3–0.5% topical.
NEBASULF: Neomycin sulph. 5 mg, bacitracin 250 U, sulfacetamide 60 mg/g oint. and powder for surface application.
POLYBIOTIC CREAM: Neomycin sulph. 5 mg, polymyxin 5,000 IU, gramicidin 0.25 mg/g cream.
NEOSPORIN: Neomycin 3400 i.u., polymyxin B 500 i.u., bacitracin 400 i.u./g oint and powder for surface application.

Uses

1. Topically (often in combination with polymyxin, bacitracin, etc.) for infected wound, ulcers, burn, external ear infections, conjunctivitis.
2. Orally for:
   (a) Preparation of bowel before surgery.
   (b) Hepatic coma: Neomycin, by suppressing intestinal flora, diminishes NH_3 production in the colon.

Adverse effects Applied topically neomycin has low sensitizing potential, however, rashes do occur.

Oral neomycin has a damaging effect on intestinal villi.

Framycetin

Obtained from *S. lavendulae,* it is very similar to neomycin. Likewise, it is too toxic for systemic administration and is used topically on skin, eye, ear in the same manner as neomycin.
SOFRAMYCIN, 1% skin cream, 0.5% eye drops or oint.

Paromomycin This aminoglycoside, related to neomycin, was introduced in the 1960s, but was discontinued soon after. It has pronounced activity against many protozoan parasites, including *Entamoeba histolytica, Giardia lamblia, Trichomonas vaginalis* and *Leishmania,* in addition to many bacteria sensitive to neomycin. Like other aminoglycosides, it is not absorbed from the gut. Paromomycin has been reintroduced orally for treatment of intestinal amoebiasis and giardiasis. Injected i.m., it is an alternative drug for treating resistant Kala-azar in India and Africa.

29
CHAPTER

Macrolide and Other Antibacterial Antibiotics

MACROLIDE ANTIBIOTICS

These are antibiotics having a macrocyclic lactone ring with attached sugars. *Erythromycin* has been in use from the 1950s. In an attempt to overcome the limitations of erythromycin, *viz.* narrow spectrum of activity, gastric irritation on oral ingestion, gastric acid lability, low oral bioavailability, limited tissue penetration and short half life, a number of semisynthetic macrolides have been produced, of which *roxithromycin*, *clarithromycin* and *azithromycin* are available.

Erythromycin

It was isolated from *Streptomyces erythreus* in 1952, and is employed mainly as an alternative to penicillin. Erythromycin is frequently prescribed in dentistry.

Mechanism of action Erythromycin is bacteriostatic at low, but can be cidal at high concentrations depending on the organism and its rate of multiplication. Sensitive gram-positive bacteria accumulate erythromycin intracellularly by active transport which is responsible for their high susceptibility to this antibiotic. Erythromycin is several fold more active in alkaline medium, because the nonionized (penetrable) form of the drug is favoured at higher pH.

Erythromycin acts by inhibiting bacterial protein synthesis. It combines with the 50S ribosome subunit and interferes with 'translocation' (*see* Fig. 28.1). After peptide bond formation between the newly attached amino acid and the nascent peptide chain at the acceptor (A) site the elongated peptide is translocated back to the peptidyl (P) site, making the A site available for the next aminoacyl tRNA attachment. This is prevented by erythromycin and the ribosome fails to move along the mRNA to expose the next codon. As an indirect consequence, the peptide chain may be prematurely terminated. Consequently, synthesis of larger proteins is specifically suppressed.

Antimicrobial spectrum It includes mostly gram-positive and a few gram-negative bacteria, and overlaps considerably with that of penicillin G. Thus, erythromycin is a narrow spectrum antibiotic. It is highly active against *Str. pyogenes*, *Str. pneumoniae*, *N. gonorrhoeae*, *Clostridia*, *C. diphtheriae*, and *Listeria*. Most penicillin-resistant *Staphylococci* and *Streptococci* have now become resistant to erythromycin as well. However, *Campylobacter*, *Legionella*, *Branhamella catarrhalis*, *Gardnerella vaginalis* and *Mycoplasma* that are not affected by penicillin are highly sensitive to erythromycin. Few others including oral anaerobes, *H. influenzae*, *H. ducreyi*, *B. pertussis*, *Chlamydia trachomatis*, *Str. viridans*, *N. meningitidis* and *Rickettsiae* are moderately sensitive. Enterobacteriaceae, other gram-negative bacilli and *B. fragilis* are not inhibited.

Resistance All cocci readily develop resistance to erythromycin, mostly by acquiring the capacity to pump it out. Resistant Enterobacteriaceae have been found to produce an erythromycin esterase enzyme. Alteration in the ribosomal binding site for erythromycin by a plasmid encoded methylase enzyme is yet another mechanism of resistance. All the above types of resistance are plasmid mediated, while change in the 50S ribosome by chromosomal mutation reduces its affinity for erythromycin.

Cross resistance with other macrolides, clindamycin and chloramphenicol occurs because the ribosomal binding sites for these antibiotics are proximal to each other.

Pharmacokinetics Erythromycin base is acid labile. To protect it from gastric acid, it is given as enteric coated tablets, from which absorption is incomplete and food delays absorption by retarding gastric emptying. The acid-stable esters of erythromycin are better absorbed.

Erythromycin is widely distributed in the body, enters into abscesses, crosses serous membranes and placenta but not blood-brain barrier. It is 70–80% plasma protein bound, partly metabolized and excreted primarily in bile in the active form. Renal excretion is minor; dose need not be altered in renal failure. The plasma t½ is 1.5 hours, but erythromycin persists longer in tissues.

Preparations and dose
Dose: 250–500 mg 6 hourly (max. 4 g/day), children 30–60 mg/kg/day.
1. Erythromycin (base): ERYSAFE 250, mg tabs, EROMED 333 mg tab, 125 mg/5 ml susp.
2. Erythromycin stearate: blood levels produced are similar to those after erythromycin base. ERYTHROCIN 250, 500 mg tab, 100 mg/5 ml susp., 100 mg/ml ped. drops. ETROCIN, ERYSTER 250 mg tab, 100 mg/5 ml dry syr.
3. Erythromycin estolate (lauryl sulfate): it is relatively acid stable and better absorbed after oral administration.

However, concentration of free and active drug in plasma may be the same as after administration of erythromycin base.
ALTHROCIN 250, 500 mg tab, 125 mg kid tab, 125 mg/5 ml and 250 mg/5 ml dry syr, 100 mg/ml ped. drops, E-MYCIN 100, 250 mg tab, 100 mg/5 ml dry syr.
4. Erythromycin ethylsuccinate: well absorbed orally; ERYNATE 100 mg/5 ml dry syr, ERYTHROCIN 100 mg/ml drops, 125 mg/5 ml syr.

Adverse effects Erythromycin base is a remarkably safe drugs, but side effects do occur.

Mild-to-severe epigastric pain, nausea is experienced by many patients after oral ingestion of erythromycin. Children are especially susceptible. Diarrhoea is occasional.

Erythromycin stimulates motilin receptors in the g.i.t.—thereby induces gastric contractions, hastens gastric emptying and promotes intestinal motility. However, contribution of this action to the g.i. side effects is not known.

Very high doses of erythromycin have caused reversible hearing impairment.

Hypersensitivity Rashes, eosinophilia and fever are infrequent.

Hepatitis with cholestatic jaundice resembling viral hepatitis or extrahepatic biliary obstruction occurs with the estolate ester (rarely with ethyl succinate or stearate ester) after 1–3 weeks. Incidence is higher in pregnant women. It clears on discontinuation of the drug, and is probably due to hypersensitivity to the estolate ester.

Though the estolate is acid stable, tasteless and better absorbed, it has been banned in some countries (but not in India).

Interaction Erythromycin inhibits hepatic oxidation of many drugs by inhibiting CYP3A4. The clinically significant interactions are—rise in plasma levels of theophylline, carbamazepine, valproate, warfarin, terfenadine, astemizole and cisapride.

Several cases of Q-T prolongation, serious ventricular arrhythmias and death have been reported due to inhibition of CYP3A4 by erythromycin/clarithromycin resulting in high blood levels of concurrently administered terfenadine/astemizole/cisapride (see p. 117). All these drugs are now banned in India.

Uses

Dental infections Because erythromycin is orally administered, safe and active against both aerobic and anaerobic gram-positive bacteria commonly infecting dental structures and mouth, it is the second choice drug to penicillins for periodontal/periapical abscesses, necrotizing ulcerative gingivitis (combine with metronidazole), postextraction infections, gingival cellulitis, etc. It is particularly valuable for patients allergic to penicillins, or those with penicillin- resistant infections. However, erythromycin is not active against gram negative anaerobes involved in polymicrobial orodental infections. Being bacteriostatic, it is less effective than penicillins in eradicating dental infections caused by penicillin-sensitive bacteria. It is a good alternative to penicillin for prophylactic uses in dentistry.

General medical uses The most common indications of erythromycin are as a substitute for penicillins in allergic patients for pharyngitis, tonsillitis and other respiratory/ENT infections, as well as for prophylaxis of rheumatic fever. It is one of the first choice drugs for atypical pneumonia caused by *Mycoplasma pneumoniae*, diphtheria (antitoxin therapy is the primary measure), early stages of whooping cough and chancroid. It is a second choice drug for Legionnaires' pneumonia, *Campylobacter* enteritis, chlamydial urogenital infections and some skin/soft tissue infections caused by penicillin resistant *Staph. aureus*, but not MRSA.

Roxithromycin

It is a semisynthetic longer-acting, acid-stable macrolide whose antimicrobial spectrum resembles closely with that of erythromycin. Improved enteral absorption and plasma t½ of 12 hours makes it suitable for twice daily dosing. Better gastric tolerance is another desirable feature.

Roxithromycin is an alternative to erythromycin for respiratory, ENT, orodental, skin and soft tissue and genital tract infections with similar efficacy.

Dose: 150–300 mg BD 30 min before meals, children 2.5–5 mg/kg BD;
ROXID, ROXIBID, RULIDE 150, 300 mg tab, 50 mg kid tab, 50 mg /5 ml liquid; ROXEM 50 mg kid tab, 150 mg tab.

Clarithromycin

The antimicrobial spectrum of clarithromycin includes bacteria sensitive to erythromycin, and in addition, it inhibits *Mycobact. avium* complex (MAC), other atypical mycobacteria and *Mycobact. leprae*. It is more active against many oral anaerobes like *Bact. melaninogenicus, Peptococcus* as well as against *Cl. perfringens* (but not *Bact. fragilis*), *Moraxella, Legionella, Mycoplasma pneumoniae* and *Helicobacter pylori*. However, bacteria that have developed resistance to erythromycin are resistant to clarithromycin as well.

Clarithromycin is more acid stable than erythromycin, and is rapidly absorbed; oral bioavailability is ~50% due to first pass metabolism. Food delays absorption. Tissue distribution is larger than that of erythromycin and it is metabolized by saturation kinetics—t½ is prolonged from 4–6 hours at lower doses to 6–9 hours at higher doses. An active metabolite is produced. About 1/3rd of an oral dose is excreted unchanged in urine. No dose modification is needed in liver disease or in mild-to-moderate kidney failure.

Clarithromycin is indicated in upper and lower respiratory tract infections, *orodental infections*, sinusitis, otitis media, atypical pneumonia, skin and skin structure infections. Used as a component of triple drug regimen (*see* p. 300) it eradicates *H. pylori* in 1–2 weeks. Clarithromycin

is a component of first line combination regimens for MAC infection in AIDS patients and a second line drug for other atypical mycobacterial diseases as well as for leprosy.
Dose: 250 mg BD for 7 days; severe cases 500 mg BD up to 14 days.

CLARIBID 250, 500 mg tab, 250 mg/5 ml dry syr; CLARIMAC 250, 500 mg tabs; SYNCLAR 250 mg tab, 125 mg/5 ml dry syr.

Side effects of clarithromycin are similar to those of erythromycin, but gastric tolerance is better. High doses can cause reversible hearing loss. Few cases of pseudomembranous enterocolitis, hepatic dysfunction or rhabdomyolysis are reported. Its safety in pregnancy and lactation is not known. Since clarithromycin also inhibits CYP3A4, the drug interaction potential is similar to erythromycin.

Azithromycin

This azalide congener of erythromycin has an expanded spectrum, improved pharmacokinetics, better tolerability and drug interaction profiles. Azithromycin is more active against *H. influenzae*, and certain anaerobes like *Peptostreptococcus*, few *Clostridia*, but less active against gram-positive cocci. High activity is exerted on respiratory pathogens—*Mycoplasma, Chlamydia pneumoniae, Legionella, Moraxella* and on others like *Campylobacter, Ch. trachomatis, N. gonorrhoeae*. However, it is not active against erythromycin-resistant bacteria. Penicillinase producing *Staph. aureus* are inhibited but not MRSA. Good activity is noted against MAC.

The improved pharmacokinetic properties are acid stability, rapid oral absorption (from empty stomach), larger tissue distribution and intracellular penetration. Absorption is decreased by food. Concentration in most tissues exceeds that in plasma; volume of distribution is ~30 L/kg. Slow release from the intracellular sites contributes to its long terminal t½ of >50 hr. It is largely excreted unchanged in bile, renal excretion is ~ 10%.

Azithromycin can be used in *orodental infections* in place of erythromycin, particularly in patients not tolerating the latter. It has better activity against oral spirochetes and gram negative anaerobes causing dental infections. Azithromycin is a second line drug for prophylaxis of postdental surgery wound infection, as well as endocarditis in predisposed patients. Because of higher efficacy, better gastric tolerance and convenient once a day dosing, azithromycin is now preferred over erythromycin as first choice drug for:

(a) *Legionnaires'* pneumonia.

(b) *Chlamydia trachomatis*: nonspecific urethritis and genital infections in both men and women and trachoma in eye.

The other indications of azithromycin are pharyngitis, tonsillitis, sinusitis, otitis media, community-acquired pneumonia, acute exacerbations of chronic bronchitis, and gonorrhoea. In combination with at least one other drug it is effective in the prophylaxis and treatment of MAC in AIDS patients.

Dose: 500 mg once daily 1 hour before or 2 hours after food, (children above 6 months 10 mg/kg) for 3 days is sufficient for most infections.

AZITHRAL 250, 500 mg cap and 250 mg per 5 ml dry syr; AZIWOK 250 mg cap, 100 mg kid tab, 100 mg/5 ml and 200 mg/5 ml susp. AZIWIN 100, 250, 500 mg tab, 200 mg/5 ml liq. Also AZITHRAL 500 mg inj.

Side effects are mild gastric upset, abdominal pain (less than erythromycin), headache and dizziness. Azithromycin has been found not to interact with hepatic CYP3A4 enzyme. Interaction with theophylline, carbamazepine, warfarin, etc. is not likely, but cannot be totally ruled out.

LINCOSAMIDE ANTIBIOTICS

Clindamycin

The distinctive feature of this lincosamide antibiotic is its high activity against a variety of anaerobic bacteria, especially *Bact. fragilis*. Otherwise, it is similar in mechanism of action (inhibits protein synthesis by binding to 50S ribosome) and spectrum of activity to erythromycin with which it exhibits partial cross resistance. Like erythromycin, it inhibits most gram-positive cocci (including penicillinase producing *Staph.*, but not MRSA), *C. diphtheriae, Nocardia, Actinomyces,* and *Toxoplasma*. Aerobic gram-negative bacilli, enterococci, spirochetes, *Chlamydia, Mycoplasma* and *Rickettsia* are not affected.

Oral absorption of clindamycin is good. It penetrates into most soft tissues and bone, but not into brain and CSF; accumulates in neutrophils and macrophages. Metabolism is extensive, and metabolites are excreted in urine as well as in bile. The t½ is 3 hr.

Side effects are rashes, urticaria, abdominal pain, but the major problem is diarrhoea and pseudomembranous enterocolitis due to *Clostridium difficile* superinfection which is potentially fatal. The drug should be promptly stopped and metronidazole (alternatively vancomycin) given to treat it.

Because of the potential toxicity, use of clindamycin is restricted to anaerobic and mixed infections, especially by *Bact. fragilis* causing abdominal, pelvic or lung abscesses, and in penetrating injuries. It is generally combined with an aminoglycoside or cephalosporin. Anaerobic streptococcal and *Cl. perfringens* infections and those involving bone and joints respond well. In AIDS patients, clindamycin is combined with pyrimethamine for toxoplasmosis, and with primaquine for *Pneumocystis* pneumonia. Topically it can be used for infected acne vulgaris.

In the treatment of *dental infections*, clindamycin is generally used as a reserve drug for those caused by anaerobic bacteria in patients who cannot be given a penicillin or a macrolide or for cases not responding to these antibiotics. Because of good penetration into bone, clindamycin is particularly suited for dentoalveolar abscesses and other bone infections caused by *Staphylococci* or *Bacteroides*. It is an alternative antibiotic for prophylaxis of endocarditis due to postextraction bacteraemia in patients with damaged heart valves or other risk factors. Because only a single dose is needed for this purpose, there is little risk of pseudomembranous enterocolitis which otherwise is the most important limitation of clindamycin.

Clindamycin, erythromycin and chloramphenicol can exhibit mutual antagonism, probably because their ribosomal binding sites are proximal; binding of one hinders access of the other to its target site.

Dose: 150–300 mg QID oral; 200–600 mg i.v. 8 hourly; DALCAP 150 mg cap; CLINCIN 150, 300 mg cap; DALCIN, DALCINEX 150, 300 mg cap, 300 mg/2 ml and 600 mg/4 ml inj.

Lincomycin
It is the forerunner of clindamycin; has similar antibacterial and toxic properties, but is less potent and produces a higher incidence of diarrhoea and colitis—deaths have occurred. Thus, it has been largely replaced by clindamycin.

GLYCOPEPTIDE ANTIBIOTICS

Vancomycin

It is a glycopeptide antibiotic discovered in 1956 as a penicillin substitute, which has later assumed special significance due to efficacy against MRSA, *Strep. viridans, Enterococcus* and *Cl. difficile*. It is bactericidal to gram-positive cocci, *Neisseria, Clostridia*, oral cavity anaerobes and diphtheroids. However, in hospitals where it has been extensively used for surgical prophylaxis, etc., vancomycin-resistant *Staph. aureus (VRSA)*, and vancomycin-resistant *Enterococcus* (VRE) have emerged. These nosocomial bacteria are resistant to methicillin and most other antibiotics as well.

Vancomycin acts by inhibiting bacterial cell wall synthesis. It binds to the terminal dipeptide 'D-ala-D-ala' sequence of peptidoglycan units—prevents its release from the bactoprenol lipid carrier so that assembly of the units at the cell membrane and their cross linking to form the cell wall cannot take place (*see* Fig. 27.2). Enterococcal resistance to vancomycin is due to a plasmid mediated alteration of the dipeptide target reducing its affinity for vancomycin.

Vancomycin is not absorbed orally. After i.v. administration, it is widely distributed, penetrates serous cavities, inflamed meninges and is excreted mainly unchanged by glomerular filtration with a t½ of 6 hours. Dose reduction is needed in renal insufficiency.

Toxicity: Systemic toxicity of vancomycin is relatively high. It can cause concentration dependent nerve deafness which may be permanent. Kidney damage is also dose related. Other oto- and nephrotoxic drugs like aminoglycosides must be very carefully administered when vancomycin is being used. Skin allergy and fall in BP during i.v. injection can occur. Vancomycin has the potential to release histamine from mast cells. Rapid i.v. injection has caused chills, fever, urticaria and intense flushing—called 'Red man syndrome'.

Uses: Given orally (125–500 mg 6 hourly), it is the second choice drug to metronidazole for antibiotic associated pseudomembranous enterocolitis caused by *C. difficile*. However, for serious cases, it may be more effective than metronidazole. Staphylococcal enterocolitis is another indication.

Systemic use (500 mg 6 hourly or 1 g 12 hourly infused i.v. over 1 hr) is restricted to serious MRSA infections for which it is the most effective drug. Vancomycin is also used as a penicillin substitute (in allergic patients) for enterococcal endocarditis along with gentamicin. Another area of its use is in dialysis patients and those undergoing cancer chemotherapy.

VANCOCIN-CP, VANCOGEN, VANCORID-CP 500 mg/vial inj; VANCOLED 0.5, 1.0 g inj. VANCOMYCIN 500 mg tab.

Use of vancomycin in *dental infections* is highly restricted to the few cases that do not respond to other safer antibiotics and are hypersensitive to penicillin. In penicillin allergic patients vancomycin 1 g (20 mg/kg) i.v. infusion is an alternative to amoxicillin for combining with gentamicin for prophylaxis of endocarditis in high-risk patients undergoing dental surgery.

Teicoplanin This later developed glycopeptide antibiotic is active against gram-positive bacteria only. The mechanism of action and spectrum of activity is similar to vancomycin. Notable features of teicoplanin are:
- It is more active than vancomycin against enterococci, and equally active against MRSA.
- Some VRE are susceptible to teicoplanin.
- It can be injected i.m. as well; is excreted by kidney; dose needs to be reduced in renal insufficiency; has a very long t½ (2–3 days); suitable for once daily dosing.
- Renal toxicity is less than vancomycin; adverse effects are rashes, fever, granulocytopenia and rarely hearing loss. Reactions due to histamine release are very rare (1 in 2500).

Teicoplanin is indicated in enterococcal endocarditis (along with gentamicin); MRSA and penicillin-resistant streptococcal infections in place of vancomycin.

Dose: 400 mg first day—then 200 mg daily i.v. or i.m.; TARGOCID, TECOCIN, TECOPLAN 200, 400 mg per vial inj. for reconstitution.

OXAZOLIDINONES

Linezolid This is the first member of a new class of synthetic AMAs 'Oxazolidinones,' useful in the treatment of resistant gram-positive coccal (aerobic and anaerobic) and bacillary infections. It is active against MRSA and some VRSA, VRE, penicillin-resistant *Strep. pyogenes*, *Strep. viridans* and *Strep. pneumoniae*. Other sensitive bacteria are *Corynebacterium*, *Listeria*, *Clostridia*, *Bact. fragilis* and *Mycobact. tuberculosis*. It is primarily bacteriostatic. Gram-negative bacteria are not affected.

Linezolid inhibits bacterial protein synthesis by acting at an early step and on a site different from that of other AMAs. It binds to the 23S fraction of the 50S ribosome and interferes with formation of the initiation complex. Binding of linezolid stops protein synthesis before it starts. As such, there is no cross resistance with any other class of AMAs.

Linezolid is rapidly and completely absorbed orally, partly metabolized nonenzymatically and excreted in urine. Plasma t½ is 5 hrs.

Linezolid given orally or i.v. can be used for skin and soft tissue infections, hospital-acquired pneumonias, bacteraemias, febrile neutropenia, wound infections and others caused by multidrug-resistant gram-positive bacteria such as VRE, vancomycin-resistant-MRSA, multiresistant *S. pneumoniae*, etc. There are no specific indications in dentistry for linezolid.

Dose: 600 mg BD, oral/ i.v.; LIZOLID 600 mg tab; LINOX 600 mg tab, 300 mg/300 ml i.v. infusion.

Side effects to linezolid have been few; mostly mild abdominal pain, taste disturbance and diarrhoea. Occasionally, rash, pruritus, headache, oral/vaginal candidiasis have been reported. Prolonged use (>2 weeks) can cause haematologic toxicity. Because linezolid is a MAO inhibitor, interactions with adrenergic/serotonergic drugs are possible.

Tedizolid It is a new oxazolidinone AMA similar to linezolid, but 4–8 times more potent and longer acting. Like linezolid, it is active only against gram +ve bacteria including MRSA, VRSA, VRE and some linezolid-resistant strains. Clinical indications of tedizolid are hospital-acquired resistant gram +ve infections, similar in range to those for linezolid.

MISCELLANEOUS ANTIBIOTICS

Quinupristin/Dalfopristin This a mixture of two semisynthetic streptogramins Quinupristin and Dalfopristin in 30:70 ratio, which together exerts rapid bactericidal effect on many gram +ve bacteria. The two antibiotics bind to adjacent sites on 50s bacterial ribosomes to exert synergistic inhibition of protein synthesis. They kill most gram +ve cocci including MRSA, VRSA, VRE, penicillin-resistant *Strep, pneumoniae*, etc. Infused i.v. over 60 min, every 8–12 hours, they are used as a reserve drug for multidrug-resistant nosocomial gram +ve infections.

SYNERCID: Quinupristin 150 mg + Dalfopristin 350 mg (total 500 mg) per vial inj.

Daptomycin This is a lipopeptide antibiotic with a unique mechanism of action. The lipoidal molecules of daptomycin get inserted in the bacterial cell membrane forming pores through which K^+ and other ions leak out and the membrane gets depolarized. Synthesis of RNA, DNA and proteins is secondarily inhibited, and the bacterial cell is killed. Cidal action is exerted only on gram +ve bacteria including MRSA, VRSA, multidrug-resistant *Streptococci*, VRE and *Corynebacteria*. Daptomycin is indicated for treatment of skin and soft tissue infections, and bacteraemia caused by resistant gram +ve bacteria. Myopathy is its specific toxicity.

DAPTOCURE 350 mg/vial, for slow i.v. injection after reconstitution.

POLYPEPTIDE ANTIBIOTICS

These are low molecular weight cationic polypeptide antibiotics. All are powerful bactericidal agents, but not used systemically due to toxicity. All are produced by bacteria. Clinically used ones are:

Polymyxin B   Bacitracin
Colistin

Polymyxin B and Colistin Polymyxin and colistin are basic polypeptides which were obtained in the late 1940s from *Bacillus polymyxa* and *B. colistinus* respectively. They are active against gram-negative bacteria only, of which all except *Proteus, Serratia* and *Neisseria* are inhibited. Both polymyxin B and colistin have very similar range of activity, but colistin is more potent on *Pseudomonas, Salmonella* and *Shigella*.

Mechanism of action Polymyxin B and colistin are rapidly acting bactericidal agents, having a detergent-like action on the cell membrane. They have high affinity for phospholipids. The peptide molecules of the antibiotic orient between the phospholipid and protein films in gram-negative bacterial cell membrane causing membrane distortion or pseudopore formation. As a result, ions, amino acids, etc. leak out. Sensitive bacteria take up more of the antibiotic.

Polymyxin B and colistin exhibit synergism with many other AMAs by improving their penetration into the bacterial cell.

Resistance Resistance to these antibiotics has never been a problem. There is no cross resistance with any other AMA.

Adverse effects Little or no absorption occurs from oral route or even from denuded skin (burn, ulcers). Applied topically, they are safe—no systemic effect or sensitization occurs. A rash is rare. Given orally, side effects are limited to the g.i.t.—occasional nausea, vomiting, diarrhoea.

Preparation and dose
Polymyxin B: (1 mg = 10,000 U)
NEOSPORIN POWDER: 5,000 U with neomycin sulf. 3,400 U and bacitracin 400 U per g.

NEOSPORIN-H EAR DROPS: 10,000 U with neomycin sulf. 3,400 U and hydrocortisone 10 mg per ml.
Colistin sulfate: 25–100 mg TDS oral;
WALAMYCIN 12.5 mg (25,000 i.u.) per 5 ml dry syr, COLISTOP 12.5 mg/5 ml and 25 mg/5 ml dry syr.

Uses
(a) *Topically* Usually in combination with other antimicrobials for skin infections, burns, otitis externa, caused by gram-negative bacteria including *Pseudomonas*.
(b) *Orally* Gram-negative bacillary (*E. coli, Salmonella, Shigella*) diarrhoeas, especially in infants and children; *Pseudomonas* superinfection enteritis.

Bacitracin It is one of the earliest discovered antibiotics from a strain of *Bacillus subtilis*. In contrast to polymyxin, it is active mainly against gram-positive bacteria (both cocci and bacilli). The sensitive gram negative bacteria are *Neisseria* and *H. influenzae*.

Bacitracin acts by inhibiting cell wall synthesis at a step earlier than that inhibited by penicillin. Subsequently, it increases the efflux of ions by binding to cell membrane. It is bactericidal.

Bacitracin is not absorbed orally. It is not injected parenterally because of high toxicity, especially to the kidney. Use is restricted to topical application for infected wounds, ulcers, eye infections—generally in combination with neomycin, polymyxin, etc.
In NEBASULF Bacitracin 250 U + neomycin 5 mg + sulfacetamide 60 mg/g powder, skin oint, eye oint; in NEOSPORIN 400 U/g powder (1 U = 26 µg).

Antitubercular and Antileprotic Drugs

ANTITUBERCULAR DRUGS

Tuberculosis is a chronic granulomatous disease and a major health problem in developing countries. About 1/3rd of the world's population is infected with *Mycobact. tuberculosis,* out of which 10–15% develop the disease over their life-time. India is the highest TB burden country in the world, where about 600 people die of TB every day. Control and treatment of TB in India is covered under the Revised National Tuberculosis Control Programme (RNTCP), which was launched in 1997, and which has successively revised the TB treatment guidelines; the last time in 2016.*.

Emergence of 'multidrug resistant' (MDR) TB which now accounts for ~20% of previously treated, and 3.3% of new TB cases worldwide is threatening the whole future of current antitubercular chemotherapy. Another complexity is added due to spread of HIV infection, because HIV patients have a high prevalence of TB/*Mycobacterium avium* complex (MAC) coinfection. Moreover, HIV patients are especially vulnerable to severe forms of TB/MAC disease, including MDR-TB.

Remarkable progress has been made in the last 75 years since the introduction of *Streptomycin* for the treatment of tuberculosis. Besides adding a number of effective drugs, strategies in the management of TB have been improved based on the understanding of biology of this infection. Clear-cut treatment guidelines have been formulated. While dentists are not called upon to treat tuberculosis, they should be familiar with important features of antitubercular drugs and the current therapeutic regimens.

According to their clinical utility, the anti-TB drugs are divided into:

First line drugs: These drugs have high antitubercular efficacy as well as low toxicity; are used routinely.

Second line drugs: These drugs have either low antitubercular efficacy or higher toxicity or both; and are used in cases with resistance to 1st line drugs, or to suppliment them.

FIRST LINE ANTITUBERCULAR DRUGS
Isoniazid (Isonicotinic acid hydrazide, H)

Isonicotinic acid hydrazide (INH, isoniazid) is an excellent antitubercular drug, and an essential component of all antitubercular regimens, unless the patient is not able to tolerate it or bacilli are resistant. It is primarily tuberculocidal. Fast multiplying organisms are rapidly killed, but quiescent ones are only inhibited. It acts on extracellular as well as on intracellular TB (bacilli present within macrophages); is equally active in acidic and alkaline medium. Isoniazid is one of

---

*RNTCP: Technical and operational guidelines for tuberculosis control in India; www.tbcindia.gov.in

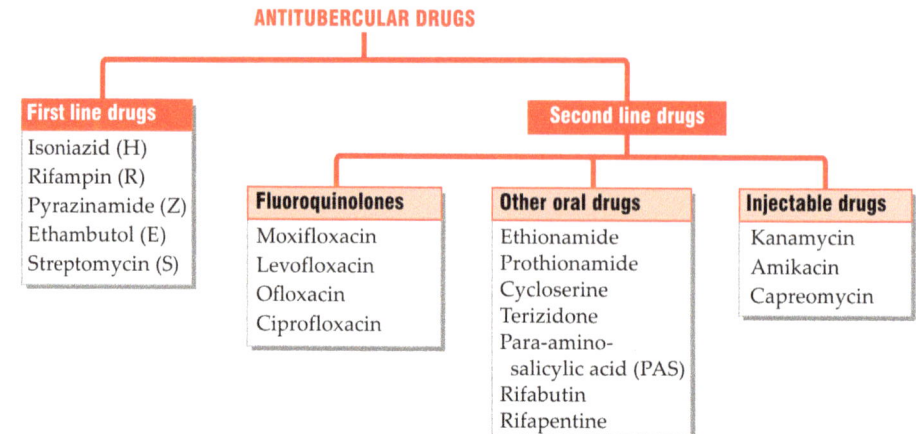

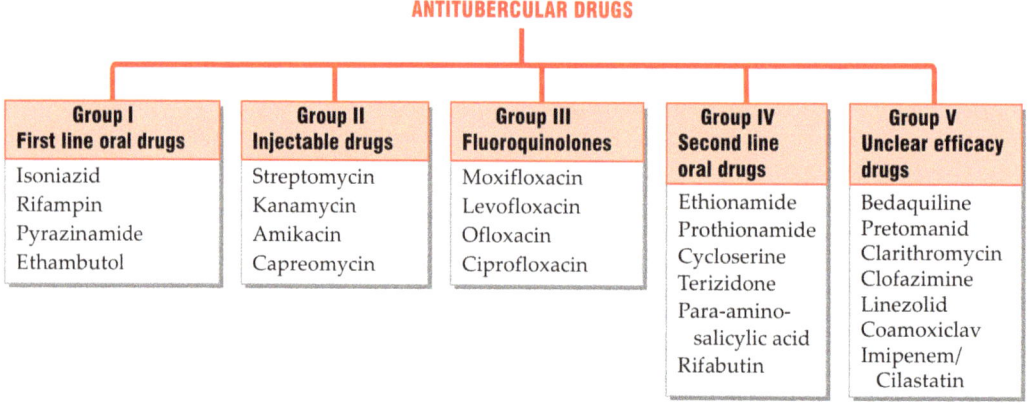

Group I: are the most potent and best tolerated oral drugs used routinely.
Group II: are potent and bactericidal, but injectable drugs which are used to supplement oral drugs, when needed.
Group III: includes fluoroquinolones which are well tolerated bactericidal oral drugs reserved for resistant TB.
Group IV: are less effective bacteriostatic/more toxic oral drugs for resistant TB.
Group V: are drugs with uncertain efficacy; not to be used for MDR-TB; but may be used as reserve drugs, and for extensively drug-resistant TB (XDR-TB).

the cheapest antitubercular drugs. However, most nontubercular mycobacteria are not inhibited by INH.

The primary mechanism of action of INH is inhibition of synthesis of *mycolic acids* which are unique fatty acid component of mycobacterial cell wall. This may explain the high selectivity of INH for mycobacteria (INH is not active against any other microorganism). The sensitive mycobacteria concentrate INH and convert it by a catalase-peroxidase enzyme into an active metabolite that interacts with '*InhA*' and *KasA* gene products involved in mycolic acid synthesis.

About 1 in 10^6 tubercle bacilli is inherently resistant to clinically attained INH concentrations. If INH is given alone, such bacilli proliferate selectively and after

2–3 months (sometimes even earlier) an apparently resistant infection emerges. The most common mechanism of INH resistance is by mutation of the catalase-peroxidase gene so that the bacilli do not generate the active metabolite of INH. Other resistant TB bacilli lose the active INH concentrating process. It is estimated that in India incidence of resistance to INH alone or in combination with other antitubercular drugs is ~18%.

Pharmacokinetics INH is completely absorbed orally and penetrates all body tissues, tubercular cavities, placenta and meninges. It is extensively metabolized in liver; most important pathway being N-acetylation by NAT2 enzyme. The acetylated metabolites are excreted in urine. The rate of INH acetylation shows genetic variation: there are slow and fast acetylators. The t½ of INH is 1 hr in fast acetylators, and 3 hours in slow acetylators. The latter have a higher risk of developing INH-related peripheral neuritis.

Adverse effects INH is well tolerated by most patients. Peripheral neuritis and a variety of neurological manifestations (paresthesias, numbness, mental disturbances, rarely convulsions) are the most important dose-dependent toxic effects. These effects are due to interference by INH with production of the active coenzyme pyridoxal phosphate from pyridoxine and its increased excretion in urine. Pyridoxine given prophylactically (10 mg/day) prevents INH neurotoxicity. INH neurotoxicity is treated by pyridoxine 100 mg/day.

Hepatitis, a major adverse effect of INH, is due to dose-related damage to liver cells. INH must be stopped at the 1st sign of hepatotoxicity, and it is reversible on stopping the drug. Other side effects are rashes, fever, acne and arthralgia.

ISONEX 100, 300 mg tabs, ISOKIN 100 mg tab, 100 mg per 5 ml liq.

Rifampin (Rifampicin, R)

It is a semisynthetic derivative of rifamycin B obtained from *Streptomyces mediterranei*. Rifampin is bactericidal to *M. tuberculosis* and many other gram-positive and gram-negative bacteria like *Staph. aureus, N. meningitidis, H. influenzae, E. coli, Klebsiella, Pseudomonas, Proteus* and *Legionella*. Against *M. tuberculosis*, it is as efficacious as INH and better than all other drugs. Rifampin acts best on slowly and intermittently (spurters) dividing bacilli. *Mycobact. leprae* is also highly sensitive, while MAC is moderately susceptible. Both extra- and intracellular organisms are affected. It has good sterilizing and resistance preventing actions.

Rifampin inhibits DNA-dependent RNA synthesis. The probable basis of selective toxicity is that mammalian RNA polymerase does not avidly bind rifampin.

Mycobacteria and other organisms develop resistance to rifampin rather rapidly. Rifampin resistance is nearly always due to mutation in the *rpoB* gene (the target of rifampin action) reducing its affinity for the drug. No cross resistance with any other antitubercular drug has been noted.

Pharmacokinetics Rifampin is well absorbed when taken on empty stomach, widely distributed in the body: penetrates cavities, caseous masses, placenta and meninges. It is metabolized in liver to an active deacetylated metabolite which is excreted mainly in bile; some in urine also. The t½ of rifampin is variable (2–5 hours).

Interactions Rifampin is a microsomal enzyme inducer, increases CYP3A4, CYP2D6, CYP1A2; enhances its own metabolism as well as that of many other drugs, including warfarin, oral contraceptives, corticosteroids, sulfonylureas, steroids, HIV protease inhibitors, ketoconazole, etc. Contraceptive failures have occurred due to concurrent rifampin medication.

Adverse effects The incidence of adverse effects is similar to that with INH.

Hepatitis, a major adverse effect, generally occurs in patients with pre-existing liver disease and is dose related.

Minor reactions are:
- '*Cutaneous syndrome*': flushing, pruritus with rash, redness and watering of eyes.
- '*Flu like symptoms*': with chills, fever, headache, malaise and bone pain.
- Abdominal cramps, nausea, vomiting, diarrhoea.

Urine and secretions may become orange-red—but this is harmless.

Other uses of rifampin are:
1. Leprosy (*see* p. 461)
2. Prophylaxis of *Meningococcal* and *H. influenzae* meningitis and carrier state.
3. Combination of doxycycline and rifampin is the first line therapy of brucellosis.

RCIN 150, 300, 450, 600 mg caps, 100 mg/5 ml susp. RIMACTANE, RIMPIN 150, 300, 450 mg caps, 100 mg/5 ml syr.; RIFAMYCIN 450 mg cap, ZUCOX 300, 450, 600 mg tabs. To be taken 1 hr. before or 2 hr. after food.

Pyrazinamide (Z)

Chemically similar to INH, pyrazinamide (Z) was developed parallel to it in 1952. It is tuberculocidal, but weaker than INH, and more active in acidic medium. Intracellularly located bacilli and those at sites showing an inflammatory response (pH is acidic at both these locations) are rapidly killed. It has good sterilizing activity and is highly effective during the first 2 months of therapy when inflammatory changes are present. Inclusion of Z has enabled duration of treatment to be shortened and risk of relapse to be reduced. Like INH, pyrazinamide has no other use, except in TB.

The mechanism of action of Z appears to be similar to that of INH. It is converted inside the mycobacterial cell into an active metabolite pyrazinoic acid which accumulates in acidic medium and inhibits mycolic acid synthesis. Mycobacterial cell membrane and its transport function are also disrupted.

Pyrazinamide is absorbed orally, widely distributed in the body, has good penetration in CSF, extensively metabolized in liver and excreted in urine; plasma t½ 6–10 hours.

Hepatotoxicity is the most important dose-related adverse effect, but it appears to be less common in the Indian population than in western countries. Hyperuricaemia is due to inhibition of uric acid secretion in kidney: gout can occur. Other adverse effects are abdominal distress, arthralgia, flushing, rashes, fever and loss of diabetes control.

PYZINA 0.5, 0.75, 1.0 g tabs, 0.3 g kid tab; PZA-CIBA 0.5, 0.75 g tabs, 250 mg/5 ml syr; RIZAP 0.75, 1.0 g tabs.

Ethambutol (E)

Ethambutol is selectively tuberculostatic and is active against MAC, but not other types of bacteria. Fast multiplying tubercle bacilli are more susceptible. Added to the triple drug regimen of RHZ, it has been found to hasten the rate of sputum conversion and to prevent development of resistance.

The mechanism of action of E is not fully understood, but it has been found to inhibit arabinogalactan synthesis, thereby interfering with mycolic acid incorporation in mycobacterial cell wall. Resistance to E develops slowly, and is due to mutation reducing affinity of the target enzyme for E. No cross resistance with any other antitubercular drug has been noted.

About 3/4th of an oral dose of E is absorbed. It is distributed widely and is briefly stored in RBCs. Less than ½ of E is metabolized. It is excreted in urine by glomerular filtration and tubular secretion; plasma t½ is ~4 hrs.

Patient acceptability of E is very good. Loss of visual acuity/colour vision, field defects due to optic neuritis is the most important dose and duration of therapy dependent toxicity, but is reversible if the drug is stopped early. Ethambutol produces few other symptoms: nausea, rashes, fever, neurological changes are infrequent.

Ethambutol is used in MAC infection as well.

MYCOBUTOL, MYAMBUTOL, COMBUTOL 0.2, 0.4, 0.6, 0.8, 1.0 g tabs.

Streptomycin (S)

The pharmacology of streptomycin is described in Ch. 28. It was the first clinically useful antitubercular drug. Streptomycin is tuberculocidal, but less effective than INH or rifampin; acts only on extracellular bacilli (because of poor penetration into cells). It penetrates tubercular cavities, but does not cross to the CSF, and has poor action in acidic medium.

Resistance develops rapidly to S. In case of S resistant infection, it must be stopped at the earliest due to risk of emergence of S-dependent bacilli. Most nontubercular mycobacteria are unaffected by S.

Because of need for i.m. injections and lower margin of safety, streptomycin is used only as a reserve/supplemental first line drug in TB.

SECOND LINE ANTI-TUBERCULAR DRUGS

These are less effective and/or less well tolerated drugs that are used only in case the bacilli are resistant to one or more first line drugs or when first line are not tolerated.

1. Kanamycin (Km), Amikacin (Am)

These are tuberculocidal aminoglycoside antibiotics (described in Ch. 28), very similar in antitubercular activity, pharmacokinetic properties and types of adverse effects to streptomycin. One of these is mostly included for streptomycin-resistant or MDR-TB during the intensive phase.

2. Capreomycin (Cm)

It is a cyclic peptide antibiotic, similar in antitubercular activity, ototoxicity and nephrotoxicity to aminoglycosides. In addition, capreomycin causes eosinophilia, rashes and injection site pain. It is used only as an alternative to aminoglycosides in MDR-TB.

3. Fluoroquinolones (FQs)

Ofloxacin, levofloxacin, moxifloxacin and *ciprofloxacin* are potent bactericidal drugs for TB, which have gained prominence as well tolerated substitutes for the first line anti-TB drugs. They are active against MAC and *Mycobact. fortuitum* as well. While moxifloxacin is the most active FQ against *M. tuberculosis*, ciprofloxacin is the most active FQ for MAC. The FQs penetrate cells and kill intracellular TB within macrophages as well. To preserve the anti-TB efficacy of these valuable drugs, their use is restricted to drug-resistant TB. The RNTCP have included levofloxacin in their standardized regimen for MDR-TB. An FQ may also be included in the regimen when either H or R or Z cannot be given due to hepatotoxicity. The FQs are described in Ch. 26.

4. Ethionamide (Etm)

It is a bacteriostatic drug of moderate efficacy which acts on extra- and intra-cellular tubercle bacilli. MAC and few other Mycobacteria are also susceptible. Similar to INH, it acts by interfering with mycolic acid synthesis. Tolerability of Etm. is relatively poor; frequent side effects are—anorexia, nausea, metallic taste, epigastric distress and hepatitis. Other adverse effects are body ache, peripheral neuritis and impotence. Pyridoxine mitigates the neurological symptoms. Etm. is used only for MDR-TB and is a component of the RNTCP standardized regimen. It is also an optional drug for MAC infection, and a reserve drug for leprosy.

Prothionamide is a similar drug, considered interchangeable with Etm.

5. Cycloserine (Cs)

This antibiotic is an analogue of D-alanine which is a component of bacterial cell wall. Accordingly, cycloserine inhibits bacterial cell wall synthesis. It is bacteriostatic against *M. tuberculosis*, MAC, some gram positive bacteria, *E. coli* and *Chlamydia*. Cycloserine is administered orally and is used only for resistant TB. It is included in the standardized regimen used by RNTCP for MDR-TB. Adverse effects of cycloserine are primarily neurological, *viz.* sleepiness, tremor, slurring of speech, altered behaviour, psychosis and convulsions. Pyridoxine reduces its neurotoxicity.

6. Terizidone

It contains 2 molecules of cycloserine, and has antibacterial properties, including mechanism of action, like cycloserine. Believed to be less neurotoxic, it is used as a substitute of cycloserine.

7. Para-amino salicylic acid (PAS)

It is chemically related to sulfonamides and acts by inhibiting folate synthase. PAS is selectively tuberculostatic and one of the least active drugs. It benefits only by preventing resistance to other drugs given concurrently. PAS frequently causes anorexia, nausea epigastric pain. It is a reserve drug for adding to the regimen for MDR-TB.

8. Rifabutin

This rifampin congener acts by the same mechanism, but is less active against *M. tuberculosis* and exhibits cross resistance with it. Rifabutin is used only as a substitute for rifampin to minimise drug interactions due to enzyme inducing property of the latter. Rifabutin is a much weaker inducer of microsomal enzymes and is less likely to interact with other drugs. Rifabutin is more active against MAC, and its primary indication is for prophylaxis and treatment of MAC infection in HIV-AIDS patients.

9. Bedaquiline

This is a novel antitubercular drug introduced recently for use in selected cases of MDR-TB. Bedaquiline inhibits mycobacterial ATP synthase enzyme, thereby limiting energy production in the mycobacterial cell, and exhibiting bactericidal action. The RNTCP have introduced it in India for use in selected cases of MDR-TB.

TREATMENT OF TUBERCULOSIS

Tuberculosis is treated with a combination of 3–5 antitubercular drugs under the *'directly observed treatment short course' (DOTS)* protocol formulated by the WHO. Under this protocol dose of all first line drugs was standardized on body weight basis, applicable to both adults and children. These are given in Table 30.1.

Table 30.1: Daily dose of 1st line antitubercular drugs on body weight basis$

Drug	Daily dose (mg/kg)
1. Isoniazid (H)	5 (4–6)
2. Rifampin (R)	10 (8–12)
3. Pyrazinamide (Z)	25 (20–30)
4. Ethambutol (E)	15 (15–20)
5. Streptomycin (S)*	15 (12–18)

$Based on WHO (2010) guidelines
*In patients above 50 years age, the maximum dose of steptomycin is 0.75 g/day.

The goals of antitubercular chemotherapy are:

(a) Kill dividing bacilli Drugs with early bactericidal action rapidly reduce bacillary load in the patient and achieve quick sputum negativity. This also affords quick symptom relief.

(b) Kill persisting bacilli To effect cure by killing all bacilli and prevent relapse.

(c) Prevent emergence of resistance so that the bacilli remain susceptible to the drugs.

The relative activity of the first line drugs in achieving these goals differs, e.g. isoniazid (H) and rifampin (R) are the most potent bactericidal drugs active against all subpopulations of TB bacilli, while pyrazinamide (Z) acts best on intracellular bacilli and those at inflamed sites—has very good sterilizing activity. Ethambutol (E) is bacteriostatic—mainly serves to prevent resistance and may hasten sputum conversion (AFB positive to AFB negative). The general principles of antitubercular chemotherapy are:

- Use of any single drug in tuberculosis results in the emergence of resistant organisms and relapse in almost 3/4th patients. A combination of two or more drugs must be used.
- Isoniazid and R are the most efficacious drugs; their combination is clearly synergistic—duration of therapy is shortened from > 12 months to 9 months. Addition of Z for the initial 2 months further reduces duration of treatment to 6 months.
- All first line antitubercular drugs (ATDs) are administered in a single daily dose.
- The response is fast in the first few weeks as the fast dividing bacilli are eliminated rapidly. Symptomatic relief is evident within 2–4 weeks. The rate of bacteriological, radiological and clinical improvement declines subsequently. Bacteriological cure takes much longer.

All anti-TB regimens have an initial *intensive phase* lasting 2–3 months with 4–6 drugs aimed to rapidly kill the bacilli and afford symptomatic relief. This is followed by a *continuation phase* with 3–4 drugs lasting 4–5 months during which the remaining bacilli are eliminated so that relapse does not occur.

Antitubercular Drugs

Antitubercular drug regimens have been devised for drug sensitive (DS) TB, as well as for various categories of drug resistant (DR) TB. The RNTCP (2016) regimens for DS-TB and for MDR-TB are described briefly.

Drug sensitive TB This is treated by 1st line ATDs as per regimens summarized in Table 30.2. The ATDs are administered once daily (the earlier thrice a week dosing has been abandoned).

Table 30.2: Treatment regimens* for new patients and previously treated patients of pulmonary TB presumed to be drug sensitive

Type of patient	Intensive phase	Continuation phase	Total duration
New	2£ HRZE	4 HRE	6£
Previously treated	2 HRZES +1 HRZE	5 HRE	8

*Based on RNTCP guidelines 2016.
£Duration of the phase/total duration in months.
H,R,Z,E,S—Standard codes for Isoniazid, Rifampin, Pyrazinamide, Ethambutol, Streptomycin.

New patients In the initial phase, 4 oral drugs, including 3 bactericidal drugs (RHZ) and one bacteriostatic drug (E), rapidly bring down the bacillary load and reduce the risk of selecting resistant bacilli. After 2 months Z is discontinued and the remaining 3 (RHE) are continued for another 4 months to eliminate the remaining bacilli from patients body.

Previously treated patients of TB who are presumed not to have DR-TB, are initially treated with all 5 first line ATDs daily for 2 months. Injected S is then stopped, and the remaining 4 (RHZE) drugs are continued for another one month. The intensive phase, therefore, is of 3 months. The continuation phase with 3 drugs (RHE) is also longer (5 months). In case of severe forms of extra-pulmonary TB, the continuation phase in both new as well as previously treated patients may be extended by 3–6 months on clinical grounds.

Multidrug-resistant (MDR) TB

MDR-TB is defined as resistance to both H and R, with or without resistance to any number of other first line drug(s). MDR-TB has a more rapid course with worse outcomes. Its treatment requires complex multiple second line drug regimens which are longer, more expensive and more toxic. In India, 3% of all new TB cases, and 12–17% of retreatment cases are MDR-TB. The general principles of treatment of MDR-TB are:

- The regimen should have at least 4 drugs certain to be effective. Often 6 drugs are started, since efficacy of some may be uncertain.
- Reliance about efficacy may be placed on drug sensitivity test (DST) results. Drugs used previously in that individual may be omitted.
- Drugs from group I to group IV (*see* p. 454) are included in a hierarchial order. Group I drugs Z and E (but not H and R) can be included + one injectable drug (group II) + one FQ (group III) + two group IV drugs. The 'standard' RNTCP regimen for MDR-TB consists of 6 drugs intensive phase lasting 6–9 months, and 4 drugs continuation phase of 18 months (*see* box).

Pyridoxine 100 mg/day is given to all patients during the whole course of therapy to prevent neurotoxicity of anti-TB drugs. However, individualized regimens can be constructed, if necessary, taking into consideration the specifics of individual patients.

Standard RNTCP regimen for MDR-TB*	
Intensive phase (6–9 months)	Continuation phase (18 months)
1. Pyrazinamide (Z)	1. Ethambutol
2. Ethambutol (E)	2. Levofloxacin
3. Kanamycin (Km)	3. Ethionamide
4. Levofloxacin (Lfx)	4. Cycloserine
5. Ethionamide (Eto)	
6. Cycloserine (Cs)	
+ Pyridoxine 100 mg/day	

*Revised National Tuberculosis Control Programme Guidelines (2016)

Extensively drug-resistant TB (XDR-TB) The MDR-TB cases who in addition are resistant to an FQ as well as to one injectable second line drug ± other drugs is designated XDR-TB. The bacilli are thus resistant to at least 4 most effective cidal drugs *viz.* H, R, FQ and one of Km/Am/Cm. The XDR-TB has a rapid course, high mortality and is very difficult to treat. The RNTCP (2016) uses a 7 drugs (all reserve drugs) regimen for treating XDR-TB..

Mycobacterium avium complex (MAC) infection

MAC is an opportunistic pathogen which causes disseminated and multifocal disease in immunocompromized (particularly HIV-AIDS) patients. Cure by eradication of MAC has not been possible by any drug. The most favoured regimen for treating MAC infection consists of 3 or 4 drug intensive phase of 2–6 months, followed by 2 drug maintenance phase for at least 12 months (*see* box).

Regimen for treatment of MAC infection

Intensive phase

1. Clarithromycin 500 mg twice daily or Azithromycin 500 mg once daily
2. Ethambutol 1000 mg (15 mg/kg) per day
3. Rifabutin 300 mg per day

±

Ciprofloxacin 500 mg twice daily or
Levofloxacin 500 mg once daily or
Moxifloxacin 400 mg once daily

Maintenance phase*

1. Clarithromycin/Azithromycin
2. Ethambutol/Rifabutin/Any one fluoroquinolone

*Doses in the maintenance phase are the same as in intensive phase

---

ANTILEPROTIC DRUGS

Leprosy, caused by *Mycobacterium leprae*, has been considered incurable since ages and bears a social stigma. Due to development of effective antileprotic drugs, it is entirely curable now, but deformities/defects already incurred may not reverse. Though certain forms of leprosy produce oral/dental lesions, chemotherapy of leprosy is not undertaken by dentists, but by leprologists. Only a brief account of the antileprotic drugs is therefore relevant here.

CLASSIFICATION

Dapsone (DDS)

It is diamino diphenyl sulfone (DDS), the simplest, oldest, cheapest, most active and the only member of the class that is used now.

Dapsone is chemically related to sulfonamides and has the same mechanism of action, i.e. inhibition of PABA incorporation into folic acid. Accordingly, its antibacterial action is antagonized by PABA. Dapsone is leprostatic at very low concentrations. Specificity for *M. leprae* may be due to difference in the affinity of its folate synthase.

Dapsone resistance among *M. leprae* was first noted in 1964. It has spread and has necessitated use of multidrug therapy (MDT). Dapsone resistant *M. leprae* have mutated folate synthase enzyme with lower affinity for dapsone. However, the peak serum concentration of dapsone after 100 mg/day dose exceeds MIC for *M. leprae* by nearly 500 times. Thus, it continues to be active against low to moderately resistant bacilli. More important is the problem of '*persister bacilli*', which though drug sensitive, become dormant and remain hidden in tissues to stage a relapse later.

Dapsone is completely absorbed after oral administration and is widely distributed in the body. It is concentrated in skin (especially lepromatous skin), muscle, liver and kidney.

Dapsone is acetylated as well as glucuronide and sulfate conjugated in liver. The plasma t½ of dapsone is variable, though often > 24 hrs. The drug is cumulative due to retention

Antileprotic Drugs

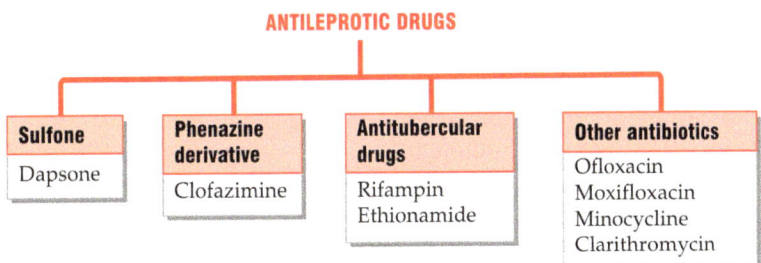

in tissues and enterohepatic circulation. Elimination takes 1–2 weeks or longer.

Dapsone is generally well tolerated at dose 100 mg/day dose or less.

Mild haemolytic anaemia is common. It is a dose related toxicity—reflects oxidising property of the drug. Patients with G-6-PD deficiency are more susceptible.

Other side effects are nausea, anorexia, headache, paresthesias, mental symptoms and drug fever.

Cutaneous reactions include allergic rashes, hypermelanosis, phototoxicity.

Lepra reaction.

Other use In combination with pyrimethamine dapsone can be used for chloroquine-resistant malaria, toxoplasmosis and *Pneumocystis jirovecii* pneumonia.

Clofazimine (Clo)

It is a dye with leprostatic and anti-inflammatory properties. The putative mechanisms of antileprotic action of clofazimine are:

- Interference with template function of DNA in *M. leprae*.
- Alteration in membrane function.
- Disruption of mitochondrial electron transport chain.

When used alone, resistance to clofazimine develops in 1–3 years.

Clofazimine is orally active. It accumulates in many tissues, especially in fat and in crystalline form. The t½ is 70 days so that intermittent therapy is possible.

Clofazimine is used as a component of multidrug therapy (MDT) of leprosy. Because of its anti-inflammatory property, it is valuable in lepra reaction.

The major disadvantage of clofazimine is reddish-black discolouration of skin, especially on exposed parts. Discolouration of hair and body secretions may also occur. Dryness of skin and itching is often troublesome. Conjunctival pigmentation may create cosmetic problem.

Enteritis with intermittent loose stools, nausea, abdominal pain, anorexia and weight loss can occur.

Rifampin (R)

This important antitubercular drug is also the most potent cidal drug for *M. leprae*. Rifampin rapidly renders leprosy patients noncontagious. Up to 99.99% *M. leprae* are killed in 3–7 days by 600 mg/day dose. Clinical effects of rifampin are very rapid; symptoms start subsiding within 2–3 weeks. However, the nerve damage already incurred is little improved. Rifampin is not satisfactory if used alone—some bacilli persist even after prolonged treatment, and resistance develops. Rifampin is included in the multidrug therapy of leprosy; serves to shorten duration of treatment. Resistance does not develop when it is used in combination with other drugs. The 600 mg monthly dose used in leprosy is nontoxic and does not induce metabolism of other drugs. It should not be given to patients with hepatic or renal dysfunction.

Ethionamide This antitubercular drug has significant antileprotic activity, but causes hepatotoxicity in ~ 10% patients. It may be used as an alternative to clofazimine.

Ofloxacin It is the most commonly tried FQ for leprosy. Used as a component of MDT, ofloxacin has been found to hasten the bacteriological and clinical response in leprosy. However, it is not included in the standard treatment protocols, but can be used in alternative regimens in case rifampin cannot be used, or to shorten the duration of treatment. Moxifloxacin and sparfloxacin are the other potent cidal FQs for leprosy.

Minocycline Because of high lipophilicity, this tetracycline penetrates into *M. leprae* and inhibits them. However, the antileprotic potency of minocycline is rated inferior to that of rifampin, but superior to that of clarithromycin. Symptomatic relief is reported in lepromatous leprosy. It is being tried in alternative MDT regimens.

Clarithromycin It is the only macrolide antibiotic with significant activity against *M. leprae*. However, it is less bactericidal than rifampin, but appears to be synergistic with minocycline and can cause symptomatic improvement in lepromatous leprosy. It has been included in alternative MDT regimens.

TREATMENT OF LEPROSY

Leprosy is a chronic granulomatous infection caused by *Mycobacterium leprae*; primarily affecting skin, mucous membranes and nerves. The National Leprosy Control Programme was launched in India in 1955, and has been upgraded to National Leprosy Eradication Programme (NLEP) in 1982. India achieved elimination of leprosy as a public health problem (prevalence rate < 1 case per 10,000 population) in Dec. 2005, but some states still have > 1 case per 10,000.

Two polar types—lepromatous (LL) and tuberculoid (TT) with 4 intermediate forms—borderline (BB), borderline lepromatous (BL), borderline tuberculoid (BT) and indeterminate (I) of the disease are recognized.

For operational purposes, leprosy has been divided into *paucibacillary* and *multibacillary* forms. The criteria used under NLEP for defining the two forms are:

Paucibacillary leprosy (PBL) Skin lesions limited to 1–5 in number with no nerve involvement or single nerve involvement, and negative skin smear at all sites. The patient has few bacilli and is noninfectious.

Multibacillary leprosy (MBL) Six or more skin lesions, or more than one nerve involved, and/or skin smear positive at any one site. The patient has large bacillary load and is infectious.

Multidrug therapy (MDT) of leprosy

Multidrug therapy with rifampin, dapsone and clofazimine was introduced by the WHO in 1981. This was implemented under the NLEP. The MDT is the regimen of choice for all cases of leprosy. Its advantages are:
- MDT is effective even in cases with primary dapsone resistance.
- MDT prevents emergence of dapsone resistance.
- MDT affords quick symptom relief and renders MBL cases noncontagious within few days. It stops disease progression and prevents further complications.
- Use of MDT reduces total duration of therapy.

For PBL cases the MDT consists of dapsone (daily) + rifampin (monthly) for 6 months. However, for MBL cases, initially the MDT consisted of dapsone + rifampin + clofazimine for 2 years or till disease inactivity was achieved. Encouraged by the very low relapse rates obtained with 2-year MDT for MBL cases, the WHO recommended shortening the duration to 1 year for the mass programme, and this has been implemented in India under NLEP. This 12 months regimen is referred to as 'fixed duration therapy-12 months (FDT-12)' and is outlined in the box.

Multidrug therapy of leprosy		
	Multibacillary	Paucibacillary
Rifampin	600 mg once a month supervised	600 mg once a month supervised
Dapsone	100 mg daily self-administered	100 mg daily self-administered
Clofazimine	300 mg once a month supervised + 50 mg daily self-administered	— —
Duration	12 months	6 months

It has been observed that some patients do not achieve disease inactivity after 1 year or even after 2-year MDT. Independent leprologists, therefore, prefer to keep the duration of therapy flexible till disease inactivity/skin smear negativity is achieved both in MBL and in PBL cases.

It may be concluded that, where feasible, treatment till cure of every individual patient should be ensured both in MBL and in PBL.

Alternative regimens Many alternative regimens incorporating newer antileprotic drugs have been tested. However, these are used only in case of rifampin resistance or when it is impossible/inadvisable to employ the standard MDT regimen. Some of these are:

- In case of refusal to accept clofazimine: ofloxacin 400 mg or minocycline 100 mg daily can be substituted for it in the standard MDT.
- Four drug regimen of rifampin 600 mg + sparfloxacin 200 mg + clarithromycin 500 mg + minocycline 100 mg daily for 12 weeks for MBL cases.
- *Intermittent RMMx*: Rifampin 600 mg + Minocycline 200 mg + Moxifloxacin 400 mg once a month: 6 doses for PBL and 12 doses for MBL, without any drug inbetween.
- *Intermittent ROM:* Rifampin 600 mg + ofloxacin 400 mg + Minocycline 100 mg once a month for 3–6 months for PBL and for 12–24 months for MBL cases, without any drug inbetween.

Reactions in leprosy

Lepra reaction It occurs in lepromatous leprosy; usually coincides with institution of chemotherapy and/or intercurrent infection. It is a Jarish Herxheimer (Arthus) type of reaction due to release of antigens from the killed bacilli. It may be mild, severe or life-threatening, i.e. erythema nodosum leprosum (ENL).

Lepra reaction is of abrupt onset; existing lesions enlarge, become red, swollen and painful; several new lesions may appear. Malaise, fever and other constitutional symptoms may be present and marked.

Clofazimine (200 mg daily) is effective in controlling the reaction (except the severe one), probably because of its antiinflammatory property.

For severe reaction, prednisolone 40–60 mg/day is started immediately, and is continued till the reaction subsides, followed by tapering of dose. Other drugs used are—analgesics, antipyretics, antibiotics, etc. according to need.

Reversal reaction This is seen in tuberculoid leprosy—is a manifestation of delayed hypersensitivity to *M. leprae* antigens. Cutaneous ulceration, multiple nerve involvement with swollen, painful and tender nerves occur suddenly. Reversal reaction is treated with clofazimine or corticosteroids.

Antifungal Drugs

ANTIFUNGAL DRUGS

These are drugs used for superficial and deep (systemic) fungal infections.

A disquieting trend after 1950s has been the emergence of more sinister type of fungal infections which are, to a large extent, iatrogenic. Fungal infections are mostly associated with the use of anticancer/ immunosuppressant drugs, corticosteroids, broad-spectrum antibiotics, *dentures*, indwelling catheters and implants, and emergence of AIDS. As a result of breakdown of host defence mechanisms by the above agents, saprophytic fungi easily invade living tissue. *Candida albicans* is normally resident in the oral cavity. It invades to cause infection when host defence is impaired or the oral flora is disturbed.

Many topical antifungals have been available since the antiseptic era. Two important antibiotics, *viz*, amphotericin B and griseofulvin as well as a number of imidazoles and triazoles have been developed for topical and/or systemic use since 1960s. Some novel antifungals, e.g. terbinafine and caspofungin have been added lately.

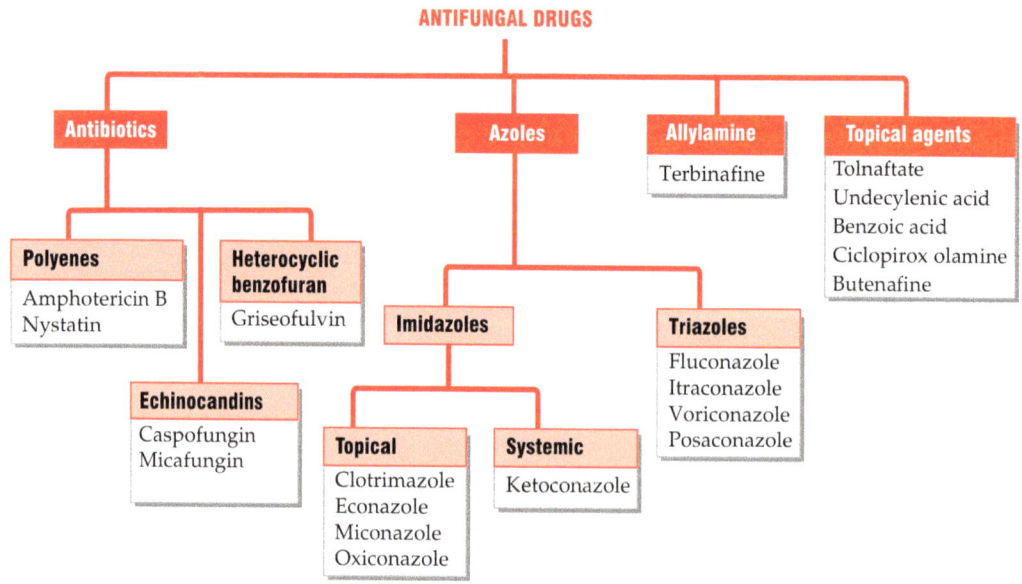

POLYENE ANTIBIOTICS

The name *polyene* is derived from their highly double-bonded structure.

Amphotericin B (AMB)

It is obtained from *Streptomyces nodosus*.

The polyenes possess a macrocyclic ring, one side of which has several conjugated double bonds and is highly lipophilic, while the other side is hydrophilic with many OH groups. All polyenes are insoluble in water and unstable in aqueous medium.

Polyene antibiotics have high affinity for ergosterol present in fungal cell membrane. They combine with it, get inserted into the membrane and several molecules together orient themselves in such a way as to form a 'micropore' through which ions, amino acids and other water-soluble substances move out (*see* Fig. 31.1). Thus, cell permeability is markedly increased.

Cholesterol, present in host cell membranes, closely resembles ergosterol; the polyenes bind to it as well, though with lesser affinity. Thus, the selectivity of action of polyenes is low, and AMB is one of the most toxic systemically used antibiotics. Bacteria do not have sterols and are unaffected by polyenes.

AMB is active against a wide range of yeasts and fungi—*Candida albicans, Histoplasma capsulatum, Cryptococcus neoformans, Blastomyces dermatitidis, Coccidioides immitis, Torulopsis, Rhodotorula, Aspergillus, Sporothrix*, etc. Dermatophytes are inhibited *in vitro*, but concentrations of AMB attained in infected skin are low and ineffective. AMB is fungicidal at high and static at lower concentrations.

Resistance to AMB is not a problem in the clinical use of the drug. AMB is also active on various species of *Leishmania* which is a protozoa.

AMB is not absorbed orally, but is active in the gut lumen and topically. Administered i.v. as a suspension made with the help of deoxycholate (DOC), it gets widely distributed in the body, but penetration in CSF is poor. It binds to sterols in tissues and to lipoproteins in plasma and stays in the body for long periods. The terminal

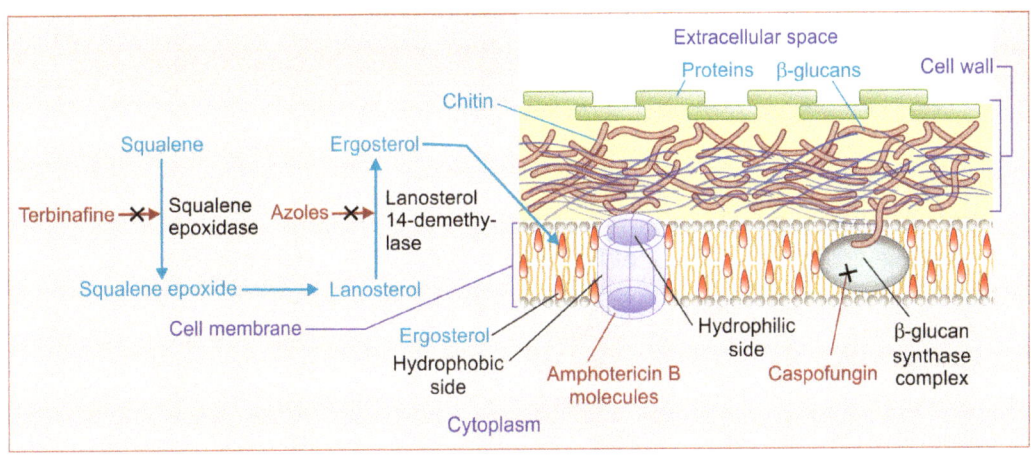

Fig. 31.1: Fungal cell wall and cell membrane along with schematic depiction of the mechanism of action of amphotericin B (AMB), caspofungin, azole antifungals and **terbinafine**
Note: The AMB molecules aggregate and orient in the fungal cell membrane to form a pore. The inner surface of the pore is formed by the hydrophilic side of AMB molecules through which ions, amino acids, etc. leak out. The outer surface of the pore is formed by the hydrophobic side of AMB molecules which are stabilized by interaction with ergosterol.

elimination t½ is 15 days. About 60% of AMB is metabolized in the liver. Excretion occurs slowly both in urine and bile.

Administration and dose Amphotericin B can be administered orally (50–100 mg QID) for intestinal moniliasis; also topically for vaginitis, otomycosis, etc.: FUNGIZONE OTIC 3% ear drops.

Amphotericin B Deoxycholate (AMB-DOC) This is the conventional preparation of AMB, which is available as dry powder along with DOC for extemporaneous dispersion before use: FUNGIZONE INTRAVENOUS, MYCOL 50 mg/vial. It is diluted to 500 ml with glucose solution and 0.3 mg/kg is infused over 4–8 hours.

The daily dose is gradually increased. The total dose needed for systemic mycosis is usually 3–4 g given over 2–3 months.

Liposomal amphotericin B (L-AMB) It has been produced to improve tolerability and to reduce toxicity of i.v. AMB, as well as to achieve targeted delivery. It consists of 10% AMB incorporated in uniform sized (60-80 nM) unilamellar liposomes made up of lecithin and other biodegradable phospholipids.

The *liposomal - AMB* produces equivalent blood levels, has similar clinical efficacy with less acute reaction and renal toxicity. It thus appears more satisfactory, can be infused at higher rates (3-5 mg/kg/day), but is many times costlier than AMB-DOC. FUNGISOME (liposomal AMB) 10 mg, 25 mg, 50 mg per vial inj.

Adverse effects The toxicity of AMB is high.

(a) *Acute reaction* This occurs with each infusion and consists of chills, fever, aches and pain all over, nausea, vomiting and dyspnoea lasting for 2–5 hours probably due to release of cytokines (IL, TNFα). Thrombophlebitis of the injected vein can occur.

(b) *Long-term toxicity* Nephrotoxicity is the most important. It occurs fairly uniformly and is dose related: manifestations are—azotaemia, reduced g.f.r., acidosis, hypokalaemia and inability to concentrate urine.

Most patients develop slowly progressing anaemia due to bone marrow depression. This is largely reversible on stopping the drug.

Uses Amphotericin B can be used topically for oral, vaginal and cutaneous candidiasis and otomycosis.

It is the most effective drug for practically all types of systemic mycoses and is the gold standard of antifungal therapy. However, because of higher toxicity of AMB, the azole antifungals are now preferred in conditions where their efficacy approaches that of AMB (see Table 31.1).

Table 31.1: Choice of drugs for systemic mycoses

Disease	Drugs	
	1st choice	2nd choice
1. Candidiasis		
oral/vaginal/cutaneous	FLU/NYS/CLO	ITR
deep/invasive	AMB/VORI	FLU/CAS/POSA
2. Cryptococcosis	AMB	FLU
3. Histoplasmosis	ITR/AMB	FLU
4. Coccidioidomycosis	AMB/FLU	ITR
5. Blastomycosis	ITR/AMB	FLU
6. Sporotrichosis (disseminated)	AMB	ITR
7. Paracoccidioidomycosis	ITR	AMB
8. Aspergillosis	AMB/VORI	ITR/CAS/POSA
9. Mucormycosis	AMB	POSA
10. Chromomycosis	ITR	TER/POSA

AMB—Amphotericin B; 5-FC—Flucytosine; KTZ—Ketoconazole; FLU—Fluconazole; ITR—Itraconazole; NYS—Nystatin; CLO—Clotrimazole; VORI—Voriconazole; CAS—Caspofungin; POSA—Posaconazole; TER—Terbinafine

Leishmaniasis: AMB is the most effective drug for resistant cases of kala azar.

Aminoglycosides, vancomycin, cyclosporine and other nephrotoxic drugs enhance the renal impairment caused by AMB.

Nystatin

Obtained from *S. noursei*, it is similar to AMB in antifungal action and other properties. However, because of higher systemic toxicity, it is used only locally for superficial candidiasis.

In dentistry, topically applied nystatin is the 2nd choice drug to clotrimazole for *oral thrush, denture stomatitis, antibiotic associated stomatitis, corticosteroid associated oral candidiasis* and *mucocutaneous candidiasis of lips*, etc. The 1 lac U (1 mg = 2,000 U) tablet is placed in the mouth to dissolve slowly 4 times a day, or the tablet can be crushed and suspended in glycerine for application on the lesions. A bitter foul taste and nausea are the side effects.

Given orally, it is not absorbed, but can be used for monilial diarrhoea. It is effective (but less than azoles) in monilial vaginitis—1 lac U tab inserted twice daily. Similarly, it is used for corneal, conjunctival and cutaneous candidiasis in the form of an ointment. No irritation or other side effect is ordinarily seen.

Candidal resistance to nystatin is not a clinical problem. It is ineffective in dermatophytosis.

MYCOSTATIN 5 lac U tab, 1 lac U vaginal tab, 1 lac U/g oint, NYSTIN EYE 1 lac U/g ophthalmic oint.

ECHINOCANDINS

These are a new class of semisynthetic cyclic lipopeptide antifungal antibiotics that are much less toxic than AMB.

Caspofungin

It is active mainly against *Candida* and *Aspergillus*, including *Candida* resistant to azole antifungals. Caspofungin acts by inhibiting synthesis of β-1,3-glucan, a unique compoent of fungal cell wall. It is not absorbed orally. Given by i.v. infusion, it diffuses into tissues; is metabolized extensively by liver and excreted in bile as well as in urine with a plasma t½ of 10 hours. Invasive/esophageal candidiasis, non-responsive aspergillosis and febrile neutropenia are its current indications.

CANCIDAS, CASPOGIN 70 mg in 10 ml and 50 mg in 10 ml inj.
Loading dose 70 mg i.v. infused over 1 hour, followed by 50 mg i.v. daily.
Rash, dyspnoea and joint pains may occur. An acute reaction is rare. Organ toxicity has not been observed.

Micafungin is another echinocandin with similar properties which is approved for use in esophageal candidiasis and candidaemia.

HETEROCYCLIC BENZOFURAN

Griseofulvin: This antibiotic obtained from *Penicillium griseofulvum* is fungistatic against most dermatophytes, including *Epidermophyton, Trichophyton, Microsporum*, etc., but not against *Candida* and other fungi causing deep mycosis. Bacteria are also insensitive. Griseofulvin interferes with mitosis—multinucleated and stunted fungal hyphae are produced as a result of its action. It also causes abnormal metaphase configurations by binding to polymerized tubulin and interfering with microtubular function. Oral absorption of griseofulvin is incomplete due to its poor aqueous solubility. It is keratophilic: gets deposited in keratin forming cells of skin and nails.

Adverse effects Toxicity of griseofulvin is low and usually not serious. Headache is the commonest complaint, followed by g.i.t. disturbances. CNS symptoms and peripheral neuritis are occasional.

Use Griseofulvin is used orally only for dermatophytosis and tinea of nails. As such, it has no utility in dentistry. It is ineffective topically. Systemic azoles and terbenafine are equally or more efficacious than griseofulvin and are preferred now for dermatophytosis and tinea of nails as well.

GRISOVIN-FP, DERMONORM 250, 500 mg tabs.

Interactions Griseofulvin induces warfarin metabolism and reduces efficacy of oral contraceptives. Phenobarbitone reduces the oral absorption and induces the metabolism of griseofulvin.

IMIDAZOLES AND TRIAZOLES (AZOLES)

These are presently the most extensively used antifungal drugs.

Four imidazoles are entirely topical, while ketoconazole is used both orally and topically. The triazoles fluconazole, itraconazole and voriconazole have largely replaced ketoconazole for systemic mycosis because of greater efficacy as well as fewer side effects and drug interactions. Posaconazole is a new triazole to be used as a reserve drug for non-responsive cases.

The azoles have broad-spectrum antifungal activity covering dermatophytes, *Candida*, other fungi involved in deep mycosis, *Nocardia* and *Leishmania*.

The mechanism of action of imidazoles and triazoles is the same. They inhibit the fungal lanosterol 14-demethylase (a cytochrome P450 enzyme) and thus impair ergosterol synthesis (*see* Fig. 31.1) leading to a cascade of membrane abnormalities in the fungus. The lower host toxicity of triazoles compared to imidazoles has correlated with their lower affinity for mammalian CYP450 enzyme and lesser propensity to inhibit mammalian sterol synthesis.

Fluconazole-resistance among *Candida* causing esophageal and other deep candidiasis has been observed, particularly in AIDS patients. However, development of fungal resistance to azoles has not so far posed any significant clinical problem in immunocompetent subjects.

Clotrimazole
It is the most commonly employed topical imidazole effective in the treatment of tinea infections like ringworm, athletes foot and otomycosis. Oral, cutaneous, and vaginal candidiasis have responded in >80% cases. Clotrimazole is the most frequently used drug for oropharyngeal candidiasis; 10 mg troche of clotrimazole is allowed to dissolve in the mouth 3 to 4 times a day, or the lotion/gel is applied/swirled in the mouth as long as possible for 7–10 days. For denture stomatitis, patients are advised to apply clotrimazole lotion/gel to the fitting surface of the denture before wearing it. Moreover, the denture should be kept overnight in sod. hypochlorite/benzalkonium/cetrimide solution, and it should be worn only when needed. Topical clotrimazole can be used to treat angular cheilitis that often is a mixed candidal, streptococcal, staphylococcal infection.

Clotrimazole is well tolerated by most patients. Local irritation with stinging and burning sensation occurs in some. No systemic toxicity is seen after topical use.

SURFAZ, CLODERM 1% lotion, cream, powder; 100 mg vaginal tab. CANDID 1% cream, mouth paint, powder, 1% ear drops with 2% lidocaine.

Econazole
It is similar to clotrimazole; and is highly effective in dermatophytosis, otomycosis, oral thrush, but is somewhat inferior to clotrimazole in vaginitis. No adverse effects, except local irritation in few is reported.

ECONAZOLE 1% oint, 150 mg vaginal tab; ECODERM 1% cream.

Miconazole
It is an alternative drug to clotrimazole for tinea, pityriasis versicolor, otomycosis, oral, cutaneous and vulvovaginal candidiasis. A single application on skin acts for a few days.

Irritation after cutaneous application is infrequent, no systemic adverse effects are seen.

DAKTARIN 2% gel, 2% powder and solution; GYNODAKTARIN 2% vaginal gel; ZOLE 2% oint, lotion, dusting powder and spray, 1% ear drops, 100 mg vaginal ovules.

Oxiconazole
A newer topical antifungal which has been used mainly for tinea and other dermatophytic infection, and in vaginal candidiasis.

OXIZON, ZODERM: Oxiconazole 1% with benzoic acid 0.25% cream and lotion.

Ketoconazole (KTZ)

It is the first orally effective broad-spectrum antifungal drug, useful in dermatophytosis, superficial candidiasis as well as in deep mycosis, but has been superseded by fluconazole and other triazoles. The oral absorption of KTZ is facilitated by gastric acidity because it is more soluble at lower pH. In the blood it is largely bound to albumin and RBCs. Hepatic metabolism is extensive; metabolites are excreted in urine and faeces. Elimination of KTZ is dose dependent: t½ varies from 4–8 hours. The usual dose is 200 mg OD or BD.

FUNGICIDE, NIZRAL, KETOVATE 200 mg tab. FUNGINOC, NIZRAL 2% oint, 2% shampoo (for dandruff), KETOVATE 2% cream.

Adverse effects Ketoconazole is much less toxic than AMB, but more side effects occur than with itraconazole or fluconazole, which have largely replaced it for systemic use.

The most common side effects are nausea and vomiting. Others are—loss of appetite, headache, paresthesia, rashes and hair loss.

Ketoconazole decreases androgen production from testes and it displaces testosterone from protein binding sites. Gynaecomastia, loss of hair and libido, and oligozoospermia may be the manifestations. Menstrual irregularities occur in some women. Hepatotoxicity is infrequent.

Interactions H_2 blockers, proton pump inhibitors and antacids decrease the oral absorption of KTZ by reducing gastric acidity.

Rifampin, phenobarbitone, carbamazepine and phenytoin induce KTZ metabolism and reduce its efficacy.

Ketoconazole inhibits CYP450, especially CYP3A4, and raises the blood level of several drugs including warfarin, sulfonylureas, phenytoin, cyclosporine, diazepam, indinavir.

Use Ketoconazole is rarely used in dental practice. Topically, it has been employed for tinea and other forms of dermal mycosis. Dandruff often responds to KTZ applied as a shampoo. Oral KTZ is effective in several forms of systemic mycosis, but fluconazole and itraconazole have largely replaced it.

Fluconazole

It is a water- soluble triazole having a wider range of antifungal activity than KTZ; indications include cryptococcal meningitis, systemic and mucosal candidiasis in both normal and immunocompromised patients, coccidioidal meningitis and some tinea infections.

Fluconazole is 94% absorbed; oral bioavailability is not affected by food or gastric pH. It is primarily excreted unchanged in urine with a t½ of 25–30 hours. Fungicidal concentrations are achieved in nails, vagina and saliva; penetration into brain and CSF is good. Dose reduction is needed in renal impairment.

Adverse effects Fluconazole produces fewer side effects; gastric tolerability is better, but dose related nausea, vomiting, abdominal pain, rash and headache may occur.

Selectivity for fungal cytochrome P450 is higher. Unlike KTZ, it does not inhibit steroid synthesis in man: antiandrogenic and other endocrine side effects have not occurred.

Fluconazole is not recommended in pregnant and lactating mothers.

Interactions Though fluconazole affects hepatic drug metabolism to a lesser extent than KTZ, increased plasma levels of phenytoin, cyclosporine, warfarin, zidovudine and sulfonylureas have been observed. Drug interaction potential is lower, but the same caution as with KTZ or itraconazole needs to be applied in coadministering other drugs.

Use Fluconazole can be administered orally as well as i.v. (in severe infections).

Oral fluconazole 150 mg/day for 2 weeks is highly effective in *Candida* infections of the mouth, but should be given only to patients not responding to topical treatment. It is a first line drug for candida esophagitis.

Most tinea infections and cutaneous candidiasis can be treated with 150 mg weekly for 4 weeks.

For disseminated candidiasis, cryptococcal/coccidioidal meningitis and other systemic fungal infections the dose is 200–400 mg/day for 4–12 weeks or longer.

An eye drop is useful in fungal keratitis.
SYSCAN, ZOCON, FORCAN, FLUZON 50, 100, 150, 200 mg caps, 200 mg/100 ml i.v. infusion.
SYSCAN 0.3% eye drops.

Itraconazole

This orally active triazole antifungal has a broader spectrum of activity than KTZ or fluconazole; includes some fluconazole-resistant candida and few moulds like *Aspergillus*. It is fungistatic, but effective in immunocompromised patients. Steroid hormone synthesis inhibition and serious hepatotoxicity are absent in itraconazole.

Oral absorption of itraconazole is variable, but is enhanced by food and gastric acid. Itraconazole is highly protein bound and metabolized in liver by CYP3A4; an active metabolite is produced which is excreted in faeces; t½ varies from 24–40 hours.

Itraconazole is well tolerated in doses below 200 mg/day. Gastric intolerance is significant at > 400 mg/day. Dizziness, pruritus, headache and hypokalaemia are the other side effects. Unsteadiness and impotence are infrequent. Hormonal adverse effects are not seen.

Drug interactions Oral absorption of itraconazole is reduced by antacids, H_2 blockers and proton pump inhibitors. Rifampin, phenobarbitone, phenytoin and carbamazepine induce itraconazole metabolism and reduce its efficacy. Itraconazole inhibits CYP3A4; drug interactions are less marked, but similar to KTZ; phenytoin, digoxin, sulfonylurea, protease inhibitors, warfarin and cyclosporine levels are increased.

Uses Itraconazole is the preferred azole for most systemic mycosis (see Table 31.1) that are not associated with meningitis. It also affords some relief in aspergillosis. It is highly effective in vaginal candidiasis, dermatophytosis and onychomycosis, but use is restricted to cases not amenable to topical therapy. Itraconazole is occasionally used in dentistry for oral candidiasis.

Dose: 100 mg OD—200 mg BD oral; 200 mg infused i.v. over 1 hour OD or BD.
SPORANOX, CANDITRAL 100 mg cap, ITASPOR 100 mg cap, 200 mg/20 ml vial.

Voriconazole

It is a second generation broad-spectrum triazole that is being utilized for difficult to treat fungal infections like invasive aspergillosis, disseminated infections caused by fluconazole resistant *Candida*, and febrile neutropenia not responding to antibacterial therapy. Voriconazole is absorbed orally, extensively metabolized, and metabolites are excreted in urine. The plasma t½ is 6 hours. The drug interaction profile is similar to itraconazole. Rashes, visual disturbances, QTc prolongation and an acute reaction on i.v. injection are the significant adverse effects.

Dose: 200 mg 1 hour before or 1 hour after meal orally; 4-6 mg/kg/slow i.v. infusion every 12 hours.
VFEND 50 mg, 200 mg tabs, 200 mg/vial for i.v. infusion; FUNGIVOR 200 mg tab.

Posaconazole

This recently introduced potent broad spectrum antifungal triazole is unique in being effective in mucormycosis. Though, active against many fungi causing deep mycosis, posaconazole is reserved for non-responsive aspergillosis, invasive candidiasis, and for febrile neutropenia. Side effects are abdominal pain, nausea, loose motions and dizziness.

Dose: 200 mg 4 times a day with meals;
NOXAFIL 200 mg/5 ml oral suspension.

ALLYLAMINE

Terbinafine

This orally as well as topically active drug against dermatophytes and *Candida* belongs to a new allylamine class of antifungals. In contrast to azoles which are primarily fungistatic, terbinafine is fungicidal. It acts as a noncompetitive inhibitor of 'squalene epoxidase', an early step enzyme in ergosterol biosynthesis by fungi (see Fig. 31.1). Accumulation of squalene within fungal cells appears to be responsible for the fungicidal action. The mammalian enzyme is inhibited only by 1000-fold higher concentration of terbinafine.

After oral absorption, terbinafine is widely distributed in the body. Because of high affinity for keratin, it is concentrated in sebum, stratum corneum of skin and into nail plates, accounting for its efficacy in tinea infection of skin and nails. Terbinafine is mainly metabolized and excreted in urine as well as in faeces. Half life after a single dose is 11–16 hours, but is prolonged upto 10 days after repeated dosing.

Side effects of oral terbinafine are gastric upset, rashes, taste disturbance. Some cases of hepatic dysfunction and haematological disorder are reported. Terbinafine does not inhibit CYP450.

Topical terbinafine can cause erythema, itching, dryness, irritation, urticaria and rashes.

Use Terbinafine applied topically as 1% cream is indicated in localized tinea pedis/cruris/corporis and in pityriasis versicolor. Oral treatment is reserved for onychomycosis, tinea capitis and for wide spread lesions.

Terbinafine is less effective against cutaneous and mucosal candidiasis: 2–4 weeks oral therapy may be used as an alternative to fluconazole.

LAMISIL, SEBIFIN, DASKIL 250 mg tab, 1% topical cream. EXIFINE 125, 250 mg tabs, 1% cream.

OTHER TOPICAL ANTIFUNGALS

All these drugs are used for dermatophytosis.

1. Tolnaftate It is an effective drug for tinea cruris and tinea corporis—most cases respond in 1–3 weeks. Because of poor penetrability, it is less effective in tinea pedis and other hyperkeratinized lesions. For the same reason, it is ineffective in tinea capitis—involving scalp and tinea unguium—involving nails.

2. Ciclopirox olamine It is effective in tinea infections, pityriasis versicolor and dermal candidiasis. Also used for vaginal candidiasis.

3. Undecylenic acid It is fungistatic used topically, generally in combination with its zinc salt. It is inferior to the drugs described above, but is still used for tinea pedis, nappy rash and tinea cruris.

4. Benzoic acid It has weak antifungal and antibacterial property in slightly acidic medium. It is a weaker fungistatic than tolnaftate, and is used in combination with salicylic acid (as Whitfield's ointment) on hyper- keratinized lesions of tinea. Irritation and burning sensation is experienced by many patients.

5. Butenafine This congener of terbinafine has the same mechanism of action, but is used only topically for tinea cruris/corporis/pedis.

Antiviral Drugs
(Non-retroviral)

Viruses are the ultimate expression of parasitism. They not only take nutrition from the host cell, but also direct its metabolic machinery to synthesize new virus particles. Viral chemotherapy, therefore, is difficult, as it would require interference with cellular metabolism in the host. However, virus directed enzymes have been identified in the infected cell and some viruses have a few enzymes of their own which may have higher affinities for some inhibitors than the regular cellular enzymes. In addition, drugs have been developed which target virus specific steps like cell penetration, uncoating, reverse transcription, virus assembly or maturation and release from host cell. Another problem in antiviral therapy is that in majority of acute infections viral replication is already at its peak when symptoms appear. To be effective, therefore, therapy has to be started in the incubation period, i.e. has to be prophylactic or preemptive.

The *application of antiviral drugs in dentistry is restricted to treatment of oropharyngeal herpes simplex and herpes labialis* that occur particularly in immunocompromised patients.

ANTI-HERPES VIRUS DRUGS

These are drugs active against the Herpes group of DNA viruses which include *Herpes simplex virus-1* (HSV-1), *Herpes simplex virus-2* (HSV-2), *Varicella-Zoster Virus* (VZV), *Epstein-Barr Virus* (EBV) and *Cytomegalovirus* (CMV).

Idoxuridine

It is 5-iodo-2-deoxyuridine (IUDR) which was the first pyrimidine antimetabolite to be used as antiviral drug. It competes with thymidine, gets incorporated in DNA so that faulty DNA is formed which breaks down easily.

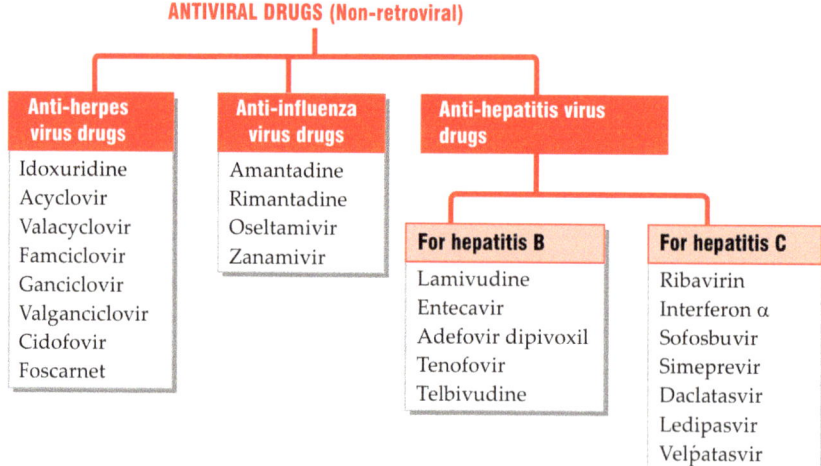

Anti-Herpes Virus Drugs

Idoxuridine is effective only against DNA viruses, and clinical utility is limited to *Herpes simplex* keratitis.

Acyclovir is an equally efficacious and better tolerated alternative.

Acyclovir

This deoxiguanosine analogue antiviral drug requires a virus specific enzyme for conversion to the active metabolite that inhibits DNA synthesis and viral replication.

Acyclovir is preferentially taken up by the virus infected cells. Because of selective generation of the active inhibitor inside the virus infected cell and its greater inhibitory effect on viral DNA synthesis, acyclovir has low toxicity for host cells : a several hundred-fold chemotherapeutic index has been noted.

Acyclovir
↓ *Herpes virus specific thymidine kinase*
Acyclovir monophosphate
↓ *Cellular kinases*
Acyclovir triphosphate
→ Inhibits herpes virus DNA polymerase competitively
→ Gets incorporated in viral DNA and stops lengthening of DNA strand. The terminated DNA inhibits DNA-polymerase irreversibly.

Acyclovir is active only against herpes group of viruses; HSV-1 is most sensitive followed by HSV-2> VZV = EBV, while CMV is practically not affected. Both *H. simplex* and *varicella-zoster* virus can develop resistance to acyclovir during therapy.

Pharmacokinetics Only about 20% of an oral dose of acyclovir is absorbed. It is little plasma protein bound and is widely distributed in the body. Acyclovir is primarily excreted unchanged in urine, plasma t½ is 2–3 hours. Renal impairment necessitates dose reduction.

ZOVIRAX 200 mg, 800 mg tab, 250 mg/vial for i.v. inj; CYCLOVIR 200 mg tab, 5% skin cream; HERPEX 200 mg tab, 3% eye oint, 5% skin cream; OCUVIR 200, 400, 800 mg tab, 3% eye oint, ACIVIR-DT 200, 400, 800 mg tab. ACIVIR EYE 3% oint.

Use Acyclovir is effective in patients with normal as well as deficient immune status.

1. *Mucocutaneous H. simplex* is a type 1 virus disease. It remains localized to lips and gums and does not usually require specific treatment. Started early, 5 times daily application of acyclovir 5% cream may abort or shorten the duration of recurrences in *herpes labialis*. Prophylactic oral acyclovir 200 mg 3 times a day therapy may prevent sun exposure related recurrences. Symptomatic improvement can occur in *acute herpetic gingivostomatitis* by acyclovir 200 mg 5 times daily for 10 days. The disease often gets disseminated in immunocompromised individuals and may be treated with oral or i.v. acyclovir (15 mg/kg/day) for 7 days, but recurrences are not prevented.

2. *Genital H. simplex* is generally caused by type 2 virus, and is treated with topical, oral or parenteral acyclovir depending upon the stage and severity of disease. Symptomatic relief is afforded, but subsequent recurrences are not prevented. Continuous oral medication is advised to ward off recurrences, if they are frequent.

3. *H. simplex encephalitis* (type 1 virus): Acyclovir injected i.v. is the drug of choice. Treatment is effective only if started early: delay precludes salutary effect on mortality and neurological complications.

4. *H. simplex (type 1) keratitis*: Acyclovir applied topically is now preferred over idoxuridine.

5. *Herpes zoster*: It is caused by VZV. Acyclovir administered i.v. or orally should be used only in immunodeficient individuals or in severe cases. It affords symptomatic relief

and faster healing of lesions, but postherpetic neuralgia is not prevented.

6. *Chickenpox* (a VZV disease): Specific antiviral therapy is not needed in patients of chickenpox with normal immunefunction. Only in patients with immunodeficiency and in neonates it calls for acyclovir therapy.

Adverse effects

Topical: stinging and burning sensation after each application.

Oral: The drug is well tolerated; headache, nausea, malaise and some CNS effects are reported.

Intravenous: rashes, sweating, emesis and fall in BP occur only in few patients.

Dose dependent decrease in g.f.r. is the most important toxicity that occurs especially in those with kidney disease. Kidney function normalises on discontinuation of the drug. Reversible neurological manifestations (tremors, lethargy, disorientation, hallucinations, convulsions and coma) have been ascribed to higher doses.

Valacyclovir It is a valyl-ester prodrug of acyclovir with improved oral bioavailability due to active transport by peptide transporters in the intestine. It is completely converted into acyclovir in the body and excreted in urine as acyclovir with a t½ of 3 hours. Orolabial herpes can be treated by single day therapy (2 g BD). In immunocompromised patient 1 g BD for 5 days is recommended.
VALCIVIR 0.5 g, 1.0 g tabs.

It can also be used for genital herpes simplex and for herpes zoster

Famciclovir It is an ester prodrug of a guanine nucleoside analogue *penciclovir* which has improved oral bioavailability and prolonged intracellular t½ of the active triphosphate metabolite. Famciclovir inhibits *H. simplex* and *H. zoster*, but not the acyclovir-resistant strains. Like acyclovir, it needs viral thymidine kinase for generation of the active DNA polymerase inhibitor. Famciclovir is used as an alternative to acyclovir for orolabial or genital herpes and herpes zoster.
Dose: Orolabial herpes 500 mg TDS for 7–10 days.
FAMTREX 250, 500 mg tabs.

Side effects are headache, nausea, loose motions, itching, rashes and mental confusion.

Ganciclovir It is an analogue of acyclovir which is most active against CMV, but also inhibits *H. simplex, H. zoster* and EBV. The mechanism of action and basis of virus selectivity is similar to acyclovir.

Systemic toxicity of ganciclovir is high (bone marrow depression, rash, fever, vomiting, neuropsychiatric disturbances) and use is restricted to severe CMV infections, especially CMV retinitis in AIDS patients or in transplant recipients.

Valganciclovir is the valyl prodrug of ganciclovir with improved oral bioavailability, which has largely replaced oral ganciclovir, and is preferred for long term treatment.

Cidofovir This monophosphate nucleotide analogue of cytidine inhibits most DNA viruses, including HSV, CMV, pox and adenoviruses. Many acyclovir-resistant HSV and ganciclovir-resistant CMV are susceptible. Cidofovir diphosphate generated intra-cellularly by cellular phosphokinases inhibits viral DNA-polymerase. Injected i.v. every week, cidofovir is used for ganciclovir-resistant CMV retinitis as well as for acyclovir-resistant mucocutaneous herpes simplex in immunosuppressed patients.

Foscarnet It is a simple straight chain phosphonate unrelated to any nucleic acid precursor, which inhibits viral DNA polymerase and reverse transcriptase. It is active against *H. simplex* (including strains resistant to acyclovir), CMV (including ganciclovir resistant ones) and HIV. Foscarnet is indicated for ganciclovir-resistant CMV retinitis and acyclovir-resistant mucocutaneous herpes simplex in AIDS patients. Toxicity of foscarnet is high.

ANTI-INFLUENZA VIRUS DRUGS

The anti-influenza virus drugs exert type and strain-specific action on influenza virus.

The influenza virus is a RNA virus, of which several types (A,B,C) are recognized. Majority of human infections and epidemics are caused by influenza A, while the B type produces sporadic seasonal cases. Several strains of influenza A characterized by its 'H' and 'N' surface glycoproteins have produced epidemics and pandemics from time-to-time. Of particular significance are the H5N1 (bird flu) and H1N1 (swine flu) strains which caused pandemic in 1997 and 2009, as well as several epidemics.

Amantadine It is a tricyclic amine, unrelated to any nucleic acid precursor, which inhibits influenza A virus, but not influenza B or the H1N1 and H5N1 strains. Amantadine acts by inhibiting the viral M2 protein, which is an ion channel. Amantadine prevents uncoating of the viral genome within the infected cell. Due to development of amantadine resistance and emergence of unresponsive strains like H5N1, use of amantadine for treatment of influenza has declined markedly. Its antiparkinsonian action is described on p. 164.

Rimantadine It is the more potent, long-acting (t½ 30 hr) methyl derivative of amantadine that has higher oral bioavailability and fewer side effects. However, it exhibits complete cross resistance with amantadine, and is ineffective against N1H1, N5H1 strains and influenza B viruses. As such, rimantadine has also gone into disuse.

Oseltamivir This is the most commonly used anti-influenza virus drug now. It has a broader-spectrum activity covering influenza A (amantadine sensitive as well as resistant), H5N1 (bird flu), H1N1 (swine flu) strains and influenza B. Oseltamivir is an ester prodrug that is rapidly and nearly completely hydrolysed during absorption in intestine and by liver to the active form *oseltamivir carboxylate* which acts by inhibiting influenza virus neuraminidase. This enzyme is needed for release of progeny virions from the infected cell. Spread of the virus in the body is thus checked.

Oseltamivir is indicated both for prophylaxis as well as treatment of influenza A, bird flu, swine flu and influenza B. Started at the onset of symptoms, it is the most effective drug in reducing severity, duration and complications of the illness. Prophylactic use within 2 days of exposure prevents illness in contacts of influenza patients.

Dose: Therapeutic—75 mg oral twice daily for 5 days; prophylactic—75 mg OD.
TAMIFLU, ANTIFLU 75 mg cap, 12 mg/ml susp; FLUVIR 75 mg cap.

Side effects are nausea, abdominal pain, headache, weakness, mood changes and insomnia.

Zanamivir Another influenza A (including amantadine resistant, H1N1, H5N1 strains) and influenza B virus neuraminidase inhibitor that is administered by inhalation as a powder due to very low oral bioavailability. The mechanism of action, clinical utility and efficacy of zanamivir are similar to that of oseltamivir. It may be effective in some oseltamivir-resistant cases, and is primarily reserved for such cases.

Dose: 10 mg through breath actuated inhaler or rotaceps, twice daily × 5 days for treatment, and once daily for prophylaxis.
RELENZA, VIRENZA 5 mg/actuation powder inhaler.

ANTI-HEPATITIS VIRUS DRUGS

Chronic viral hepatitis is mainly caused by two viruses—*hepatitis B virus (HBV)* and *hepatitis C virus (HCV)*. While HBV is a DNA virus which, like retroviruses, integrates into host chromosomal DNA to establish permanent infection, the HCV is a RNA virus which does not integrate into chromosomal DNA, does not establish noncurable infection, but frequently causes chronic hepatitis. Some antiviral drugs (e.g. ribavirin, interferon α) used mainly for viral hepatitis are nonselective, and inhibit several other viruses as well.

Drugs for Hepatitis B

Since the hepatitis B virus cannot be eradicated from the body, treatment is aimed at suppression of the virus and its inflammatory–hepatocyte damaging effect. This results in improved liver function and reduction of risk for development of cirrhosis and hepatic carcinoma. Combination therapy of HBV has not proven superior; drugs are generally used sequentially.

Lamivudine This nucleoside analogue is active against HBV as well as HIV, and is described with anti-retroviral drugs on p. 480–81.

Entecavir This guanosine nucleoside analogue is currently the most active 1st line option for treating chronic hepatitis B. It is activated intracellularly by phosphorylation and inhibits HBV-DNA polymerase. Entecavir brings down HBV titer rapidly and profoundly resulting in clinical, biochemical and histological improvement. The response is well sustained, and resistance is infrequent. Side effects are dyspepsia, nausea, diarrhoea and disturbed sleep. Lactic acidosis can develop in patients with cirrhosis.

Adefovir dipivoxil It is a mono-phosphate analogue of AMP that is active against HBV and some other DNA and RNA viruses, but is used only for HBV hepatitis. On entering cells, adefovir is phosphorylated to the diphosphate which inhibits HBV-DNA polymerase. Adefovir itself gets incorporated in the viral DNA resulting in termination of the DNA chain. Adefovir dipivoxil is indicated in chronic hepatitis B, including lamivudine-resistant cases, but is slower acting and less effective. Therefore, it is not a first-line drug. Side effects are sore throat, headache, weakness, abdominal pain and flu syndrome. Nephrotoxicity can occur.

Tenofovir disoproxil fumarate (TDF) It is a monophosphate nucleotide related to AMP, and is active against HBV as well as HIV. Tenofovir released from the prodrug TDF is diphosphorylated by cellular kinases, and preferentially inhibits HBV-DNA polymerase, as well as HIV-reverse transcriptase (*see* p. 481). It also gets incorporated in the viral DNA to cause chain termination.

Administered once daily, TDF has produced good clinical and virological response in chronic hepatitis B, including lamivudine-resistant cases. Tenofovir-resistance has not developed during treatment of chronic hepatitis B, and it is a first line drug for HBV hepatitis. Side effects are mostly limited to g.i. tract—nausea, flatulence, abdominal discomfort and headache. Renal injury or chronic renal disease is a risk.

Telbivudine This newer anti-HBV drug is a thymidine nucleoside analogue which is phosphorylated intracellularly to generate the active triphosphate nucleotide. Telbivudine triphosphate inhibits HBV-DNA polymerase, and itself gets incorporated into the HBV-DNA resulting in chain termination. It causes faster and more complete suppression of HBV-DNA titer than lamivudine, but resistance often develops, resulting in the return of viraemia. As such, it is not a first-line drug for chronic hepatitis B. Tolerability of telbivudine is good; side effects are abdominal pain, diarrhoea, cough, dizziness and myalgia.

Drugs for Hepatitis C

Since HCV does not integrate into host DNA to establish permanent infection, the aim of treatment in chronic hepatitis C is to attain *Sustained viral response (SVR)*, which is defined as undetectable HCV-RNA in blood for at least 6 months after completion of therapy. If this is achieved, only ~5% patients relapse. Oral ribavirin combined with injected peginterferon α (Peg-INFα) has been the standard therapy for HCV infection, but over the past 10 years several novel specific oral antiviral drugs have been introduced, which have revolutionized the treatment of hepatitis C.

Ribavirin This purine nucleoside analogue has broad-spectrum antiviral activity, including that against HCV, influenza A, B, respiratory syncytial virus, many other DNA and RNA viruses. Its mono- and triphosphate derivatives generated intracellularly inhibit GTP synthesis and viral RNA synthesis. They have other sites of action as well. No viral resistance to ribavirin has yet been observed.

The most common use of oral ribavirin is in chronic hepatitic C, in which it is combined with injected peginterferon for 6–12 months. This combination is active against all genotypes of HCV and achieves SVR in 50–80% cases. Nebulized ribavirin is used for respiratory syncytial virus bronchiolitis in infants and children.

Interferon α

Interferons are low molecular weight glycoprotein cytokines produced by host cells in response to viral infections and some other inducers. They have nonspecific antiviral as well as other complex effects on immunity and cell proliferation. Interferons bind to specific cell surface receptors and affect viral replication at multiple steps, *viz.* viral penetration, synthesis of viral mRNA, assembly of viral particles and their release, but the most widespread effect is direct or indirect suppression of viral protein synthesis. Interferon receptors are JAK-STAT tyrosine protein kinase receptors which on activation phosphorylate cellular proteins. These proteins then induce transcription of 'interferon-induced proteins' which exert antiviral effects.

Interferons inhibit many RNA and DNA viruses, but they are host specific, i.e. those produced by another species have poor activity in man. Three types of human interferons (α, β and γ) have antiviral activity. Only interferon $α_{2A}$ (INF$α_{2A}$) and INF $α_{2B}$ produced by recombinant DNA technology are clinically used. More active pegylated (polyethylene glycol complexed) interferons have been produced, which can be injected s.c. at weekly intervals.

Uses

1. Chronic hepatitis B: Peg INF$α_{2A}$ once weekly for 24–48 weeks produces sustained response in some patients.
2. Chronic hepatitis C: Peg INF$α_{2A}$ injected s.c. weekly + oral ribavirin has been the standard therapy, achieves SVR in 50–80% cases.
3. AIDS-related Kaposi's sarcoma (but not to treat HIV as such).
4. Condyloma acuminata caused by papilloma virus refractory to podophyllin.

Clinical utility of s.c. or i.m. injected interferon is limited by substantial adverse effects.
- Flu-like symptoms—fatigue, aches and pains, malaise, fever, dizziness, anorexia, taste and visual disturbances: develop a few hours after each injection.
- Neurotoxicity—numbness, neuropathy, tremor.
- Myelosuppression (dose limiting); neutropenia, thrombocytopenia.

New specific anti-HCV drugs

Several novel anti-HCV drugs are now available which target specific nonstructural (NS) viral proteins that play essential role in the replication of HCV inside hepatocytes. All of them are used in combination, either among themselves or with ribavirin ± PegINFα, because of lower efficacy and early development of resistance if used as monotherapy. Used in combination, the newer drugs have achieved SVR of up to 99%, and have shortened the duration of therapy to 12–24 weeks. They are also much less toxic than ribavirin or INFα. However, drug interactions are important. The specific anti-HCV drugs may be grouped according to their target NS proteins into:

1. *NS5B polymerase inhibitor:* Sofosbuvir
2. *NS3 protease inhibitor:* Simeprevir
3. *NS5A inhibitor:* Daclatasvir, Ledipasvir, Velpatasvir.

NS5B polymerase inhibitor

Sofosbuvir It is a uridine analogue prodrug which is converted within hepatocytes into its triphosphate nucleotide that inhibits HCV-NS5B. The NS5B is a HCV-RNA polymerase—hence replication of HCV is interfered, and the RNA chain is terminated. Sofosbuvir is active against all (1–6) genotypes of HCV, espicially genotype 1. It is always used in combination, either with simeprevir or one of the NS5A inhibitors or with ribavirin ± PegINFα. Such combinations have achieved 85–99% SVR after 12–24 weeks therepy. Adverse effects are abdominal pain, fatigue, agitation and anaemia.

NS3/4A protease inhibitor

Simeprevir This new drug is a HCV protease NS3 inhibitor which blocks the cleavage of HCV polyprotein complex so that functional viral RNA is not formed, and viral replication is halted. Simeprevir is active against HCV genotype 1 and 4. It is used along with sofosbuvir or with ribavirin +PegINFα. The simeprevir-sofosbuvir combination has achieved SVR in 83–97% noncirrhotic HCV patients after 12 weeks therapy, and in cirrhotics after 24 weeks therapy.

Simeprevir inhibits the efflux transporter Pgp and interacts with many drugs. Adverse effects are nausea, dyspnoea, rashes and photosensitivity.

NS5A inhibitors

NS5A is a multifunctional protein that serves essential role in the replication of HCV. Three orally active NS5A inhibitors—*Daclatasvir, Ledipasvir* and *Velpatasvir* are available, which block HCV-RNA replication and assembly of progeny virions. All NS5A inhibitors are used only in combination with the NS5B polymerase inhibitor sofosbuvir. The combinations are highly effective. In noncirrhotic chronic hepatitis C patients, the combinations have achieved SVR in 90–99% cases after 12 weeks therapy, and in cirrhotics after 24 weeks therapy. All three NS5A inhibitors are well toterated by majority of patients; usual side effects are headache, fatigue, abdominal pain, weakness and anaemia. The three NS5A inhibitors differ in pharmacokinetic properties and drug interaction profile.

Daclatasvir is metabolized by CYP3A and effluxed by Pgp. The dose needs to be halved in patients receiving CYP3A inhibitors, and increased in those taking CYP3A inducers.

Ledipasvir absorption is dependent on gastric acid; it is impaired in patients taking H_2 blockers or proton pump inhibitors (PPIs). Ledipasvir should not be used in patients being treated with Pgp inducers.

Velpatasvir absorption is also impaired in patients receiving acid suppressant drugs (H_2 blockers, PPIs). It should not be given to patients receiving CYP3A and Pgp inducers, because they lower blood levels and efficacy of velpatasvir.

Anti-Retrovirus Drugs
(Anti-HIV Drugs)

These are drugs active against human immunodeficiency virus (HIV), which is a retrovirus. They are useful in prolonging life, improving its quality and postponing complications of acquired immunodeficiency syndrome (AIDS) or AIDS-related complex (ARC), but do not cure the infection. The clinical efficacy of antiretrovirus drugs is monitored primarily by plasma HIV-RNA assays and CD4 lymphocyte count carried out at regular intervals.

The first antiretrovirus (ARV) drug *Zidovudine* was developed in 1987. Over the past 30 years, large number of drugs belonging to 3 major classes, *viz.* nucleoside reverse transcriptase inhibitors (NRTIs), non-nucleoside reverse transcriptase inhibitors (NNRTIs) and protease inhibitors (PIs) have been produced and are used as first line drugs. In addition, the integrase inhibitors are also now first line drugs; while the entry inhibitor and CCR-5 receptor inhibitor are reserve drugs. In India, the control and treatment of HIV-AIDS is covered under the National AIDS Control Programme (NACP) and is implimented by the National AIDS Control Organization (NACO).

Dentists run the risk of accidental exposure to HIV infection during dental procedures, and should be well informed about its prophylaxis.

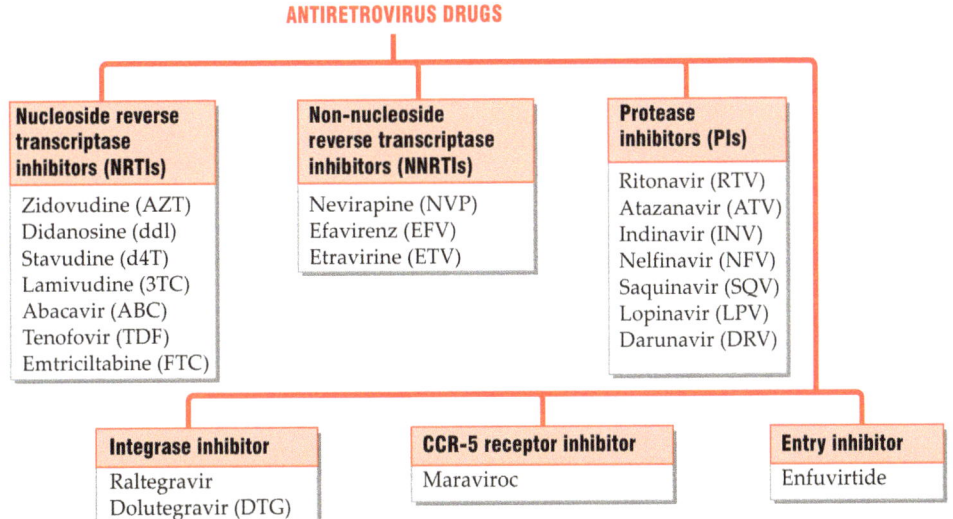

Nucleoside reverse transcriptase inhibitors (NRTIs)

Zidovudine (AZT) It is a thymidine analogue (azidothymidine), the first and the prototype NRTI. After phosphorylation in the host cell—zidovudine triphosphate selectively inhibits viral reverse transcriptase (RNA-dependent DNA polymerase) in preference to cellular DNA polymerase.

Single-stranded viral RNA
↓ Virus directed reverse transcriptase (inhibited by zidovudine triphosphate)
Double-stranded proviral DNA

On the template of single-stranded RNA genome of HIV, a double-stranded DNA copy is produced by viral reverse transcriptase. This DNA translocates to the nucleus and is integrated with chromosomal DNA of the host cell (by *viral integrase* enzyme) which then starts transcribing viral genomic RNA as well as mRNA. Under the direction of viral mRNA, viral regulatory and structural proteins are produced. Finally, viral particles are assembled and matured by involving a *viral protease* enzyme. Zidovudine thus prevents infection of new cells by HIV but has no effect on proviral DNA that has already integrated into the host chromosome. It is effective only against retroviruses. Zidovudine itself gets incorporated into the proviral DNA and terminates chain elongation. Resistance to AZT occurs by point mutations which alter reverse transcriptase enzyme. In the past, when AZT was used alone, >50% patients became nonresponsive to AZT within 1–2 years therapy due to growth of resistant mutants.

Pharmacokinetics The oral absorption of AZT is rapid, but bioavailability is ~65%. It is quickly cleared by hepatic glucuronidation (t½ 1 hr); 15–20% of the unchanged drug along with the metabolite is excreted in urine.

Adverse effects Anaemia and neutropenia are the most important and dose-related adverse effects.
Nausea, anorexia, abdominal pain, headache, insomnia and myalgia are common at the start of therapy but diminish later.
Myopathy, lactic acidosis, hepatomegaly are infrequent.

Interactions Paracetamol increases AZT toxicity, probably by competing for glucuronidation. Azole antifungals also inhibit AZT metabolism. Stavudine and zidovudine exhibit mutual antagonism by competing for the same activation pathway.

Use Zidovudine is used in HIV-infected patients only in combination with at least 2 other ARV drugs. However, it is no longer included in the preferred 1st line WHO (2016) as well as NACO (2018) regimens.

Didanosine This purine nucleoside analogue NRTI is infrequently used now due to higher toxicity, mainly peripheral neuropathy.

Stavudine It is also a thymidine analogue which utilizes the same thymidine kinase for activation as AZT. However, due to serious metabolic complications like lipodystrophy, lactic acidosis and peripheral neuropathy, stavudine has been phased out by NACO and WHO; and is rarely used now.

Lamivudine (3TC) This deoxycytidine analogue is phosphorylated intracellularly and inhibits HIV reverse transcriptase as well as HBV-DNA polymerase (*see* p. 475–76). Its incorporation into viral DNA results in chain termination. Human DNA polymerases are not affected and systemic toxicity of lamivudine is low. Point mutation in HIV-reverse transcriptase and HBV-DNA polymerase gives rise to rapid lamivudine resistance.

Lamivudine is used in combination with other anti-HIV drugs. It synergises with most other NRTIs, and is an essential component of all 1st line triple drug WHO as well as NACO regimens. It is also frequently used for chronic hepatitis B. HBV-DNA titre is markedly reduced and biochemical as well as histological indices of liver function improve. However, viral titres rise again after discontinuation. Even with continued medication HBV viraemia tends to return after 1 year due to emergence of resistant mutants.

Lamivudine is generally well tolerated, because of which it is accorded high priority in use. Side effects are headache, fatigue, nausea, anorexia, abdominal pain. Pancreatitis and neuropathy are rare.

Abacavir (ABC) This guanosine analogue is a potent antiretroviral (ARV) drug that acts after intracellular conversion to carbovir triphosphate. Resistance to ABC develops slowly, and it exhibits little cross resistance with other NRTIs. Hypersensitivity reactions such as rashes, fever, flu-like symptoms are the major problems. Abacavir is a component of 1st line regimens as an alternative to tenofovir.

Tenofovir (TDF) This nucleotide (not nucleoside) analogue is active against both HIV and HBV, and has been described on p. 476. Because of its good tolerability profile, tenofovir is now included in first line anti-HIV regimens prescribed by NACO and WHO.

Emtricitabine (FTC) It is a fluorinated cytidine analogue that is converted intracellularly into its triphosphate which inhibits HIV reverse transcriptase. Its action resembles that of lamivudine, and partial cross-resistance occurs between these two NRTIs. Like lamivudine it is also active against HBV, but is not advised for HIV-HBV coinfected patients. Toxicity of emtricitabine is low; side effects are headache, fatigue, diarrhoea and discolouration of exposed skin. Emtricitabine is a 1st line ARV drug, marketed only in combination with tenofovir or with tenofovir + efavirenz.

Non-nucleoside reverse transcriptase inhibitors (NNRTIs)

Nevirapine (NVP) and Efavirenz (EFV) These are nucleoside unrelated compounds which directly inhibit HIV reverse transcriptase without the need for intracellular phosphorylation. Their locus of action on the enzyme is different, and they are non-competitive enzyme inhibitors. They are more potent than AZT on HIV-1, but do not inhibit HIV-2. Viral resistance to these drugs develops by point mutation, and cross resistance is common between NVP and EFV, but not with NRTIs or PIs. A patient failing any NNRTI containing regimen should not be treated with another NNRTI.

The NNRTIs are used mostly in combination with two NRTIs; almost all 1st line regimens include either EFV or NVP. Both NVP and EFV are enzyme inducers and cause auto-induction of their own metabolism. Nevirapine dose is doubled after 2 weeks because of fall in its level due to autoinduction, but this is not needed in case of EFV. Rifampin induces NVP metabolism to render it ineffective, but not EFV. Rashes, nausea, headache are the usual side effects. Fever and hepatic impairment can occur with nevirapine, while efavirenz can cause a variety of neuropsychiatric symptoms.

Etravirine This is a 2nd generation NNRTI which is active against HIV-1 mutants resistant to NPV/EFV. Etravirine is indicated in adults and children > 6 years who have already been treated with another NNRTI, or are intolerant to them. It is completely metabolized by CYP isoenzymes, and induces CYP3A4, but inhibits CYP2C9. Clinically significant interactions occur with many drugs. Major adverse effect is skin reactions, including serious Stevens-Johnson syndrome. Etravirine is used only as a reserve drug.

Retroviral protease inhibitors (PIs)

An aspartic protease enzyme encoded by HIV is involved in the production of structural proteins and enzymes (including reverse transcriptase and integrase) of the virus.

A large viral polyprotein is synthesized in the infected cell and is broken into various functional components by this enzyme. This protease acts at a late step in HIV replication, i.e. maturation of the new virus particles when the RNA genome acquires the core proteins and enzymes. The protease inhibitors—*ritonavir, atazanavir, indinavir, nelfinavir, saquinavir, lopinavir* and *darunavir* bind to the protease molecule and interfere with its cleaving function. The PI inhibitors are more effective antiviral drugs than AZT. Because they act at a late step of viral cycle, they are effective in both newly as well as chronically infected cells. Under their influence, HIV-infected cells produce immature noninfectious viral progeny—hence prevent further rounds of infection.

All PIs are extensively metabolized by CYP3A4, except nelfinavir which, is metabolized by CYP2C19. Most PIs (especially ritonavir) are inhibitors of CYP3A4—interact with many drugs. Among the drugs used in dentistry whose plasma levels are increased by PIs are metronidazole, lidocaine, midazolam and carbamazepine. The CYP3A4 inhibitory action of ritonavir is utilized to reduce the dose of other PIs. A low dose (100 mg) of ritonavir is combined with the other PI. By reducing first-pass metabolism, ritonavir increases bioavailability, and by slowing systemic metabolism it decreases clearance of the companion PI. This 'boosted PI' regimen permits reduction in the number/frequency of tablets to be taken each day. Only boosted PIs are used now. Nelfinavir and ritonavir induce their own metabolism.

Because different PIs either inhibit or induce specific CYP isoenzymes to different extents, drug interactions with them are frequent and often unpredictable. Rifampin and other enzyme inducers enhance the metabolism of PIs and render them ineffective.

If used as monotherapy, viral resistance develops against PIs over months due to selection of resistant mutants in a stepwise manner. Current recommendation is to combine a PI with two NRTIs or one NRTI + one NNRTI. However, PIs are avoided in first line regimens and are reserved for failure cases. Large tablet load, metabolic derangement, poor patient acceptability and risk of drug interactions also restrict their use.

The most prominent adverse effects of PIs are metabolic complications like abnormal distribution of body fat, dyslipidaemia, insulin resistance and worsening of diabetes. Other side effects are gastrointestinal intolerance, asthenia headache, dizziness and parasthesias.

Integrase inhibitors

The HIV intergase enzyme enters the host cell along with the genomic RNA. After the HIV-proviral DNA is transcripted in the host cell cytoplasm, this enzyme translocates to the nucleus along with the proviral DNA, nicks host chromosomal DNA, integrates the proviral DNA with it and reseals it. Thus, the cell gets permanently infected. Interference with this virus-specific function provides an important target of action for ARV drugs.

Raltegravir This integrase inhibitor is active against both HIV-1 and HIV-2, and exhibits no cross-resistance with other classes of ARV drugs. Raltegravir rapidly clears HIV-RNA from circulation in treatment-naive as well as previously treated AIDS patients. It is orally active and produces few side effects like nausea, headache and loose motions. Myopathy is a potential toxicity. Because of high efficacy and good tolerability, raltegravir combined with 2 NRTIs is being used in first line regimens in some countries. However, in India, due to higher cost, NACO is utilizing it only in 2nd line regimens for treatment failure cases.

Dolutegravir This is a 2nd generation integrase inhibitor with activity similar to raltegravir. In addition, it retains some activity against raltegravir-resistant HIV. Dolutegravir combined with 2 NRTIs has yielded superior results than raltegravir containing regimens. It is well tolerated; adverse effects are rashes, hypersensitivity reactions and occasionally liver damage. Given its potent activity, good tolerability and once a day dosing, dolutegravir along with 2 NRTIs is gaining popularity as a 1st line treatment option for new HIV cases, if cost is not a constraint. By doubling the dose, it can also be used in raltegravir-resistant cases.

Entry (fusion) inhibitor

Enfuvirtide is a synthetic peptide that acts by binding to HIV-1 envelope glycoprotein '*gp41*' which is involved in fusion of viral and cellular membranes. Entry of the virus into the cell is blocked. Enfuvirtide is not active against HIV-2. It is a reserve drug for multiresistant HIV.

CCR5 receptor inhibitor

Maraviroc is an anti-HIV drug which blocks the host CD4 cell receptor labelled *CCR5*. This chemokine receptor of host CD4 cells anchors the the HIV through its glycoprotein *gp120*. Entry of the viral genome into the CD4 cell is thus interfered.

Treatment of HIV infection

The treatment of HIV infection and its complications is complex, lifelong, needs expertise, strong motivation and commitment of the patient, resources and is expensive. However, in India ARV drugs are provided free under the National AIDS Control Programme (NACP).

Because of rapid development of resistance to monotherapy with any ARV drug and inevitable therapeutic failure, it is now mandatory to treat HIV infection with a combination of 3 or more ARV drugs belonging to at least two different classes.

It has been realized that even with 3 drug antiretroviral therapy (ART) which rapidly kills > 99% virions, a small number survive within the resting CD4 lymphocytes and invariably give rise to relapse when treatment is discontinued. Even on continued therapy with the same drugs, relapse may occur due to development of resistance to one or all the drugs used. As the disease progresses in the individual (and several ARV drugs are used), the HIV population becomes genetically complex and diverse with respect to susceptibility to drugs.

Since none of the currently available regimens can eradicate HIV from the body of the patient, the goal of therapy is to maximally and durably inhibit viral replication so that the patient can attain and maintain effective immune response towards potential microbial pathogens. Greater the suppression of viral replication, lesser is the chance of emergence of drug resistant virus.

The current WHO (2016) and NACO (2018) guidelines recommend that ART should be started in all adults, including pregnant and breast feeding women, and children as soon as the diagnosis of HIV infection is confirmed. Treatment has to be life-long, irrespective of disappearance of detectable viraemia, normalization of CD4 cell count and the clinical status. With adequate adherence to current 3 drug ART, the life-expectancy of HIV infected subjects approaches that of uninfected subjects.

Therapeutic regimens

When ART is instituted, it should be aggressive with at least 3 anti-HIV drugs. The optimum response is reduction of plasma HIV-RNA to undetectable level and restoration of CD4 cell count to near normal within 6 months. The immune status improves and opportunistic infections subside. There is a sense of wellbeing and patients gain weight.

First-line regimens The first-line regimens universally include 2 NRTIs + 1 NNRTI. Considering relative efficacy and tolerability, the preferred NRTIs are—lamivudine, tenofovir, abacavir and emtricitabine. Efavirenz is the preferred NNRTI over nevirapine, because the latter is potentially hepatotoxic. The 1st line regimens recommended by NACO (2018) are given in the box. PIs are not used in the 1st line regimens

First-line antiretroviral regimens for HIV-1 infected adults and adolescents (>10 years age)*	
ART regimens	Recommended for
• $^{\$}$Tenofovir + Lamivudine + Efavirenz	• First-line ART regimen for all ARV-naive PL-HIV of age >10 years and body weight >30 kg
• Abacavir + Lamivudine + Efavirenz	• First-line regimen for all patients with abnormal serum creatinine, or with body weight <30 kg.
• Tenofovir + Lamivudine + Lopinavir/r (800/200 mg)	• First-line ART regimen for all women with single dose Nevirapine exposure in a past pregnancy • All confirmed HIV-2, or HIV-1 + HIV-2 coinfected patients$^{£}$
• Zidovudine + Lamivudine + Nevirapine/ Efavirenz	• All patients who are already on these first-line regimens need to be continued on the same regimen unless failing.
• Tenofovir + Lamivudine + Nevirapine OR • Abacavir + Lamivudine + Nevirapine	• Other alternative regimens when preferred regimen cannot be used

* Recommended by NACO (2018) guidelines.
$^{\$}$ To be taken as one FDC (300 mg + 300 mg + 600 mg) tablet at bed time. 2–3 hours after dinner, avoiding fatty food.
$^{£}$ Because NNRTIs are not effective against HIV-2

Response to and durability of a regimen depends largely on adherence of the patient to it. Use of combined drug formulations (FDCs) greatly improves convenience and patient compliance, lowers cost and pill burden, ensures that no component of the regimen is missed, minimizes chances of developing resistance leading to treatment failure. The NACO provides 1st line drugs as FDC tablets.

All drugs must be used in their recommended doses. In case of intolerance/toxicity, or drug interaction of any drug, it should be '*substituted*' by another drug (usually of the same class). No dose reduction should be tried.

Second-line regimens Failure (loss of efficacy) of any regimen is due to development of resistance to one or more components of the regimen. When it occurs, all 3 drugs of the regimen should be changed. This is called '*Switch*' of the entire regimen. However, lamivudine, even if administered in the failed regimen, may be continued in the 2nd line regimen, because it can exert residual antiviral activity and has the potential to reduce viral fitness, as well as improve viral sensitivity to zidovudine and tenofovir. A boosted PI, e.g. atazanavir/r or lopinavir/r is nearly always included in the 2nd line regimens along with 2 NRTIs (usually lamivudine + one NRTI not used earlier), or with an integrase inhibitor (raltegravir/dolutegravir).

Post-exposure prophylaxis (PEP) of HIV infection

Dentists and other healthcare workers who get accidentally exposed to the risk of HIV infection by needle-stick or other sharp injury, or contact with blood/biological fluid of HIV patients, or blood transfusion should be considered for PEP. Requirement of PEP depends on the assessment of risk of HIV

Prophylaxis of HIV Infection

infection, which is governed by nature of exposure and the HIV status of the source patient. Categories of exposure, grading the risk of infection are given in the box. The aim of PEP is to suppress local viral replication prior to dissemination, so that the infection is aborted.

> **Catagories of exposure for assessment of risk of HIV transmission***
>
> **Mild exposure**
> Exposure to mucous membranes / eyes / non-intact skin (e.g. superficial erosion) with small volumes, or subcutaneous injections following small bore needles.
>
> **Moderate exposure**
> Exposure to mucous membranes / non-intact skin with large volumes OR percutaneous superficial exposure with solid needle, e.g. a cut or needle-stick injury penetrating gloves.
>
> **Severe exposure**
> Percutaneous exposure with large volume, e.g. an accident with high calibre needle (>18 G) contaminated with visible blood, OR a deep wound (haemorrhagic wound), transmission of a significant volume of blood, OR an accident with material that has been previously used intravenously or intra-arterially.

*Based on NACO (2018) guidelines.

A 4 week regimen of at least 2 ARV drugs (mostly 2 NRTIs) has been found to significantly reduce the risk of HIV infection, if started soon after exposure. The current NACO (2018) guidelines recommend a minimum 2 NRTI-ARV drug regimen, preferably with added 3rd drug of a different class, for 28 days (*see* box).

If the source HIV patient has already received one or more ART regimens, it is likely that he/she be harbouring drug resistant virus. In such a case alternative PEP regimens may be required. If the drugs received by the source person are known, the PEP regimen may be individualized to include at least 2 drugs that the source has not received, and is unlikely to be resistant to. Nevirapine is not recommended for PEP in adults and in children ≥2 years due to its hepatotoxic potential.

When indicated, PEP should be started as soon as possible, preferably within 1–2 hours of exposure. The likelihood of preventing infection declines with the delay; most guidelines, including NACO (2018), do not recommend starting it beyond 72 hours of exposure.

> **NACO (2018) recommended HIV post-exposure prophylaxis regimens***
>
> **For adults and adolescents**
> - Tenofovir (TDF) 300 mg + Lamivudine (3TC) 300 mg one FDC tab once daily ±
> - Lopinavir 200 mg + Ritonavir 50 mg two FDC tabs twice daily
>
> [if Lopinavir/r not available/cannot be used, give TDF (300 mg) + 3TC (300 mg) + Efavirenz (600 mg) one FDC tab once daily]
>
> **For children (Age >3 years and weight >10 kg)**
> - Zidovudine (AZT) OR Abacavir (only if AZT contraindicated) + Lamivudine ±
> - Lopinavir/r OR EFV (only if LPV/r not available/cannot be used)
> (dose of drugs as per body weight band)
>
> **Duration of regimens: 4 weeks**

Prophylaxis after sexual exposure The same PEP regimen as for needle-stick may be employed after sexual exposure of HIV. In USA, a 28-day regimen of tenofovir + emtricitabine (as FDC once daily) + raltegravir (400 mg twice daily) is most popular.

Antiprotozoal Drugs

ANTIMALARIAL DRUGS

These are drugs used for prophylaxis, treatment and prevention of relapses of malaria.

Malaria, caused by 4 species of the protozoal parasite *Plasmodium*, is endemic in most parts of India and other tropical countries. It is one of the major health problems. In India, the control and treatment of malaria is covered under the 'National Vector-borne Disease Control Programme" (NVBDCP).

Objectives and use of antimalarial drugs

The aims of using drugs in relation to malarial infection are:

- To prevent clinical attack of malaria (prophylactic).
- To treat clinical attack of malaria (clinical curative).
- To completely eradicate the parasite from the patient's body (radical curative).
- To cut down human-to-mosquito transmission (gametocidal).

These objectives are achieved by attacking the parasite at its various stages of life cycle in the human host (*see* Fig. 34.1). Antimalarials that act on erythrocytic schizogony are called *erythrocytic schizontocides*, those that act on preerythrocytic as well as exoerythrocytic (occurs in *P. vivax*) stages in liver are called

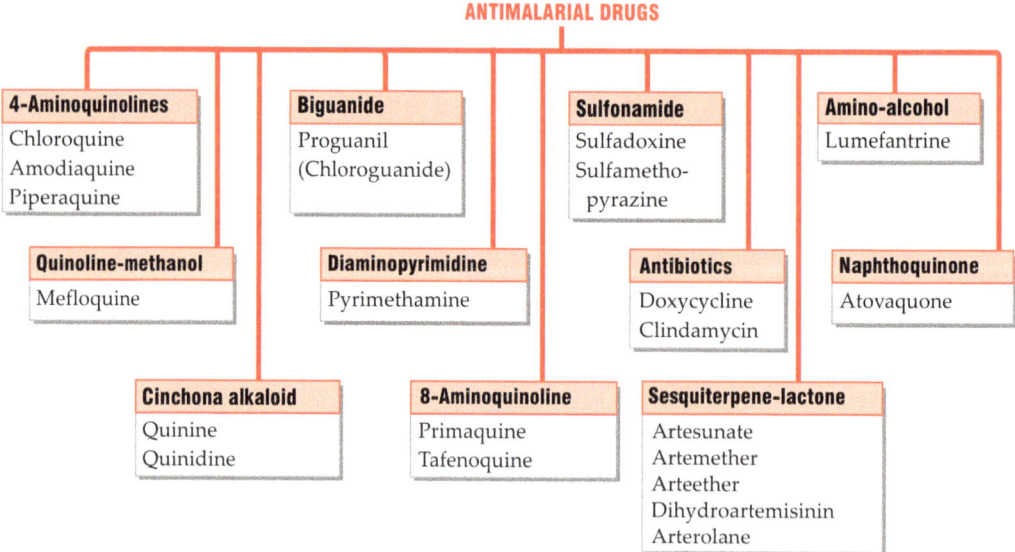

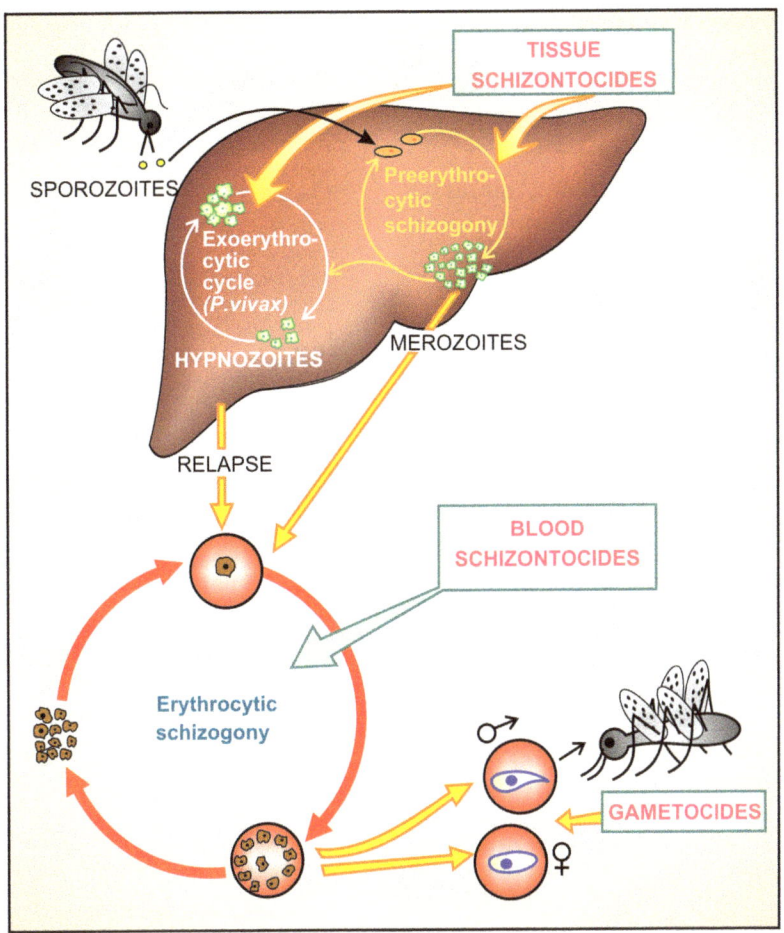

Fig. 34.1: The life cycle of malarial parasite in man. Stages and forms of the parasite at which different types of antimalarial drugs act are indicated

tissue schizontocides, while those which kill gametocytes in blood are called *gametocides*. Antimalarial drugs exhibit considerable stage selectivity of action. Primaquine is a tissue schizontocide: acts on pre- as well as exo-erythrocytic stages, but has little action on erythrocytic stage. All others are erythrocytic schizontocides and have no effect on liver stages, except proguanil which can also kill preerythrocytic forms of *P. falciparum*. Antimalarial therapy is given in the following forms.

1. **Causal prophylaxis** The preerythrocytic phase (in liver), which is the *cause* of malarial infection and clinical attacks, is the target for this purpose. Proguanil is a causal prophylactic primarily for *P. falciparum*, but is not very effective against *P. vivax*. Since both *P. vivax* and *P. falciparum* infections occur in majority of areas, proguanil is not used as prophylactic. Primaquine is a causal prophylactic for all species of malaria, but has not been used in mass programmes because of its toxic potential.

Chapter 34: Antiprotozoal Drugs

2. Suppressive prophylaxis The schizontocides which suppress the erythrocytic phase and thus attacks of malarial fever can be used as prophylactics. Though the exoerythrocytic phase in case of vivax and other relapsing malarias continues, clinical disease does not appear. Chloroquine, proguanil, mefloquine and doxycycline have been used for suppressive prophylaxis. Due to spread of chloroquine resistance among *P. falciparum*, it is no longer used in India. Mefloquine and doxycycline are used for malaria prophylaxis by travellers visiting endemic areas.

3. Clinical cure The erythrocytic schizontocides are used to terminate an episode of malarial fever. The available drugs can be divided into:

(a) High-efficacy drugs: Artemisinins, chloroquine, amodiaquine, quinine, mefloquine, lumefantrine, atovaquone. These drugs can be used singly to treat attacks of malarial fever, but are combined now.

(b) Low-efficacy drugs: Proguanil, pyrimethamine, sulfonamides, tetracyclines and clindamycin. They are used only in combination for clinical cure.

The faster acting drugs are preferred. The exoerythrocytic phase of vivax (hypnozoites) persists even after clinical cure, and can cause *relapses* subsequently without reinfection. Thus, the erythrocytic schizontocides are radical curatives for falciparum but not for vivax malaria. *Recrudescences* occur in falciparum infection if the blood is not totally cleared of the parasites by the drug.

The drugs and regimens used for treatment of uncomplicated falciparum and vivax malaria are listed in the box. Only oral drugs are used for uncomplicated malaria.

Treatment of uncomplicated malaria

A. Vivax (also ovale, malariae) malaria

1. Chloroquine 600 mg (10 mg/kg) followed by 300 mg (5 mg/kg) after 8 hours and then for next 2 days (total 25 mg/kg over 3 days) + Primaquine 15 mg (0.25 mg/kg) daily × 14 days

   In occasional case of chloroquine resistance

2. Quinine 600 mg (10 mg/kg) 8 hourly × 7 days + Doxycycline 100 mg daily × 7 days or Clindamycin 600 mg 12 hourly × 7 days + Primaquine (as above)

   or

   Artemisinin-based combination therapy (except sulfa-pyrimethamine based ACT) + Primaquine (as above)

B. Chloroquine-sensitive falciparum malaria[£]

1. Chloroquine (as above) + Primaquine 45 mg (0.75 mg/kg) single dose (as gametocidal) on day 2, is an option

C. Chloroquine-resistant falciparum malaria

1. Artesunate 100 mg BD (4 mg/kg/day) × 3 days + Mefloquine 750 mg (15 mg/kg) on 2nd day and 500 mg (10 mg/kg) on 3rd day.

   or

2. Artemether 80 mg + Lumefantrine 480 mg twice daily × 3 days (child 25–35 kg BW ¾ dose; 15–25 kg BW ½ dose; 5–15 kg BW ¼ dose)

   or

3.* Artesunate 100 mg BD (4 mg/kg/day) × 3 days + Sulfadoxine 1500 mg (25 mg/kg) + Pyrimethamine 75 mg (1.25 mg/kg) single dose

   or

4. Arterolane (as maleate) 150 mg + Piperaquine 750 mg once daily × 3 days

   or

5.[$] Quinine 600 mg (10 mg/kg) 8 hourly × 7 days + Doxycycline 100 mg daily × 7 days or Clindamycin 600 12 hourly × 7 days

*First line ACT under NVBDCP, except in Northeastern states where FDC of artemether-lumefantrine is used.
[£]In India (including under NVBDCP) all P.f. cases, irrespective of CQ-resistance status, are treated with artemisinin-based combination therapy (ACT) + Primaquine (0.75 mg/kg) single dose on the 2nd day (as gametocidal).
[$]Falciparum malaria during 1st trimester of pregnancy should be treated with a 7 day course of quinine + clindamycin.

4. Radical cure In the case of vivax and ovale malaria, drugs which attack the exoerythrocytic stage (hypnozoites) given together with a clinical curative achieve total eradication of the parasite from the patient's body. A radical curative is needed in relapsing malaria, while in falciparum malaria—adequate treatment of clinical attack leaves no parasite in the body.

Drug of choice for radical cure of vivax malaria is primaquine 15 mg daily for 2 weeks immediately following 3 day chloroquine (or other schizontocide) therapy. However, it is contraindicated in G-6-PD deficient subjects. Tafenoquine, a new long acting radical curative, has been recently approved for single dose antirelapse treatment of vivax malaria.

5. Gametocidal This refers to the elimination of male and female gametes of *Plasmodia* formed in the patient's blood. Gametocidal action is of no benefit to the patient being treated, but will reduce transmission to mosquito.

Primaquine is gametocidal to all species of *Plasmodia*, while chloroquine and quinine are active against vivax but not falciparum gametes.

- A single 45 mg (0.75 mg/kg) dose of primaquine is employed immediately after clinical cure of falciparum malaria.

Chloroquine (CQ)

It is a rapidly acting erythrocytic schizontocide against all species of *Plasmodia* except chloroquine (CQ) resistant *P. falciparum*. It controls most clinical attacks in 1–2 days with disappearance of parasites from peripheral blood. However, it has no effect on pre- and exoerythrocytic phases of the parasite — does not prevent relapses in vivax malaria.

Chloroquine is actively concentrated by sensitive intraerythrocytic plasmodia. By accumulating in the acidic vesicles of the parasite and because of its weakly basic nature, it raises the vesicular pH and thereby interferes with degradation of haemoglobin by parasitic lysosomes. Polymerization of toxic heme to nontoxic parasite pigment haemozoin is inhibited. Heme then damages the plasmodial membranes.

Chloroquine resistance among *P. vivax* has been slow in developing. However, *P. falciparum* has acquired considerable CQ resistance, and CQ-resistant strains have become wide spread. Some of these have become multidrug resistant. Resistance in *P. falciparum* is associated with a decreased ability of the parasite to accumulate CQ.

Other actions Chloroquine is active against *Entamoeba histolytica* and *Giardia lamblia* also.

It has anti-inflammatory, local irritant and local anaesthetic (on injection), weak smooth muscle relaxant, antihistaminic and antiarrhythmic properties.

Oral absorption of CQ is excellent. It is partly metabolized by liver and slowly excreted in urine. The plasma t½ varies from 3–10 days or more. Because of tight tissue binding, small amounts persist in the body for months.

Toxicity of CQ is low, but side effects are frequent and unpleasant: nausea, vomiting, anorexia, uncontrollable itching, epigastric pain, uneasiness, difficulty in accomodation and headache. Prolonged use of high doses may cause loss of vision due to retinal damage.

Uses

1. Chloroquine is the drug of choice for clinical cure of vivax malaria and CQ sensitive falciparum malaria. However, in India, due to spread of CQ resistance among *P. falciparum*, it is no longer used for any case of falciparum malaria, irrespective of

CQ resistance status, but continues to be the standard treatment of vivax malaria.
2. Extraintestinal amoebiasis.
3. Rheumatoid arthritis
4. Discoid lupus erythematosus—very effective; less valuable in systemic LE.
5. Lepra reactions.
6. Photogenic reactions.

Amodiaquine It is almost identical to CQ in properties and is less bitter. It can be used as an alternative to CQ for clinical cure of uncomplicated malaria, but is not recommended for prophylaxis. Amodiaquine is active against CQ resistant *P. falciparum* and is used in combination with artesunate as artemisinin combination therapy (ACT) for resistant falciparum malaria.

Piperaquine It is a bisquinoline congener of chloroquine developed in China as a long acting (t½ 2-3 weeks) erythrocytic schizontocide with a slower onset of action. Piperaquine is active against CQ-resistant *P. falciparum* and is combined with dihydroartemisinin or arterolane as ACT for treating falciparum malaria.

Mefloquine

Mefloquine is a rapidly acting erythrocytic schizontocide, but slower than chloroquine or quinine due to slow absorption after oral ingestion. It is effective against CQ-sensitive as well as resistant plasmodia. It controls fever and eliminates circulating parasites in infections caused by *P. falciparum* or *P. vivax*. However, like CQ, relapses occur subsequently in vivax malaria. It is also an efficacious suppressive prophylactic for multiresistant *P. falciparum* and other types of malaria.

Mefloquine is bitter in taste. Common side effects are dizziness, nausea, vomiting, diarrhoea, abdominal pain and sinus bradycardia. Major concern in the use of mefloquine is a variety of neuropsychiatric reactions occurring in some recipients.

Use Mefloquine is used in combination with artesunate as ACT for uncomplicated CQ-resistant falciparum malaria. It is also utilized for malaria prophylaxis in travellers visiting malaria endemic areas.

Quinine

Quinine is the levo rotatory alkaloid obtained from cinchona bark. Its *d*-isomer quinidine is used as an antiarrhythmic (and for malaria as well in some countries).

Quinine is an erythrocytic schizontocide for all species of *Plasmodia*; less effective and more toxic than CQ, but is active against CQ and multidrug resistant strains of *P. falciparum*. However, even quinine resistance has been encountered in some countries, but is sporadic in India, particularly along Myanmar border. Quinine has no effect on preerythrocytic stage and on hypnozoites of relapsing malaria.

The current indications of quinine are:
1. Uncomplicated CQ-resistant falciparum malaria: a 7 day course of oral quinine + doxycycline or clindamycin is prescribed.
2. Severe and complicated falciparum malaria: Quinine is given by slow i.v. infusion every 8 hours.
3. Nocturnal muscle cramps.

Quinine has many other actions. It is intensely bitter and irritant: orally causes nausea, vomiting and epigastric discomfort. Gastric secretion is stimulated. Weak analgesic, antipyretic actions, impairment of hearing and vision are produced at higher doses. Cardiodepressant, antiarrhythmic and hypotensive actions are similar to those of quinidine. Quinine stimulates uterine contractions, but reduces skeletal muscle contractility. Hypoglycaemia can occur on i.v. injection of quinine.

Proguanil (Chloroguanide)

It is a slow acting erythrocytic schizontocide. In addition, it inhibits pre-erythrocytic stage of *P. falciparum*. Proguanil is cyclized in the body to a triazine derivative (cycloguanil) which inhibits plasmodial dihydrofolate reductase (DHFRase) in preference to the mammalian enzyme. Resistance to proguanil develops rapidly due to mutational changes in the plasmodial DHFRase enzyme.

Proguanil is very well tolerated; side effects are less compared to chloroquine.

Currently in India, proguanil is not being used either for prophylaxis or for clinical cure of malaria. In some countries its combination with atovaquone is used for treating CQ resistant falciparum malaria.

Sulfonamide-Pyrimethamine (S/P) combination

Like trimethoprim, pyrimethamine is a directly acting inhibitor of DHFRase, but has high affinity for the plasmodial DHFRase compared to the bacterial or mammalian enzyme. Pyrimethamine gradually stops schizogony of malarial parasite in blood, but has little effect on pre- or exo-erythrocytic schizogony. Thus, it is a slow acting erythrocytic schizontocide. While sulfonamides are weak antimalarial drugs in their own right, they form supra-additive synergistic combination with pyrimethamine due to sequential block. Though both components are slow acting, the S/P combination acts faster, so that it can be employed as a clinical curative for *P. falciparum*. Activity against *P. vivax* is low. By the addition of sulfonamide, development of resistance to pyrimethamine is retarded.

Sulfadoxine and sulfamethopyrazine are ultra-long acting sulfonamides—attain low blood concentrations, but are able to synergise with pyrimethamine which also has long t½. The combination has the potential to cause serious cutaneous reactions (exfoliative dermatitis, Stevens-Johnson syndrome, etc.) due to the sulfonamide component. Therefore, its use is restricted to single dose treatment of uncomplicated CQ-resistant (as well as CQ sensitive) *P. falciparum* malaria. Presently, the single dose sulfadoxine + pyrimethamine combination is used along with 3 day artesunate to treat uncomplicated falciparum malaria. It is the first line ACT regimen used under NVBDCP in India, except in North-eastern states.

Primaquine

In contrast to other antimalarial drugs, primaquine is a poor erythrocytic schizontocide. It has weak action on *P. vivax*, but blood forms of *P. falciparum* are totally insensitive. Primaquine differs from all other available antimalarials in having a marked effect on primary as well as secondary hepatic phases of the malarial parasite. Therefore, it is a causal prophylactic and radical curative, but not a clinical curative. Primaquine is highly active against gametocytes and hypnozoites.

Adverse effects The usual doses of primaquine produce only abdominal pain, g.i. upset, weakness or uneasiness in chest as side effect.

The most important toxic potential is dose-related haemolysis, methaemoglobinaemia, tachypnoea and cyanosis. These effects are due to the oxidant property of primaquine. In normal individuals, doses < 60 mg (base) produce little haemolysis. Subjects with G-6-PD deficiency are highly sensitive, and haemolytic anaemia can occur with 15–30 mg/day dose. The incidence of G-6-PD deficiency is low among Indians, except in some tribal people. Passage of dark urine is an indication of haemolysis.

Use The primary indication of primaquine is for radical cure of relapsing (vivax) malaria. A 14 day course with 15 mg/day is given after spot test for G-6-PD status shows no deficiency.

Falciparum malaria: A single 45 mg dose of primaquine is given with the curative dose of artemisinin based combination therapy (ACT) to kill the gametes and cut down transmission to mosquito.

Tafenoquine

It is a new long-acting 8-aminoquinoline which has been recently approved as single dose radical curative for vivax malaria. It has a long (14–19 day) plasma t½ (contrast 6–8 hours plasma t½ of primaquine). Thus, tafenoquine continues to act for weeks after a single dose. Up to 100% relapse prevention has been achieved in vivax malaria by single dose tafenoquine (800 mg) given along with the standard 3 day course of CQ.

Tetracycline / Doxycycline

These antibiotics have slow and weak erythrocytic schizontocidal action against all plasmodial species. However, they are never used alone to treat malaria, but are combined with quinine for the treatment of chloroquine-resistant falciparum malaria (*see* box on p. 488).

Doxycycline 100 mg/day is used as a prophylactic for short term (<6 weeks) travellers to chloroquine-resistant *P. falciparum* areas.

Clindamycin

It has action similar to tetracyclines, and is used in place of doxycycline in pregnant women and in children (*see* box on p. 488), because tetracyclines are contraindicated in them.

Artemisinin derivatives

Artemisinin is the active principle of the plant *Artemisia annua* used in Chinese traditional medicine as 'Quinghaosu'. It is a sesquiterpene lactone active against *P. falciparum* resistant to all other antimalarial drugs as well as sensitive strains. Potent and rapid blood schizontocide action is exerted eliciting quicker defervescence and parasitaemia clearance (in 24–48 hr) than chloroquine or any other drug. However, it does not kill primary liver forms and vivax hypnozoites.

Artemisinin is poorly soluble in water as well as in oil. Several derivatives have been produced, of which *Artemether* is soluble in oil, while *Artesunate* (sod.) is water soluble. Both can be given orally as well as i.m., but artesunate sod. can be injected i.v. as well. Another injectable (i.m.) compound *Arteether* was developed in India, and lately a synthetic oral compound *Arterolane* has been introduced. All these are collectively referred to as *Artemisinins*. So far no resistance among *P. falciparum* patients to artemisinin has been noted.

The mechanism of action of artemisinins is not clearly known. However, it is believed that the endoperoxide bridge of artemisinin molecule interacts with the heme moiety in the parasite, releasing a highly reactive free radical species which damages the parasite.

Because artemisinins are short-acting drugs, monotherapy with them needs to be extended beyond the disappearance of the parasites to prevent recrudescence. Recrudescence can be totally prevented by combining 3 day artesunate with a long-acting drug which acts by a different mechanism.

Adverse effects Artemisinins produce few adverse effects; most are mild: nausea, vomiting, abdominal pain, itching and drug fever. Abnormal bleeding, dark urine, S-T segment changes, Q-T prolongation have been rarely noted, which subside when the patient improves or the drug is stopped. Intravenous artesunate is much safer than i.v. quinine.

Use Oral artemisinins are to be used only for treating acute attacks of *uncomplicated falciparum malaria* (both chloroquine sensitive as well as resistant). To preserve their powerful antimalarial activity and to contain recrudescences, it is mandatory that artemisinins be used only in combination with a long acting schizontocide like mefloquine/piperaquine/amodiaquine/lumefantrine or S/P. Such artemisinin-based combination therapy (ACT) is highly effective and has been found to reduce the prevalence of malaria as well as to check the spread of drug-resistant strains. Under the National policy, use of oral artemisinins alone is prohibited. It is mandated that all uncomplicated falciparum malaria cases be treated with one of the ACT combinations. The currently available ACT regimens are given in the box.

For vivax malaria, artemisinins (as ACT other than artesunate-S/P) are indicated only in rare cases of CQ resistant infection when quinine + doxycycline/clindamycin also cannot be used.

Severe and complicated falciparum malaria: Parenteral artemisinin *viz.* artesunate (i.v. or i.m.)/artemether (i.m.)/arteether (i.m.) given till the patient is fit to take oral medication, followed by 3 day ACT is highly effective, better tolerated and is now preferred over i.v. quinine.

Lumefantrine is an orally active aminoalcohol having erythrocytic schizontocidal activity comparable to mefloquine. Lumefantrine kills *P. falciparum* resistant to CQ as well as S/P. It is long acting, well tolerated, and has not shown cardiotoxicity in contrast to its predecessor halofantrine. It is combined with artemether for treatment of falciparum malaria as ACT.

Atovaquone This synthetic naphthaquinone is a rapidly acting erythrocytic schizontocide for *P. falciparum* and other plasmodia. Proguanil potentiates its antimalarial action and prevents emergence of resistance. A fixed dose oral combination of the two drugs is used for 3 day treatment of uncomplicated chloroquine-resistant *P. falciparum* malaria in some countries.

ACT regimens for uncomplicated falciparum malaria*

1. *Artemether-lumefantrine (1:6)$^{£, \$}$*
   Artemether (80 mg BD) + lumefantrine (480 mg BD) × 3 days
   COARTEM, COMBITHER, LUMETHER (artemether 20 mg + lumefantrine 120 mg tab.) to be taken with fatty meal.
   Adult and child >35 kg 4 tab BD; child 25–35 kg 3 tab BD; 15–25 kg 2 tab BD; 5–15 kg 1 tab BD, all for 3 days.
   FALCIMAX PLUS, ARTE PLUS (artemether 80 mg + lumefantrine 480 mg tab) 1 tab BD × 3 days for adults.

2. *Artesunate-mefloquine (AS/MQ)$^{£, \$}$*
   Artesunate 100 mg BD (4 mg/kg/day) × 3 days + mefloquine 750 mg (15 mg/kg) on 2nd day and 500 mg (10 mg/kg) on 3rd day (total 25 mg/kg).
   MEFLIAM PLUS: Artesunate 100 mg + mefloquine 200 mg pack of 6 FDC tabs; LARINATE-MF Kit: Artesunate 200 mg (3 tabs) + mefloquine 250 mg (6 tabs) kit; FALCIGO PLUS kit (Artesunate 50 mg tab + Mefloquine 250 mg tab kit)

3. *Artesunate-amodiaquine (AS/AQ)$^{\$}$*
   Artesunate 200 mg (4 mg/kg) + amodiaquine 600 mg (10 mg/kg) per day × 3 days
   Artesunate 25 mg/50 mg/100 mg + amodiaquine 67.5 mg/135 mg/270 mg fixed dose combination tablets;
   ASAQ, FALCINIL-Aq: 25 + 67.5 mg, 50 + 135 mg, 100 + 270 mg FDC tabs.

4. *Artesunate-sulfadoxine + pyrimethamine (AS-S/P)$^{£, \$}$*
   Artesunate 100 mg BD (4 mg/kg/day) × 3 days + sulfadoxine 1500 mg (25 mg/kg) and pyrimethamine 75 mg (1.25 mg/kg) single dose.
   ZESUNATE kit, MASUNATE kit, FALCIART kit (Artesunate 100 mg × 6 tab + sulfadoxine 500 mg/pyrimethamine 25 mg × 3 tab kit)

5. *Dihydroartemisinin-piperaquine (DHA/PPQ 1:8)$^{£, \$}$*
   DHA 120 mg (2 mg/kg) + piperaquine 960 mg (16 mg/kg) daily × 3 days; for children < 25 kg body weight, DHA not less than 2.5 mg/kg + piperaquine 20 mg/kg daily × 3 days.
   PALUDOSE PLUS: Dihydroartemisinin 40 mg + piperaquine 320 mg tab.; DYSURE: DHA 80 mg + piperaquine 640 mg per 5 ml suspension.

6. *Arterolane-piperaquine$^{\$}$*
   Arterolane (as maleate) 150 mg + piperaquine 750 mg daily × 3 days (approved only for adults).
   SYNRIAM (arterolane 150 mg + piperaquine 750 mg) cap, 1 cap OD × 3 days

* All drugs are administered orally
$^{£}$ WHO approved ACTs; $^{\$}$ Approved in India

Chapter 34: Antiprotozoal Drugs

ANTIAMOEBIC DRUGS

These are drugs useful in infection caused by the protozoa *Entamoeba histolytica*.

Amoebiasis occurs by faecal contamination of food and water. Amoebic cysts reaching the intestine transform into trophozoites which either live on the surface of colonic mucosa as commensals—form cysts that pass into the stools (luminal cycle) and serve to propagate the disease, or invade the mucosa—form amoebic ulcers (Fig. 34.2) and cause acute dysentery (with blood and mucus in stools) or chronic intestinal amoebiasis (with vague abdominal symptoms, amoeboma).

Occasionally, the trophozoites pass into the blood-stream, reach the liver *via* portal vein and cause amoebic liver abscess. Other organs like lungs, spleen, kidney and brain are rarely involved. In the tissues, only trophozoites are present; cyst formation does not occur. Tissue phase is always secondary to intestinal amoebiasis, which may be asymptomatic.

Metronidazole Metronidazole and other nitroimidazoles are the first line drugs for all forms of amoebiasis. They are also active against other protozoa (*Trichomonas vaginalis, Giardia lamblia*) as well as against many anaerobic bacteria, and are described in Ch. 26.

Emetine
It is an alkaloid from *Cephaelis ipecacuanha*. Emetine is a potent amoebicide—kills trophozoites but has no effect on cysts.

In acute dysentery, the stool is rapidly cleared of the trophozoites and symptomatic relief occurs in 1–3 days. It is highly efficacious in amoebic liver abscess also.

Emetine cannot be given orally because it will be vomited out. It is administered by s.c. or i.m. injection.

Toxicity of emetine is high, the most prominent of which is nausea, vomiting, abdominal cramps, myocarditis, ECG changes, heart failure, hypotension and myositis. It is now rarely used for severe intestinal or hepatic amoebiasis; only in patients allergic to metronidazole or not responding to it.

Chloroquine

Chloroquine kills trophozoites of *E. histolytica* and is highly concentrated

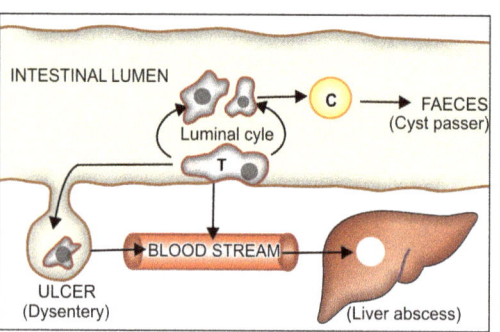

Fig. 34.2: The luminal cycle and invasive forms of amoebiasis. T—trophozoite; C—cysts

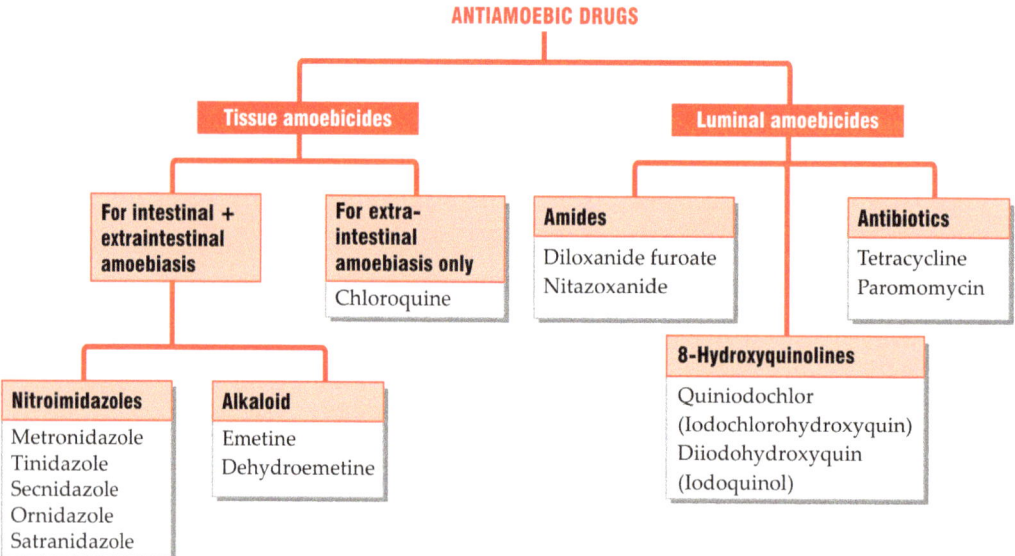

in liver. Therefore, it is used in hepatic amoebiasis only. Because it is largely absorbed from the upper intestine (only small amount reaches colonic lumen), and not much concentrated in the intestinal wall—it is neither effective in invasive dysentery nor in controlling the luminal cycle (cyst passers).

For amoebic liver abscess, chloroquine has to be given for 2–3 weeks, and this produces unpleasant side effects. It is employed mainly in patients allergic to metronidazole. It may also be used as additional drug following a course of emetine or metronidazole.

Diloxanide furoate

It is a highly effective luminal amoebicide: directly kills trophozoites responsible for production of cysts. The furoate ester is hydrolysed in intestine and the released diloxanide is largely absorbed, but no systemic antiamoebic activity is evident. The furoate ester is more active than diloxanide as such.

Diloxanide furoate is less effective in invasive amoebic dysentery. However, it has produced high cure rates in mild intestinal amoebiasis and in asymptomatic cyst passers.

Diloxanide furoate is very well tolerated; the only side effects are flatulence, occasional nausea, itching and rarely urticaria.

Nitazoxanide
This congener of the antitapeworm drug niclosamide has been introduced for the treatment of cryptosporidiasis and giardiasis, but is useful in amoebic dysentery as well. The active metabolite of nitazoxanide acts by inhibiting the enzyme pyruvate: ferredoxin oxidoreductase (PFOR) in the parasite. Thus, its mechanism of action resembles that of metronidazole. Side effects are mild.

8-Hydroxyquinolines

The 8-hydroxyquinolines *viz.* quiniodochlor and diiodohydroxyquin were widely employed in the past, but are infrequently used now. Both have similar properties; are active against *Entamoeba, Giardia, Trichomonas,* some fungi (dermatophytes, *Candida*) and some bacteria. They kill the cyst forming trophozoites in the intestine, but do not have tissue amoebicidal action. Like diloxanide furoate, the 8-hydroxyquinolines are not very effective in acute amoebic dysentery but afford relief in chronic intestinal amoebiasis. Their efficacy in eradicating cysts from asymptomatic carriers is rated lower than that of diloxanide furoate and they are totally valueless in extraintestinal amoebiasis.

The 8-hydroxyquinolines are partially absorbed from intestines, and are well tolerated: produce few side effects—nausea, transient loose and green stools, pruritus, etc., but carry toxic potential if used inappropriately.

Prolonged/repeated intake of relatively high doses of quiniodochlor caused a neuropathic syndrome called 'subacute myelo-optic neuropathy' (SMON) in Japan in an epidemic form, affecting several thousand people in 1970. However, despite widespread use in the past, only sporadic and unconfirmed cases have been reported from India. The 8-hydroxyquinolines have been banned in Japan and few other countries; but in India, they are prohibited only for pediatric patients, because their use for chronic diarrhoeas in children has caused blindness.

The 8-hydroxyquinolines may be employed in intestinal amoebiasis as alternative to diloxanide furoate. Other uses are—giardiasis; local treatment of monilial and trichomonas vaginitis, fungal and bacterial skin infections.

Chapter 34: Antiprotozoal Drugs

Tetracyclines Tetracyclines have modest direct inhibitory action on *Entamoeba*. Tetracycline and oxytetracycline are incompletely absorbed in the small intestine, reach the colon in large amounts and inhibit the bacterial flora with which *Entamoebae* live symbiotically. Thus, tetracyclines indirectly reduce proliferation of entamoebae in the colon and are specially valuable in chronic, difficult to treat cases who only have the luminal cycle with little mucosal invasion. Tetracyclines have an adjuvant role in conjunction with a more efficacious luminal amoebicide. They are not good for acute dysentery and for hepatic amoebiasis.

Paromomycin It is an aminoglycoside antibiotic closely resembling neomycin, which inhibits many protozoa including *Entamoeba, Giardia, Trichomonas* and *Leishmania*. Oral paromomycin is an efficacious luminal amoebicide which can be used to treat chronic amoebic colitis. For acute amoebic dysentery, it can be combined with metronidazole. Intramuscular paromomycin is an alternative drug for visceral leishmaniasis (kala-azar).

35

CHAPTER

Antiseptics, Disinfectants and Other Locally Acting Drugs

ANTISEPTICS AND DISINFECTANTS

The terms *antiseptic* and *disinfectant* connote an agent which inhibits or kills microbes on contact. Conventionally, agents used on living surfaces (patient's mouth, dentist's hands, etc.) are called *antiseptics* while those used for inanimate objects (instruments, working surfaces, water supply, privies, etc.) are called *disinfectants*. There is considerable overlap and many agents are used in either way. A practical distinction between the two on the basis of a *growth inhibiting* action on one hand, and a *direct lethal* action on the other is futile because these are often concentration dependent actions. The term *Germicide* covers both category of drugs.

There, however, is difference between 'disinfection' and 'sterilization'. While sterilization means complete killing of all forms of microorganisms, including spores, disinfection refers to reduction in the number of viable pathogenic microbes to a level that they do not pose a risk to individuals with normal host defence. The terms *'sanitization'* (used for environment and inanimate surfaces), and *'decontamination'* also have similar connotation. Thus, in ordinary usage, disinfectants do not eliminate all microbes. Application of a disinfectant to the dentists working platform does not make it totally germ free.

Antiseptics and disinfectants are routinely used in dentistry to check cross infection as well as to prevent and treat some infective conditions. Many instruments are sterilized by autoclaving, but certain instruments, working surfaces and operating light handles, etc. cannot be autoclaved. They have to be sanitized by disinfectants.

The era of antiseptics and disinfectants was heralded by Semmelweiss (washing of hands in chlorinated lime) and Lister (antiseptic surgery by the use of phenol) in the 19th century. These germicides differ from systemically used antimicrobials by their low parasite selectivity. They are too toxic for systemic use. However, many systemic antimicrobials are applied topically as well, and some antibiotics (bacitracin, neomycin) are restricted to topical use, but are generally not enumerated with the antiseptics. A strict distinction is thus impossible.

A good antiseptic/disinfectant should be:
- Chemically stable.
- Cheap.
- Nonstaining with agreeable colour and odour.
- Cidal and not merely static, destroying spores as well.
- Active against all pathogens—bacteria, fungi, viruses, protozoa.
- Able to spread through organic films and enter folds and crevices.
- Active even in the presence of blood, pus, exudates and excreta.
- Require brief time of exposure.

A disinfectant in addition should not corrode or rust instruments and be easily washable.
An antiseptic in addition should be:
(i) Rapid in action and afford sustained protection.

Chapter 35: Antiseptics, Disinfectants and Other Locally Acting Drugs

(ii) Nonirritating to tissues, should not delay healing.
(iii) Nonabsorbable, produce minimum toxicity if absorbed.
(iv) Nonsensitizing (no allergy).
(v) Compatible with soaps and other detergents.

Spectrum of activity of majority of antiseptic-disinfectants is wide, reflecting nonselectivity of action. However, some are relatively selective, e.g. hexachlorophene, chlorhexidine, quaternary ammonium antiseptics, gentian violet and acriflavin are more active on gram-positive than on gram-negative bacteria; silver nitrate is highly active against gonococci and benzoyl peroxide against *P. acnes*.

Mechanisms of action of germicides are varied, but can be grouped into:
(a) Oxidation of bacterial protoplasm.
(b) Denaturation of bacterial proteins including enzymes.
(c) Detergent like action increasing permeability of bacterial membrane.

Factors which modify the activity of germicides are:
- Temperature and pH.
- Period of contact with the microorganism.
- Nature of microbe involved.
- Size of innoculum.
- Presence of blood, pus or other organic matter.

Potency of a germicide is generally expressed by its *phenol coefficient* or *Rideal Walker coefficient*, which is the ratio of the minimum concentration of the test compound required to kill a 24 hour culture of *B. typhosa* in 7.5 minute at 37.5 C to that of phenol under similar conditions. This test has only limited validity, particularly in relation to antiseptics which have to be tested on living surfaces.

Therapeutic index of an antiseptic is defined by comparing the concentration at which it acts on microorganisms with that which produces local irritation, tissue damage or interference with healing.

CLASSIFICATION

1. *Phenol derivatives*: Phenol, Cresol, Chloroxylenol, Hexachlorophene, Triclosan.
2. *Oxidizing agents*: Pot. permanganate, Hydrogen peroxide, Benzoyl peroxide.
3. *Halogens*: Iodine, Iodophores, Chlorine, Chlorophores.
4. *Biguanide*: Chlorhexidine.
5. *Quaternary ammonium (Cationic)*: Cetrimide, Cetylpyridinium chloride, Benzalkonium chloride.
6. *Soaps*: of Sod. and Pot.
7. *Alcohols*: Ethanol, Isopropanol.
8. *Aldehydes*: Formaldehyde, Glutaraldehyde.
9. *Acids*: Boric acid.
10. *Metallic salts*: Silver nitrate, Zinc sulfate, Calamine, Zinc oxide.
11. *Dyes*: Gentian violet, Acriflavine, Proflavine.
12. *Furan derivatives*: Nitrofurazone.

1. PHENOLS

Phenol (Carbolic acid) It is one of the earliest used antiseptics and still the standard for comparing other germicides. It is a relatively weak agent (static at 0.2%, cidal at >1%, has poor action on bacterial spores). Phenol is a general *protoplasmic poison*, injuring microbes and tissue cells alike. At higher concentrations it causes skin burns and is a caustic. It acts by denaturing bacterial proteins. Organic matter diminishes its action slightly while alkalies and soaps do so profoundly (carbolic soaps are not more germicidal than soap itself). It is now seldom employed as an antiseptic, but being cheap, it is used to disinfect urine, faeces, pus, sputum of patients and is sometimes included in antipruritic preparations because of its mild local anaesthetic action.

Cresol It is methyl-phenol; more active (3–10 times) and less damaging to tissues. It is used for disinfection of utensils, excreta and for washing hands.
LYSOL is a 50% soapy emulsion of cresol.

Triclosan It is a chlorinated bisphenol having broad spectrum activity against most oral bacteria. Denaturation of membrane bound enzymes is primarily responsible for its bactericidal action. Triclosan is nonirritating, does not stain teeth and its sensitization potential is negligible.

The hydroalcoholic solution of a mixture of phenolic volatile oils thymol, menthol, eucalyptol along with benzoic acid is a popular mouthwash LISTERINE. It is widely used for bad breath, dental plaque and gingivitis.

Chloroxylenol It has a phenol coefficient of 70; does not coagulate proteins, is noncorrosive, nonirritating to intact skin, but its efficacy is reduced by organic matter. Chloroxylenol is poorly water soluble; the commercial 4.8% solution (DETTOL) is prepared in 9% terpinol and 13% alcohol and is used for surgical antisepsis. A 0.8% skin cream and soap, 1.4% lubricating obstetric cream (for vaginal examination, use on forceps, etc.) and a mouthwash (DETTOLIN 1% with menthol 0.45%) are also available. These preparations have very low contact sensitization potential, but lose activity if diluted with water and kept for some time.

Hexachlorophene This potent chlorinated phenol acts by inhibiting bacterial enzymes and (in high concentration) causing bacterial lysis. It is odourless, nonirritating and does not stain. Its activity is reduced by organic matter but not by soap. Hexachlorophene is commonly incorporated in soap and other cleansing antiseptics for surgical scrub. Activity against gram-positive bacteria is high, but poor against gram-negative organisms (*P. acnes*) and spores. The degerming action is slow but persistent due to deposition on the skin as a fine film that is not removed by rinsing with water. Incorporated in toilet products, it is a good deodorant.

2. OXIDIZING AGENTS

Potassium permanganate It occurs as purple crystals, highly water soluble, liberates oxygen which oxidizes bacterial protoplasm. The available oxygen and germicidal capacity is used up if much organic matter is present, and the solution gets decolourised. A 1:4000 to 1:10,000 solution (condy's lotion) is used for gargling, douching, irrigating cavities, urethra and wounds. The antiseptic action is rather slow. Higher concentrations cause burns and blistering—popularity therefore has declined.

Potassium permanganate has also been used to disinfect water (wells, ponds) and for stomach wash in alkaloidal poisoning. It promotes rusting and is not good for surgical instruments.

Hydrogen peroxide It liberates nascent oxygen which oxidizes necrotic matter and bacteria. A 3% solution produces 10 volumes of oxygen, much of which escapes in the molecular form. Catalase present in tissues speeds decomposition resulting in foaming. This helps in loosening and removing slough, ear wax, etc. Hydrogen peroxide has poor penetrability and a weak, transient antiseptic action. The potency declines further on keeping. Use therefore is much restricted.

Hydrogen peroxide mouthwash has been employed in acute necrotizing gingivitis because of predominance of anaerobic bacteria in this condition. Though efficacy in reducing plaque formation is marginal, H_2O_2 mouthwash has been advocated in periodontal disease. A 20-30% solution in water or ether has also been used as a bleaching agent on the teeth. Frequent use of 3% H_2O_2 rinse can produce oral ulcers.

Benzoyl peroxide It is specifically active against *P. acnes*, and is used on acne vulgaris.

3. HALOGENS

Iodine It is a rapidly acting, broad spectrum (bacteria, fungi, viruses) microbicidal agent that has been in use for more than a century. It acts by iodinating and oxidizing microbial protoplasm. A 1 : 20,000 solution kills most vegetative forms within 1 min. Even bacterial spores are killed with higher concentration/longer contact. Organic matter retards, but does not nullify its germicidal action.

Iodine crystals are corrosive, stronger solutions (> 5%) cause burning and blistering of skin. *Tincture iodine* (2% in alcohol) stings on abrasions and cuts. It is used on cuts, for degerming skin before surgery, and to treat ring worm. *Mandel's paint* (1.25% iodine dissolved with the help of Pot. iodide forming soluble I_3-ions) is applied on sore throat. A *nonstaining iodine ointment* (IODEX 4%) is popular as antiseptic and counterirritant. Some individuals are sensitive to iodine—rashes and systemic manifestations occur in them.

Iodophores These are soluble complexes of iodine with large molecular organic compounds that serve as carriers and release free iodine slowly. The most popular—*Povidone (Polyvinylpyrrolidone) iodine*: is nonirritating, nontoxic, nonstaining and exerts prolonged germicidal action. Treated areas can be bandaged or occluded without risk of blistering. Povidone iodine is extensively used in a variety of ways, e.g., on boils, furunculosis, burns, otitis externa, ulcers, tinea, monilial/trichomonal/nonspecific vaginitis and for surgical scrubbing, disinfection of endoscopes and instruments. In dentistry, 1% povidone iodine oral rinse is employed for gingivitis.

BETADINE 5% solution, 5% ointment, 7.5% scrub solution, 200 mg vaginal pessary; PIODIN 10% solution, 10% cream, 1% mouthwash; RANVIDONE AEROSOL 5% spray with freon propellant.

Chlorine A highly reactive element and a rapidly acting, potent germicide, 0.1–0.25 ppm kills most pathogens (but not *M. tuberculosis*) in 30 sec. However, the degerming action is soon exhausted and it lacks substantivity. It is used to disinfect urban water supplies. Organic matter binds chlorine, so that excess has to be added to obtain free chlorine concentration of 0.2–0.4 ppm. This is known as the 'chlorine demand' of water. Chlorine is more active in acidic or neutral medium.

Chlorophores These are compounds that slowly release hypochlorous acid (HOCl). Because of ease of handling, they are used in preference to gaseous chlorine.

(i) Chlorinated lime (bleaching powder) It is obtained by the action of chlorine on lime (CaO) resulting in a mixture of calcium chloride and calcium hypochlorite. On exposure, it decomposes releasing 30–35% W/W chlorine. Bleaching powder is used as disinfectant for drinking water, swimming pools and sanitizer for privies, etc. The bleaching action is occasionally utilized for removing stains from teeth and for their cosmetic whitening.

(ii) Sodium hypochlorite solution Contains 4–6% sodium hypochlorite. It is a powerful disinfectant used in dairies for milk cans and other equipment, infant feeding bottles, etc. It is unstable and too irritant to be used as antiseptic, except for *root canal therapy in dentistry*. Irrigation of root canal with 2% sod. hypochlorite solution loosens and dissolves dead tooth pulp in addition to exerting rapid antisepsis.

4. BIGUANIDE

Chlorhexidine It is a powerful, nonirritating, cationic antiseptic that disrupts bacterial cell membrane. Denaturation of intracellular proteins occurs as a secondary action. It is relatively more active against gram positive bacteria. Like hexachlorophene it persists on the skin for a long time. Present in SAVLON (*see* below), it is extensively used for surgical scrub, neonatal bath, mouthwash, obstetrics and as general skin antiseptic.

Chlorhexidine is the most widely employed antiseptic in dentistry, mainly in the form of oral rinse (0.12–0.2%) or toothpaste (0.5–1%). It is one of the most effective antiplaque and antigingivitis agents (*see* p. 507). Good results have been obtained in acute necrotizing gingivitis. Rinsing before the procedure, chlorhexidine solution prevents infections following periodontal and other forms of oral surgery. Twice daily chlorhexidine rinse markedly reduces oral infections in immuno-compromised patients including those with AIDS. Major disadvantage of intraoral use of chlorhexidine is brownish discolouration of teeth and tongue, an unpleasant after-taste, alteration of taste perception and occasionally oral ulceration.

CHLODIN, FLUDENT-CH, HEXIL, REXIDIN 0.2% mouthwash.

5. QUATERNARY AMMONIUM (CATIONIC) ANTISEPTICS

These are detergents; cidal to bacteria, fungi and viruses. However, many gram-negative bacteria (specially *Pseudomonas*), *M. tuberculosis* and bacterial spores are relatively resistant. They act by altering permeability of cell membranes. Soaps, being anionic, neutralize their action, while alcohol potentiates them. They spread through oil and grease, have cleansing and emulgent properties. These antiseptics are nonirritating and mildly keratolytic. However, the germicidal action is rather slow and bacteria may thrive under a film formed by them on the skin. Pus, debris and porous material like cotton, polyethylene reduce their germicidal activity. Sensitization occurs occasionally. These disadvantages not withstanding, they are widely used as sanitizers, antiseptic and disinfectant for surgical instruments, gloves, etc., but should not be considered sterilizing.

Cetrimide It is a soapy powder with faint fishy odour. Used as 1–3% solution, it has good cleansing action, efficiently removing dirt, grease, tar and congealed blood from road side accident wounds. Alone or in combination with chlorhexidine, cetrimide is one of the most popular hospital antiseptic and disinfectant for surgical instruments, utensils, baths, etc.

CETAVLON CONCENTRATE: Cetrimide 20%
SAVLON LIQUID ANTISEPTIC: Chlorhexidine gluconate 1.5% + Cetrimide 3%.
SAVLON/CETAVLEX CREAM: Chlorhexidine HCl 0.1% + Cetrimide 0.5%.
SAVLON HOSPITAL CONCENTRATE: Chlorhexidine gluconate 7.5% + Cetrimide 15%.

Cetylpyridinium chloride It is similar to cetrimide, has been included in mouth washes and lozenges to reduce plaque formation. However, it leaves a bad taste and can cause oral ulceration.

Benzalkonium chloride It is highly soluble in water and alcohol. A 1:1000 solution is used for sterile storage of instruments and 1 in 5000 to 1 in 10,000 for douches, irrigation, etc.

6. SOAPS

Soaps are anionic detergents with weak antiseptic action. They affect only gram positive bacteria. Their usefulness primarily resides in their cleansing action. Washing hands and other surfaces with soap and warm water is an effective method of preventing transmission of infection by removing/diluting pathogenic bacteria. Soaps can also be medicated by other antiseptics.

7. ALCOHOLS

Ethanol It is an effective antiseptic and cleansing agent at 40–90% concentration. The rapidity of action increases with the concentration up to 70% and decreases above

90%. It acts by precipitating bacterial proteins. A cotton swab soaked in 70% ethanol rubbed on the skin kills 90% bacteria in 2 min. This has been used before hypodermic injection and on minor cuts. After a soap and water wash, rubbing hands with 70% alcohol is the method of choice for decontaminating hands. Alcohol is irritant; should not be applied to mucous membranes or to delicate skin (scrotum), ulcers, etc. Applied to open wounds, it produces a burning sensation, injures the surface and forms a coagulum under which bacteria could grow.

Usefulness of alcohol in dentistry is limited; effective concentrations cannot be applied on gums or oral mucosa. Low concentration (5–10%) present in many mouth rinses (as solvent for essential oils, etc.) has no antiseptic efficacy. However, alcohol enhances the antiseptic activity of iodine and chlorhexidine when employed as solvent for these. Because alcohol evaporates without leaving any residue and has good cleansing property, it is often employed to sanitize working surfaces in dentistry, but it is a poor disinfectant for instruments, because it does not kill spores and promotes rusting.

Isopropanol It is less volatile, and can be used in place of ethanol, particularly for hand sanitization.

8. ALDEHYDES

Formaldehyde It is a pungent gas which is sometimes used for fumigation. A 37% aqueous solution called *Formalin* is diluted to 4% and used for hardening and preserving dead tissues because of its astringent and wide spectrum germicidal action. It denatures proteins and is a general protoplasmic poison, but acts slowly. Use of formaldehyde as antiseptic is restricted by its irritating nature and pungent odour. Low concentrations of formaldehyde are included in some desensitizing toothpastes, but the desensitizing action is weak. Use as mummifying agent for root canal treatment is outmoded. It is occasionally employed to disinfect instruments and excreta. Those who handle formalin can develop eczematoid reactions.

Glutaraldehyde It is less volatile, less pungent, less irritating and better sterilizing agent than formalin. Broad-spectrum activity against bacteria, viruses and fungi is exerted, but it needs to be activated by alkalinization of the solution. Organic matter does not inactivate it, and its 2% solution is often used in dentistry as an immersion disinfectant for instruments that cannot be autoclaved, but prolonged contact is needed. Glutaraldehyde should not be used to disinfect working surfaces because repeated inhalation of its vapours can induce asthma. Repeated application on skin can cause sensitization. The alkalinized solution has a short shelf-life (2 weeks) unless stablilizing agents are added.

9. ACIDS

Boric acid It is only bacteriostatic and a very weak antiseptic. But being nonirritating even to delicate structures, saturated aqueous solutions (4%) have been used as mouthwash, douche, etc., and to irrigate eyes. Boroglycerine paint (30% in glycerine) is used for stomatitis and glossitis. A 10% ointment (BOROCIDE) is available for cuts and abrasions. It is included in prickly heat powders and ear drops. However, boric acid is not innocuous; systemic absorption causes vomiting, abdominal pain, diarrhoea, visual disturbances and kidney damage.

10. METALLIC SALTS

Silver compounds These are astringent and caustic; react with SH, COOH, PO_4 and NH_2 groups of proteins.

Silver nitrate rapidly kills microbes, action persisting for long periods because of slow release of Ag⁺ ions from silver proteinate formed by interaction with tissue proteins. Tissues get stained black due to deposition of reduced silver. Silver nitrate touch is used for hypertrophied tonsillitis and aphthous ulcers. It is highly active against gonococci—1% solution is used for ophthalmia neonatorum.

Zinc salts They are astringent and mild antiseptics.
(i) Zinc sulfate is highly water soluble, 0.1–1% is used for eye wash and in eye/ear drops (Zinc-boric acid drops— in ZINCO-SULFA 0.1% eye drop). Applied to skin, it decreases perspiration.
(ii) Calamine and zinc oxide are insoluble. In addition to being mildly antiseptic, they are popular dermal protectives and adsorbants.

11. DYES

Gentian violet (crystal violet) This rosaniline dye is active against staphylococci, other gram-positive bacteria and fungi, but gram-negative organisms and mycobacteria are insensitive. Aqueous or alcoholic solution (0.5–1%) is used on furunculosis, bed sores, chronic ulcers, infected eczema, thrush, Vincent's angina, ringworm, etc. It has become unpopular due to deep staining.

Acriflavine and Proflavine These are orange-yellow acridine dyes active against gram-positive bacteria and gonococci. Their efficacy is not reduced by organic matter and is enhanced in alkaline medium. Solutions lose efficacy on exposure to light. They should be stored in amber coloured bottles. They are nonirritant and do not retard healing; therefore, particularly suitable for chronic ulcers and wounds. Bandage impregnated with acriflavine-vaseline is used for burn dressing;
ACRINOL 0.1% acriflavine cream.

12. FURAN DERIVATIVE

Nitrofurazone (Nitrofural) It is cidal to both gram-positive and gram-negative, aerobic and anaerobic bacteria, but activity is reduced in the presence of serum. It acts by inhibiting enzymes necessary for carbohydrate metabolism in bacteria. Nitrofurazone is highly efficacious in burns and for skin grafting. Its local toxicity is negligible, but sensitization occurs frequently.
FURACIN 0.2% cream, soluble ointment, powder.

Use and selection of antiseptics/disinfectants in dentistry

Purposes	Preferred agents
1. Cleaning and disinfection of working surfaces, instrument trays, operating light handles, etc.	Alcohols NH_4^+ antiseptics
2. Cold sterilization of certain instruments and storage of sterilized equipment.	Glutaraldehyde NH_4^+ antiseptics
3. Decontamination of the dentist's and assistant's hands.	Soaps, alcohol Chloroxylenol NH_4^+ antiseptics
4. Prevention and treatment of dental plaque and periodontal disease.	Chlorhexidine NH_4^+ antiseptics Triclosan
5. Treatment of ANUG, aphthous ulcers and other infective oral conditions.	Povidone iodine Chlorhexidine Hydrogen peroxide Boric acid Silver nitrate
6. Root canal therapy.	Hypochlorite Na⁺
7. Preoperative preparation of oral mucosa by reducing bacterial load so as to minimise local as well as distant infection.	Chlorhexidine Povidone iodine
8. As an ingredient of certain dentifrices.	Chlorhexidine NH_4^+ antiseptics, Triclosan

NH_4^+: Quaternary ammonium
ANUG: Acute necrotizing ulcerative gingivitis.

Antiseptics and disinfectants in dentistry

Antiseptics and disinfectants are used extensively in dentistry. The main purposes for which they are employed along with the commonly used agents are given in the box.

LOCALLY ACTING DRUGS

A variety of drugs applied topically to the skin or mucous membranes produce therapeutic effects localized to the site of application. They act primarily by virtue of their physical/mechanical/chemical or biological attributes. Some of these relevant to dentistry are:

Demulcents Demulcents are inert substances which sooth inflamed or denuded mucosa or skin by preventing contact with air/irritants in the surroundings. They are, in general, high molecular weight substances and are applied as thick colloidal/viscid solutions in water.

Glycyrrhiza, the sweet tasting root of liquorice, is used to sooth the throat. It is also a flavouring/sweetening agent. *Glycerine* is a clear, sweet, viscous liquid that is used as vehicle for gum/throat paints and as emollient on dry/cracked lips. Undiluted glycerine is dehydrating and produces a warm sensation in the mouth. It also has mild antiseptic property. *Methylcellulose, gum acacia* and *propylene glycol* are other demulcents.

Emollients Emollients are bland oily substances which sooth and soften skin. They form an occlusive film over the skin, preventing evaporation and drying, thus restoring elasticity of cracked and dry skin. *Olive oil, arachis oil, sesame oil, hard and soft paraffin, liquid paraffin, wool fat, bees wax* and *spermaceti* are the commonly employed emollients. They are also used as vehicles for topically applied medicaments and as ointment bases.

Adsorbants and protectives Adsorbants are finely powdered, inert and insoluble solids capable of binding to their surface (adsorbing) noxious and irritant substances. They are also called protectives because they afford physical protection to the skin or mucosa. Other protectives form a continuous, adherent and flexible occlusive coating on the skin. Demulcents and emollients also serve as protectives.

Magnesium stearate, zinc stearate, talc, calamine, zinc oxide, starch, collodion, Aloe vera gel, dimethicone and *sucralfate* are used as protectives.

Aloe vera gel can be used as protective on oral ulcers. Sucralfate is an aluminium salt of sulfated sucrose that has been employed as peptic ulcer protective. It is also formulated as a topical gel to be applied on aphthous ulcers; serves to facilitate healing by covering the denuded surface. Sucralfate gel can be applied on burns, bedsores, excoriated skin, diabetic ulcers as well.

Astringents Astringents are substances that precipitate proteins, but do not penetrate cells, thus affecting the superficial layer only. They are intended to toughen the surface making it mechanically stronger and decrease exudation.

Tannic acid obtained from nutgalls and *tannins* found in tea, catechu, betelnut are vegetable astringents. Glycerine of tannic acid (30%) is used as a paint on bleeding gums. Mouthwashes/gum paints containing tannic acid (1–5%) have been applied to strengthen swollen and spongy gums. Efficacy however, is dubious.

Heavy metal salts have astringent property. Zinc chloride, zinc sulfate, aluminium chloride, ferric chloride, strontium chloride are included in several mouthwashes and dental gels to afford symptomatic relief and promote healing of oral lesions, as well as to reduce dentine sensitivity and gum bleeding.

Alcohol is a potent astringent, but is unsuitable for use in mouth because it produces burning sensation. It is rubbed on skin to prevent bedsores. Other uses of astringents are in bleeding piles and as antiperspirant/deodorant.

Caustics These are corrosive chemicals that cause local tissue destruction and sloughing. Concentrated solutions of *silver nitrate, zinc chloride, phenol, trichloroacetic acid* and *podophyllum resin* are caustic and have been used to remove moles, warts, papillomas and necrotic material. They are to be applied carefully on the lesions only so as to avoid ulceration of normal mucosa/skin.

The use of caustics in dentistry is very limited; occasionally applied on aphthous ulcers. Silver nitrate painted on exposed necks of teeth can reduce dentine sensitivity, but is not favoured because of black staining. Carefully applied trichloracetic acid can reduce pain of pericoronitis.

Drugs and Aids with Specific Application in Dental Disorders

Most of the common problems affecting teeth, gums and oral mucosa are managed primarily by various professionally carried out dental procedures, often aided by some specific drugs/agents which have little application outside dentistry. Selected dental conditions and specific agents are briefly described in this chapter.

ANTIPLAQUE AND ANTIGINGIVITIS AGENTS

Plaque Dental plaque is a tenaciously adherent soft deposit on the tooth surface, composed mainly of bacterial aggregates embedded in a matrix of polysaccharides and glycoproteins, that resists removal by ordinary brushing and rinsing. Plaque is the primary causative factor in both dental caries and periodontal diseases.

Dental plaque tends to develop spontaneously unless teeth are cleaned thoroughly and regularly. The salivary glycoproteins get adsorbed on the tooth surface and form a thin membrane-like *pellicle* over it within minutes after brushing. With time, the glycoprotein molecules cross-link and form an insoluble coating over the tooth. The resident oral bacteria anchor on this coating and gradually develop into a plaque. The bacterial composition of the plaque is dynamic (changes with time). As the plaque grows and ages, gram negative and anaerobic bacteria predominate. Bacterial products like lactic acid, ammonia, hydrogen sulfide and other toxic metabolites generated in the plaque irritate gingival margins and produce inflammation (gingivitis). The gums become edematous, swollen and develop subgingival pockets. Mediators released by the inflammatory reaction perpetuate the condition producing *chronic gingivitis*. Enzymes like hyaluronidase and collagenase produced by the pathogens damage the connective tissue support to the teeth; gums become spongy and periodontal disease develops.

Periodontal disease can be prevented as well as treated by inhibiting plaque formation and removing it mechanically before it produces inflammatory changes. Regular brushing of teeth by correct technique is the most effective method of inhibiting plaque. However, this may not be practical in all individuals. Plaque on some parts of the teeth is left behind after brushing by most people. Periodic professional scaling of the teeth may be required in susceptible individuals. This may be supplemented by use of antiplaque agents.

Since bacteria are the major component of plaque, *antibacterial drugs* are the most important antiplaque agents.

Effective therapy of plaque requires that the drug applied as mouth rinse, gels or toothpaste remains at the site without being washed away to exert sustained antimicrobial effect. As such, the two most

Antiplaque Agents
1. Chlorhexidine
2. Quaternary ammonium antiseptics
Cetylpyridinium chloride
Benzalkonium chloride
3. Phenols
Triclosan
Listerine
4. Oxygenating agents
Hydrogen peroxide
Sodium perborate
5. Zinc citrate
6. Stannous fluoride
7. Sanguinarine

important properties of an antiplaque agent are *antimicrobial spectrum* covering the relevant microbes, and *'substantivity'* which refers to persistence of the substance on the surface of teeth/gums due to initial binding and subsequent slow release.

Chlorhexidine It exerts high antiplaque activity, largely because of its substantivity in the mouth, rather than due to any unique spectrum of activity on oral microbes, which nevertheless are inhibited. Chlorhexidine binds electrostatically to the acidic groups of the surface proteins affording the substantivity. Though it can also bind to hydroxyapatite of the teeth, this is less important for the antiplaque activity. The amount of chlorhexidine retained on the oral mucosa/tooth surface depends on the volume as well as concentration of the rinse solution. Lowering the pH (acidification) of rinse solution markedly decreases retention of chlorhexidine on oral mucosa. Calcium ions inhibit chlorhexidine binding as well as displace already bound drug. Accordingly, toothpastes containing calcium salts reduce substantivity of chlorhexidine if rinsing is done within 30-60 min of brushing with such a toothpaste. Optimum benefits appear to be obtained by twice daily mouth rinsing for 1-3 min with 10–15 ml of 0.12–0.2% chlorhexidine solution. Such rinsing achieves marked reduction in the number of oral bacteria (85% reduction in 24 hours and 95% reduction after 5 days). With long-term use, bacterial counts tend to increase again, but approximately 70% reduction is maintained till rinsing is continued. Resistance to chlorhexidine by bacteria is not clinically significant.

Twice daily oral rinse with 0.2% chlorhexidine consistently reduces dental plaque and prevents onset of gingivitis. Long-term regular use protects against periodontal diseases in susceptible individuals and improves gingival health. However, it should be employed only as adjuvant to other oral hygienic measures and professional care. The main disadvantage of chlorhexidine oral rinse is brown staining of teeth and tongue. Heavy tea/coffee consumption intensifies the staining effect. A lingering bitter aftertaste and occasional mucosal ulceration are the other side effects.

CHLODIN, CLOHEX, ORAHEX, REXIDIN, HEXIL 0.2% mouth wash.

Quaternary ammonium antiseptics such as *cetrimide, cetylpyridinium chloride* and *benzalkonium chloride* are other effective antiplaque agents, but are inferior to chlorhexidine. Being cationic, they also exhibit considerable substantivity, but their retention on oral mucosa after rinsing is less persistent than that of chlorhexidine. Since they are more active against gram positive bacteria than against gram negative, they are better suited for prophylaxis of plaque than for treatment of aged plaque/gingivitis. Adverse effects are burning sensation in the mouth, bad taste, discolouration of teeth and oral ulcers. They are alternative antiplaque agents.

Cetrimide: 0.1% in STOLIN gum paint.
Benzalkonium chloride: 0.02% in ZYTEE gel; 0.01% in DENTOGEL gel.

Phenolic antiseptics like *triclosan* and LISTERINE are another class of germicides that have antiplaque activity and are employed in mouth washes, tooth pastes/tooth powders and gum paints. Triclosan is active against both gram positive and negative bacteria. The binding of triclosan itself to gingival tissues and dental plaque is relatively weak (has lesser substantivity than chlorhexidine). However, certain polyvinyl copolymers and zinc salts included with it in toothpastes and dentifrices prolong its substantivity to nearly 12 hours. As such, these are common ingredients of proprietary toothpastes and toothpowders intended to prevent and treat plaque formation and gingivitis. The nonstaining, nonirritating nature of triclosan, and that it does not impart bad taste or odour favours its use.

Triclosan: 0.3% in REXIDIN PLUS gel; TRIGUARD, MAGDENT-KF, THERMOBEST tooth pastes.

Oxygenating agents *Hydrogen peroxide* (1.5-3%) and *sodium perborate* (3-6%) used as oral rinse release molecular oxygen and particularly inhibit anaerobic microbes. As such, they are often used in ANUG in which anaerobes play a major role. Though regular rinsing with H_2O_2 may reduce plaque scores, efficacy is limited due to its transient action. Frequent rinsing may cause oral ulceration.

Zinc citrate/chloride Included in some tooth pastes and gum paints, zinc citrate (2-4%) or zinc chloride (1%) have been found to decrease plaque formation, probably due to activity against gram positive cocci which predominate in early stage plaque. Its mild astringent action on gums may also help. However, it has utility only as an adjuvant antiplaque agent.

Zinc chloride: 0.09% in DENTOMAX gel, TRIGUARD mouth wash; 1.0% in STOLIN gum paint.

Stannous fluoride Daily oral rinsing with stannous fluoride (0.1–0.3%) significantly reduces dental plaque. Both tin and fluoride ions are mildly antibacterial, and appear to contribute to the antiplaque activity. Stannous ions reduce the adhesion of gram-positive bacteria to the tooth surface and alter their metabolism, while fluoride ions inhibit bacterial glycolytic enzymes and glucose transport. However, long term antiplaque efficacy of stannous fluoride is much inferior to chlorhexidine. Staining of teeth may discourage its use. Some toothpastes contain stannous fluoride.

Sanguinarine It is an alkaloid from the blood-root plant with high in vitro activity against many periodontal pathogens and high affinity for dental plaque. The antibacterial action has been ascribed to inhibition of sulfhydryl enzymes of the bacteria. Sanguinarine requires low pH (below 5.5) to transform into the active quaternary ammonium configuration. Accordingly, sanguinarine oral rinse solution and toothpaste are formulated at low pH. However, this low pH may not be maintained in the oral fluid for long.

Though some trials have shown modest short term antiplaque and gingivitis reducing action of sanguinarine, others have found marginal overall efficacy. One explanation offered for the discrepancy between high *in vitro* antibacterial activity and poor clinical efficacy is its tight binding to the oral tissues with minimal subsequent release to act on the pathogens. It produces few side effects, but the taste is found disagreeable by many individuals.

ANTIBIOTICS IN PERIODONTAL DISEASE

The causative role of bacterial pathogens in all forms of periodontal disease suggests that specific antibiotics should have major therapeutic value. However, in majority of cases antibiotics are unable to afford long-term benefit or modify course of the disease. The reason may be that the causative bacteria are derived from the resident oral flora which can, at best, be suppressed by antibiotics only temporarily. Recolonization occurs once the drug is stopped, or even during long-term use due to development of resistance. As such, antibiotics have only adjuvant role, and that too only in certain types of periodontal disease. Plaque removal supplemented by appropriate periodontal surgical procedures, followed by oral hygienic and plaque control measures are the primary therapeutic interventions.

Though many antibiotics like penicillins, erythromycin, vancomycin, etc. have been tried, none is now recommended. Only *tetracyclines* and *metronidazole* have established adjuvant therapeutic value in severe/rapidly progressing or refractory forms of periodontitis. In such cases, tetracycline (1 g/day)/doxycycline (200 mg/day) therapy favourably alters the subgingival flora by eliminating spirochetes and gram-negative bacilli with less effect on gram positive bacteria. Additional mechanisms of benefit of tetracyclines proposed are halting of periodontal connective tissue breakdown by inhibition of Ca^{2+} dependent collagenases and free radical scavenging (*see* p. 435).

Oral *metronidazole* when combined with conventional local measures affords clear-cut additional benefit in advanced periodontitis with pocket formation and connective tissue loss, as well as in juvenile periodontal disease. The benefit is ascribed to its specific activity against anaerobic pathogens. Metronidazole has also been used by local application to the gums in combined gel formulation with chlorhexidine. The dramatic therapeutic effect of metronidazole in ANUG is described on p. 412.

REXIDIN-M, ORAHEX-M, METROHEX: Metronidazole 1% + chlorhexidine 0.25% gel.

ANTICARIES DRUGS

Dental caries is localized loss of tooth tissue due to bacterial action resulting in formation of cavity in tooth. The cariogenic bacteria, mainly *Streptococcus mutans*, *Lactobacilli* and others present in dental plaque breakdown dietary sugars to produce lactic acid on the tooth surface. Sucrose is most easily converted into acids by plaque bacteria and is the most cariogenic sugar. The acid remaining in contact with tooth enamel for sufficient time destroys hydroxyapatite crystals causing demineralization and loss of tooth substance.

Anticaries drugs help only to prevent dental caries, since no drug can restore already formed caries cavity. The drugs are:
1. Fluoride makes tooth more resistant to caries and has weak antibacterial action.
2. Antiplaque agents (mainly chlorhexidine and triclosan) reduce the population of cariogenic bacteria.

Other preventive measures for caries are:
(a) Restriction of sugar containing food
(b) Frequent brushing of teeth
(c) Prevention of xerostomia by good hydration and other measures, since dryness of mouth promotes caries.

Fluoride

The carioprotective role of fluoride was realized when high incidence of dental caries among children in certain geographical areas was related to the low fluoride levels in the local water supply. Systematic epidemiological studies and the beneficial effect of fluoride supplementation on caries have confirmed this relationship.

Mechanism of action

The hardness of tooth enamel is primarily due to its hydroxyapatite crystals; but these are readily dissolved by the action of acid over a period of time. Fluoride radical being highly reactive exchanges with hydroxyl radical forming fluorapatite. The fluorapatite is a more compact, harder and less acid labile substance than hydroxyapatite. As a result teeth become less prone to caries.

Moreover, fluoride enhances remineralization of enamel that has been attacked by acid. Free fluoride ions released from fluorapatite by the action of acid raise the local fluoride ion concentration and facilitate remineralization of damaged enamel.

Fluoride is mildly antibacterial. However, plaque bacteria bind fluoride with high affinity, so that fluoride concentration in plaque is several times higher than its salivary concentration: significant intraplaque bacteriostasis may be exerted. Fluoride ions inhibit acid forming enzyme of plaque bacteria providing another mechanism of carioprotection.

Fluoride therapy

To reduce the incidence of dental caries, particularly among children, fluoride can either be administered systemically or applied locally to the teeth.

Systemic fluoride

Systemic administration of fluoride is indicated only in areas with established fluoride deficient water supply. It is considered that a concentration of 0.7–1.0 p.p.m. fluoride is optimum for health. Both low as well as high fluoride content of drinking water is harmful. Fluoride supplementation is needed only to the extent that deficit in drinking water is made good. This can be done in several ways.

1. *Fluoridation of water supply* This is practical in urban areas with common piped water supply to the masses, but not in communities drawing water from separate sources (like wells, ponds, etc). The amount of fluoride to be added must be determined by frequently measuring the content in natural water and adjusting it to achieve a final level of 0.5–1.0 p.p.m. The optimum level is lower in tropical countries and in summer because the volume of daily water consumption is higher. Failure to adjust the fluoride content to the optimum level can expose the population to the risk of fluorosis.

2. *Fluoridation of common salt* This is another way of supplementing fluoride intake. In Europe, table salt has been fortified with 200–350 mg/kg of salt in deficient areas.

3. *Sodium fluoride tablets/lozenges/drops* Infants and children in deficient areas where no mass fuoridation (of water or salt) is done, may be protected against high incidence of caries by administering sodium fluoride tablets (0.55 and 1.1 mg), lozenges (2.2 mg) or drops (0.55 and 1.1 mg per drop) daily till the age of 16 years. Lozenges and drops also provide local application to the teeth. However, to avoid risk of fluorosis, use of these supplements must be guided by measurement of fluoride in the local drinking water.

Topical fluoride

Fluoride is effective in enhancing resistance to caries even when applied directly to the tooth surface. Since there is little risk of systemic as well as dental fluorosis by topical fluoride, it can be employed without regard to the fluoride content of drinking water or food. The permeation and uptake of topically applied fluoride into the outer layers of tooth enamel depends on the fluoride salt used, its concentration and the time for which it remains in contact with the tooth surface. Low concentration of fluoride can be applied by the subject himself (daily), or fluoride may be applied at high concentration by the dentist once a while (generally every 6 months).

1. *Fluoride toothpastes* This is the easiest and most frequently employed method of fluoride application. Most of the commercially marketed toothpastes now contain fluoride. The commonest salt added is *sodium monofluorophosphate* (MFP) at a concentration of 0.76%. Other salts used earlier have some limitations. Calcium salts included as abrasives in certain dentifrices inactivate sodium fluoride, while stannous fluoride can stain teeth. Some other compounds and co-polymers

have been included in toothpastes to improve retention of fluoride on the tooth. Care must be exercised to avoid ingestion of fluoridated toothpastes (especially by infants and young children) to prevent systemic toxicity. Thorough rinsing of the mouth is advised after brushing with fluoridated toothpaste.

2. *Fluoride mouth rinse* Sodium fluoride (0.055%) or stannous fluoride (0.1%) solution have been used as daily mouth rinse by susceptible individuals to prevent caries. The rinse solution is held in the mouth for 1–3 min. and swished around. It is then discarded and food/drink are avoided for the next 30 min to minimise washing away of fluoride that is in contact with the teeth. Though stannous fluoride is more effective than sodium fluoride, it can stain the teeth.

3. *Professionally applied fluoride* Caries protective effect of fluoride can also be obtained by providing brief intensive exposure to the teeth by the dentist at relatively long intervals. High concentrations of sodium fluoride and stannous fluoride have disadvantages and are no longer used.

    (a) *Acidulated phosphate fluoride (APF)* This fluoride system suitable for application to the teeth by the dentist has been specifically developed to achieve high fluoride permeation into the enamel and thus afford prolonged caries protection. Formulated as a solution or gel, it contains 1.23% fluoride and 0.1M orthophosphoric acid; the pH is adjusted to about 3.0. This acidic medium enhances fluoride diffusion into the enamel while orthophosphoric acid prevents enamel dissolution. Applications are generally repeated at 6 month intervals and the optimal duration of each application is 4 min. Because of the high fluoride concentration, it can produce nausea, vomiting and acute fluoride toxicity if swallowed. Precautions taken to avoid ingestion are—use of disposable tray applicator, upright position during application, instruction not to swallow the solution/gel, constant suction of saliva during application and wiping the teeth and gums dry after the application.

    (b) *Fluoride varnishes* These are non-aqueous preparations which are not washed off by saliva and are retained on the teeth for longer period. A 2% sodium fluoride lacquer in resin base or a polyurethane varnish containing 0.7% fluoride is painted over the teeth or applied to the cavity. The efficacy of these preparations is variable and they are less popular.

Fluoride toxicity

Chronic fluoride toxicity The condition is called *fluorosis* and occurs due to excess fluoride content of drinking water, or occasionally due to industrial exposure or ingestion of fluoride supplements/toothpastes, etc. over a period of time. Low levels of excess fluoride (>2 p.p.m.) in drinking water produce dental fluorosis in children, while higher levels (>8 p.p.m.) produce skeletal fluorosis in children as well as in adults.

Dental fluorosis It occurs in children due to relatively low excess fluoride exposure from birth to 14 years of age when teeth are developing and erupting. There is hypomineralization of enamel while its protein content increases. White flecks appear on the teeth. Later there is brown discolouration, pitting, hypoplasia and deformity of dentition.

Skeletal fluorosis is a crippling disorder producing rigidity of spine, kyphosis, thoracic and pelvic deformity; limb bones become thick but brittle, spontaneous fractures occur and ligaments calcify.

Fluorosis can be prevented by changing the source of drinking water or defluoridation of water by adsorption on activated alumina/charcoal, or by avoiding other sources of excess fluoride, as the case may be. Once fluorosis has developed, it can only be halted but not reversed.

Acute fluoride toxicity Ingestion of gross overdose of fluoride causes acute toxicity; especially in children; $\geq$ 5 mg/kg sodium fluoride is considered lethal. The toxic manifestations are nausea, vomiting, abdominal pain, gastric erosion, muscle weakness, spasms and tetany due to hypocalcaemia, acidosis, hypotension and cardiac arrhythmia.

Treatment consists of gastric lavage, calcium gluconate infusion (i.v.) to precipitate excess fluoride and to counteract hypocalcaemia, correction of acidosis and fluid/electrolyte imbalance, and other supportive measures.

Antiplaque agents for caries

The crucial role of dental plaque in the causation of caries has already been described. As such, antiplaque measures including use of orally applied germicides can clearly reduce the incidence of caries and add to the protection afforded by fluoride. The antiplaque agents have been considered earlier (*see* p. 506). The two most commonly used agents are:

Chlorhexidine Used mainly as a mouth rinse or gel, it reduces the population of *Streptococcus mutans* and other cariogenic bacteria. The risk of caries occurrence is reduced, but regular use causes staining of teeth.

Triclosan Because it is nonirritant, tasteless and nonstaining, it is included along with other active ingredients in many anticaries and antiplaque toothpastes and gels.

DESENSITIZING AGENTS

Desensitizing agents are those which applied to the teeth mitigate *dentine sensitivity* (also called dentine hypersensitivity), i.e. shooting pain triggered from sensitive tooth by thermal (hot and cold), mechanical (touch, chewing, blast of air) or chemical (sour and sweet food) stimuli. Dentine may get exposed to external stimuli due to enamel damage caused by chewing hard substances, age related tooth attrition, erosion at the crown by acidic food, or due to denudation of root as a result of gingival recession of old age, faulty brushing, periodontal disease, etc. Dentine is traversed by numerous fine fluid-filled dentinal tubules. When these tubules are exposed, mechanical and thermal stimuli cause abnormal perturbations of the fluid in the tubules and activate the nerve endings at their inner mouth or in the pulp. Soluble chemicals (acids/sugars in food) diffuse through the tubules and act on the sensory nerves—all producing sharp pain.

The desensitizing agents aim to interrupt this pain-inducing process by either creating a plug in the dentinal tubules, or by sealing their mouth at the tooth surface, or by modulating the generation of painful nerve impulses. Most desensitizing agents are self-applied by the patient 1–3 times daily, while some are applied by the dentist once a while. Though it is desirable that the desensitizing agent produces rapid relief, in reality, most agents act slowly – need regular application over several days to weeks for optimum relief.

The commonly used desensitizing agents are:

1. *Potassium nitrate* At a concentration of 5%, it is the most frequently included active ingredient of desensitizing toothpastes. The paste is to be applied on the sensitive teeth and left in place for ~ 5 minutes before brushing lightly and then rinsing it off. This is repeated 2–3 times daily. Potassium nitrate is

believed to obliterate the dentinal tubules by precipitation. It may also dampen the pain inducing nerve impulses.

Potassium nitrate 5%: in MICRODENT-K, SENSODENT-KF, AQUADENT-K, EMOFORM, TRIGUARD, MAGDENT-KF, THERMOSEAL toothpastes.

2. *Strontium chloride* It is a salt of alkali-earth metal that precipitates proteins in the dentinal tubular fluid and thus tends to limit/obstruct the easy displacement of fluid by the pain inducing stimuli. Calcification of the bony component of tooth is believed to be hastened by strontium ions providing another mechanism of desensitizing action. Many desensitizing toothpastes and gels contain 10% strontium chloride.

Strontium chloride 10%: in SENOLIN gel; in SENSOFORM, FLODENT, STOLIN, THERMODENT toothpastes.

3. *Potassium oxalate* It diffuses into the dentinal tubules, reacts with ionic calcium in the fluid there to produce calcium oxalate which being insoluble deposits as crystals. These crystals hinder fluid movement in the tubules induced by external stimuli, thereby lessening the pain.

4. *Fluoride* Fluoride compounds like sodium monofluorophosphate, sodium/stannous fluoride are included in many multi-ingredient desensitizing toothpastes. These may react with calcium and produce calcium fluoride crystals in the dentinal tubules. Stannous fluoride may deposit fine layers of tin particles in the tubules creating partial obstruction. In the long-term fluoride ion accelerates secondary dentine formation which may reinforce the tubules and reduce dentine sensitivity. However, the contribution of the fluoride salt to the short-term desensitizing action of these toothpastes is uncertain.

Sodium monofluorophosphate 0.7%: in MICRODENT-KF, MAGDENT-KF, SENSODENT-KF, TRIGUARD, THERMO-BEST toothpastes.

Fluoride iontophoresis Quick diffusion of fluoride ions into the dentinal tubules is obtained by applying electrical current through 2% sodium fluoride solution. It causes rapid desensitization of sensitive tooth, but requires special equipment and expert application. It is therefore expensive and often needs several repetitions.

5. *Formaldehyde* At a concentration of 1-1.5%, it is a weak desensitizing agent. Its most prominent action is denaturation and precipitation of proteins. Such action within the dentinal tubules may underlie its desensitizing property. However, it has disagreeable taste and smell, and is not favoured now.

Formaldehyde 0.25%: in STOLIN toothpaste with strontium chloride 10% (any contribution of this low (0.25%) concentration to the desensitizing action is uncertain).

6. *Dentine bonding agents* Certain acrylic bonding agents (like hydroxy ethyl methacrylate), some resins, composites, varnishes, etc. have been developed which can be burnished on the exposed root or sensitive part of crown to seal off the external openings of the exposed dentinal tubules. After suitable preparation of the sensitive tooth and use of primers, the bonding agent is applied and allowed to dry. A long lasting bonding with dentine occurs rapidly—so that stimuli which induced pain earlier are blocked from reaching the pulpal nerve endings. The treatment may have to be repeated at suitable intervals.

OBTUNDANTS

Obtundants are almost obsolete drugs which when applied to the teeth and gums produce a kind of numbness that could dampen toothache due to cavity formation and other causes, as well as pain of excavation. They penetrate poorly and do not relieve deep seated or sharp pain. Obtundants act by:

1. *Stimulation followed by desensitization of nerve endings*: Clove oil, Thymol, Menthol, Camphor, Phenol.

Majority of these are essential oils or stearoptenes (volatile solids) which have a characteristic pleasant smell and which irritate sensory nerve-endings. They have counter-irritant property and produce relative numbness due to desensitization of sensory nerves lasting one to few hours. Clove oil has been used as a household remedy for tooth ache, but can stain the tooth.

2. *Astringent action*: Stannous chloride, Zinc chloride, Paraformaldehyde.

   They precipitate surface proteins and may interfere with the function of pain receptors. The pain-relieving action is mild.

Local anaesthetics have rendered obtundants redundant.

MUMMIFYING AGENTS

Mummification connotes hardening of dead tissue and rendering it resistant to microbial attack and degradation. Mummifying agents used earlier in dentistry are protoplasmic poisons having astringent and preservative properties. Before the availability of modern root canal filling materials, they were used during root canal therapy to kill the tissues in tooth pulp, make it hard and dry so that it does not get infected later. Commonly used mummifying agents were:

1. *Formaldehyde* or *Paraformaldehyde* (*Paraform*) mixed with zinc oxide or zinc sulfate + creosote and made into a paste for filling in the root canal. Paraformaldehyde releases formaldehyde slowly which destroys all living tissues in the pulp, hardens it and makes it resistant to future infection. A local anaesthetic like lidocaine or benzocaine was included by some, especially when formaldehyde was used, to prevent pain caused by the filling.

2. *Iodoform + Phenol* made into a paste with glycerine. To improve the smell of the paste, eugenol and cinnamon oil were generally added. The liberated iodine as well as phenol kept the pulp uninfected.

3. *Tannic acid* mixed with some of the above additives was also used.

Apart from the possibility of systemic toxic effects due to absorption of the mummifying agents, the major disadvantage was that the dead tooth pulp was retained, albeit in a dry and hard condition, but chances of future infection/inflammation could not be ruled out.

The modern technique of root canal therapy is to perform pulpectomy, achieve a tissue free dry canal and obliterate it by packing with *gutta-percha points* (a tough material made from latex), *silver points* or *epoxy resin canal sealant*. These are inert, impervious, nonirritant materials which preclude risk of reinfection and do not cause any complication.

BLEACHNG AGENTS

These are agents used to remove stains from teeth or to improve their whiteness. Most of the bleaching agents act by oxidizing the stain/yellowish coating on the enamel, but few reducing agents also have stain removing action.

1. *Oxygen releasing agents* They release oxygen which reacts with the organic pigment to decolourise it and loosen it from tooth surface. It is then washed off to expose the white enamel.

Hydrogen peroxide is the primary oxygenating agent. While the dilute (3%) mouth wash is occasionally used as an antiseptic/antiplaque agent (*see* p. 499), the concentrated solution (20–30%) in water (called *perhydrol*) or ether (named *pyrozone*) may be applied carefully to the stained teeth and wiped off for cosmetic whitening. Burning sensation, erythema, inflammation and sloughing may occur if it comes in contact with gingival/oral mucosa.

Carbamide peroxide is an equimolar complex of hydrogen peroxide with urea which acts as a carrier and releases hydrogen peroxide on reacting with water. Some tooth whiteners contain 10% carbamide peroxide.

Sodium peroxide is water soluble, releases oxygen in solution and may be used for bleaching teeth. *Sodium perborate* is insoluble but slowly releases oxygen on coming in contact with water. It is present in some tooth powders.

2. *Chlorine releasing agent* Bleaching powder (chlorinated lime) slowly releases chlorine which acts as an oxidizing agent and decolourises many dyes. Addition of acetic acid to bleaching powder immediately before application accelerates its decomposition and hastens stain removal.

Excessive use of any oxidizing bleaching agent can damage the tooth enamel and even affect dentine. Tooth sensitivity and weakening of crown may result. The oral microbial flora may also be disturbed.

3. *Reducing agent* Sodium thiosulfate is a reducing agent which is used for removing certain stains, e.g. iodine stain. Sequential application of an oxidizing agent followed by a reducing agent may be needed for silver stain.

4. *Silica* It is a nonabrasive adsorbent which is included in some whitening toothpastes and tooth powders.

Use of *laser* for whitening the teeth is increasing.

DISCLOSING AGENTS

Dyes used to facilitate clear visualization of dental plaque are called *disclosing agents*. By staining the bacterial plaque deeply, they increase the contrast between plaque and the gums. Dyes selected for the purpose are those which:
- have higher affinity for the bacterial plaque than for oral mucosa/teeth.
- are not bad tasting, irritating or toxic.
- diffuse uniformly and stain all supragingival plaque.
- are easily washed off by rinsing after plaque removal.

Dyes used as disclosing agent are:
1. *Erythrosine* It is the most commonly used disclosing agent. This red dye is bland tasting, nontoxic and stains the plaque deeply, but the gums and oral mucosa also take light stain. The residual stain goes after repeated rinsing.
2. *Fluorescein* It is a yellow dye which fluoresces under ultraviolet light; is selectively taken up by the bacterial plaque, but not by oral soft tissue. As such, after rinsing with an aqueous solution of fluorescein, the plaque can be demarcated clearly, but needs ultraviolet light. However, it is nonirritating and nontoxic.
3. *Two-tone dye* It is used to differentiate the older and thicker part of plaque from the thinner, newer plaque. A mixture of red and green dye is used; the mature plaque appears blue while the fresh plaque appears red.

The disclosing agents may be applied either by rinsing the mouth with a dilute solution of the dye, or it may be painted on the teeth with a brush/cotton swab. If the dye is available in tablet form, it may be chewed, swished around in the mouth followed by rinsing. The plaque is then removed by scaling or other techniques.

DENTIFRICES

These are powders, pastes, gels or creams used as hygiene aids for routine dental care during brushing. Dentifrices facilitate cleaning of teeth and gums, improve their appearance and control bad breath. They may be medicated to impart specific preventive and therapeutic properties. The usual ingredients present in dentifrices may be grouped into the following.
1. *Abrasives* Finely powdered inert and poorly soluble solids having smooth particles are used as dental abrasives, e.g. *prepared chalk, silicates, calcium phosphate,*

magnesium carbonate, aluminium oxide, magnesium oxide. Silica used in gel toothpastes has mild abrasive action. *Sodium bicarbonate* is another mild abrasive which on reacting with slightly acidic saliva releases some CO_2 that facilitates foaming during brushing. It also reduces oral bacteria that thrive in the acidic medium. Coarse particles like charcoal, pumice powder should not be used routinely because they may scratch and damage the enamel. Limited use may however be made carefully for strong abrasive action. Generally toothpastes are less abrasive than tooth powders.

2. *Detergents* These are surface acting agents (surfactants) which reduce surface tension between oil and water and produce foam on brushing. They emulsify fats and help in suspending fine particles. This action promotes cleaning of teeth and gums and removal of food particles sticking to the teeth. The foam also provides lubrication during brushing. *Sodium lauryl sulfate* has been a popular detergent in toothpastes, because it promotes penetration of fluoride into dentine, can loosen plaque and has antibacterial action. However, it can irritate oral mucosa; regular use can produce sore mouth. It is being replaced by nonirritating agents like *lauryl sarcosinate*. Other detergents present in dentifrices are *dioctyl sodium sulfosuccinate, ammonium lauryl sulfate, dodecyl benzene sulfonate*, etc.

3. *Humectants and binding agents* Humectants like *glycerine (glycerol), sorbitol* and *propylene glycol* retain moisture and prevent drying of the toothpaste. Glycerine (~10%) is most commonly included because it is sweet, nongreasy and adds thickness, softness and smoothness to the paste. Binding agents like *methyl cellulose, bentonite, mucilage of tragacanth* swell in the presence of water and hold together the solid and liquid phases of the paste. They also give thick consistency to the paste.

4. *Sweetening agents* Saccharine is an artificial sweetener, about 500 times more sweet than sugar. Small amount is added to the dentifrices to mask their blandness, improve their taste and make them acceptable even to children. It is noncariogenic as are other less commonly used sweeteners like *sorbitol* and *glycerol*.

5. *Flavouring agents* Essential (volatile) oils with a characteristic pleasant aroma are added to dentifrices to improve their flavour and acceptability. They also counteract halitosis (bad breath). *Menthol* is very commonly used, because it produces a cooling sensation in the mouth and imparts a feeling of freshness. Other flavouring agents are *thymol, eugenol, camphor, clove oil*.

6. *Colouring agents* Many dentifrices are white, but some are brightly coloured blue, green or cherry red to make them look attractive by the addition of *methylene blue, chlorophyll* and *liquor rubri* or other permitted colours.

7. *Medicated dentifrices* Certain medications are added to the toothpastes and tooth powders so as to empower them with prophylactic/therapeutic activity against specific dental conditions. These are:
Fluoride: Sodium monofluorophosphate or sodium fluoride for caries prevention. Most toothpastes contain a fluoride.
Antiseptics: Chlorhexidine, triclosan or benzalkonium chloride for prevention and treatment of dental plaque. A copolymer is often included with triclosan to prolong its substantivity.
Desensitizing agents: Potassium nitrate or strontium chloride are mostly added to treat dentine sensitivity.
Bleaching agents: Carbamide peroxide is the commonest bleaching agent added to stain-removing dentifrices.

Some dentifrices contain more than one medicament and have broader spectrum of utility.

Management of Medical Emergencies in Dental Office
(Emergency Drug Tray)

Dental surgeons should realise that medical emergencies can and do develop occasionally in their patients while they are in the dentist's office. Medical emergencies are most likely to occur during and after local anaesthesia, especially while performing tooth extraction or an endodontic procedure. Dentists and their staff should be prepared to provide first hand treatment promptly and efficiently; and should have expert medical backup, which may be summoned at short notice. Many emergencies can be prevented by eliciting thorough medical history of the patient, and if needed, prior consultation with the patient's treating physician.

Surveys have shown that 'syncope' or fainting is the most common emergency faced by the dentists. Other emergencies that have usually been encountered in the dentist's office are listed in the box.

Medical emergencies in dentist's office

- Syncope; postural hypotension
- Acute allergic reactions/anaphylaxis
- Angina pectoris/myocardial infarction (MI)
- Cardiac arrest/ventricular fibrillation (VF)
- Severe asthmatic attack/bronchoconstriction
- Hypoglycaemia
- Seizures/status epilepticus

The most important aspect of tiding over medical emergencies is to prevent and correct deficient oxygenation of the brain and heart. Dentists should have received training to provide basic life support directed to maintaining the patient's vital functions and to deal with the immediate crisis. The ABCs of cardiopulmonary resuscitation (CPR) are assessment and treatment, if needed, of:
A. Airway (maintain patency)
B. Breathing (respiratory movements)
C. Circulation (heart beat and blood pressure) in that order.

Use of any emergency drugs is considered only after attending to these ABCs. The steps of basic life support by CPR are summarized in the box.

Cardiopulmonary Resuscitation

- Lay the patient flat on the dental chair or on the floor and raise the foot end to facilitate venous return of blood to the heart. Turn the head to one side and lift the chin to prevent falling of tongue in the throat. Start suction and suck out any secretion from the throat to ensure a clear airway.
- If the patient is not breathing, provide artificial ventilation, preferably using a tight-fitting face mask and an Ambu bag connected to oxygen cylinder.
- If no pulse is felt (carotid pulse is most reliable), begin external cardiac massage by pressing on the lower sternum with one palm kept over the other at a rate of 60–70 times per minute. Continue this till the heart starts beating and a good volume pulse returns.
- Medical help should be summoned and the patient shifted to a hospital for expert care.

Emergency drug tray/kit

Since medical emergencies occur unpredictably, and may sometimes rapidly evolve into a life-threatening situation, the dental surgeon and his team should be prepared to act swiftly and at all times. All medicines and equipment needed to deal with the emergency should be available in ready-to-use condition at an easily accessible location in the office, so that no time is wasted in searching for them. An *emergency drug tray or kit* containing a limited number of medicines sufficient for tackling common emergencies should be maintained. The dentist should have knowledge about the actions, doses, method of administration, type of formulation, indications and contraindications, etc. of these emergency medicines. There is no point in stocking an array of drugs in the emergency tray with which the dentist is not familiar, or is not trained to use. The emergency drugs should be periodically checked. A log book of the drugs in the tray should be kept and reviewed every month. Soon to expire drugs and those used up should be replaced.

A core (basic) emergency medicine list, along with their type of preparations, dose, route of administration and indications is presented in Table 37.1. The marketed preparations and leading trade names of these medicines are listed below.

Preparations

1. **Adrenaline:** ADRENALINE 1 mg/ml inj, ADRENA (as bitartrate) 2 mg/2 ml inj.
2. **Chlorpheniramine:** PIRITON, CADISTIN 4 mg tab
3. **Cetirizine:** CETZINE, ALERID 10 mg tab

Table 37.1: Core (basic) emergency drug tray for dental office

Drug		Dose and Route	Indication
1. Adrenaline (Epinephrine)	1 mg/ml inj	0.3–0.5 ml i.m.	Anaphylactic shock, Bronchospasm, Angioedema of larynx
2. Chlorpheniramine or Cetirizine	4 mg tab 10 mg tab	4 mg oral 10 mg oral	Allergic reaction, urticaria, itching, flushing, lip swelling
3. Pheniramine or Promethazine	22.5 mg/ml inj 25 mg/ml inj	22.5–45 mg i.m./i.v. 25–50 mg i.m./i.v.	Allergic reaction (severe), Anaphylaxis
4. Hydrocortisone sod. succinate	100 mg/ml inj	100–200 mg i.v.	Anaphylaxis, severe allergic reaction
5. Glyceryl trinitrate (Nitroglycerine)	0.5 mg subling. tab or 0.4 mg/puff spray	0.5–1.0 mg subling. 0.4–0.8 mg oral spray	Angina pectoris, M.I.
6. Aspirin	75 mg, 300 mg dis. tab	300 mg oral	M.I.
7. Oxygen in steel cylinder		7–10 L/min inhalation	M.I., severe asthma, anaphylaxis, along with CPR in cardiac arrest
8. Salbutamol	100 µg/puff inhaler	2 puff by inhalation	Asthma, bronchospasm
9. Sugar as cubes/crystals or Dextrose powder		20–30 g in 1 glass water oral 20–50% injectable solution 50–100 ml i.v.	Hypoglycemia
10. Lorazepam or Diazepam	4 mg/ml inj 10 mg/ml inj	4 mg i.v. 10 mg i.v.	Status epilepticus
11. Morphine	10 mg/ml inj	3 mg i.v., 5 mg i.m.	M.I.

4. **Pheniramine:** AVIL 22.5 mg/ml inj 2 ml amp., 10 ml vial
5. **Promethazine:** PHENERGAN 25 mg/ml inj
6. **Hydrocortisone sod. succinate:** EFCORLIN SOLUBLE 100 mg inj., LYCORTIN-S 100 mg (3 ml), 200 mg (5 ml) inj.
7. **Glyceryl trinitrate (Nitroglycerine):** ANGISED 0.5 mg subling. tab, GTN-SPRAY 0.4 mg/puff oral spray.
8. **Aspirin:** ASPIRIN DISPERSIBLE 75 mg tab (4 tabs)
9. **Salbutamol:** ASTHALIN, DERIHALER 100 µg/puff inhaler
10. **Lorazepam:** LORA 2 mg/ml, 2 ml inj.
11. **Diazepam:** CALMPOSE, PLACIDOX 10 mg/2 ml inj.
12. **Morphine sulfate:** MORPHINE SULPHATE 10 mg/ml inj.

The first hand management of some of the likely medical emergencies in dental office is outlined below.

1. Syncope (fainting)

Fainting occurs due to transient insufficiency of blood supply to the brain resulting in loss of consciousness. The commonest cause is a *vaso-vagal attack*, i.e. sudden reflex vagal stimulation producing marked bradycardia and fall in blood pressure. Severe pain or emotional stress is the usual trigger. Syncope is more likely to occur in a patient who is unduly anxious before the dental procedure. The symptoms and signs of syncope are—the patient feels sick and a sense of fainting, dizziness, nausea, looks pale, cold sweat breaks out, may yawn, pulse is weak and slow, muscles twitch, blood pressure falls and pupils may dilate.

Management consists of laying the patient flat on the dental chair or on the ground. The foot end should be raised a little to improve blood flow to the brain, provided there is no breathlessness. Any tight clothing around the neck should be loosened.

Mostly, no medication is needed and the patient regains consciousness soon. The traditional method of making the patient smell ammonia or putting a drop of alcohol into the nose is outmoded. The patient should then be reassured and given a cup of tea or coffee with sugar, or a fruit juice.

Postural hypotension Fainting could also be due to orthostatic hypotension. In the dental office, it occurs mostly as a consequence of getting up abruptly from a reclining position on the dental chair after a procedure. Elderly patients, diabetics, those who have bled, those receiving an α adrenergic blocking drug or other antihypertensive medication are especially prone to develop postural hypotension. In such predisposed subjects, fainting can be avoided by bringing them to upright posture gradually, asking them to keep sitting for a couple of minutes and then getting up slowly. The symptoms and management of postural hypotension are the same as that of vasovagal attack.

2. Acute allergic reaction

An immediate or Type-1 allergic reaction (*see* p. 71) can develop to any medication, including the local anaesthetic administered by the dentist, or to a dental material, or even to the latex gloves of the dentist. The reaction may manifest as itching, flushing, feeling of warmth, urticaria, swelling of lips/face due to angioedema which becomes life-threatening if larynx gets involved, bronchoconstriction and even anaphylactic shock. The reaction may sometimes develop within minutes. More rapidly developing reaction tends to be more severe. As a routine preventive measure, all dental patients must be asked about any history of allergy or sensitivity to a medication. Medicines to which the patient has reacted in the past should not be administered.

Atopic patients are at a higher risk of developing a reaction or anaphylaxis.

The treatment of allergic reactions is described on p. 72 and 118. Briefly:
- Mild nonlife-threatening reactions like urticaria, rashes, swelling only of lips,

may be treated with an oral antihistaminic like chlorpheniramine 4 mg or cetirizine 10 mg.
- For a rapidly developing reaction, a parenteral antihistaminic like pheniramine 20–50 mg or promethazine 25–50 mg may be injected i.m. When bronchoconstriction is prominent, it can be counteracted by salbutamol inhalation through a spacer device.
- For bronchospasm, laryngeal edema and anaphylaxis, only adrenaline 0.5 mg i.m repeated as required, is life saving. A parenteral antihistaminic and i.v. hydrocortisone (100–200 mg) have adjuvant value. Simultaneously started oxygen inhalation is very important. After overcoming the crisis, urgent arrangement should be made to shift the patient to a hospital for further management.

3. Angina pectoris and myocardial infarction (MI)

Angina is due to ischaemic heart disease and is characterized by sudden onset substernal pain which may radiate to left shoulder and arm; occasionally also to the lower jaw and teeth. In the dental office, angina may be precipitated by the anxiety attending the dental surgery. The patient may have had attacks of angina in the past and will recognise the symptoms himself. Angina pectoris and antianginal drugs are described in chapter 11.

An anginal attack is treated by administering 0.5 mg glyceryl trinitrate (GTN) tablet sublingually, or one/two puffs of GTN oral spray (0.4 mg/puff) in the mouth and then closing the mouth. A patient who had anginal attacks in the past may be carrying his medication, but it must be kept in the emergency drug tray of the dental office. Tablets of GTN have a short shelf life of 2–3 months after opening the container, because GTN is a volatile liquid which evaporates away slowly from the tablets. Care should be taken to ensure that the tablets are active when administered. It is preferable to use the spray formulation which has a predictable shelf life and acts faster than the sublingual tablets. The patient should be put in the sitting posture to reduce cardiac preload by favouring pooling of blood in the legs. Anxiety should be allayed by reassuring the patient. Majority of angina attacks subside with one dose of GTN; those not relieved can be given another dose after 10 min.

Myocardial infarction (MI) The pain of MI is similar to that of angina, but generally more severe, more prolonged, and is not fully relieved even by 2 doses of GTN. It is not advisable to administer more than 2–3 doses of GTN, because this may cause hypotension and accentuate myocardial ischaemia. Other features which distinguish MI from angina are:
- MI is often accompanied by a sinking sensation.
- Skin is often pale and clammy in MI.
- Breathlessness is common in MI.
- Nausea and vomiting may occur in MI.

The drug therapy of MI is outlined on p. 203–04, but what a dentist could do is:

Put the patient in a comfortable position (not necessarily lying flat) and call for medical assistance. Administer oxygen through a face mask. If breathing is inadequate, ventilatory support should be provided as mentioned above under CPR. One dispersible 300 mg tablet, or four 75 mg tablets of aspirin should be put in a cup of water and given to drink immediately. The purpose is to prevent progression of the thrombus by the antiplatelet aggregatory action of aspirin. If possible, 3 mg morphine should be injected i.v. slowly to relieve pain and anxiety, keeping watch on respiration and BP. Older patients are more susceptible to the respiratory depressant and hypotensive actions of morphine. The i.m. route for morphine is not suitable in this setting, because absorption of morphine from the i.m. site may be delayed due to hypotension and reflex vasoconstriction. Further measures are not within the perview or competence of a dental surgeon.

4. Cardiac arrest and ventricular fibrillation (VF)

In the dental office, cardiac arrest or VF (pulseless non-synchronized ventricular contractions) are mostly a consequence of acute MI. However, anaphylactic reaction, complete heart block or adrenal crisis may also be causative. When cardiac arrest or VF occurs, the patient collapses and becomes unconscious, pulse cannot be felt, heart beat cannot be felt or heard. Breathing stops and the skin looks pale or gray (if cyanosis develops); pupils dilate a little later.

Cardiac arrest or VF is a medical catastrophe. Immediate institution of CPR, as described above, is critical. Time is the essence of management because brain suffers irreversible damage if its blood supply is cutoff for more than 3 minutes. Medical help should be sought without wasting any time, and CPR is continued till spontaneous heart beat is restored or till expert help arrives.

Though in case of cardiac asystole, i.v. injection of adrenaline can help in restoring heart beat, it is not advisable in the dental office setting. Firstly, in case of MI, adrenaline can worsen cardiac ischaemia by increasing cardiac oxygen demand, and is contraindicated. Secondly, it may not be possible for the dentist to differentiate cardiac asystole from VF, and VF is perpetuated by adrenaline. The only measure which can terminate VF and restore heart beat is application of electric shock delivered from a defibrillator through padded thoracic electrodes. But dentists are not trained to use defibrillator. Amiodarone, an antiarrhythmic drug, injected i.v. has been used to prevent recurrences of VF; but this is not in the purview of a dentist.

5. Bronchospasm / asthmatic attack

The treatment of mild to severe asthmatic attack, as well as that of status asthmaticus is outlined on p. 321. Asthmatic patients may develop an attack of acute asthma during their visit to the dental office. The stress of the dental procedure may precipitate an attack. In both asthmatic and non-asthmatic subjects bronchoconstriction may occur as a consequence of allergic reaction.

Most asthmatic subjects carry their own bronchodilator inhaler, and should use it when an attack occurs. Otherwise, salbutamol 100 µg/puff metered dose inhaler (MDI) kept in the dentist's emergency drug tray should be made available. Inhalation of 2 puffs, repeated if necessary after 10 minutes, usually suppresses the attack. If the patient is unable to use the MDI correctly, further puffs are given through a large volume spacer device. If the bronchoconstriction is still not reversed, nebulized salbutamol + ipratropium bromide solution should be administered through an oxygen mask. However, nebulizers are not generally kept in the dental office. In that case the patient should be given oxygen inhalation and sent to a hospital urgently. For life-threatening asthma, 0.5 mg adrenaline can be injected i.m., along with hydrocortisone 100 mg i.v. (as for anaphylaxis) and medical help is summoned.

6. Hypoglycaemia

Hypoglycaemia is highly unlikely to develop in a nondiabetic patient coming to a dental clinic for treatment. Only when a diabetic who has taken insulin injection or other hypoglycaemic medication and has missed the meal before coming for dental treatment is likely to suffer hypoglycaemia. The symptoms, signs and treatment of hypoglycaemia are described on p. 236. Most diabetics recognise the symptoms of hypoglycaemia and are instructed to carry glucose, sugar or some sweets along with them to mitigate unanticipated hypoglycaemia. However, the behaviour and mentation of the patient may be grossly affected by hypoglycaemia. The dentist should be able to recognise hypoglycaemia and be prepared to correct it by administering 4–6 teaspoons of sugar/glucose dissolved in a glass of water. A packet of crystalline sugar or sugar cubes or dextrose powder should be kept in the emergency drug tray. Improvement is seen within 15–30 min. Only when the patient is unconscious, or is unable to drink sugar solution, should i.v. glucose administration be considered.

7. Seizures, status epilepticus

Occurrence of seizure in an epileptic is unpredictable. Therefore, an attack is possible in the dental office or even during a dental procedure. Generally, epileptics do not voluntarily inform the dentist about it, unless specifically asked for. The dentists should routinely elicit history of all past and present illnesses before undertaking any treatment. The precaution dentists should take in an epileptic patient and the management of seizures as well as status epilepticus occurring in their office is described on p. 160–61.

Drug Interactions

Drug interaction refers to modification of response to one drug by another when they are administered simultaneously or in quick succession. The modification is mostly quantitative, i.e. the response is either increased or decreased in intensity, but sometimes it is qualitative, i.e. an abnormal or a different type of response is produced. The possibility of drug interaction arises whenever a patient concurrently receives more than one drug, and the chances increase with the number of drugs taken.

Many medical/dental conditions are treated with a combination of drugs. The components of the combination are so selected that they complement each other's action, e.g. an antibiotic is used along with an analgesic to treat a painful infective condition; adrenaline is added to lidocaine for dental anaesthesia; mixed aerobic-anaerobic bacterial infections, including many orodental infections, are treated with a combination of antimicrobials (e.g. metronidazole + amoxicillin). More commonly, multiple drugs are used to treat a patient who is suffering from two or more diseases at the same time (e.g. diabetes and hypertension). The chances of unintended or adverse drug interactions are greater in this later situation because an assortment of different drugs may be administered to a patient depending on his/her diseases/symptoms.

Several drug interactions are desirable and deliberately employed in therapeutics, e.g. the synergistic action of ACE inhibitors + diuretics to treat hypertension, or sulfamethoxazole + trimethoprim to treat bacterial infection, or furosemide + amiloride to prevent hypokalaemia. These are well-recognized interactions and do not pose any undue risk to the patient. The focus of attention in this chapter are drug interactions which may interfere with the therapeutic outcome, or be responsible for adverse effects, or may even be fatal (bleeding due to excessive anticoagulant action).

The severity of drug interactions in most cases is highly unpredictable. Because the dentist prescribes and administers certain drugs, he/she must know which drugs are not to be prescribed concurrently. More importantly, a large section of dental patients are elderly, who are especially likely to be receiving one or several drugs for

Regular medication drugs
(Likely to be involved in drug interactions)

1. Antidiabetics
2. Antihypertensives
3. Antianginal drugs
4. Antiarthritic drugs
5. Antiepileptic drugs
6. Antiparkinsonian drugs
7. Oral contraceptives
8. Anticoagulants
9. Antiasthmatics
10. Psychopharmacological agents
11. Antipeptic ulcer drugs
12. Corticosteroids
13. Antitubercular drugs
14. Anti-HIV drugs

their chronic medical conditions like hypertension, diabetes, arthritis, etc. (*see* box for regular medication drug classes employed commonly). The dentist may prescribe certain drugs which may interact with those already being taken by the patient and result in adverse consequences. It is, therefore, imperative for the dentist to elicit a detailed medical history of the patient and record all the medication that he/she is currently taking. The list of potential adverse drug interactions is already quite long and constantly growing. It is practically impossible for anyone to know/remember all possible drug interactions. Fortunately, the clinically important and common drug interactions that may be encountered in dental practice are relatively few. These are listed in Table 38.1. More exhaustive compilations and documentation are available in specialized books, monographs, review articles and computer database on the subject, but these also need constant updating.

Certain types of drugs (*see* box) can be identified that are most likely to be involved in clinically important drug interactions. The dentist may take special care and pay attention to the possibility of drug interactions when the patient is receiving one or more of such medications or when he/she intends to prescribe any of such drugs. Consultation with the physician treating the medical condition is advised.

Types of drugs most likely to be involved in clinically important drug interactions

- Drugs with narrow safety margin, e.g. aminoglycoside antibiotics, digoxin, lithium
- Drugs affecting closely regulated body functions, e.g. antihypertensives, antidiabetics, anticoagulants
- Highly plasma protein bound drugs like NSAIDs, oral anticoagulants, sulfonylureas
- Drugs metabolized by saturation kinetics, e.g. phenytoin, theophylline

MECHANISMS OF DRUG INTERACTIONS

Drug interactions can be broadly divided into *pharmacokinetic* and *pharmacodynamic* interactions. In certain cases, however, the mechanisms are complex and may not be well understood. Few interactions take place even outside the body when drug solutions are mixed before administration.

Pharmacokinetic interactions

These interactions alter the concentration of the object drug at its site of action (and consequently the intensity of response) by affecting its absorption, distribution, metabolism or excretion.

Pharmacokinetic interactions

- Alteration of absorption or first-pass metabolism
- Displacement of plasma protein bound drug
- Alteration of drug binding to tissues affecting volume of distribution and clearance
- Inhibition/induction of metabolism
- Alteration of excretion

Absorption Absorption of an orally administered drug can be affected by other concurrently ingested drugs. This is mostly due to formation of insoluble and poorly absorbed complexes in the gut lumen, as occurs between tetracyclines and calcium/iron salts, antacids or sucralfate. Phenytoin absorption is decreased by sucralfate due to binding in the g.i. lumen. Such interactions can be minimized by administering the two drugs with a gap of 2–3 hours so that they do not come in contact with each other in the g.i.t. Ketoconazole absorption is decreased by H_2 blockers and proton pump inhibitors, because gastric acidity needed for dissolution and absorption of ketoconazole is reduced by these drugs. Antibiotics like ampicillin, tetracyclines, cotrimoxazole markedly reduce gut flora that normally deconjugates oral contraceptive steroids secreted in the bile as glucuronides and permits their enterohepatic circulation. Several instances of contraceptive failure have been reported with concurrent use of these antibiotics due to lowering of the contraceptive blood levels. Alteration of

Table 38.1: Clinically important drug interactions in dentistry

Precipitant drug*	Object drug£	Likely interaction and comments
1. Ampicillin, Amoxicillin	Oral contraceptives	Interruption of enterohepatic circulation of the estrogen → failure of contraception; Advise alternative contraception
	Warfarin	Inhibition of gut flora → decreased vit K production in gut → risk of bleeding; Monitor INR and reduce warfarin dose if needed.
2. Probenecid	Penicillin, Ampicillin, Cephalosporins	Inhibition of tubular secretion → prolongation of antibiotic action; Desirable interaction utilized for single dose therapy.
3. Allopurinol	Ampicillin	Increased incidence of rashes; Avoid concurrent use.
4. Carbenicillin, Ticarcillin	Aspirin and other antiplatelet drugs	Perturbation of surface receptors on platelets → additive platelet inhibition → risk of bleeding; Avoid concurrent use
5. Ceftriaxone, Cefoperazone	Warfarin	Additive hypoprothrombinaemia → bleeding; Monitor INR and reduce dose of warfarin.
6. Sulfonamides, Cotrimoxazole	Phenytoin	Displacement$ + inhibition of metabolism → phenytoin toxicity; Avoid concurrent use
	Warfarin	Displacement + inhibition of metabolism + decreased production of vit K in gut → risk of bleeding; Monitor INR and reduce dose of warfarin
	Sulfonylureas	Displacement + inhibition of metabolism → hypoglycaemia; Avoid concurrent use
7. Metronidazole, Tinidazole, Cefoperazone	Alcohol	Disulfiram-like or bizarre reactions; warn the patient not to drink alcohol
8. Metronidazole, Tinidazole	Lithium salts	Decreased excretion → Li$^+$ toxicity; Monitor Li$^+$ level and reduce lithium dose
	Warfarin	Inhibition of metabolism → risk of bleeding; Avoid concurrent use
9. Ciprofloxacin, Norfloxacin, Pefloxacin	Theophylline, Warfarin	Inhibition of metabolism → toxicity of object drug; Monitor and reduce dose of object drug
10. Erythromycin, Clarithromycin, Ketoconazole, Itraconazole, Fluconazole, HIV-protease inhibitors	Phenytoin, Carbamazepine, Warfarin, Sulfonylureas, Diazepam, Theophylline, Cyclosporine, HIV protease inhibitors, Statins	Inhibition of metabolism by CYP3A4 → toxicity of object drug; Avoid concurrent use or readjust dose of object drug Inhibition of metabolism, higher risk of myopathy; Avoid concurrent use.
11. Tetracyclines	Oral contraceptives	Interruption of enterohepatic circulation of the estrogen → failure of contraception; Advise alternative contraception
	Lithium salts	Rise in plasma Li$^+$ level due to decreased excretion; Avoid use of tetracycline or monitor and reduce dose of lithium

Contd...

* Precipitant drug is the drug, which alters action/pharmacokinetics of the other drug
£ Object drug is the drug whose action/pharmacokinetics is altered
$ Displacement of plasma protein bound drug

Contd..

Precipitant drug*	Object drug	Likely interaction and comments
12. Iron salts Calcium salts Antacids Sucralfate	Tetracyclines Fluoroquinolones	Decreased absorption due to formation of complexes in g.i.t. → failure of antibiotic therapy; stager drug administration by 2–3 hours
13. Furosemide	Minocycline Aminoglycoside antibiotics	Watch for additive ototoxicity and nephrotoxicity
14. Tetracyclines Chloramphenicol Macrolide antibiotics	Penicillins Cephalosporins	Bactericidal action of penicillins and cephalosporins may be antagonized by the bacteriostatic antibiotics; Avoid concurrent use, consult the physician
15. Clindamycin	Erythromycin Clarithromycin Azithromycin Chloramphenicol	Mutual antagonism of antibacterial action due to proximal binding sites on bacterial ribosomes; Avoid concurrent use
16. Phenobarbitone Phenytoin Carbamazepine Rifampin	Metronidazole Doxycycline Chloramphenicol Warfarin	Induction of metabolism → failure of antimicrobial therapy; Avoid concurrent use or increase antibiotic dose with monitoring
17. Chloramphenicol	Warfarin Phenytoin Sulfonylureas	Inhibition of metabolism → toxicity of the object drug; Avoid concurrent use or monitor and reduce dose of object drug
18. NSAIDs	Ciprofloxacin and other fluoroquinolones	Enhanced CNS toxicity, seizures; Caution in concurrent use
19. Aspirin and other NSAIDs	Sulfonylureas Phenytoin Valproate Methotrexate	Displacement and/or reduced elimination → toxicity of object drug; Avoid concurrent use/substitute NSAID with paracetamol
	Warfarin Heparin	Enhanced risk of bleeding due to antiplatelet action and gastric mucosal damage; Avoid concurrent use
	ACE inhibitors β blockers Thiazide diuretics	Reduced antihypertensive effect due to inhibition of renal PG synthesis; Avoid concurrent use
	Furosemide	Reduced diuretic action due to PG synthesis inhibition in kidney; Avoid concurrent use
	Alcohol Corticosteroids	Increased risk of gastric mucosal damage and gastric bleeding; Concurrent use contraindicated
20. Aspirin	Spironolactone	Reduced K^+ conserving action due to decreased tubular secretion of canrenone (active metabolite of spironolactone); Avoid concurrent use
21. Chronic alcoholism	Paracetamol	Hepatotoxic dose of paracetamol is reduced; doses ≤ 3 g/day are safe
22. Chlorpromazine Imipramine and other TCAs	Morphine Pethidine Codeine	Enhanced CNS and respiratory depression; Avoid concurrent use
23. TCAs	Adrenaline (added to local anaesthetic)	Potentiation due to neuronal uptake inhibition → rise in BP; Use plain local anaesthetic solution

Contd..

Pharmacodynamic Interactions

Contd..

Precipitant drug*	Object drug^f	Likely interaction and comments
24. Promethazine Alcohol Opioids Antipsychotics	Diazepam and other benzodiazepines	Additive CNS and respiratory depression, motor impairment; Avoid concurrent use
25. Cimetidine Isoniazid	Diazepam and other benzodiazepines	Inhibition of metabolism → exaggerated CNS depression; Avoid concurrent use, or reduce benzodiazepine dose
26. Lidocaine	β-blockers	Enhanced bradycardia and hypotension; Avoid concurrent use
	Quinidine and other antiarrhythmic drugs	Exaggerated cardiac depression, precipitation of arrhythmias; Avoid concurrent use

NSAIDs: Nonsteroidal anti-inflammatory drugs
TCAs: Tricyclic antidepressants

gut motility by atropinic drugs, tricyclic antidepressants, opioids and prokinetic drugs like metoclopramide can also affect drug absorption.

Distribution Interactions involving drug distribution are primarily due to displacement of one drug from its binding sites on plasma proteins by another drug. Drugs highly bound to plasma proteins that have a relatively small volume of distribution like coumarin anticoagulants, sulfonylureas, certain NSAIDs and antiepileptic drugs are particularly liable to displacement interactions. Another requirement is that the displacing drug should bind to the same sites on the plasma proteins with higher affinity. Displacement of bound drug will initially raise the concentration of the free and active form of the drug in plasma that may result in toxicity. However, such effects are usually brief because the free form rapidly gets distributed, metabolized and excreted so that steady-state levels are only marginally elevated. The clinical outcome of displacement interactions is generally significant only when displacement extends to tissue binding sites as well, or is accompanied by inhibition of metabolism and/or excretion. Quinidine has been shown to reduce the binding of digoxin to tissue proteins as well as its renal and biliary clearance by inhibiting the efflux transporter P-glycoprotein, resulting in nearly doubling of digoxin blood levels and toxicity.

Metabolism Certain drugs reduce or enhance the rate of metabolism of other drugs. They may thus affect the bioavailability (if the drug undergoes extensive first pass metabolism in liver) and the plasma half-life of the drug (if the drug is primarily eliminated by metabolism). Inhibition of drug metabolism may be due to competition for the same CYP 450 isoenzyme or cofactor, and attains clinical significance mostly for drugs that are metabolized by saturation kinetics. Macrolide antibiotics, azole antifungals, chloramphenicol, omeprazole, cimetidine, HIV-protease inhibitors, ciprofloxacin and metronidazole are some important inhibitors of metabolism of multiple drugs. Because lidocaine metabolism is dependent on hepatic blood flow, propranolol has been found to prolong its t½ by reducing blood flow to the liver.

A number of drugs induce microsomal drug metabolizing enzymes and enhance biotransformation of several drugs (including their own in many cases). Induction involves gene mediated increased synthesis of certain CYP450 isoenzymes, which takes ~2 weeks of medication with the inducer to produce maximal effect (contrast inhibition of metabolism which develops quickly) and regresses gradually over 1–3 weeks after discontinuation of the inducer. Barbiturates, phenytoin, carbamazepine, rifampin, cigarette smoking, chronic alcoholism and certain pollutants are important microsomal enzyme inducers. Contraceptive failure and loss of therapeutic effect of many other drugs have occurred due to enzyme induction. On the other hand, the toxic dose of paracetamol is lower in chronic alcoholics and in those on enzyme inducing medication because one of the metabolites of paracetamol is responsible for its overdose hepatotoxicity.

Excretion Interaction involving excretion are important mostly in case of drugs actively secreted by tubular transport mechanisms, e.g. probenecid inhibits tubular secretion of penicillins and cephalosporins and prolongs their plasma t½. This is particularly utilized in the single dose treatment of gonorrhoea. Aspirin blocks the uricosuric action of probenecid and decreases tubular secretion of methotrexate. Change in the pH of urine can also affect excretion of weakly acidic or weakly basic drugs. This has been utilized in the treatment of poisonings. Diuretics and to some extent tetracyclines, ACE inhibitors and certain NSAIDs have been found to raise steady-state blood levels of lithium by promoting its tubular reabsorption.

Pharmacodynamic interactions

These interactions derive from modification of the action of one drug at the target site by another drug, independent of a change in its concentration. This may result in an enhanced response (synergism), an attenuated response (antagonism) or an abnormal response. The phenomena of synergism and antagonism are described in Chapter 3, and are intentionally utilized in therapeutics for various purposes. Of clinical significance are the inadvertent concurrent administration of synergistic or antagonistic pair of drugs with adverse consequences. Some examples are:

1. Excessive sedation, respiratory depression, motor incoordination due to concurrent administration of a benzodiazepine (diazepam), a sedating antihistaminic (promethazine), a neuroleptic (chlorpromazine), an opioid (morphine) or drinking alcoholic beverage while taking any of the above drugs.
2. Excessive fall in BP and fainting due to concurrent administration of α_1 adrenergic blockers, vasodilators, ACE inhibitors, high ceiling diuretics and cardiac depressants.
3. Additive prolongation of prothrombin time and bleeding by administration of ceftriaxone or cefoperazone to a patient on coumarin anticoagulants.
4. Excessive platelet inhibition resulting in bleeding due to simultaneous use of aspirin/clopidogrel and carbenicillin.
5. Precipitous fall in BP and myocardial ischaemia due to use of sildenafil by patients receiving organic nitrates, because nitrates increase generation of cGMP, while sildenafil prevents its degradation by inhibiting PDE 5.
6. Blunting of K^+ conserving action of spironolactone by aspirin, because it inhibits the tubular secretion of canrenone (an active metabolite of spironolactone).
7. Antagonism of bactericidal action of β-lactam antibiotic by combining it with a bacteriostatic drug like tetracycline.
8. Mutual antagonism of antibacterial action of macrolides, clindamycin and chloramphenicol due to interference with each other's binding to the bacterial 50S ribosome.
9. Attenuation of antihypertensive effect of ACE inhibitors/β blockers/diuretics

by NSAIDs due to inhibition of renal PG synthesis.

10. Blockade of antiparkinsonian action of levodopa by neuroleptics and metoclopramide having antidopaminergic action.

Abnormal responses sometimes result from pharmacodynamic interaction between certain drugs, e.g. metronidazole and cefoperazone produce bizarre distressing symptoms if the patient drinks alcohol. The basis of certain interactions is not explained, e.g. ampicillin has produced high incidence of skin rashes in patients treated with allopurinol.

Drug interactions before administration

Certain drugs react with each other and get inactivated if their solutions are mixed before administration. In combined oral or parenteral formulations the manufacturers take care that such incompatibilities do not take place. In practice situations these *in vitro* interactions take place when injectable drugs are mixed in the same syringe or infusion bottle. Some examples are:

- Penicillin G or ampicillin mixed with gentamicin or another aminoglycoside antibiotic.
- Thiopentone sodium when mixed with succinylcholine or morphine.
- Heparin when mixed with penicillin/gentamicin/hydrocortisone.
- Noradrenaline when added to sodium bicarbonate solution.

In general, it is advisable to avoid mixing of any two or more parenteral drugs before injecting.

Comment Not all patients taking interacting drugs experience adverse consequences, but it is advisable to take due precautions to avoid mishaps in all cases where interactions are possible. That two drugs have the potential to interact does not necessarily contraindicate their concurrent use. In many cases, knowledge of the nature and mechanism of the possible interaction may permit their concurrent use provided appropriate dose adjustments are made or other corrective measures are taken. A list of clinically significant and common drug interactions that may be encountered in dental practice is given in Table 38.1, along with the suggested corrective measure. However, it is a good practice to consider the possibility of drug interaction whenever two or more drugs are prescribed to a patient, or any drug is added to what the patient is already taking.

Index

A

Abacavir, 479, 481, 484
Abciximab, 290
Abrasives, 515
Absorption of drugs, 19-22
Acarbose, 238, 242
Acebutolol, 107, 109
Aceclofenac, 359
Acenocoumarol, 286
Acetaminophen. *See* Paracetamol
Acetazolamide, 224, 226
Acetylation of drugs, 28
Acetylcholine (ACh), 82-83
Acetylcholinesterase (AChE), 84
Acetylcysteine, 315, 361
Acetylsalicylic acid. *See* Aspirin
Acid neutralizing capacity (ANC), 298-99
Acidulated phosphate fluoride (APF), 511
Acriflavine, 503
Acromegaly, 230, 231
ACTH (Adrenocorticotropic hormone), 228, 232, 244
Actinomycin D, 335
Action potential (AP): local anaesthetic on, 378
Activation of drugs, 26
Active transport of drugs, 18-19
Acute necrotizing ulcerative gingivitis (ANUG), 396, 412, 418, 420
Acyclovir, 473
Addiction: to drugs, 73
Adefovir dipivoxil, 476
Adenosine, 215-16

Adenylyl cyclase: cAMP pathway, 47, 48
Adrenaline (Adr), 48, 94, 96, 98-101, 103, 104, 380, 383, 386, 387
Adrenergic
 blockers, 104-11, 193, 210
 drugs, 98-104
 receptors, 95, 97, 99
 transmission, 94-98
Adrenochrome monosemicarbazone, 279
Adrenocorticosteroids. *See* Corticosteroids
Adsorbants, 504
Adverse drug effects, 68-75
Affinity, 44
Agonist, 43, 44, 45
AIDS: drugs for, 479-85
Akathisia, 170
Alcohol, ethyl, 35, 151-53, 501-02, 503, 504
Alcoholism: dental implications, 153
Aldosterone, 211, 225, 224
Aldosterone antagonist, 193, 211, 224-26
Alendronate, 273
Alfa adrenergic blockers, 98, 104-07, 193-94
Alfa tocopherol (vit E), 323, 324-25
Alfacalcidol, 272
Alfuzosin, 107
Aliskiren, 188
Alkaloids, 5
Alkylating agents, 329, 332-33
Allergic reaction (acute), 70-72, 417, 517, 519-20
Allergy: to drugs, 70-72

Allylestrenol, 256
Alprazolam, 144, 149, 181
Alprostadil (PGE$_1$), 126
Alteplase (rt-PA), 288
Altretamine, 329
Aluminium hydroxide, 299
Amantadine, 164, 475
Ambroxol, 315
Amikacin (Am), 439, 444, 457
Amisulpiride, 166
Aminoglycoside antibiotics, 439-44
 common properties, 439
 mechanism of action, 439-40
 shared toxicities, 440-41
 use in dentistry, 442
Aminopenicillins, 420-21
5-Aminosalicylic acid (5-ASA). *See* Mesalazine
Amiodarone, 215, 521
Amitriptyline, 174, 176, 177
Amlodipine, 188, 190, 197
Amodiaquine, 490
Amoxapine, 180
Amoxicillin, 300, 401, 402, 420-21
Amphetamine, 102, 103
Amphotericin B (AMB), 464-67
 deoxycholate (AMB-DOC), 466
 liposomal (L-AMB), 466
Ampicillin, 401, 420-21
Amrinone, 211
Anabolic steroids, 252
Anaemia: drugs for, 274-79, 328
Anaesthesia: general, 128-36
 complications of, 136
 general: in dentistry, 128
 local *vs* general, 378

local: in dentistry, 386-87
mechanism of (general), 128-29
stages of, 129
techniques of: local, 384-86
Anakinra, 343
Analgesic nephropathy, 350
Analgesics, 347-63, 364-76
combinations, 362-63
definition, 347
in dentistry, 362
nonopioid, 347-62
opioid, 364-71
Anaphylactic reaction, 71, 519
Anaphylactic shock: treatment of, 72, 520
Anastrozole, 255, 256
Androgens, 251-52
Aneurine. See Thiamine
Angina pectoris, 110, 190, 197-203, 520
Angiotensin (Ang II), 183-85
converting enzyme (ACE) inhibitors, 185-87, 192, 209-10
receptor, 184
receptor blockers (ARBs), 187-88
Anorectic drugs, 103
Antacids, 298-99
combinations, 299
Antagonism, 57-58
Antagonist: competitive, 57, 58
Anterior pituitary hormones, 229-31
Anthraquinone purgatives, 306, 307
Antiamoebic drugs, 494-96
Antiandrogens, 252
Antianginal drugs, 110, 197-203
Antianxiety drugs, 181-82
Antiarrhythmic drugs, 211-16
Antibiotic, 388
in periodontal disease, 435, 508-09
Anticancer: drugs, 329-39
general principles in use of, 337-39
general toxicity, 330-31

oral complications of, 331-32
Anticaries drugs, 509-11
Anticholinergic drugs, 89-93, 301, 319
Anticholinesterases, 86-89
poisoning, 88-89
Anticoagulants, 283-87
and dental surgery bleeding, 282-83
Anticonvulsants, 154-61, 173
Antidepressants, 174-80
atypical, 179-80
Antidiabetic drugs, 233-44
Antidiarrhoeal drugs, 310-13
Antiemetic drugs, 301-05
Antiepileptic drugs, 154-61
dental implications, 160-61
Antiestrogen, 255
Antifibrinolytic drugs, 288
Antifungal drugs, 464-71
Antigingivitis agents, 506-09
Antihaemophilic factor, 281
Anti-herpes virus drugs, 472-74
Antihistamines, 315-19
H_1 blockers, 115-19
H_2 blockers, 114, 194-96, 297-98
second generation (H_1), 116, 117-18
Anti H. pylori drugs, 295, 300-01
Antihypertensive drugs, 186, 188, 191-97
Antileprotic drugs, 460-63
Antimalarial drugs, 486-93
causal prophylactics, 487
clinical curatives, 488
for chloroquine-resistant falciparum malaria, 488, 492, 493
gametocidal, , 489
radical curative, 489
suppressive prophylactics, 488
Antimetabolites, 329, 333-34, 342-43
Antimicrobial agent, 388
choice of, 394-98
combinations, 398-400

failure of therapy with, 402
history of, 388-89
in liver disease, 395
in pregnancy, 396
in renal insufficiency, 395
mechanisms of action, 390
prophylactic use of, 400-02
prophylaxis in dentistry, 400-02
synergism among, 398, 399
Antineoplastic. See Anticancer
Antioxidant vitamin, 325
Antiparkinsonian drugs, 161-63
Antiplaque agents, 506-08
Antiplatelet drugs, 288-90
Antiprogestin, 257-58
Antipsychotic drugs, 166-69
Antipyretic-analgesics, 347-63
Antiretrovirus drugs, 479-85
Antiseptics, 497-503
definition, 497
desirable properties, 497-98
factors modifying activity of, 498
in dental plaque and periodontal disease, 501, 507-08
in dentistry, 503, 507-08
Antithrombotic. See Antiplatelet drugs
Antithymocyte globulin (ATG), 344
Antithyroid drugs, 265-66
Antitubercular drugs, 453-60
Antitussives, 315
Antiviral drugs, 472-78
nonretroviral, 472-78
retroviral, 479-85
Aphthous ulcers, 257, 360, 503
Apixaban, 283, 286-87
Aprepitant, 305
Arecoline, 86
Argatroban, 285
Aripiprazole, 167, 169, 171, 174
Arteether, 492
Artemether, 488, 492, 493
Artemisinin derivatives, 492-93
Arterolane, 488, 492, 493,

Artesunate, 488, 492, 493
Articaine, 384, 387
Ascorbic acid, 323, 327-28
Aspirin, 288-89, 349, 350-54
 and dental surgery
  bleeding, 349, 351, 353
Asthma: bronchial, 92, 104,
 126, 249, 316-21
Astringents, 504
 in dentistry, 504
Atenolol, 110
Atorvastatin, 291
Atovaquone, 493
Atracurium, 30, 140,
Atrial fibrillation (AF), 209,
 212, 215
Atrial flutter (AFl), 209, 212
Atropine, 84, 89, 90-93, 216
Atropine methonitrate, 92
Attention deficit hyperkinetic
 disorder (ADHD), 104,
 180
Atypical antidepressants, 176,
 179-80
Atypical antipsychotics, 166,
 169, 170, 174
Autacoids: definition, 112
A-V block, 104, 212, 216
Azathioprine, 313, 333, 342-43
Azelastine, 116, 118,
Azithromycin, 446, 448
AZT (Azidothymidine). See
 Zidovudine
Aztreonam, 429

B

Bacitracin, 444, 452
Baclofen, 142-43
Bacteriological sensitivity
 testing, 397
Bacteriostatic AMAs, 390, 397
Balsalazide, 310, 312
Barbiturates, 145-47, 154
Basiliximab, 339, 343
Beclomethasone dipropionate,
 320
Bedaquiline, 454, 458
Belladonna poisoning, 88, 93
Bendamustine, 329

Benidipine, 190
Benign hypertrophy of
 prostate (BHP): drugs
 for, 106, 253
Benserazide, 57, 163
Benzalkonium chloride, 501,
 507
Benzathine penicillin, 400,
 417, 418
Benzhexol. See
 Trihexyphenidyl
Benzocaine, 384
Benzodiazepines (BZDs), 135,
 144, 147-50
 antagonist, 148, 150-51
 receptor, 147, 148
Benzoic acid, 471
Benzothiadiazines. See
 Thiazides
Benzoyl peroxide, 500
Benzthiazide, also See Thiazide
 diuretics
Beta adrenergic blockers, 107-
 11, 182, 193, 202, 210-11,
 267
Beta carotene, 322, 323
Beta-lactam antibiotics, 414-30
Beta-lactamase inhibitors,
 422-23
Betamethasone, 248, also See
 Corticosteroids
Bethanechol, 85, 86
Bezafibrate, 291, also See
 Fibrates
Bicalutamide, 252, 337
Bimatoprost, 126, 127
Bioavailability, 21-22
Bioequivalance, 21-22
Biological membrane, 15-16
Biological response modifiers,
 339
Biotechnological drugs
 (products), 6
Biotransformation, 26-32
Biperiden, 92
Bipolar disorder, 165, 171-74
Bisacodyl, 307
Bishydroxycoumarin, 286
Bismuth: colloidal, 300
Bisoprolol, 109, 210
Bisphosphonates (BPNs),
 272-73

Bivalirudin, 285
Bleaching agents, 514-15, 516
Bleaching powder, 500, 515
Bleomycin, 331, 335
Blood-brain barrier, 23-24
Boric acid, 502, 503
Bran, 306
Bretylium, 98
Broad spectrum antibiotics,
 390, 431-38
Bromhexine, 315
Bromocriptine, 163, 231
Bronchial asthma: drugs for,
 316-21
Bronchodilators, 101, 103, 316,
 317-19
Budesonide, 320
Bumetanide, 221
Bupivacaine, 382, 383-84, 387
Buprenorphine, 372, 375
Bupropion, 180
Buspirone, 120, 182
Busulfan, 332
Butamben, 384
Butenafine, 471
Butorphanol, 374
Butyrycholinesterase (BuChE).
 See Pseudocholinesterase

C

Cabergoline, 231
Caffeine, 317, 318
Calamine, 503, 504
Calciferol, 271, 323
Calcitonin, 268, 270
Calcitriol, 268, 270, 271, 272,
 323
Calcium, 267-69
 carbonate, 269
 citrate, 269
 daily allowance, 269
 gluconate, 269
Calcium channel blockers
 (CCBs), 188-91, 192
Camphor, 5, 513, 516
Canagliflozin, 238, 242
Cancer chemotherapy. See
 Anticancer drugs

general principles in, 337-39
oral complications of, 331-32
Capecitabine, 334
Capreomycin (Cm), 457
Capsules, 7
Captopril, 185, 186
Carbachol, 85, 86
Carbamazepine, 157, 160, 173
Carbamide peroxide, 514-15, 516
Carbapenems, 429-30
Carbenicillin, 421
Carbidopa, 57, 163, 164
Carbimazole, 265, 266
Carbocisteine, 315
Carbolic acid. *See* Phenol
Carbonic anhydrase (CAse), 218
  inhibitors, 224
Carbonyl iron, 276
Carboplatin, 333
Carboprost, 126, 127
Carcinogenicity, 75, 331
Cardiac arrest, management of, 104, 518
Cardiac glycosides, 205-09
Cardiopulmonary resuscitation, 517
Cardiotonic drugs. *See* Digitalis
Carisoprodol, 142
Carrier transport, 17-19
Carvedilol, 111, 193
Cascara sagrada, 307
Caspofungin, 466, 467
Catecholamines (CAs), 94, 95, 96, *also See* individual drugs
Caustics, in dentistry, 505
Cefaclor, 425
Cefadroxil, 424
Cefazolin, 424
Cefdinir, 426
Cefepime, 427
Cefixime, 426
Cefoperazone, 426
Cefotaxime, 425
Cefpirome, 427
Cefpodoxime proxetil, 426

Cefprozil, 425
Ceftaroline fosamil, 424, 427
Ceftazidime, 426
Ceftibuten, 426
Ceftizoxime, 425
Ceftopiprole medocaril, 424, 427
Ceftriaxone, 425
Cefuroxime, 425
Cefuroxime axetil, 425
Celecoxib, 360
Centchroman, 261
Centrally acting muscle relaxants, 142-43
Cephalexin, 424
Cephalosporins, 424-29
  in dental infections, 428
Cetirizine, 116, 118
Cetrimide, 501, 507
Cetylpyridinium chloride, 501, 507
Cheese reaction, 106, 175
Chemotherapy. *See* Antimicrobial
  definition, 4, 388
  failure of, 402
  of cancer, 329-39
Child dose calculation, 61
Chlophedianol, 315
Chlorambucil, 332
Chloramphenicol, 436-38
  in dental infections, 438
  palmitate, 437
Chlordiazepoxide, 144, 181
Chlorhexidine, 500-01, 503
  in caries, 512
  in dental plaque and periodontal disease, 507
Chlorinated lime (bleaching powder), 500
Chlorine, 500, 515
Chlormezanone, 142
Chloroguanide. *See* Proguanil
Chlorophores, 500
Chloroprocaine, 378, 379
Chloroquine, 488, 489-90
Chloroxylenol, 499
Chlorpheniramine, 116, 518, 520
Chlorpromazine (CPZ), 166-70

Chlorthalidone, 191, 220, *also See* Thiazides
Chlorzoxazone, 142
Cholestyramine, 292
Choline esters, 85, 86
Cholinergic
  Antagonists, 89-93
  drugs, 85-86
  transmission, 82-84
Cholinesterase reactivators, 89
Cholinesterase, 84
Cholinoceptors, 84
Cholinomimetic alkaloids, 85, 86
Chronic obstructive pulmonary disease (COPD), 92, 316, 319, 320, 321
Ciclesonide, 320
Ciclopirox olamine, 471
Cidofovir, 474
Cimetidine, 294-95, *also See* H_2 antagonists
Cimetropium bromide, 89, 92
Cinacalcet, 269
Cinnarizine, 116, 119
Ciprofloxacin, 407, 408-09, 457, 460, *also See* Fluoroquinolones
Cisplatin, 331, 333
Citalopram, 174, 176, *also See* Selective serotonin reuptake inhibitors
Citrovorum factor. *See* Folinic acid
Clarithromycin, 447-48, 460, 462
Clavulanic acid, 422
Clearance of drug (CL), 35
Clemastine, 116
Clidinium, 92
Clindamycin, 401, 449, 488, 492
  in dentistry, 449
Clinical pharmacology, 4
Clobazam, 158
Clofazimine (Clo), 461, 463
Clomiphene citrate, 255
Clomipramine, 176, 180
Clonazepam, 158, 181

Clonidine, 194
Clopamide, 220, *also See* Thiazide diuretics
Clopidogrel, 289, 290
Clorgyline, 174
Clotrimazole, 468
Clove oil, 5, 513, 514, 516
Cloxacillin, 419
Clozapine, 167, 168, 169
Coagulants, 279-81
Cobra bite, 88
Cocaine, 380, 381, 382-83
Codeine, 311, 315, 363
Colestipol, 292
Colistin, 451, 452
Collodion, 504
Colloidal bismuth subcitrate (CBS), 300
Competitive: antagonism, 57, 58
  enzyme inhibition, 42
COMT inhibitors, 98, 164
Congestive heart failure (CHF), 208, 209
  drugs for, 208, 209
  effect on drug kinetics, 65
  treatment of, 209-11
Conscious sedation (in dentistry), 132, 135, 136-37
Constipation: treatment of, 306, 307, 308,
Contraceptives, 258-61
  emergency (postcoital), 259-60
  hormonal, 258-61
  injectable, 260
Controlled release tablet/capsule, 38
Coronary steal, 190
Corticosteroids (glucocorticoids), 244-50, 320-21
  implications in dentistry, 250
Corticotropin, 232 *See* ACTH
Cortisol. *See* Hydrocortisone
Cotransmission, 82
Cotrimoxazole, 405-06
Cough: drugs for, 119, 314-15

COX-I/COX-2 (cyclooxygenase) isoenzymes, 122
COX-2 (cyclooxygenase-2) inhibitors, 122, 348, 359-60
Cresol, 499
Cretinism, 263, 264, 265
Cromoglycate sod (Cromolyn sod), 320
Cross resistance, 393
Cross tolerance, 66-67
Cumulation, 66
Curare, 137, *also See* Tubocurarine
Cyanide poisoning, 201-02
Cyanocobalamin, 277-78 *See* Vit. B_{12}
Cyclic AMP (cAMP), 41, 126, 241, 318, 373
Cyclic GMP (cGMP), 114, 199, 200, 318
Cyclooxygenase (COX), 121, 122
  inhibitor, 122, 348-50, *also See* Nonsteriodal antiinflammatory drugs
  isoforms, 348
Cyclopentolate, 92
Cyclophosphamide, 332, 343
Cycloserine (Cs), 457
Cyclosporine, 313, 341-42
Cyproheptadine, 116
Cyproterone acetate, 252
Cytarabine, 331, 334
Cytochrome P450 (CYP) isoenzymes, 27, 28, 30
Cytotoxic drugs, 329, 330, 331-35, 342-43

D

Dabigatran, 287
Dacarbazine, 331, 332
Daclatasvir, 472, 478
Danaparoid, 285
Danazol, 252
Dantrolene, 141
Dapagliflozin, 238, 242
Dapoxetine, 174, 180

Dapsone (DDS), 460-61, 463
Daptomycin, 451
Darifenacin, 89, 92
Darunavir, 479, 482
Dasatinib, 330, 336
Daunorubicin (Rubidomycin), 335
DDS. *See* Dapsone
Decamethonium (C10), 138
Deflazacort, 248
Dehydroemetine, 494
Demeclocycline, 433, 434
Demulcents, 504
  pharyngeal, 314
Dental plaque; antiseptics in, 499, 501, 503, 507-08
Dentifrices, 503, 515-16
Dentine bonding agents, 513
Dentine sensitivity, 505, 512-13, 516
Depot preparations, 13, 14, 21
Depression (of function), 40
  mental, 164, 174, 180
Dermojet, 13
Desensitization, 53
Desensitizing agents, 512-13
Desflurane, 131, 133
Desipramine, 174
Desloratadine, 118
Desmopressin, 281, 282
Desogestrel, 256, 258, 259
Detergents, 516
Dexamethasone, 248, *also See* Corticosteroids
Dexchlorpheniramine, 116
Dexrabeprazole, 297
Dextromethorphan, 315
Diabetes
  implications in dentistry, 243
  insipidus, 223, 435
  mellitus, 233-44
Diarrhoea: treatment of, 309-13
  antimicrobials in, 310-11
  antimotility drugs in, 311-12
  antisecretory drugs in, 311
Diazepam, 135, 141, 142, 147, 148, 158, 160, 161, 178
Dibucaine, 384

Diclofenac sod, 358, 362
Dicumarol. *See* Bishydroxycoumarin
Dicyclomine, 92, 301
Didanosine, 480
Dietary fibre, 306
Diffusion: of drugs, 16-17
Diffusion hypoxia, 130, 131
Digitalis, 205, 208
  toxicity, 207-08
Digoxin, 205-09, *also See* Digitalis
  antibodies, 208
Dihydroartemisinin, 486, 493
Dihydroergotamine (DHE), 105
Dihydroergotoxine, 106
Dihydrofolate reductase (DHFRase) inhibitors, 313, 333, 343
  bacterial, 405
  protozoal, 491
Dihydropyridines (DHPs), 188, 189, 190, 192
Dihydrotestosterone, 251, 252, 253
Diiodohydroxyquin, 495
Diloxanide furoate, 495
Diltiazem, 189, 190, 191, 208, 215
Dimenhydrinate, 116, 302
Dinoprost (PGF$_2$), 126
Dinoprostone (PGE$_2$), 126
Dioctyl sodium sulfosuccinate (DOSS). *See* Docusates
Diphenhydramine, 116, 302
Diphenoxylate, 311, 371
Dipyridamole, 289
Direct renin inhibitor, 185, 188
Direct thrombin inhibitor, 285
Disclosing agents, 515
Disinfectants, 497-503
  definition, 497
  desirable properties of, 497
  in dentistry, 503
Disopyramide, 213
Dissociative anaesthesia, 135
Distribution of drugs, 22-26
Diuretic therapy:
  complications of, 223
Diuretics, 191-93, 209, 219-27
Divalproex, 158, 173
DMPA (Depot medroxyprogesterone acetate), 260
Dobutamine, 102, 211
Docetaxel, 334
Docusates, 307, 309
Dofetilide, 215
Dolutegravir, 479, 483
Domperidone, 304
Donepezil, 88
DOPA, 94, 162
Dopamine (DA), 94, 102
Doripenem, 430
Dosage forms of drugs, 4, 5, 7-9
Dose: of drug, 36, 61-67
  child, 61
  for elderly, 62
  loading, 38
  maintenance, 38, 65
Dose-response relationship, 53-54, 143
Dothiepin, 176
Doxacurium, 140
Doxazosin, 106, 194
Doxepin, 176
Doxorubicin, 335
Doxycycline, 433, 434, 488, 492, 526
Doxylamine, 302
Dronabinol, 305
Dronedarone, 215
Drops, 8
Drug
  absorption, 19-22, 527
  abuse, 74
  action and drug effect, 45, 48
  activation, 26
  addiction, 73
  adverse effects, 68-75
  allergy, 70-72, 118
  antagonism, 57-59
  combinations (fixed dose), 60-61
  definition, 4
  dependence, 73-74
  diffusion, 16-17
  distribution, 22-25
  dosage, 59-60
  dosage forms of, 7-9
  efficacy, 54-55
  enterohepatic circulation of, 33
  excretion, 32-34
  factors modifying action of, 61-67
  habituation, 74
  induced diseases, 75
  interactions, 523-29
    before administration, 529
    in dentistry, 525-27
    mechanism of, 524, 527, 528
  mechanisms of action, 40-51
  metabolism, 26-32
  nomenclature, 6
  non-prescription, 9
  penetration into brain, 23-24
  potency, 54-55
  prescription, 9
  resistance, 67, 391-93
  routes of administration, 10-14
  selectivity, 55-56
  sources of, 5-6
  storage (in the body), 25
  synergism, 56-57
  transport, 15-19
  vesicular transport, 19
  withdrawal reactions, 74
Duloxetine, 179
Dydrogesterone, 256
Dyflos, 87, *also See* Organophosphates
Dynorphins, 372, 376

E

Ebastine, 116, 117
Echothiophate, 86
Econazole, 468
EDRF (Endothelium dependent relaxing factor), 85, 113, *also See* Nitric oxide
Edrophonium, 87

Index

Efavirenz, 481, 484, 485
Eicosanoids, 120-25
Elimination rate constant (K), 36
Elixirs, 8
Emergency contraception, 258, 259, 260
Emergency drug tray/kit, 517-18
Emesis, 301, 302
Emetine, 494
Emollients, 504
Emtricitabine (FTC), 479, 481
Enalapril, 185, 186, *also See* Angiotensin converting enzyme inhibitors
Endocytosis, 19
Endogenous (major) depression: treatment, 180
Endorphins (β-END), 372, 376
Enfuvirtide, 483
Enkephalins, 372, 376
Entacapone, 164
Entecavir, 472, 476
Enteric nervous system, 80
Entero-hepatic circulation of drugs, 33
Enzyme
  induction, 30-31, 42
  inhibition, 41-42
  stimulation, 41-42
Ephedrine, 102
Epidural anaesthesia, 385
Epilepsies, 154
  during dental procedures, 160-61
  treatment of, 159-61
Epinephrine. *See* Adrenaline
Eplerenone, 211, 226
Epoprostenol, 126
Epsilon amino caproic acid (EACA), 288
Eptifibatide, 289, 290
Ergot alkaloids, 106
Ergotamine, 106
Ergotoxine, 106
Ertapenem, 430
Erythrityl tetranitrate, 201
Erythromycin, 445-47
  in dental infections, 447

Erythrosine, 515
Escitalopram, 176, *also See* Selective serotonin reuptake inhibitors
Eserine, 87, *also See* Physostigmine
Eslicarbazepine, 154, 157
Esmolol, 110, 197, 215
Esomeprazole, 295, *also See* Proton pump inhibitors
Estradiol, 253, *also See* Estrogens
Estramustine, 330, 335
Estrogens, 253-55, *also See* Oral contraceptives
Eszopiclone, 144, 150
Etanercept, 343
Ethambutol (E), 456-57, 458, 459, 460
Ethamsylate, 281
Ethanol. *See* Alcohol ethyl
Ether 130, 131, 132
Ethinylestradiol, 253, 259, *also See* Oral contraceptives
Ethinylestranol, 256, *See* Lynestrenol
Ethionamide (Etm), 457, 459
Ethosuximide, 157, 160
Ethyl alcohol. *See* Alcohol ethyl
Ethyl biscoumacetate, 286
Etidronate, 273
Etodolac, 347, 359
Etoposide, 331, 335
Etoricoxib, 347, 359, 360
Etravirine, 479, 481
Eutectic lidocaine/prilocaine, 383
Everolimus, 339, 342
Excretion: of drugs, 32-34
Exemestane, 255, 256
Exenatide, 237, 241
Exocytosis, 19, 81
Expectorants, 314-15
Ezetimibe, 293

F

Facilitated diffusion, 18
Factors modifying drug action, 61-67

Fainting, management of, 517, 519
Famciclovir, 474
Famotidine, 296, *also See* H_2 antagonists
Faropenem, 430
Felodipine, 190
Fenofibrate, 291, *also See* Fibrates
Fentanyl, 135-36, 369
  transdermal, 369
Ferric
  ammonium citrate, 275
  carboxy-maltose, 276
  hydroxide, 275
Ferrous
  fumarate, 275
  gluconate, 275
  succinate, 275
  sucrose, 276
  sulphate, 275
Fexofenadine, 116, 118
Fibrates (Fibric acid derivatives), 291, 292
Fibrin, 282
Fibrinogen, 281
Fibrinolytic drugs, 287-88
Filtration: of drugs, 17
Finasteride, 253, 337
First dose effect, 106, 194
First order kinetics, 35, 36, 37
First pass metabolism, 31-32
Fixed dose combinations (FDCs), 60-61
Flavoxate, 92
Flecainide, 213, 214
Fluconazole, 466, 469
  in oral candidiasis, 469
Fludarabine, 334
Flumazenil, 147, 148, 150-51
Fluorescein, 515
Fluoride, 509-12, 516
Fluoroquinolones (FQs), 406-10, 457, 460, 462
Fluorosis, 511, 512
5-Fluorouracil (5-FU), 334, 339
Fluoxetine, 176, *also See* Selective serotonin reuptake inhibitors
Flupenthixol, 167

Fluphenazine, 167, 168, 170
Flurazepam, 149
Flurbiprofen, 355
Flutamide, 252, 253, 337
Fluticasone propionate, 316, 320
Fluvoxamine, 176, *also See* Selective serotonin reuptake inhibitors
Folic acid, 278-79, 323
   antagonists. *See* Dihydrofolate reductase inhibitor
Folinic acid (THFA), 279, 323, 333, 334, 339
Follicle stimulating hormone (FSH), 228, 229
Fondaparenux, 283, 285
Formalin (Formaldehyde), 502
Formoterol, 317
Foscarnet, 474
Fosinopril, 185
Fosphenytoin, 157, 161
Framycetin, 444
Frusemide. *See* Furosemide
Fulvestrant, 255, 337
Furosemide, 193, 203, 209, 219-21, 226, *also See* High ceiling diuretics

G

GABA$_A$-benzodiazepine receptor, 145, 147, 148
Gabapentin, 159, 160
Ganciclovir, 474
Gastric acid secretion: regulation of, 294, 296
Gastric hurrying agent, 303, *also See* Prokinetic drugs
Gastroesophageal reflux disease (GERD), 294, 298
   drugs for, 298
Gelatin foam, 282
Gels, 9
Gemcitabine, 329, 334
Cemeprost, 126
Gemfibrozil, 291, *See* Fibrates
Gemifloxacin, 409, 410
General anaesthetics (GA), 128-36

Genetics: and drug action, 63
Gentamicin, 440, 442-43, *also See* Aminoglycoside antibiotics
   in dentistry, 442
Gentian violet, 503
Germicide, 497-98
Gestodene, 256
Glaucoma: drugs for, 88, 111, 127, 224
Glibenclamide, 239, *also See* Sulfonylureas
Gliclazide, 239
Glimepiride, 239
Glipizide, 239
Glucagon-like peptide-1 (GLP-1) receptor agonists, 237
Glucocorticoid receptor, 52, 247
Glucocorticoids, (Corticosteroids), 244-50, 320-21
   antagonist, 258
Glucuronide conjugation, 27
Glutaraldehyde, 502
Glutathione conjugation, 29
Glyburide. *See* Glibenclamide
Glycerol (Glycerine), 516
Glyceryl trinitrate (GTN), 199-201, *also See* Nitrates
Glycopeptide antibiotics, 449-50
Glycoprotein (GP) II$_b$/III$_a$ antagonists 290
Glycopyrrolate, 92
Glycosides, 5
   cardiac, 205-09
Glycyrrhiza, 504
GnRH agonists, 231-32, 252
Goiter, 265, 266
Gonadotropins (Gns), 231
Goserelin, 229, 231
G-proteins, 46, 47, 48, 49
Granisetron, 305
Graves' disease, 232, 265, 266
Gray baby syndrome, 438
Griseofulvin, 467
Growth hormone (GH), 228, 229-30
Guaiphenesin, 314
Guanethidine, 98

H

H$_1$ antagonists, 115-19
H$_2$ antagonists, 119, 294-96, 297-98
Habituation, 74
Haematinics, 274-78
Haemophilia, drugs for, 281, 282
Haemostasis in dentistry, 281-83
Haemostatics: local, 281-82
Half life (t½), 35-36
Haloperidol, 167, 168, 174
Halothane, 131, 132-33, 136
Heart block. *See* A-V block
Heparin, 283-85, 287
   antagonist, 285
   low molecular weight, 284
Heroin, 368
Herpes simplex: drugs for, 472-74
   mucocutaneous, 473
Hexachlorophene, 499
Hexamethonium, 83, 84
High-ceiling diuretics, 193, 209, 219-21, 223, 224, 528
Histamine, 112-15
   receptors, 113
HIV infection: drugs for, 479-83
   postexposure prophylaxis, 484-85
   treatment of, 483-84
HMG-CoA reductase inhibitors (Statins), 291-92
Hofmann elimination, 30, 140
Homatropine, 92
Hormonal contraceptives, 258-61
Hormone: definition, 228
Hormones regulating calcium, 267-72
Hormone replacement therapy (HRT), 254-55, 257
Humectants, 516
Hydralazine, 195, 210
Hydrochlorothiazide, 191-92, 220, *also See* Thiazide diuretics

Hydrocortisone, 244, 247, 248, also See Corticosteroids
Hydroflumethiazide, 220, also See Thiazide diuretics
Hydrogen peroxide, 499, 508, 514
Hydrolysis: of drugs 27
Hydroxocobalamin, 277, also See Vit B$_{12}$
Hydroxyprogesterone caproate, 255
8-Hydroxyquinolines, 495
5-Hydroxytryptamine (5-HT), 119-20
  receptor subtypes, 120
Hydroxyurea, 335
Hydroxyzine, 116, 182
Hyoscine, 89, 91, 92, 301
  butyl bromide, 92
Hypersensitivity (allergic) reactions, 70-72
  to penicillin, 395, 402, 417
Hypertension: drugs for, 106, 110, 186-87, 190, 191-95, 223
Hypertensive emergencies/urgencies, 196-97
Hyperthyroidism. See Thyrotoxicosis
Hypervitaminosis A, 324
Hypervitaminosis D, 272
Hypnotics, 144-51
  definition, 144
Hypoglycaemia, management of, 236, 521-22
Hypoglycaemic drugs, 233-44 See Antidiabetic drugs
Hypolipidaemic drugs, 291-93
Hypothyroidism, 263, 265, 266, 267

I

Ibandronate, 273
Ibuprofen, 355, 357, 362
Ibutilide, 215
Idarubicin, 330
Idiosyncrasy, 70
Idoxuridine, 472-73
Ifosfamide, 329
Imatinib, 336

Imipenem, 429, 430
Imipramine, 175, 176, 177, 180, 526
Immunosuppressants, 313, 339-44
Implants, 13
Inamrinone, 211, See Amrinone
Indapamide, 193, 220, also See Thiazide diuretics
Indinavir, 469, 482
Indomethacin, 124, 357
Induction of drug metabolism, 30-31, 527
Infertility: drugs for, 231, 255
Infliximab, 339, 343
INH. See Isoniazid
Inhaled steroids, 249, 317, 320-21
Inhalation of drugs, 10, 13
Inhalational anaesthesia, 130, 131, 132
Inhibition of drug metabolism, 30, 527
Injections, 8, 13
Inodilator, 211
Insulin, 233-37
  analogues, 235-36
  aspart, 235
  detemir, 236
  glargine, 236
  glulisine, 236
  human, 235
  lispro, 235
  preparations, 234-36
  reactions to, 236-37
  receptor, 234, 235
Insulin-like growth factors (IGFs), 230
Integrase inhibitor, 479, 482-83, 484
Interferon, 477
Intolerance, 70
Intraarterial injection, 10
Intradermal injection, 14
Intramuscular injection (i.m.), 13-14
  absorption from, 21
Intravenous anaesthetics, 134-35

Intravenous injection (i.v.), 14
Intrinsic activity, 44, 57
Inverse agonists, 44, 148, 150
Iodide. sod./pot., 266
Iodine, 266, 500
  radioactive (^{131}I), 266, 267
Iodochlorohydroxyquin. See Quiniodochlor
Iodoform, 514
Iodophores, 500
Ion channels as targets of drug action, 43
Ipratropium bromide, 92, 319, 321
Irinotecan, 335
Iron, 274-77
  absorption, 274-75
  deficiency: oral manifestations, 274
  dextran, 276
  hydroxy polymaltose, 275
  isomaltoside-1000, 276
Irritation, 40
Isoflurane, 131, 133
Isoniazid (INH; H), 453-55, 458, 459
Isoprenaline (Iso), 96, 98, 100, 104
Isopropanol, 502
Isosorbide dinitrate, 201
Isosorbide mononitrate, 201
Isoxsuprine, 101
Ispaghula, 306, 308
Itraconazole (ITR), 466, 470
Itopride, 304
Ivabradine, 203

K

Kanamycin (Km), 440, 443, 457, 459
Ketamine, 135
Ketoconazole (KTZ), 466, 468-69
Ketoprofen, 355
Ketorolac, 356-57, 362
Ketotifen, 320
Kidney disease and drugs, 64, 395
Kinetics of drug elimination, 35-39

Index

L

Labetalol, 111, 193, 197
Lacidipine, 190
Lacosamide, 159, 160
Lactitol, 306, 308
Lactulose, 306, 308, 309
Lamivudine, 475, 480-81, 484, 485
Lamotrigine, 159, 160, 173
Lansoprazole, 295, 301, *also See* Proton pump inhibitors
L-Asparaginase, 335, 338
Latanoprost, 124, 127
Laxatives, 305-09
L-Dopa. *See* Levodopa
Ledipasvir, 472, 478
Lepra reaction, 463
Leprosy: drugs for, 460-63
   alternative regimens for, 463
   multidrug therapy (MDT) in, 462
Lercanidipine, 190
Letrozole, 255-56
Leucovorin. *See* Folinic acid
Leukotrienes (LTs), 125, 319
   antagonists, 126, 319-20
   receptors, 126
Leuprolide, 229, 231
Levarterenol, 101, *also See* Noradrenaline
Levetiracetam, 159, 160
Levobupivacaine, 384
Levocetirizine, 116, 118
Levodopa, 162-63, 164
Levofloxacin, 409, 410, 457, 459, 460
Levonorgestrel, 256, 258, 259,
Levosimendan, 211
Lidocaine, 214, 377, 381, 382, 383, 384, 386-87
Ligand, 44
Lignocaine. *See* Lidocaine
Lincomycin, 449
Linezolid, 451
Liothyronine, 265, *also See* Triiodothyronine
Liquid paraffin, 307, 309, 504

Liquorice, 504
Liraglutide, 237, 241
Lisinopril, 186, *also See* Angiotensin converting enzyme inhibitors
Listerine, 499, 507
Lithium, 171-73
   alternatives to, 173-74
Liver disease and drugs, 64, 395
Loading dose: of drug, 38
Local anaesthesia, 377-87
   compared to general anaesthesia, 378
   in dentistry, 386-87
   techniques of, 384-86
Local anaesthetics (LAs), 377-387
   mechanism of action, 378-79
   with adrenaline, 380
Local routes of administration, 10
Lomustine, 331, 332
Loperamide, 311, 312
Lopinavir, 482, 484, 485
Loratadine, 118
Lorazepam, 135, 149, 159, 160, 161, 518
Losartan, 184, 187-88, *also See* Angiotensin antagonist
Lotions, 8
Lovastatin, 291, *also See* Statins
Loxapine, 167
Lozenges, 7
Lubiprostone, 306, 307
Lumefantrine, 488, 493
Luteinizing hormone (LH), 229, 231
Lynestrenol, 256

M

MAC (*Mycobacterium avium* complex): drugs for, 460
Macrolide antibiotics, 445-48
Mafenide, 404-05
Magaldrate, 299
Magnesium

   hydroxide, 299, 306
   sulphate, 306
   trisilicate, 299
Maintenance dose (of drug), 38
Malignant hyperthermia, 133, 141
Malignant neuroleptic syndrome, 170
Mania, 157, 158, 165, 171-74
Mannitol, 227
Maraviroc, 483
Mast cell stabilizers, 320
Maturation factors, 277-79
Mechanism of drug action, 40-52
Meclozine (meclizine), 116, 302
Medical emergencies in dental office, 517-22
Medroxyprogesterone acetate, 256, 260
Mefloquine, 488, 490, 492, 493
Meglitinide analogues, 239, 240, 243
Melatonin, 151
Meloxicam, 359
Melphalan, 332
Menadione, 281, 323
Menthol, 499, 513, 516
Meperidine. *See* Pethidine
Mephenamic acid, 356
Mephenesin, 142
Mephentermine, 103
Mercaptopurine (6-MP), 333
Meropenem, 429-30
Mesalazine (5-ASA, Mesalamine), 312
Metabolism, 26-32, *See* Biotransformation
Metabolism: presystemic (first pass), 31, 32, 64
Metformin, 233, 240-41, *also See* Biguanides
Methacholine, 85, 86
Methadone, 369, 370
Methamphetamine, 101
Methandienone, 252
Methicillin, 419

Index

Methicillin resistant *Staph. aureus* (MRSA), 416, 419, 427
  drugs for, 427, 449, 450, 451
Methimazole, 265
Methocarbamol, 142, 143
Methotrexate (Mtx), 279, 313, 331, 333, 339, 343
Methoxamine, 103
Methylation of drugs, 28
Methyl cellulose, 516
Methyldopa, 194-95
Methylprednisolone, 247
Methylxanthines, 317-19
Metoclopramide, 303-04
Metolazone, 220
Metoprolol, 109, 110, 210
Metronidazole, 152, 153, 311, 411-12, 494
  in orodental infections, 412, 509
Mexiletine, 214
Mianserin, 179
Miconazole, 468
Microsomal enzymes, 29
  induction, 30-31, 527-28
Midazolam, 135, 161
Mifepristone, 257-58, 259
Miglitol, 242
Milk: excretion of drugs in, 32
Milrinone, 209, 211
Mineralocorticoid, 244, 248
Minimal alveolar concentration (MAC), 128, 131
Minimum bactericidal concentration (MBC), 397
Minimum inhibitory concentration (MIC), 397
Minocycline, 431, 432, 433, 462, 463
Miotic, 88, 91
Mirtazapine, 179-80
Misoprostol, 126, 298, 350
Mivacurium, 140, 141
Mizolastine, 116
Moclobemide, 175
Monoamine oxidase (MAO), 96, 97, 98, 113, 174
  inhibitors (MAOI), 97, 163-64, 174-75

Monobactam, 429
Montelukast, 319, *also See* Leukotriene antagonists
Mood stabiliser. *See* Bipolar disorder
Morning sickness, 301, 302, 303
Morphine, 364-68, 370, 372
  dependence, 367
  in dental pain, 370
  poisoning, 367
Mosapride, 304
Motion sickness: drugs for, 92, 118, 302, 303
Moxifloxacin, 409, 410, 457, 462, 463
Multidrug resistant tuberculosis (MDR-TB), 454, 457, 459-60
Muromonab CD3, 340, 344
Muscarine, 83, 85, 86
Muscarinic,
  actions, 85, 86, 89, 116
  antagonists, 89-93, *also See* Anticholinergic drugs
  receptor, 84, 85, 89, 296
Muscle relaxants, 137-43
  centrally acting, 142-43
Mushroom poisoning, 86, 92
Mutagenicity of drugs, 75
Myasthenia gravis, 88, 249, 343
Mycobacterium avium complex (MAC) infection, 457, 458, 460
Mycophenolate mofetil, 343
Mydriatics, 90, 91, 92, 103
Myocardial infarction (MI):
  drugs for, 110, 187, 201, 203-04
Myxoedema, 265, *also See* Hypothyroidism

N

Nabumetone, 357
N-acetylcysteine, 315, 361
Nafarelin, 231
Nalbuphine, 373, 374
Nalidixic acid, 406, 407
Nalorphine, 372, 374

Naloxone, 367, 372, 375,
Naltrexone, 375-76
Nandrolone, 252
Naproxen, 355
Nasal administration of drugs, 13
Nasal decongestants, 103, 104
Nateglinide, 239, 240
Nebivolol, 110
Nefopam, 362
Nelfinavir, 482
Neomycin, 444
Neostigmine, 87, 88, 138, 139, 141
Nerve block anaesthesia, 385
Netilmicin, 444
Neurohumoral transmission, 79-82
Neuroleptic drugs. *See* Antipsychotic drugs
Neuromuscular blocking agents, 137-41
Neuroses, 165
Nevirapine, 481, 484
Niacin (Vit B_3), 323, 326
Nicardipine, 188, 190, 196
Nicorandil, 202
Nicotinamide. *See* Niacin
Nicotine, 83, 93
  chewing gum, 93
  transdermal, 93
Nicotinic acid (Vit B_3), 292-93, 323, 326
Nicotinic actions, 85, 86
Nicotinic receptors, 84, 88, 138
Nicoumalone. *See* Acenocoumarol
Nifedipine, 43, 189, 190
Nimesulide, 358, 362
Nitazoxanide, 495
Nitrates, 199-201
Nitrate tolerance, 200
Nitrazepam, 149
Nitrendipine, 190
Nitric oxide (NO), 85, 110, 199, 200
Nitrofurazone, 503
Nitroglycerine. *See* Glyceryl trinitrate
Nitroimidazoles, 411-13, 494

Nitroprusside sod., 195, 196, 210
Nitrous oxide (N$_2$O), 132
Nomegestrol, 256
Non-benzodiazepine hypnotics, 149-50
Noncompetitive antagonism, 58-59
Noncompetitive enzyme inhibition, 42
Nonmicrosomal enzymes, 29
Nonnucleoside reverse transcriptase inhibitors (NNRTIs), 481, 484
Nonprescription drugs, 9
Nonsedating antihistamines. See Antihistamines: second generation
Nonsteroidal antiinflammatory drugs (NSAIDs), 347-62
  and dental surgery bleeding, 349
  and gastric mucosal damage, 350
  and PG synthesis inhibition, 348-50
  drug interactions with, 355
  in dentistry, 355, 362
  shared toxicities, 349, 354
Noradrenaline (NA), 94, 96, 99, 100, 101
Norepinephrine. See Noradrenaline
Norethisterone. See Norethindrone
Norethindrone, 256, 259, 260
  enanthate (NEE), 260
Norfloxacin, 310, 409, 525
Norgestimate, 256
Nortriptyline, 176
Noscapine, 315, 364
Nucleoside reverse transcriptase inhibitors (NRTIs), 479, 480-81, 484
Nystatin, 467
  in oral candidiasis, 467

O

Obtundants, 513
Octreotide, 230
Ofloxacin, 409, 410, 457, 462

Oils, 5
  fixed (nonvolatile), 5
  volatile (essential), 5
Ointments, 8-9
Olanzapine, 167, 169, 171, 174
Omeprazole, 296-97, *also See* Proton pump inhibitors
Ondansetron, 304-05, 339
On-off effect, 163
Opioid
  agonist-antagonists, 371, 373-75
  analgesics, 364-71
  antagonists (pure), 375-76
  antidiarrhoeals, 311-12
  antitussives, 314, 315
  in dental pain, 376
  in preanaesthetic medication, 371
  peptides, 376
  receptors, 371-73
Opium, 364
Oral
  absorption of drugs, 20
  anticoagulants, 283, 285-87
  antidiabetic drugs, 238-44
  contraceptives (OCs), 258-61
  hypoglycaemic drugs. See Oral antidiabetic drugs
  iron preparations, 275-76
  rehydration salt/solution (ORS), 309
  route of administration, 10-11
Organophosphates, 87, 88
Organophosphate poisoning, 89
Ornidazole, 411, 413
Oseltamivir, 475
Osmotic diuretics, 227
Osmotic (saline) purgatives, 307-08, 309
Osteomalacia, 272
Osteoporosis, 249, 252, 255, 269, 271, 272, 273
  anabolic steroids in, 252
  bisphosphonates in, 273
  calcium in, 269
  raloxifene in, 255
  vit D in, 271, 272

Oxaliplatin, 333
Oxazepam, 144, 181
Oxazolidinone antimicrobial, 451
Oxcarbazepine, 157, 160
Oxethazaine, 384
Oxiconazole, 468
Oxidation of drugs, 27
Oxidized cellulose, 282
Oximes, 89
Oxybutynin, 92
Oxymetazoline, 103
Oxymetholone, 252
Oxyphenonium, 92
Oxytetracycline, 433, 434, 496
Oxytocin, 228

P

Paclitaxel, 334
Palonosetron, 305
Pamidronate, 273
Pancuronium, 140, 141
Pantoprazole, 297, *also See* Proton pump inhibitors
Para aminosalicylic acid (PAS), 457
Paracetamol, 4, 360-61, 362
  Poisoning, 361
Paraffin, liquid, 307, 309, 504
Paraformaldehyde (Paraform), 514
Parasympathetic system, 79, 80, 84
Parasympathomimetic drugs. See Cholinergic drugs
Parathyroid hormone (PTH), 268, 269, 270
Parecoxib, 359, 360
Parenteral routes, 13-14
Parkinsonism, drugs for, 92, 161-64
Paromomycin, 444, 496
Paroxetine, 176, *also See* Selective serotonin reuptake inhibitors
Paroxysmal supraventricular tachycardia (PSVT), 209, 211, 215
Partial agonist, 44, 58, 109, 368, 370, 372

Pastes, 9, 515, 516
Pefloxacin, 409-10
Pellet implantation, 13
Pemetrexed, 333
Penicillinase, 416
   resistant penicillins, 419
Penicillins, 414-22
   acid resistant, 418-19
   benzathine, 417
   benzyl (G), 416-18
   extended spectrum, 419-20
   in dental infections, 418, 420
   penicillinase resistant, 419
   phenoxymethyl (V), 418-19
   procaine, 417
   semisynthetic, 418-22
Pentaerythritol tetranitrate, 201
Pentazocine, 370, 372, 374
Peptic ulcer: drugs for, 294-300
Perindopril, 185, 186, *also See* Angiotensin converting enzyme inhibitors
Periodontal disease, 506
   antibiotics in, 508-09
   antiseptics in, 503
   drugs for, 506-09
   tetracyclines in, 435, 509
Peripheral decarboxylase inhibitors, 163
Pernicious anaemia, 277, 278
Pethidine, 368, 369, 370
P-glycoprotein, 19, 23
Pharmaceutics, 4
Pharmacodynamics, 3, 40-59
Pharmacogenetics, 63
Pharmacogenomics, 63
Pharmacokinetics, 3-4, 15-38
Pharmacology: definition, 3
   relevance to dentistry, 3
Pharmacotherapeutics, 4
Pharmacy: definition, 4
Pheniramine, 116, 518, 519
Phenobarbitone, 145, 146, 154-55, 156, 160, 161, *also See* Barbiturates
Phenol, 498, 505, 514
   coefficient, 498
Phenothiazines, 167, 168

Phenoxybenzamine, 105, 106
Phenoxymethyl penicillin, 418
Phentolamine, 106
Phenylephrine, 103, 104
Phenytoin, 155-56, 160
Pheochromocytoma, 106, 111, 197
Pholcodine, 315, 368
Phospholipase C:IP$_3$-DAG pathway, 47-48, 49
Photosensitivity, 72-73
Phylloquinone, 280-81, 323 *See* vit. K
Physical dependence, 73
Physostigmine, 57, 86, 88, 93
Phytonadione (vit K$_1$), 281, 323
Pilocarpine, 86, 88
Pimozide, 167, 168
Pindolol, 109, 110
Pioglitazone, 239, 242, 243
Pipecuronium, 140
Piperacillin, 421, 423
Piperaquine, 490, 492, 493
Piroxicam, 356, 359
Pitavastatin, 291
pKa, 16, 17, 23
Placebo, 64
Placental transfer of drugs, 24
Plaque (dental), 153, 499, 503, 506, 507, 508, 509, 512
Plasma half life (t½), 4, 35-36
Plasma protein binding, 24-25
Plateau principle, 37
Podophyllum resin, 505
Poisoning, 69-70
Polyene antibiotics, 465-66
Polymyxin B, 451-52
Polypeptide antibiotics, 451-52
Posaconazole, 466, 470
Postantibiotic effect (PAE), 397, 408, 440
Postpartum haemorrhage, 127
Postural hypotension, management of, 519
Potassium
   channel openers, 202
   iodide, 266
   nitrate, 512-13
   oxalate, 513

   permanganate, 499
   sparing diuretics, 224-26
Potentiation, 56-57
Povidone iodine, 500, 503
Powders, 7
Pramipexole, 163
Prasugrel, 289-90
Pravastatin, 291
Prazosin, 106, 194
Preanaesthetic medication, 92, 119, 135, 371
Prednisolone, 247, 248, 313, *also See* Corticosteroids
Preferential COX-2 inhibitors, 358-59
Pregabalin, 159
Pregnancy: and drugs, 62, 74, 75
   category of drugs, 75
Prescription drugs, 9
Pressor agents, 101, 103
Presystemic (first pass) metabolism, 31-32
Pretomanid, 454
Prilocaine, 383
Primaquine, 488, 489, 491
Primidone, 155
Prinzmetal's angina, 198, *See* Variant angina
Probenecid, 34, 39, 43, 224, 417, 525
Probiotics, 311
Procainamide, 213
Procaine, 381, 383
Procarbazine, 331, 332
Prochlorperazine, 303
Procyclidine, 92, 161
Prodrug, 26
Progesterone, 256, *also See* Progestins
Progestins, 256-258, *also See* Oral contraceptives
Proguanil (Chloroguanide), 491
Prokinetic drugs, 298, 303-04
Prolactin (Prl), 228, 229, 230-31
Prolonging drug action, 38
Promethazine, 115, 116, 119, 302, 518
Propafenone, 214

Propantheline, 92
Proparacaine, 384
Propionic acid derivatives, 354-56, *also See* Nonsteroidal anti-inflammatory drugs
Propofol, 134, 137
Propranolol, 107-11, 182, 202, 208, 214, 267
Propylthiouracil, 263
Propyphenazone 357-58
Prostacyclin (PGI$_2$), 122, 123, 125, 348
Prostaglandins (PGs), 120-27
 synthesis inhibitors, 124, 348, See Nonsteroidal anti-inflammatory drugs
Prostanoid receptors, 125-26
Protamine sulfate, 285
Protease inhibitors (PIs); retroviral, 481-82
Protectives, 504
Proton pump inhibitors (PPIs), 296-98, 300
Prulifloxacin, 410
Pseudocholinesterase (BuChE), 84
 deficiency/atypical, 63, 139, 140
Psychological dependence, 73
Psychopharmacological agents (Psychotropic drugs), 165-82
Psychoses, 165
Psyllium, 306
Purgatives, 305-09
 bulk forming, 306, 309
 mechanism of action, 306, 307
 osmotic, 307-08
 stimulant, 307
Purine antagonists, 333-34
Pyrazinamide (Z), 456, 458, 459
Pyridostigmine, 87
Pyridoxine (Vit B$_6$), 323, 327, 455, 459
Pyrimethamine, , 491, 493
Pyrimethamine-sulfonamide combination, 488, 491, 493
Pyrimidine antagonists, 334

Q

Quaternary ammonium antiseptics, 501, 503, 507
Quetiapine, 167, 169, 171, 174
Quinidine, 213, 527
Quinine, 142, 488, 490
Quiniodochlor, 495
Quinolones, 406-10
Quinupristin/Dalfopristin, 451

R

Rabeprazole, 297, 298, *also See* Proton pump inhibitors
Racecadotril, 311
Raloxifene, 255
Raltegravir, 482, 483, 384
Ramelteon, 144, 151
Ramosetron, 301, 305
Ramipril, 185, 186, *also See* Angiotensin converting enzyme inhibitors
Ranitidine, 114, 295, 296, *also See* H$_2$ antagonists
Ranolazine, 202-03
Rasagiline, 164
Receptors, 41, 43-53
 desensitization, 53
 functions of, 53
 G-protein coupled, 46-49
 ion channel, 46, 49-50
 nature of, 44-45
 occupation theory, 44
 regulating gene expression 51, 52
 regulation, 51, 53
 subtypes, 45
 transducer mechanisms, 45-51
 transmembrane enzyme linked, 50
 transmembrane JAK-STAT binding, 50-51
Rectal administration, 11
'Red man' syndrome, 450
Redistribution, 23, 146
Reduction of drugs, 27
Reflux esophagitis. *See* Gastroesophageal reflux
Remifentanil, 132, 136

Renal excretion of drugs, 32-33
Renin: Angiotensin system (RAS), 183-85
Repaglinide, 239, 240
Replacement therapy, 40, 254, 265
Reserpine, 95, 98
Resistance: to AMAs, 67, 391-93, 399
Reteplase, 288
Retinoic acid, 324
Retinol, 322-24
Retroviral protease inhibitors (PIs), 481-82
Reversal reaction: in leprosy, 463
Reverse transcriptase inhibitors, 479-81
Reversible inhibitors of MAO-A (RIMAs), 174-75
Reye's syndrome, 352, 362
Rheumatic fever, 249, 353, 400, 418, 447
Rheumatoid arthritis, 249, 341, 343, 353, 355, 357
Ribavirin, 476
Riboflavin (vit B$_2$), 323, 326
Rickets, 271, 272
Rideal-Walker coefficient, 498
Rifabutin, 458, 460
Rifampin (Rifampicin, R), 455-56, 458, 459
Rifapentine, 454
Rifaximin, 310
Rimantadine, 475
rINN (recommended International Nonproprietary Name), 6
Risedronate, 273
Risk-benefit ratio, 56
Risperidone, 167, 169
Ritonavir, 482, 484
Rivaroxaban, 286
Rivastigmine, 88
Rocuronium, 140, 141
Ropinirole, 163
Ropivacaine, 384, 387
Rosuvastatin, 291, 292

Routes of administration, 10-14
Roxatidine, 295, *also See* H$_2$ antagonists
Roxithromycin, 447
Rupatadine, 116

S

Salbutamol, 55, 98, 317, 319, 321, 518
Salicylates, 350-53
Salmeterol, 317
Sanguinarine, 508
Saquinavir, 482
Satranidazole, 411, 413
Saxagliptin, 240
Schizophrenia, 165, 170-71
    drugs for. *See* Antipsychotic drugs
Scopolamine. *See* Hyoscine
Scurvy, 328
Secnidazole, 411, 413
Second gas effect, 130
Secondary effects, 69
Sedative, 144-51
    definition, 144
Seizures, management of, 159-61, 522, *also See* Epilepsy, treatment
Selective COX-2 inhibitors, 348, 359-60
Selective estrogen receptor down regulator (SERD), 253, 255, 337
Selective estrogen receptor modulators (SERMs), 253, 255, 337
Selective serotonin reuptake inhibitors (SSRIs), 176, 178-79
Selectivity of drugs, 55-56
Selegiline, 163-64, 174
Senna, 307, 308, 309
Serotonergic receptors, 119-20
Serotonin. *See* 5-Hydroxytryptamine
Serotonin and noradrenaline reuptake inhibitors (SNRIs), 176, 179

Sertraline, 176, *also See* Selective serotonin reuptake inhibitors
Sevoflurane, 131, 133-34
Sex hormones, 251-58
Sibutramine, 103
Side effects, 69
Silver nitrate, 498, 502-03
Silver sulfadiazine, 405
Simeprevir, 472, 477-78
Simvastatin, 291, *also See* Statins
Sirolimus, 341-42
Sitagliptin, 239, 240, 241
Skeletal muscle relaxants, 137-43
Sleep, 144-45, 150, 151
SMON, 63, 495
Sodium
    bicarbonate, 299
    citrate, 299
    cromoglycate, 320
    fluoride, 510, 511, 516
    hypochlorite solution, 500
    monofluorophosphate (MPF), 513
    nitroprusside, 195, 196, 210
    perborate, 508, 515
    peroxide, 515
    phosphate, 306
    pot. tartrate, 306
    sulphate, 306
    valproate. *See* Valproic acid
Sofosbuvir, 472, 477, 478
Solifenacin, 89, 92
Somatostatin, 230
Somatropin, 230
Sorafenib, 330, 336
Sotalol, 110, 215
Sources of drugs, 5-6
Spinal anaesthesia, 385
Spironolactone, 193, 211, 224-26
Stannous chloride, 514
Stannous fluoride, 508, 511, 513
Stanozolol, 252
Statins (HMG-CoA reductase inhibitors), 291-92

Status asthmaticus, 320, 321, 521
Status epilepticus, 155, 160, 161, 522
Stavudine, 480
Stimulation, 40
Stokes-Adams syndrome, 104
Streptokinase, 288
Streptomycin (S), 440, 443, 457, 458, 459
Strontium chloride, 513
Styptics, 281-82
Subcutaneous injection (s.c.), 13
    absorption from, 21
Sublingual administration, 11
Substantivity, 507, 508
Succinylcholine (SCh), 138, 140, 141
Sucralfate, 300, 504, 526
Sulbactam, 422-23
Sulfacetamide sod., 404, 405
Sulfadiazine, 403, *also See* Sulfonamides
Sulfadoxine, 404, 488, 491, 493
Sulfamethoxazole, 404, 405, *also See* Cotrimoxazole
Sulfamethopyrazine, 404, 491
Sulfanilamide, 403
Sulfasalazine, 312, 404
Sulfonamides, 403-05
Sulfonamide-pyrimethamine (S/P), 491
Sulfone, 460, *also See* Dapsone
Sulfonylureas, 238-40, 243, 525
Sultamicillin tosylate, 423
Superactive GnRH agonists, 231-32, 252, 337
Superinfection (Suprainfection), 393-94, 435, 449
Supersensitivity, 51, 194
Suppositories, 7, 11
Surface anaesthesia, 383, 384
Sustained release tablets, 7, 38
Suvorexant, 144, 151
Suxamethonium. *See* Succinylcholine

Sweetening agents, 516
Sympathetic nervous system, 79, 80
Sympathomimetics, 98-104
  directly acting, 98
  indirectly acting, 98
Syncope (fainting), 519
Synergism, 56-57
  among antimicrobials, 398-99

T

Tablets, 7
Tachyphylaxis, 67
Tacrolimus, 341, 342
Tafenoquine, 486, 489, 492
Talc, 504
Tamoxifen citrate, 255, 337
Tamsulosin, 106, 107
Tannic acid/Tannins, 504, 514
Tapentadol, 370
Tardive dyskinesia, 170
Targeted anticancer drugs, 336
Target level strategy, 37, 60
Tazobactam, 422, 423
Tedizolid, 451
Teicoplanin, 450
Telbivudine, 476
Telmisartan, 187, 188
Temazepam, 149
Tenecteplase, 204, 288
Teneligliptin, 238, 240
Tenofovir, 476, 481, 484, 485
Tenoxicam, 356
Teratogenicity, 74-75
Terazosin, 106, 194
Terbinafine, 466, 470-71
Terbutaline, 103, 317, 321
Terfenadine, 117
Teriparatide, 269
Terizidone, 454, 457
Testosterone, 251-52
Tetracaine, 383
Tetracyclines, 431-36
  in chronic periodontitis, 435, 509
Thalidomide, 74, 75
Theophylline, 317-19, 321

Therapeutic index, 55, 498
Thiamine (vit B_1), 323, 325-26
Thiazide diuretics, 191-93, 221-24, 226
Thiazolidinediones, 239, 242
Thiocolchicoside, 143
6-Thioguanine (6-TG), 331, 333, 339
Thiopentone sod., 23, 134, 141
Thioridazine, 167, 168, 169
Thrombolytics. *See* Fibrinolytic drugs
Thromboxane A2 (TXA2), 121, 123, 124, 125, 288, 289
Thymol, 5, 513, 516
Thyroid disease and drugs, 65
Thyroid hormones, 262-65
Thyroid inhibitors, 265-67
Thyroid stimulating hormone (TSH), 232, 263
Thyrotoxicosis (Hyperthyroidism), 111, 265
  drugs for, 111, 265-67
Thyrotropin. *See* Thyroid stimulating hormone
Thyroxine (T_4), 262, 263, 264, 265
Tiagabine, 154, 160
Tibolone, 253
Ticagrelor, 289, 290
Ticarcillin, 421
Ticlopidine, 289
Tigecycline, 431, 436
Timolol, 110, 111
Tinidazole, 411, 412-13, 494
Tiotropium bromide, 92, 319
Tirofiban, 289, 290
Tissue plasminogen activator (rt-PA, Alteplase), 288
Tizanidine, 143
Tobramycin, 440, 443
Tolbutamide, 239
Tolcapone, 98, 164
Tolerance, 31, 66-67
Tolnaftate, 471
Tolterodine, 92
Topical application, 10
Topiramate, 159, 160
Topotecan, 335

Torasemide, 221
Toxic effects, 69-70
Toxicology: definition, 4
Tramadol, 172, 369-70
Trandolapril, 185
Tranexaemic acid, 282, 288
Tranquillizer, 166
Transdermal therapeutic systems (TTS), 11, 12
Transducer mechanisms, 45-52
Transporters (drug), 17-19, 23, 41
  as targets of drug action, 43
Traveller's diarrhoea, 310, 312
Travoprost, 126, 127
Trazodone, 176, 179
Triamcinolone, 247, 248
Triamterene, 226
Triazolam, 149
Trichloroacetic acid, 505
Triclofos, 144, 151
Triclosan, 499, 503, 507-08, 512
Tricyclic antidepressants (TCAs), 175-78, 180
Trifluoperazine, 167, 168
Trifluperidol, 167
Triflupromazine, 167
Trigeminal neuralgia, 155, 156, 157
Trihexyphenidyl, 92, 164
Triiodothyronine (T_3), 262, 263, 264
Trimetazidine, 202
Trimethoprim + sulfamethoxazole, 405-06, *also See* Cotrimoxazole
Trimipramine, 176
Tripotassium dicitratobismuthate, 300
Triptorelin, 231
Triprolidine, 116, *also See* H_1 antagonists
Tropicamide, 92
Tuberculosis, 453
  extensively drug resistant (XDR), 460
  multidrug resistant (MDR), 453, 457, 458
  treatment of, 458-60

Index

Tubocurarine (d-TC), 83, 84, 138, 139, 140
Tubular reabsorption/secretion of drugs, 32, 33, 34
Two tone dye, 515
Tyramine, 98, 175

U

Ulcerative colitis: drugs for, 250, 312-13, 343
Ulcer protective, 300
Ulipristal, 258, 259
Unstable angina, 198, 202, 290
Urinary pH and excretion of drugs, 33
Urokinase, 288

V

Valacyclovir, 474
Valethamate, 92
Valproic acid (Sodium valproate), 157-58, 160, 173
Valsartan, 187, 188
Vancomycin, 402, 449-50
 in dentistry, 450
Variant angina, 190, 198, 199, 201
Vasodilators, 195, 210
Vasomotor reversal, 100, 104, 107

Vecuronium, 140, 141
Velpatasvir, 472, 477, 478
Venlafaxine, 176, 179
Ventricular fibrillation (VF), 212, 215, 521
Verapamil, 189, 190, 191, 215
Vildagliptin, 239, 240, 241
Vinblastine, 331, 334
Vinca alkaloids, 334
Vincristine, 334
Vinorelbine, 334
Visual cycle: vit A in, 323-24
Vitamins, 322-28
 definition, 322
 fat soluble, 322-25
 vit A, 322-24
 vit B complex, 325-27
 vit B_{12} 277-78, 323
 vit C, 323, 327-28
 vit D, 271-72, 323
 vit E, 323, 324-25
 vit K, 280-81, 323
 water soluble, 323, 325-28
Voglibose, 242
Volume of distribution (V), 22, 23, 35
Voriconazole, 470

W

Warfarin sod., 286, *also See* Oral anticoagulants

Withdrawal reactions, 74, 149, 367
Wool fat, 9, 504

X

Xipamide, 220
Xylometazoline, 101, 103

Y

Yohimbine, 98, 106

Z

Zafirlukast, 126, 319-20, 321
Zaleplon, 150
Zanamivir, 475
Zero order kinetics, 36, 37, 152
Zidovudine (AZT), 480, 484, 485
Zinc
 citrate/chloride, 508
 oxide, 503, 504, 514
 stearate, 504
 sulphate, 503, 514
Ziprasidone, 167, 169
Zoledronate, 273
Zollinger-Ellison syndrome, 298
Zolpidem, 150
Zonisamide, 159, 160
Zopiclone, 150

EU GSPR Authorised Reprsentative
Logos Europe, 9 rue Nicolas Poussin
1700, La Rochelle, France
Phone: +33 (0) 6 67 93 73 78
E-mail: contact@logoseurope.eu

www.ingramcontent.com/pod-product-compliance
Ingram Content Group UK Ltd.
Pitfield, Milton Keynes, MK11 3LW, UK
UKHW050430150426

5217IPUK00019B/1317